Nursing Research

Methods, Critical Appraisal, and Utilization

Nursing Research

Methods, Critical Appraisal, and Utilization

Fourth Edition

With 44 illustrations

Geri LoBiondo-Wood, PhD, RN
Associate Professor
University of Texas Health Science Center—Houston
School of Nursing
Houston, Texas

Judith Haber, PhD, APRN, CS, FAAN
Visiting Professor
Director of Master's and Post-Master's Certificate Program
New York University
Division of Nursing
New York, New York

Private Practice
Stamford, Connecticut

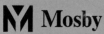 Mosby

St. Louis Baltimore Boston Carlsbad
Chicago Minneapolis New York Philadelphia Portland
London Milan Sydney Tokyo Toronto

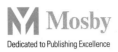

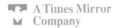

Vice President and Publisher: Nancy L. Coon
Editor: Loren S. Wilson
Associate Developmental Editor: Aimee E. Loewe
Project Manager: John Rogers
Senior Production Editor: Lavon Wirch Peters
Designer: Yael Kats
Manufacturing Manager: Linda Ierardi

Fourth Edition
Copyright © 1998 by Mosby–Year Book, Inc.

Previous editions copyrighted 1986, 1990, 1994

Printed in the United States of America
Composition by Graphic World, Inc.
Printing/binding by R.R. Donnelly & Sons Company

Mosby–Year Book, Inc.
11830 Westline Industrial Drive
St. Louis, Missouri 63146

Library of Congress Cataloging-in-Publication Data
Nursing research : methods, critical appraisal, and utilization /
 [edited by] Geri LoBiondo-Wood, Judith Haber. — 4th ed.
     p.   cm.
   Includes bibliographical references and index.
   ISBN 0-8151-2390-6 (softcover)
   1. Nursing—Research.   I. LoBiondo-Wood, Geri.   II. Haber,
Judith.
   [DNLM: 1. Nursing Research.   WY 20.5 N97445 1997]
 RT81.5.N8665   1997
 610.73′072—dc21
 DNLM/DLC
 for Library of Congress   97-33347
                                                            CIP

97 98 99 00 01 / 9 8 7 6 5 4 3 2 1

Contributors

Ann Bello, MA, RN
Professor of Nursing
Norwalk Community College
Norwalk, Connecticut
Chapter 14

Betty J. Craft, MPN, RN
Assistant Professor
University of Nebraska Medical Center
College of Nursing
Omaha, Nebraska
Chapter 17

Harriet R. Feldman, PhD, RN
Dean and Professor
Lienhard School of Nursing
Pace University
Pleasantville, New York
Chapter 5

Margaret Grey, DrPH, RN, FAAN
Independence Foundation Professor of
Nursing
Associate Dean for Research and Doctoral
Studies
Yale University School of Nursing
New Haven, Connecticut
Chapters 7, 12, and 15

Judith Haber, PhD, APRN, CS, FAAN
Visiting Professor
Director of Master's and Post-Master's
Certificate Program
New York University
Division of Nursing
New York, New York
Private Practice
Stamford, Connecticut
Chapters 1, 2, 3, 8, 10, 11, and 13

Judith A. Heermann, PhD, RN
Associate Professor
University of Nebraska Medical Center
College of Nursing
Omaha, Nebraska
Chapter 17

Barbara Krainovich-Miller, EdD, RN
Consultant
Garden City, New York
Chapters 2 and 4; Critical Thinking Challenges

Patricia R. Liehr, PhD, RN
Associate Professor
University of Texas Health Science Center—
Houston
School of Nursing
Houston, Texas
Chapter 9

Geri LoBiondo-Wood, PhD, RN
Associate Professor
University of Texas Health Science Center—
Houston
School of Nursing
Houston, Texas
Chapters 1, 2, 6, 8, 13 and 16

Marianne Taft Marcus, EdD, RN, FAAN
Professor and Chairperson, Nursing Systems
and Technology
University of Texas Health Science Center—
Houston
School of Nursing
Houston, Texas
Chapter 9

Helen J. Streubert, EdD, RN
Associate Professor and Director,
Nursing Program
College Misericordia
Dallas, Pennsylvania
Chapter 18

Marita G. Titler, PhD, RN
Associate Director of Nursing Research
University of Iowa Hospitals and Clinic
Iowa City, Iowa
Chapter 19

Foreword

A meaningful overview of the evolution of nursing research with excellent "real world" examples sets the stage for the fourth edition of *Nursing Research: Methods, Critical Appraisal, and Utilization* by LoBiondo-Wood and Haber. The authors tackle the enormously complex issues of how to incorporate the knowledge generated by means of the research process into care of patients, families, and communities, citing both successes and challenges for the 1990s. A combination of models for research utilization, with practical illustrations, is particularly useful for the student, clinician, researcher, educator, or administrator who is serious about the value and importance of research and its application in practice. A rich overview of the strategies that have been developed and used provides an incentive for the reader to absorb the content. Health care reform brings an enormous challenge to the discipline. Utilization of research findings generated by means of sound theoretical and methodological methods can only strengthen the effectiveness of practice and, therefore, outcomes to which nursing is committed.

The wider community of "world" is another focus of the book, and rightfully so. As the globe shrinks and health problems become world health problems, nursing must take its place in grappling with the enormous discrepancies between industrialized, developing, and third-world countries. The work by LoBiondo-Wood and Haber has proven its value as a superb guide in international collaboration. Having had the opportunity to live and teach in highly diverse countries (e.g., Finland, India, Greece, and Thailand), this writer has found that *Nursing Research: Methods, Critical Appraisal, and Utilization* serves as an excellent resource for both faculties and students. Out of these international opportunities has developed a strong belief that appreciation of cultural differences is the only basis for meaningful collaboration. Health care systems, political and economic structures, and most importantly, the health of societies are enormously diverse. It follows that the purposes and foci of nursing research in different countries are widely discrepant. Thus, global collaboration will be effective only to the extent that there is a commitment to fully understand differences between particular cultures and strive to research the needs and find methods and solutions that have the potential to be effective.

In this extremely timely work, LoBiondo-Wood and Haber address the urgent needs of quality, cost, and outcomes of care. The book is designed specifically to provide the baccalaureate student with the essential knowledge and skills to evaluate critically the findings from studies pertaining to all three issues. The ability of our "entry-level consumers" of research to critically evaluate their practice and participate in the research process may be a determining factor in the survival of nursing as a profession.

Excellent examples of studies of growing populations are provided. The list is extensive: the chronically ill, the aged, persons with Alzheimer's disease, persons with AIDS, and vulnerable groups (e.g., the abused, single parents, children with marginal or no health care, and families who struggle to provide care). LoBiondo-Wood and Haber point to the importance of new information acquired by sound methodologies, which must be the cornerstone for testing theories and models of care relevant to the growing numbers in these groups. Both associate degree and baccalaureate-prepared nurses must be involved in the research process as the only legitimate route by which we learn about the specific needs of these populations, design care, and evaluate its effectiveness by means of sound studies of outcomes. Further, the authors have provided a state-of-the-art guide to the literature review. As computer technology becomes a part of every facet of care, so too does it provide an entre to the most current information for any discipline.

Finally, a major strength of the book is the infectious enthusiasm of the authors. The writing style invites the interest of the reader, and the content serves as a genuine inspiration for its intended audience.

Carol Noll Hoskins, PhD, RN, FAAN
Professor
Division of Nursing
School of Education
New York University

Preface

The foundation of the fourth edition of *Nursing Research: Methods, Critical Appraisal, and Utilization* continues to be the belief that nursing research is integral with all levels of nursing education and practice. As we move toward the twenty-first century, more and more nurses are conducting and using research that shapes clinical practice, education, and public policy. Nurses are involved in using research data to influence the nature and direction of health care delivery and document outcomes related to the quality and cost-effectiveness of patient care. As nurses continue to develop a unique body of nursing knowledge through research, decisions about clinical nursing practice will be increasingly research based.

As editors we believe that all nurses need not only to understand the research process but also to know how to critically read, evaluate, and apply research findings in practice. We know that understanding research is a challenge for every student. However, we believe that the challenge can be accomplished in a stimulating, lively, and learner-friendly manner.

We agree that the kind of research knowledge appropriate to different levels of education varies. Consistent with this perspective is the belief that nursing research must be an integral dimension of baccalaureate education. Its presence must be evident not only in the undergraduate nursing research course but also threaded throughout the curriculum. The research role of the baccalaureate graduate calls for the skills of critical appraisal—that is, the nurse should be a competent research consumer. Preparing students for this role involves developing their understanding of the research process, their appreciation of the role of the critiquer, and their ability to critique research and use the findings in clinical practice. An undergraduate course in nursing research should develop this basic level of competence in baccalaureate graduates, an essential requirement for full integration of research into clinical practice. This is in contrast to the focus of a graduate level research course in which the emphasis is on carrying out research, as well as understanding and appraising it.

The primary audience of this textbook remains undergraduate students who are learning the steps of the research process, learning how to critique published research literature, and learning when and how to apply research findings in clinical practice. This book is also a valuable resource for students at the master's and doctoral levels who want a concise review of the basic steps of the research and critiquing process. Furthermore, it is an important research utilization resource for practicing nurses who strive to use research findings as the basis for clinical decision making and development of research-based policies, protocols, and procedures rather than tradition, authority, or trial and error. It is also an important resource for nurses who collaborate with nurse-scientists in the conduct of clinical research.

Building on the success of the third edition, the fourth edition of *Nursing Research: Methods, Critical Appraisal, and Utilization* prepares nursing students and practicing nurses to become knowledgeable nursing research consumers by:

- Addressing the role of the nurse as a research consumer, thereby facilitating the movement of research into the mainstream of nursing.
- Demystifying research, which is sometimes viewed as a complex process.
- Teaching the fundamentals of the research process and critical appraisal process in a logical, systematic progression that is user friendly. This approach promotes a lively spirit of inquiry and encourages critical thinking and development of clinical judgment skills that will promote enthusiasm on the part of students and nurses about expanding their research knowledge base.
- Elevating the critiquing process and the use of research to a position of importance comparable to that of producing research. Before becoming research producers, students need to become knowledgeable research consumers.
- Stimulating thoughtful practice that is both creative and innovative through the use of nursing research.
- Emphasizing the role of research utilization as the basis for clinical decision making and research-based clinical nursing practice that demonstrates quality and cost-effective outcomes of nursing care delivery.
- Developing critical thinking and critical reading skills that facilitate mastery of the critiquing process.
- Developing computer-related research consumer competencies that prepare students and nurses to effectively locate and manage research information.
- Presenting numerous examples of recently published research studies that illustrate and highlight each research concept in a manner that brings abstract ideas to life for students new to the research and critiquing process. The examples are a critical link for reinforcement of the research and critiquing processes.
- Showcasing vignettes by renowned nurse researchers whose careers exemplify the link between research, education, and practice.
- Providing numerous pedagogical chapter features, including *learning outcomes; key terms; critical thinking decision paths; technology highlights; helpful hints; numerous tables, figures, boxes, and critiquing criteria; and key points and critical thinking challenges at the end of each chapter.*

The text is organized into two parts that are preceded by an introductory section. The introductory section contains Chapter 1, *The Role of Research in Nursing*, which provides an exciting overview of roles, approaches, and issues in nursing research. It introduces the importance of the nurse's role as a research consumer and provides a futuristic perspective about research and research utilization principles that shape clinical practice into the next millennium. Part One focuses on the integration of the research and critiquing processes. Chapter 2, which speaks directly to students, provides an overview of Part One that highlights critical thinking and critical reading concepts and strategies that facilitate student understanding of the research process and its relationship to the critiquing process. The style and content of this chapter are designed to make subsequent chapters more user friendly to students. Chapter 3 through 16 delineate each step of the research process, with published clinical research studies used to illustrate each step. The interrelatedness of the steps is examined in relation to the total research process. Both qualitative and quantitative designs are presented. Critical thinking is stimulated by presentation of the potential strengths and weaknesses in each step of the research process. Critical thinking is also enhanced by new chapter features that include *Critical Thinking Decision Paths, Helpful Hints,* and *Critical Thinking Challenges* that promote development of research consumer decision making skills. Computer-related research consumer competencies that prepare students and nurses to effectively locate and manage research information are showcased in Chapter 4, *Literature Review,* and are highlighted by technology icons in many chapters throughout the text. Consistent with previous editions, each chapter includes a section describing the critiquing process related to the focus of that chapter, as well as lists of *Critiquing Criteria* that are designed to stimulate a systematic and evaluative approach to reading research literature.

Part Two focuses on critique and application. In this section, the whole process of critical thinking, critical reading, critiquing, and utilization is synthesized. Chapters 17 and 18 provide summary *Critiquing Guidelines* for each step of both quantitative and qualitative research methods. These guidelines are used to evaluate several recently published quantitative and qualitative research articles, including their applicability to clinical nursing practice. Chapter 19, *Research Utilization,* provides an exciting conclusion to this text through its vibrant presentation about the application of nursing research in clinical practice using a research utilization framework.

The accompanying *Instructor's Resource Manual,* written by Harriet Feldman and Rona Levin, and the revised *Test Bank,* developed by Deborah Sherman, complement the textbook and provide chapter-by-chapter cooperative learning activities and strategies that promote the development of critical thinking, critical reading, and computer-related skills designed to develop the competencies necessary to produce informed consumers of nursing research. The Student *Study Guide,* written by Mary Jo Gorney Moreno and Kathy Rose-Grippa, including a new *CD-ROM* instruction component for student review and reinforcement, is a new cutting-edge, self-paced teaching/learning resource designed to enhance student learning outcomes.

The development of a scientific foundation for clinical nursing practice remains an essential priority for the future of professional nursing practice. The fourth edition of *Nursing Research: Methods, Critical Appraisal, and Utilization* will help students develop a basic level of competence in understanding the steps of the research process that will enable them to critically analyze research studies, judge their merit, and judiciously apply research findings in clinical practice. To the extent that this goal is accomplished, nursing will have a cadre of clinicians who derive their practice from theory and research specific to nursing.

Acknowledgments

No major undertaking is accomplished alone. There are those who contribute directly and those who contribute indirectly to the success of a project. We acknowledge with our warmest thanks the help and support of the following people:

- Our students, particularly the nursing students at the University of Texas—Houston Health Science Center School of Nursing and the Division of Nursing at New York University, whose interest and lively curiosity sparked ideas for revisions in the fourth edition.
- Our chapter contributors, whose expertise, cooperation, and punctuality made them a joy to have as colleagues.
- Our vignette contributors, whose willingness to share evidence of their research wisdom makes a unique contribution to this project.
- Our foreword contributor, Carol Noll Hoskins, our former research professor and a chapter contributor to the first edition of this text, whose insightful introduction to the fourth edition lends special meaning to this text.
- Our colleagues, who have taken time out of their busy professional lives to offer feedback and constructive criticism that has assisted us in preparing the fourth edition.
- Our editors, Loren Wilson and Aimee Loewe, for their willingness to listen to yet another creative idea about teaching research in a meaningful way and for their help with manuscript production and last-minute details.
- Our production editor, Lavon Peters, for her skilled assistance with the editing and last-minute details.
- Our families, Brian Wood and Lenny and Andrew Haber and Laurie and Bob Goldberg, for their unending love, faith, understanding, and support throughout what is inevitably a consuming but exciting experience.

Geri LoBiondo-Wood
Judith Haber

Student Preface

We invite you to join us on an exciting nursing research adventure that begins as you turn the first page of the fourth edition of *Nursing Research: Methods, Critical Appraisal, and Utilization*. The adventure is one of discovery! You will discover that the nursing research literature sparkles with pride, dedication, and excitement about this dimension of professional nursing practice. Whether you are a student or a nurse whose goal is to use research as the foundation of your practice, you will discover that nursing research positions our profession at the cutting edge of change. You will discover that nursing research is integral with meeting the challenge of providing quality biopsychosocial physical and mental health care in partnership with clients, their families/significant others, and the communities in which they live. Finally, you will also discover the cutting edge "Who," "What," "Where," "When," "Why," and "How" of nursing research and research utilization, developing a foundation of knowledge and skills that will equip you for clinical practice today as well as in the new millennium, the twenty-first century!

We think you will enjoy reading this text. Your nursing research course will be short but filled with new and challenging learning experiences that will develop your research consumer skills. The fourth edition of *Nursing Research: Methods, Critical Appraisal, and Utilization* reflects "cutting edge" trends for developing competent consumers of nursing research. The two-part organization and use of numerous special features contained in this text are designed to help you develop your critical reading, critical thinking, and clinical decision making skills while providing a "user friendly" approach to learning that expands your competence to deal effectively with these new and challenging experiences.

Remember that research consumer skills are used in every clinical setting and can be applied to every client population or clinical practice issue. Irrespective of whether your clinical practice involves primary care or specialty care and provides inpatient or outpatient treatment in a hospital, clinic, or home, you will be challenged to apply your research consumer skills and use nursing research as the foundation of your clinical practice. The fourth edition of *Nursing Research: Methods, Critical Appraisal, and Utilization* will guide you through this exciting adventure where you will discover your ability to play a vital role in contributing to the building of research-based professional nursing practice!

Geri LoBiondo-Wood
Judith Haber

Contents

Introduction, 1

From Research to Practice, 2
Nancy Bergstrom

Chapter 1 **The Role of Research in Nursing, 5**
Geri LoBiondo-Wood, Judith Haber

Key Terms, 5
Learning Outcomes, 5
Significance of Research in Nursing, 6
Research: Linking Theory, Education, and Practice, 7
Roles of the Nurse in the Research Process, 9
Historical Perspective, 11
Future Directions—The 1990s and Beyond, 20
Key Points, 26
Critical Thinking Challenges, 27
References, 27
Additional Readings, 32

Part One Research Process, 35

Importance of Research to Nursing Practice, 36
Cheryl Tatano Beck

Chapter 2 **Overview of the Research Process, 39**
Geri LoBiondo-Wood, Judith Haber, Barbara Krainovich-Miller

Key Terms, 39
Learning Outcomes, 39
Critical Thinking and Critical Reading Skills, 40
Process of Critical Reading, 41
Perceived Difficulties and Strategies for Critiquing Research, 47
Research Articles: Format and Style, 48
Key Points, 55
Critical Thinking Challenges, 56
References, 56
Additional Readings, 57

Chapter 3 **Research Problems and Hypotheses, 59**
   Judith Haber
Key Terms, 59
Learning Outcomes, 59
Developing and Refining a Research Problem, 60
Final Problem Statement, 65
Statement of the Problem in Published Research, 71
Purpose Statement, 72
Developing the Research Hypotheses, 73
Relationship Between the Hypothesis and the Research Design, 82
Research Questions, 82
Critiquing the Research Problem and Hypotheses, 84
Key Points, 89
Critical Thinking Challenges, 90
References, 90
Additional Readings, 91

Chapter 4 **Literature Review, 93**
   Barbara Krainovich-Miller
Key Terms, 93
Learning Outcomes, 93
Review of the Literature: Purposes, 95
Review of the Literature for Quantitative Studies: Conductor of Research Perspective, 99
Review of the Literature: Consumer of Research Perspective, 100
Scholarly Literature, 102
Primary and Secondary Sources, 106
Conducting a Search as a Consumer of Research, 110
Types of Resources, 110
Performing a Computer Search, 119
Literature Review Format: What to Expect, 123
Critiquing Criteria for a Review of the Literature, 124
Key Points, 127
Critical Thinking Challenges, 127
References, 128
Additional Readings, 130

Chapter 5 **Theoretical Framework, 133**
   Harriet R. Feldman
Key Terms, 133
Learning Outcomes, 133
Ways of Knowing—Sources of Knowledge, 134
Relationship Between Theory and Research, 144
Relationship Between Theory and Method, 146
Theory—What and Whose, 147
Critiquing the Theoretical Framework, 148
Key Points, 150

Critical Thinking Challenges, 150
References, 151
Additional Readings, 153

Chapter 6 **Introduction to Design, 155**
   Geri LoBiondo-Wood
Key Terms, 155
Learning Outcomes, 155
Purpose of Research Design, 157
Objectivity in the Problem Conceptualization, 157
Accuracy, 158
Feasibility, 159
Control, 159
Quantitative Control and Flexibility, 163
Internal and External Validity, 163
Critiquing the Research Design, 169
Key Points, 171
Critical Thinking Challenges, 171
References, 172
Additional Readings, 172

Chapter 7 **Experimental and Quasiexperimental Designs, 175**
   Margaret Grey
Key Terms, 175
Learning Outcomes, 175
True Experimental Design, 176
Quasiexperimental Designs, 183
Evaluation Research and Experimentation, 188
Critiquing Experimental and Quasiexperimental Designs, 189
Key Points, 191
Critical Thinking Challenges, 192
References, 192
Additional Readings, 193

Chapter 8 **Nonexperimental Designs, 195**
   Geri LoBiondo-Wood, Judith Haber
Key Terms, 195
Learning Outcomes, 195
Descriptive/Exploratory Survey Studies, 197
Interrelationship/Difference Studies, 199
Causality in Nonexperimental Research, 205
Additional Types of Designs, 206
Critiquing Nonexperimental Designs, 210
Key Points, 212
Critical Thinking Challenges, 212
References, 213
Additional Readings, 214

Chapter 9 **Qualitative Approaches to Research, 215**
Marianne Taft Marcus, Patricia R. Liehr
Key Terms, 215
Learning Outcomes, 215
Quantitative and Qualitative Research Approaches, 216
Qualitative Approach and Nursing Science, 220
Four Qualitative Research Methods, 221
Qualitative Approach: Nursing Methodology, 234
Issues in Qualitative Research, 234
Critiquing Qualitative Research, 240
Key Points, 241
Critical Thinking Challenges, 242
References, 242

Chapter 10 **Sampling, 247**
Judith Haber
Key Terms, 247
Learning Outcomes, 247
Sampling Concepts, 248
Types of Samples, 251
Sample Size, 263
Sampling Procedures, 266
Critiquing the Sample, 267
Key Points, 271
Critical Thinking Challenges, 272
References, 273
Additional Readings, 273

Chapter 11 **Legal and Ethical Issues, 275**
Judith Haber
Key Terms, 275
Learning Outcomes, 275
Ethical and Legal Considerations in Research: An Historical Perspective, 276
Evolution of Ethics in Nursing Research, 282
Protection of Human Rights, 284
Scientific Fraud and Misconduct, 297
Product Testing, 298
Legal and Ethical Aspects of Animal Experimentation, 298
Critiquing the Legal and Ethical Aspects of a Research Study, 299
Key Points, 303
Critical Thinking Challenges, 303
References, 304
Additional Readings, 306

Chapter 12 **Data Collection Methods, 307**
Margaret Grey
Key Terms, 307
Learning Outcomes, 307
Measuring Variables of Interest, 308
Data Collection Methods, 311
Construction of New Instruments, 320
Critiquing Data Collection Methods, 321
Key Points, 324
Critical Thinking Challenges, 325
References, 325
Additional Readings, 326

Chapter 13 **Reliability and Validity, 327**
Geri LoBiondo-Wood, Judith Haber
Key Terms, 327
Learning Outcomes, 327
Reliability, Validity, and Measurement Error, 328
Validity, 331
Reliability, 337
Critiquing Reliability and Validity, 345
Key Points, 348
Critical Thinking Challenges, 348
References, 348
Additional Readings, 350

Chapter 14 **Descriptive Data Analysis, 351**
Ann Bello
Key Terms, 351
Learning Outcomes, 351
Levels of Measurement, 352
Frequency Distribution, 355
Measures of Central Tendency, 357
Normal Distribution, 361
Interpreting Measures of Variability, 362
Correlation, 364
Critiquing Descriptive Statistics, 365
Key Points, 367
Critical Thinking Challenges, 367
References, 368
Additional Readings, 368

Chapter 15 **Inferential Data Analysis, 369**
Margaret Grey
Key Terms, 369
Learning Outcomes, 369

Descriptive and Inferential Statistics, 370
Hypothesis Testing, 370
Probability, 372
Type I and Type II Errors, 374
Tests of Statistical Significance, 376
Critiquing Inferential Statistical Results, 383
Example of the Use and Critique of Inferential Statistics, 384
Key Points, 385
Critical Thinking Challenges, 386
References, 386
Additional Readings, 387

Chapter 16 **Analysis of the Findings, 389**
  Geri LoBiondo-Wood
Key Terms, 389
Learning Outcomes, 389
Findings, 390
Critiquing the Results and Discussion, 398
Key Points, 400
Critical Thinking Challenges, 400
References, 401
Additional Readings, 401

Part Two **Critique and Application, 403**
Intangible Benefits of Nursing Research, 404
  Dorothy Brooten

Chapter 17 **Evaluating Quantitative Research Studies, 407**
  Judith A. Heermann, Betty J. Craft
Key Terms, 407
Learning Outcomes, 407
Stylistic Considerations, 408
- **Critique of Research Study: Sample No. 1, 412**
- **A Comparison of the Effects of Jaw Relaxation and Music on Postoperative Pain, 413**
Method, 415
Results, 418
Discussion, 420
Introduction to Critique No. 1, 423
- **Critique of Research Study: Sample No. 2, 428**
- **Problem-Focused Coping in HIV-Infected Mothers in Relation to Self-Efficacy, Uncertainty, Social Support, and Psychological Distress, 429**
Review of Literature, 430
Framework for the Study, 430
Methodology, 431

Results, 434
Discussion, 434
Conclusion, 436
Introduction to Critique No. 2, 438
Critical Thinking Challenges, 444
References, 444
Additional Readings, 444

Chapter 18 Evaluating the Qualitative Research Report, 445
 Helen J. Streubert
Key Terms, 445
Learning Outcomes, 445
Stylistic Considerations, 446
Application of Qualitative Research Findings in Practice, 447
■ **Critique of a Qualitative Research Study, 449**
■ **The Lived Experience of Women Military Nurses in Vietnam During the Vietnam War, 450**
Research Approach, 451
Data Collection, 451
Data Analysis, 451
Findings, 453
Discussion, 459
Introduction to the Critique, 461
Critical Thinking Challenges, 465
References, 465

Chapter 19 Use of Research in Practice, 467
 Marita G. Titler
Key Terms, 467
Learning Outcomes, 467
Overview of Research Utilization, 468
Steps of Research Utilization, 479
Implementing a Research Utilization Program, 491
Future Directions, 494
Critical Thinking Challenges, 495
References, 495

Appendix A A Comparison of Three Wound Dressings in Patients
 Undergoing Heart Surgery, 499
 Karin Wikblad, Beth Anderson

Appendix B Healing of Adult Male Survivors of Childhood Sexual
 Abuse, 509
 Claire Burke Draucker, Kathleen Petrovic

Appendix C Patient Outcomes for the Chronically Critically Ill: Special
 Care Unit Versus Intensive Care Unit, 521
 Ellen B. Rudy, Barbara J. Daly, Sara Douglas, Hugo D. Montenegro, Rhayun Song, Mary Ann Dyer

Appendix D **Concerns About Analgesics Among Patients and Family Caregivers in a Hospice Setting, 537**
Sandra E. Ward, Patricia Emery Berry, Hollis Misiewicz

Glossary, 549

Index, 563

Nursing Research

Methods, Critical Appraisal, and Utilization

Introduction

Research Vignette
**From Research
to Practice**

Chapter 1
**The Role of Research
in Nursing**

Research Vignette

FROM RESEARCH TO PRACTICE

When I began collaborating with Dr. Barbara Braden on the development of a tool to predict pressure sore risk in nursing home patients, our hope was that we could improve the care of patients in the nursing home where we were doing our research. The knowledge generated in our program of research has, after many years of work, exceeded our initial expectations. Public policy has been influenced, and change in clinical practice has reduced the incidence of pressure sores in many settings.

We began work on the Braden Scale for Predicting Pressure Sore Risk in 1983. This tool is composed of six subscales (Mobility, Activity, Sensory Perception, Moisture, Friction and Shear, and Nutrition) that address the major conceptually defined risk factors for pressure ulcers. Each subscale quantifies the level of a specific factor placing the patient at risk for pressure ulcers. The total score is used to determine if the patient is at risk. We learned through studies in many settings that this tool has very good sensitivity and specificity; that is, it helps us identify with a high degree of accuracy who will or who will not develop pressure sores. Once we know this, we can use the subscale scores to plan care specifically tailored to the individual's needs. It is also important to know, as we can with the Braden Scale, who is unlikely to develop pressure sores so that we don't needlessly use nursing care time or special resources on individuals who do not require this care.

It has been interesting to learn through our studies that even experienced nurses benefit from using formal risk assessment. Most nurses can tell who is at high risk, because the risk factors are usually fairly obvious. Likewise, most nurses can tell who is at no risk, but those patients at moderate or low risk are most likely to slip through the cracks. When nurses do not know patients are at risk they do not initiate preventive strategies. In fact, our studies showed that a high number of patients who were at high risk did not have nursing or medical orders for turning or support surfaces when formal risk assessment was not part of routine care.

Predicting pressure sore risk is only the first step in prevention. The Braden Scale serves as the basis for developing an overall plan of care for each patient. It is important that this plan of care is also based on the best possible research and that it is carried out faithfully. The Agency for Health Care Policy and Research (AHCPR) helped nurses and other health care providers by identifying and synthesizing research related to pressure ulcer prevention. Guidelines for the Prediction and Prevention of Pressure Ulcers were written and disseminated. These guidelines recommend that all patients who are bedfast or chairfast should be evaluated for pressure ulcer risk (using the Braden or Norton Scale) on admission to a health care facility. Those individuals at risk are to be placed on protocols that manage the amount and duration of pressure to which the patient is exposed, decrease exposure of the skin to moisture, and promote more adequate nutritional status. More than 2.5 million copies of the guidelines were distributed.

On a very positive note, there are many practice changes based on the AHCPR guidelines and the requirements of surveyors, payors, and accreditors for risk assessment and management. Most often practice changes come about when skin care teams within clinical settings decide that they need to reduce the incidence of pressure ulcers in their settings. They evaluate the literature and create a protocol to reduce risk factors, they make decisions based on research and guideline recommendations, they collect before and after data to determine if their efforts are effective, and they educate all health care providers who will be working with patients. The results of implementing such protocols have been very exciting; the incidence of pressure ulcers has been decreasing, and savings in health care dollars are being reported.

Nancy Bergstrom, PhD, RN, FAAN
Professor and Interim Associate Dean
University of Nebraska Medical Center
College of Nursing
Omaha, Nebraska

The Role of Research in Nursing

Geri LoBiondo-Wood ∎ Judith Haber

Key Terms

applied research
basic research
consumer
critique
research
research utilization
theory

Learning Outcomes

After reading this chapter the student should be able to do the following:

- State the significance of research to the practice of nursing.
- Identify the role of the consumer of nursing research.
- Discuss the differences in trends within nursing research before and after 1950.
- Describe the way research, education, and practice relate to each other.
- Evaluate the nurse's role in the research process as it relates to the nurse's level of educational preparation.
- Identify the future trends in nursing research.
- Formulate the priorities for nursing research for moving into the twenty-first century.

As you begin to read the first chapter of this book you may be wondering, "Why on earth is a research course part of my course curriculum?" You may be asking yourself what research has to do with nursing. You may also wonder how nursing research will help you practice nursing in a better way or how it will help your patients. In answer to such questions, the research course you are taking has everything to do with the practice of professional nursing. As you develop the ability to appraise research studies knowledgeably, your critical thinking skills will become sharper. This, in turn, will help you fine tune your clinical judgment and decision-making skills; the ultimate beneficiary will be your patients! As you may have guessed, many nurses do share the belief that a knowledge of and involvement in nursing research can have a significant effect on the depth and breadth of the professional practice of every nurse. The purpose of this chapter is to help you begin to develop an appreciation of the significance of research in nursing and the research roles of nurses through a historical and futuristic approach.

SIGNIFICANCE OF RESEARCH IN NURSING

The health care environment is changing at an unprecedented pace. Pender (1992) states that "to thrive nursing as a profession must not only keep up with the pace but set the pace for the future of health care." Nurses are challenged to expand their "comfort zone" by offering creative approaches to old and new health problems, designing new and innovative programs that truly make a difference in the health status of our American citizens. This challenge can best be met by integrating rapidly expanding knowledge about biological, behavioral, and environmental influences on health into nursing practice. Nursing research provides a specialized scientific knowledge base that empowers the nursing profession to anticipate and meet these constantly shifting challenges and maintain our societal relevance.

You can think of **research utilization** as the actual systematic implementation of a scientifically sound, research-based innovation in a health care setting with an accompanying process to assess the outcome(s) of change (Titler et al, 1994). Through research utilization efforts, knowledge obtained from research is transformed into clinical practice, culminating in nursing practice that is research based. For example, to help you understand the importance of research utilization, think about the study by Rudy et al (1995) (see Appendix C), which sought to determine whether there would be any differences in patient outcomes of length of stay, mortality, readmission, complications, satisfaction, and cost when chronically critically ill patients were cared for in a low-technology special care unit (SCU) using a nursing case management delivery system versus a traditional high-technology environment such as an intensive care unit (ICU) and primary nursing care delivery system. Findings from this 4-year clinical trial demonstrated that few significant differences were found between the two groups in terms of satisfaction, length of stay, mortality, or complications. However, the findings showed significant cost savings in the SCU group in the charges accrued during the study period and in the charges and costs to produce a survivor. The average total cost of delivering care was $5000 less per patient in the SCU than in the traditional ICU. In addition, the cost to produce a survivor was $19,000 less in the SCU. These findings provide nurses with quality and cost-effectiveness outcome data that confirm that care managed by nurses working with collaboratively derived medical protocols produces outcomes that are equal to or exceed those of patients whose care is managed by residents and interns in the routine ICU setting. Such data support scientifically based clinical decisions about making changes in nursing care delivery models rather than adherence to traditional models of delivering care to long-term critically ill patients. Although the data from this research study have definite potential for utilization in practice, changes in hospital policy will not and should not occur as a result of one study. Replication of this study is necessary to build an adequate knowledge base for implementation in practice, one that has been systematically evaluated over time.

Today more than ever before, nurses are required to be accountable for the quality of patient care they deliver. In an era of consumerism that is questioning the quality of health care and high health care costs, consumers and employers, the purchasers of health insurance, are asking health professionals to document the effectiveness of their services. Essentially they are asking, "How do nursing services make a difference?" The message can hardly be clearer; how consumers and employers perceive the value of nurses' contributions will determine the profession's role in any future delivery system (Buerhaus, 1996). Public and private sector reimbursement groups, including insurance companies, managed care organizations, and governmental agencies using capitated and prospective payment systems (e.g., Medicare and Medicaid) are also requiring accountability for services provided. Health care report cards that document outcomes related to quality and cost are increasingly common (ANA, 1994). The Joint Commission on Accreditation of Healthcare Organizations (JCAHO) 1995 standards require health care agencies to implement outcomes management programs that demonstrate the link between quality care and cost-effective patient outcomes.

The Commission on Nursing Research of the American Nurses Association (ANA, 1989) has recognized the need for research skills at all levels of professional nursing. The Cabinet proposes that all nurses share a commitment to the advancement of nursing science through the conduct of research and utilization of research findings in practice. Scientific investigation promotes accountability, one of the hallmarks of a profession and a fundamental concept of the ANA (1985) Code for Nurses. There is a general consensus that the research role of the baccalaureate graduate calls for the skills of critical appraisal. That is, the nurse must be a knowledgeable consumer of research, one who can **critique** research and use existing standards to determine the merit and readiness of research for utilization in clinical practice (ANA, 1989). The remainder of this book is devoted to helping you develop that consumer expertise.

RESEARCH: LINKING THEORY, EDUCATION, AND PRACTICE

Research links **theory,** education, and practice. Theoretical formulations supported by research findings may potentially become the foundations of theory-based practice in nursing. The educational setting provides an environment in which students can learn about the research process. In this setting they can also explore different theories and begin to evaluate them in light of research findings.

A classic research study by Brooten et al (1986) illustrates a theory-based investigation that has societal relevance, is clinically oriented, is interdisciplinary, and provides research experience for student research assistants. The study sought to determine the safety, efficacy, and cost savings of early hospital discharge of very-low-birth-weight infants. One group of infants ($n = 40$) was discharged according to routine nursery criteria (weight above 2200 g). Those in the early discharge group ($n = 39$) were discharged before they reached this weight if they met a standard set of conditions. For families of infants in the early discharge group, education, counseling, home visits, and on-call availability of a hospital-based nurse specialist for 18 months were provided. The two groups did not differ in specific outcome criteria, including the number of rehospitalizations and acute care visits and measures of physical and mental growth. The average hospital cost for the early discharge group was 27% less than that for the standard discharge group, and the average physician cost was 22% less. The average cost of the home follow-up care was $576, yielding a net savings of $18,560 for each infant in the early discharge group. Brooten et al (1986) stated that if only half of the 36,000 very-low-birth-weight infants born in the United States each year were discharged according to the protocol tested, the annual health care savings could be as much as $334 million, with no adverse effect on the infants or their families. These findings have had enormous implications not only for nursing practice but also for related health care disciplines, all of which compose the interdisciplinary health care team involved in the care of very-low-birth-weight infants. Using the team's quality-cost model, Brooten and other researchers have extended their work to three additional patient groups—women with unplanned cesarean births, women with antepartum and postpartum diabetes, and women who have had hysterectomies (Brooten et al, 1988; Brooten et al, 1989; Cohen, Hollingsworth, and Rubin, 1989; Graff et al, 1992).

Another study examined the healing process of adult male survivors of childhood sexual abuse. The descriptive data obtained from interviews with male survivors who had experienced healing from the trauma of childhood sexual abuse provided the basis for constructing a four-stage theoretical framework titled "Escaping the Dungeon: The Journey to Freedom" (Draucker and Petrovic, 1996). This framework illustrates how men experienced the process of healing from childhood sexual trauma. The data reveal that the men engaged in a journey from captivity to freedom: living in the dungeon, breaking free, living free, and freeing those left behind. The metaphor of "dungeon" reflects the men's experiences of powerlessness, isolation, silence and darkness, shame, and pain from their abuse. Healing involved a struggle against an internal force, emotional pain, and against an external force, the sociocultural prescription that men should not be victims. The findings of this study highlight the need for nurses to consider and acknowledge the unique and pervasive effects of childhood sexual abuse experiences on male survivors; develop treatment programs not based on societal stereotypes, but sensitive to gender differences; and address the context of their healing in a society where the victimization of men is often invalidated, seeking treatment is often discouraged, and the expression of painful feelings by males is often squelched (e.g., "Real men don't cry").

The preceding examples provide the answer to a question you may have been asking: How will the theory and research content of your course relate to your nursing practice? The data from each study have clearly demonstrated societal and practice implications. The study by Brooten et al (1986) provided data that illustrated an innovative nursing intervention protocol with very-low-birth-weight infants that was cost-effective and maintained high-quality infant outcomes. In an era of continuing concern about health care costs, empirically supported programs that are cost-effective without compromising quality are essential. Given the national concern about the long-term individual and family effects of trauma and the physical, emotional, and financial sequelae often experienced, the study by Draucker and Petrovic (1996) provided important data about a four-stage theoretical framework for understanding the healing experience of male survivors of childhood sexual abuse. This model can be used to plan treatment that addresses the gender specific needs of male survivors in a manner that facilitates the healing process.

At this point you may logically ask how education in nursing research links theory and practice. The answer is twofold. First, it will provide you with an appreciation and an understanding of the research process such that you will become a participant in research activities. Second, it must help you become an intelligent consumer of research. A **consumer** of research uses and applies research in an active manner. To be a knowledgeable consumer, a nurse must have a knowledge base about the relevant subject matter, the ability to discriminate and evaluate information logically, and the ability to apply the knowledge gained. It is not necessary to conduct studies to be able to appreciate and use research findings in practice. Rather, to be intelligent consumers, nurses must understand the research process and develop the critical evaluation skills needed to judge the merit and relevance of findings before applying them in practice.

ROLES OF THE NURSE IN THE RESEARCH PROCESS

There are many roles for nurses in research. One of the marks of success in nursing research is the delineation of research activities geared for nurses prepared in different types of educational programs (McBride, 1988; Wheeler, Fasano, and Burr, 1995).

Graduates of associate degree nursing programs should demonstrate an awareness of the value or relevance of research in nursing. They may assist in identifying problem areas in nursing practice within an established structured format, assist in data collection activities, and in conjunction with the professional nurse, appropriately use research findings in clinical practice (ANA, 1989).

Nurses with a baccalaureate education must be intelligent consumers of research; that is, they must understand each step of the research process and its relationship to every other step. Such understanding must be linked with a clear idea about the standards of satisfactory research. This comprehension is necessary when critically reading and understanding research reports, thereby determining the validity and merit of reported studies. Through critical appraisal skills that use specific criteria to judge all aspects of the research, a professional nurse interprets, evaluates, and determines the credibility of research findings. The nurse discriminates between an idea that is interesting but requires further investigation before implementation in practice and findings that have sufficient support to be considered for utilization (ANA, 1989; Beyea, Farley, and Williams-Burgess, 1996; Buckwalter, 1992).

In this context, understanding the research process and acquiring critical appraisal skills open a broad realm of information that can contribute to the professional nurse's body of knowledge and that can be applied judiciously to practice in the interest of providing scientifically based care (Batey, 1982; Duffy, 1987). Thus the role of the baccalaureate graduate in the research process is primarily that of a knowledgeable consumer, a role that promotes the integration of research and clinical practice.

Lest anyone think that this is an unimportant role, let us assure you that it is not. Fawcett (1984) states that we are all aware of those who assert that research is the bailiwick of "ivory tower" investigators. She goes on to state, however, that it is the staff nurse who is ultimately responsible for utilization of the findings of nursing and other health-related research in clinical practice. To use such research findings appropriately, nurses must understand and critically appraise them. Thus if nursing as a profession is ever to have a genuine theory-based practice, it will be in large part up to nurses in their role as consumers of research to accomplish this task.

Baccalaureate graduates also have a responsibility to identify nursing problems that require investigation and to participate in the implementation of scientific studies (ANA, 1989). It is often clinicians who generate research ideas or questions from hunches, gut-level feelings, intuition, or observations of patients or nursing care. These ideas are often the seeds of further research investigations. For example, a nurse working on a psychiatric unit observed that a certain percentage of discharged patients were readmitted to the unit within 2 months of discharge. She noted that there were differences in the discharge procedure and wanted to find out whether the type of aftercare treatment made a difference in the readmission rate. Of particular interest was the variation related to whether the patient was connected to the aftercare therapist or facility before discharge and how this influenced the readmission rate. The presence and support of an expert nurse researcher in the clinical setting can often provide leadership and direction for staff nurses in the systematic investigation of such an idea in an onsite clinical research project. Systematic collection of data about a clinical problem contributes to the refinement and extension of nursing practice.

Baccalaureate graduates may also participate in research projects as members of an interdisciplinary or intradisciplinary research team. The nurse may participate in one or more phases of such a project. For example, a staff nurse may work on a clinical research unit where a particular type of nursing care is part of an established research protocol, such as for decubitus ulcers (pressure sores) or urinary incontinence. In such a situation the nurse administers the care according to the format described in the protocol. The nurse may also be involved in the collection and recording of data relevant to the administration of and patient response to the nursing care.

Promotion of ethical principles of research, especially the protection of human subjects, is another essential responsibility of baccalaureate prepared nurses. For example, a nurse caring for a patient who is beginning an antinausea chemotherapy research protocol would make sure that the patient had signed the informed consent and had all his or her questions answered by the research team before beginning the protocol. A nurse who observed the patient having an adverse reaction to the medication protocol would know that his or her responsibility would be not to administer another dose before notifying an appropriate member of the research team (see Chapter 11).

As members of a profession, it is also incumbent on baccalaureate graduates to share research findings with colleagues. This may involve collaborative dissemination of the findings of a study that you have participated in through development of an article or presentation for a research or clinical conference, or it may involve sharing with colleagues the findings of a research report that you have critiqued and have found to have merit and potential applicability in your practice. In a more formal way, it may involve joining your health care agency's research committee or its quality assurance (QA) or quality improvement (QI) committee where research articles from literature reviews are evaluated for evidence-based clinical decision making.

Nurses who are educationally prepared at the master's and doctoral levels must also be sophisticated consumers of research. However, they are also being prepared to conduct research as either a coinvestigator or a primary investigator.

At the master's level, nurses are prepared to be active members of research teams. They are able to assume the role of clinical expert, collaborating with an experienced researcher in proposal development, data collection, data analysis, and interpretation (ANA, 1989). Master's prepared nurses enhance the quality and relevance of nursing research by providing clinical expertise about problems and by providing knowledge about the way the clinical services are delivered. They facilitate the investigation of clinical problems by providing a climate favorable to conducting research. This includes collaborating with others in investigations and enhancing nursing's access to patients and data. At the master's level, nurses conduct research investigations for the purpose of monitoring the quality of the practice of nursing in a clinical setting. They provide leadership by assisting others in applying scientific knowledge in nursing practice (ANA, 1989).

Doctorally prepared nurses have the greatest amount of expertise in appraising, designing, and conducting research. They develop theoretical explanations of phenomena relevant to nursing. They develop methods of scientific inquiry and use analytical and empirical methods to discover ways to modify or extend existing knowledge so that it is relevant to nursing. Two types of research are conducted by doctorally prepared nurses: **basic research** and **applied research.** Table 1-1 provides a definition and an example of each type of research. In addition to their role as producers of research, doctorally prepared nurses act as role models and mentors who guide, stimulate, and encourage other nurses who are developing their research skills. They also collaborate with and serve as consultants to social, educational, or health care institutions or governmental agencies in their research endeavors. Doctorally prepared nurses are charged with dissemination of their research findings to the scientific community, to clinicians, and, as appropriate, to the lay public. Scientific journals, professional conferences, and the news media are among the mechanisms for dissemination (ANA, 1989; Brink 1995; Downs, 1991).

The most important implication of the delineation of research activities according to educational preparation is the necessity of having a collaborative research relationship within the nursing profession. Not all nurses must or should conduct research. However, all nurses can play some part in the research process. Nurses at all educational levels, whether they are consumers or producers of research or both, need to view the research process as something of integral value to the growing professionalism in nursing.

Professionals need to take the time to read research studies and to evaluate them using the standards congruent with scientific research. The critiquing process is used to identify the strengths and weaknesses of each study. Nurses should keep in mind that no study is perfect; although the limitations should be recognized, nurses may extrapolate from the study whatever is sound and relevant evidence to be considered for potential use in clinical practice.

HISTORICAL PERSPECTIVE

The history of nursing research comprises many changes and developments. The groundwork for what has blossomed was laid in the late nineteenth century and the first half of the twentieth century. To capture the essence of the development of nursing research and the works of so many excellent researchers, especially in the 1980s and 1990s, is beyond the scope of this chapter. A review of the many nursing journals available provides further support of the ef-

Table 1-1

Types of Nursing Research

TYPE OF RESEARCH	DEFINITION	EXAMPLE
Basic research	Theoretical or pure research that generates, tests, and expands theories that describe, explain, or predict the phenomenon of interest to the discipline without regard to its later use (Silva, 1986).	Barrett's (1989, 1990) Power Theory is based on a postulate of Rogers' Science of Unitary Human Beings (i.e., that humans can knowingly participate in change). Barrett proposed that power is the way humans knowingly participate in change, creating their reality by actualizing some potentials for change rather than others. The methodological focus of Barrett's research concerned development of an instrument to measure the theoretical power construct.
Applied research	"Answers questions related to the applicability of basic theories in practical situations" (Donaldson and Crowley, 1978); tests the practical limits of descriptive theories but does not examine the efficacy of actions taken by practitioners.	Ward, Berry, and Misiewicz's study (1996) of concerns about analgesics among patients and family caregivers in a hospice setting examined the comparison of patients and caregivers in relation to concerns about reporting pain and using analgesics and whose concerns are more strongly associated with hesitancy to report pain and use analgesics.

forts of nursing researchers. Box 1-1 highlights key events that have set the stage for the richness of the current nursing research efforts.

Nineteenth Century—After 1850

In the mid-nineteenth century, nursing as a formal discipline began to take root with the ideas and practices of Florence Nightingale. Her concepts have contributed to and are congruent with the present priorities of nursing research. The promotion of health, prevention of disease, and care of the sick were central ideas of her system. Nightingale believed that the systematic collection and exploration of data were necessary for nursing. Her collection and analysis of

Box 1-1   Historical Perspective

Nineteenth Century—After 1850

1852   Nightingale wrote *Cassandra*.

1855   Nightingale studied and calculated mortality rates of British in Crimean War and on basis of data developed plans to decrease military overcrowding.

1859   Nightingale's *Notes on Matters Affecting the Health, Efficiency and Hospital Administration of the British Army;* and *Notes on Hospitals* published.

1859   Nightingale's *Notes on Nursing* published.

1860   Nightingale founded St. Thomas's Hospital School of Nursing in England.

1861   Nightingale developed cost accounting system for Army Medical Services.

1872   First nursing schools in the U.S. began: New England Hospital for Women & Children, Boston; Women's Hospital, Philadelphia.

1893   Lillian Wald and Mary Brewster established Henry Street Visiting Nurse Service.

1899   International Council of Nurses organized.

Twentieth Century—Before 1950

1900-1909

1902   Lavinia Dock reported school health experiment begun by Lillian Wald for free child health care.

1900   *American Journal of Nursing* publication began.

1909   Nursing programs began at Columbia University Teacher's College and University of Minnesota.

1909   "Visiting Nursing in the United States" conducted by Waters.

1910-1919

1912   American Nurses Association established.

1914   Metropolitan Life Insurance Company contracted nurses to collect data on health problems and tuberculosis.

1920-1929

1923   Goldmark Report published.

1923   Yale and Case Western Reserve universities' nursing programs began.

1924   First nursing doctoral program began at Teacher's College, Columbia University.

1926   From 1926 to 1934 Committee on Grading of Nursing Schools convened.

1927   Edith S. Bryan became the first nurse to receive a Ph.D. in psychology and counseling from The Johns Hopkins University.

1930-1939

1934   Nursing doctoral program established at New York University.

1934   Nightingale International Foundation established.

1936   Sigma Theta Tau, National Honor Society for Nursing, began nursing research funding.

Continued

Box 1-1   Historical Perspective—cont'd

1940-1949

1948   *Nurses for the Future—The Brown Report* was published.

1948   United States Public Health Service Division of Nursing conducted nursing surveys and published manuals for the conduct of nursing research.

Twentieth Century—After 1950

1950-1959

1950   American Nurses Association established a Master Plan for Research, 1951-1956.

1952   National League for Nursing was established.

1952   *Nursing Research* publication began.

1953   *Nursing Outlook* publication began.

1953   Institute of Research & Service in Nursing Education was established at Teacher's College, Columbia University.

1955   American Nurses' Foundation was formed.

1956   United States Public Health Service began awarding grants for nursing research.

1956   Predoctoral fellowships for nursing research were first awarded.

1957   Department of Nursing Research was established at Walter Reed Army Hospital.

1957   Western Council on Higher Education in Nursing (WCHEN) sponsored Western Interstate Commission for Higher Education (WICHE) to augment graduate nursing education, especially in nursing research.

1958   Abdellah and Levine study of nursing personnel was published.

1959   National League for Nursing (NLN) Research & Studies Service was established.

1959   First faculty research grants awarded to University of Washington and University of California at Los Angeles.

1960-1969

1962   American Nurses Association Blueprint for Nursing Research was issued.

1962   Nurse Scientist Graduate Training Grants Program was initiated.

1962   *Nursing Forum* publication began.

1963   *International Journal of Nursing Studies* publication began.

1963   *Surgeon General's Consultant Group on Nursing* report was issued.

1963   Lydia Hall published study of chronically ill at Loeb Center.

1965   American Nurses Association began sponsoring conferences for nursing research.

1969   Wayne State University College of Nursing established the first nursing research center.

1970-1979

1970   *Abstract for Action—Lysaught Report* was published.

1971   American Nurses Association Council of Nurse Researchers was organized.

1974   Western Council on Higher Education in Nursing set 5-year goal to triple nursing research.

1974   American Nurses Association Commission on Nursing Research proposed involvement of various levels of students in research and a clinical thrust for research.

Box 1-1   Historical Perspective—cont'd

1975   American Nurses Association testified at President Gerald Ford's Panel on Biomedical Research.

1976   *Research in Nursing: Toward a Science of Health Care* published by ANA—Report of nursing research trends.

1976   National League for Nursing set criteria for undergraduate nursing research course in B.S.N. programs.

1978   *Research in Nursing & Health* publication began.

1978   *Advances in Nursing Science* publication began.

1979   *Western Journal of Nursing Research* publication began.

1979   Haller, Reynolds, and Horsley published research utilization criteria.

1980-1989

1980   Commission on Nursing Research of the American Nurses Association set research priorities for 1980s.

1983   Institute of Medicine completed report of *Nursing & Nursing Education: Public and Private Action.*

1986   National Center for Nursing Research established at the National Institutes of Health.

1987   *Scholarly Inquiry for Nursing Practice* and *Applied Nursing Research* publications began.

1988   *Nursing Science Quarterly* and *Nursing Scan in Research* publications began.

1988   Conference on Research Priorities in Nursing Science (CORP No. 1) set research priorities known as National Nursing Research Agenda.

1989   National Center for Health Services Research became Agency for Health Care Policy and Research (AHCPR).

1990s

1991   National Pressure Ulcer Advisory Panel gives its first award to Nancy Bergstrom.

1991   *Qualitative Health Research* publication began.

1992   Kathleen McCormick calls for outcome research efforts.

1992   Conference on Research Priorities in Nursing Science (CORP No. 2) met to set updated research priorities.

1992   Clinical Practice Guidelines: *Urinary Incontinence in Adults, Acute Pain Management,* and *Pressure Ulcers in Adults* were published by AHCPR.

1992   *Healthy People 2000* was published by the Public Health Service.

1993   Report was released of a proposed multiyear funding mechanism by National Center for Nursing Research to increase the integration of biological and nursing sciences.

1993   National Center for Nursing Research becomes National Institute of Nursing Research (NINR).

1993   Online Journal of Knowledge Synthesis published by Sigma Theta Tau International.

1993   Online Computer Library established by Sigma Theta Tau International.

1996   ANA established the Nursing Information and Data Set Evaluation Center (NIDSEC).

data on the health status of British soldiers during the Crimean War led to a variety of reforms in health care (Palmer, 1977). Nightingale also noted the need for measuring outcomes of nursing and medical care (Nightingale, 1863), and she had an expertise in statistics and epidemiology. Nightingale stated, "Statistics are history in repose, history is statistics in motion" (Keith, 1988).

Other than Nightingale's work, there seems to have been little research during the early years of nursing's development, perhaps in part because schools of nursing had just begun to be established in the United States, schools were unequal in ability to educate, and nursing leadership had just begun to develop.

Twentieth Century—Before 1950

Nursing research in the first half of the twentieth century focused mainly on nursing education, but some patient- and technique-oriented research was evident. The early efforts in nursing education research were made by such leaders as Lavinia Dock (1900), Anne Goodrich (1932), Adelaide Nutting (1912, 1926), Isabel Hampton Robb (1906), and Lillian Wald (1915). Nutting's *The Education and Professional Position of Nurses* (1907) and Nutting and Dock's *A History of Nursing* (1907) were the earliest studies of nursing and nursing education. These pioneering works consist of documentation gathered for the purpose of reforming education in nursing and establishing it as a viable profession.

The continued need for reform in nursing education was met by the Nursing and Nursing Education in the United States Landmark Study, known as the Goldmark Report (1923). Sponsored by the Rockefeller Foundation, the Committee on Nursing and Nursing Education was funded to survey on a national level the educational preparation of the faculty and the clinical experiences of the administrators, private duty nurses, public health nurses, and nursing students. The report identified multiple deficiencies and disparate educational backgrounds at all levels of nursing. This study and others in the first half of the century recommended reorganization of nursing education and, most important, its movement into the university setting.

Clinically oriented research emerged in the early half of the century and mainly centered on the morbidity and mortality rates associated with such problems as pneumonia and contaminated milk (Carnegie, 1976). A few of these projects were instrumental in the development of patient care protocols and the employment of nurses in community settings. An experimental project by Wald and Dock conducted in 1902 led to the employment of school nurses in the New York City school system and subsequently in other cities (Roberts, 1954). Although Linda Richards, the first trained American nurse at Bellevue Hospital, did not perform formal research, she was the first nurse to keep written documentation of patient care. This documentation was used by the medical profession for its investigations (Carnegie, 1976).

In 1913 the Committee on Public Health Nursing of the National League of Nursing Education (NLNE) studied such concerns as infant mortality, blindness, and midwifery. The committee called for nursing to distinguish its role in the prevention of disease and the promotion of health through the knowledge and use of the scientific approach.

The 1920s saw the development and teaching of the earliest nursing research course because of the influence of Isabel M. Stewart (Henderson, 1977). The course "Comparative

Nursing Practice," first taught by Smith and later by Henderson, introduced students to the scientific method of investigation. Students were encouraged to question all aspects of nursing care and to do laboratory experiments on such topics as measuring the oxygen content in an oxygen tent during a patient's bed bath to assess whether it dropped below a therapeutic level. Also during this period, case studies appeared in the *American Journal of Nursing* (AJN). These were used as a teaching tool for students and as a record of patient progress (Gortner and Nahm, 1977). Scientific criteria were applied to assess the appropriateness of the methodology used (Gortner and Nahm, 1977).

Other practice-related research focused on improving nursing techniques (Clayton, 1927), handwashing procedures (Broadhurst et al, 1927), and thermometer disinfecting techniques (Ryan and Miller, 1932), among others. Clinical investigations similar to these and subsequent studies of nurses and nursing education were made through the first part of the century.

Social change and World War II affected all aspects of nursing, including research. There was an urgent need for more nurses: increased hospital admissions and military needs created a shortage of personnel. In 1943 the U.S. Cadet Nurses Corps was created after the Nurse Practice Act of 1943 was passed. The Corps provided assistance for nurses and after the war offered information that assisted in planning for nursing education. During the war, investigations focused on hospital environments, nursing status, nursing education, and nursing shortages.

After the war, nursing, like the rest of the world, began to reassess itself and its goals. In 1948 *Nursing for the Future* by Esther Lucille Brown was published. This was the culmination of a 3-year study funded by the Carnegie Foundation. This report reemphasized the inconsistencies in educational preparation and the need to move into the university setting, and it included an updated description of nursing practices. An outgrowth of Brown's report was a number of studies on nursing roles and needs. Also during the immediate postwar period many states carried out studies on nursing needs and resources (Simmons and Henderson, 1964).

Twentieth Century—1950 through 1980

The 1950s saw the blossoming of nursing research. The developments of the 1950s laid the groundwork for nursing's current level of research skill. Nursing schools at the undergraduate and graduate levels were growing in number, and graduate programs were including courses related to research. The worth and benefit of research were appreciated by nursing leadership and were beginning to filter to the various levels of nursing. This period saw the inception of the *Journal of Nursing Research,* which was dedicated to the promotion of research in nursing. In 1955 the American Nurses' Foundation was chartered as a center for research; the audience for its publications consisted of receivers and administrators of research monies. Also at the national level of the ANA a standing Committee on Research and Studies was formed in 1954. This committee was charged with planning, promoting, and guiding research and studies relating to the functions of the Association (See, 1977). A secondary function of the committee was to collect and unify nursing information that could be used to advise the ANA Board regarding periodic inventories of nurses. Concurrently in 1955 the Commonwealth Fund endowed the NLN with monies for the support of research education and training. Throughout the 1950s these organizations and others, such as the U.S. Public Health Service, put forth funds and personnel to study the characteristics of nursing members and students; the supply, organization, and distribution of nursing services; and job satisfaction.

The first nursing unit for practice-oriented research was set up at the Walter Reed Army Institute of Research. This unit was geared toward chemical research. Although research during this period was focused on nurses and their characteristics, the fields of psychiatric nursing and maternal-child health care received monies from federal grants to develop nursing content and educational programs at the master's and doctoral levels. Grants were also conferred on individuals who studied the social context of psychiatric facilities and its influence on relations between staff and patients (Greenblatt et al, 1955; Stanton and Schwartz, 1954) and the role of the nurse with single mothers (Donnell and Glick, 1954).

In the late 1950s nursing studies began to address clinical problems. In a guest editorial featured in *Nursing Research* (1956), Virginia Henderson commented that studies about nurses outnumber clinical studies 10 to 1. She stated that "the responsibility for designing its methods is often cited as an essential characteristic of a profession."

Thus in the 1960s there began a reordering of research priorities and a targeting of practice-oriented research. These priorities were supported by the American Nurses' Foundation and other major nursing organizations. However, even with this support, research did not flourish. This may be partly attributed to the lack of educational preparation of nurses in research. Where research education did exist, nurses had not yet developed sufficient expertise in research design and methodology to teach their own research courses. Therefore nurses were, until recently, dependent on others from related disciplines such as psychology, education, and sociology who had this expertise to teach these courses. Today this is not usually the case.

Consistent with this need for guidance, many of the studies during the 1950s and 1960s were coinvestigated by individuals from the social sciences and medicine. Another reason for the paucity of research was the small number of nurses with baccalaureate and higher degrees. Although enrollment in these programs had increased by 1960, fewer than 2% of the employed registered nurses held master's degrees and fewer than 7% held baccalaureate degrees (ANA, 1960).

During the 1960s, studies on nurses and nursing continued, but at the same time the pioneers in the development of nursing theories and models, such as Ida Jean Orlando (1961), Hildegarde Peplau (1952), and Ernestine Wiedenbach (1964), called for the development of nursing practice based on theory. Although their theories and those of others have only begun to be tested, the early development of those theories has spurred nurses into a more critical level of thinking regarding nursing practice.

Collaborative efforts in the 1960s on practice-oriented research led to follow-up research by Diers and Leonard (1966) and Dumas and Leonard (1963). These studies done at Yale University explored the effects of nurse-patient teaching and communication on such events as hospitalization, surgery, and the labor experience. Another classic study, the culmination of 8 years of work by Glaser and Strauss (1965), explored various aspects of thanatology among dying patients and their caretakers.

A review of the nursing research studies published during the 1960s reveals that clinical studies were beginning to predominate. These studies investigated a wide gamut of nursing care issues such as infection control, alcoholism, and sensory deprivation. Lydia Hall (1963) published the results of a 5-year study that looked at alternatives to hospitalization for a select group of elderly clients. This study gave rise to a totally nurse-run care facility, the Loeb Center in New York City, which is still in operation and run by nurses today.

The rich history of nursing was also recognized during the 1960s. Nursing archives at Boston University's Mugar Library were established through a federally funded grant with the goal of promoting nursing research. In 1967 the First Nursing Research Conference of the ANA was held. A group of nurses and nursing faculty gathered to report on research and critique the findings presented.

The opening of the 1970s saw the publication of the National Committee for the Study of Nursing and Nursing Education Report or the Lysaught Report (1970). This report, conducted with the support of the ANA, NLN, and other private foundations, surveyed nursing practice and education. It offered the conclusions that more practice-oriented and education-oriented research was necessary and that these data must be applied to the improvement of educational organizations and curricula. The call for clinically oriented study was becoming a reality. Carnegie (1976) noted that the majority of research published in the nursing journals was clinically oriented.

The 1970s also saw new growth in the number of master's and doctoral programs for nursing. These programs, along with the ANA, NLN, Sigma Theta Tau, and Western Interstate Council for Higher Education in Nursing, clearly supported nurses learning the research process as well as producing research that could be used to enhance care quality. In the 1970s newer journals such as *Advances in Nursing Sciences, Research in Nursing and Health,* and *The Western Journal of Nursing Research* that promoted the generation of nursing theory and research were established.

The 1980s

The decade of the 1980s was exciting and productive for research in nursing. The period saw extended growth among upper-level programs in nursing, especially at the doctoral level. By 1989 more than 5000 of the doctorally prepared nurses held their doctorate in nursing. Consistent with the increased numbers of nurses with advanced training, federal funding and support for research increased not only in universities but also in practice settings. Many centers for nursing research exist in educational settings and in hospitals. A number of these centers have programs joining education and practice that provide support and guidance for research efforts.

Mechanisms for communicating research have also increased. A number of journals and reviews now provide additional forums for communicating research. Most nursing organizations also have research sections that serve to foster the conduct and use of research.

Public Law 99-158, which was enacted in 1985, allowed for the establishment of the National Center for Nursing Research (NCNR). Established in 1986, NCNR provided funding programs that focus on studies related to health care outcomes.

The efforts of the 1980s were aimed at the refinement and development of research and the utilization of research findings in clinical practice. The developments and strides in the area of research made in the 1980s suggested that nursing was ready to rise to the societal and professional demands that now confront the discipline in the 1990s.

FUTURE DIRECTIONS—THE 1990S AND BEYOND

During the 1990s, nursing research continues to grow and flourish. There are 54 nursing doctoral programs in the United States and 25 nursing doctoral programs outside the United States, and additional programs are under development (Sigma Theta Tau International, 1995a, 1995b). At the conduct level a major focus of nurse researchers is the development of clinically based outcome studies that provide the foundation for evidence-based practice. Recognition of the value of qualitative research studies that increase our understanding of clinical phenomena and provide direction for defining programs of research will expand. The mechanisms for outcomes management and the utilization of the research produced also are being refined and identified as priorities (see Chapter 19). Research-based practice guidelines and protocols will become benchmarks for cost-effective quality clinical practice.

Nurse researchers and nurse leaders are visibly involved at the national level, participating in policy making, representing nursing on expert panels and by providing testimony at Congressional hearings, and lobbying for needed funding dollars. A review of the twentieth century reveals that nursing has truly risen to the challenges of the development of nursing science with the ultimate goal of improving health care. Nursing's research efforts now have further recognition. In June 1993, the National Institutes of Health (NIH) reauthorization bill gave the NCNR institute status. NCNR is now the NINR. Hereafter in the text, NCNR will be referred to as NINR.

Promoting Depth in Nursing Research

In a complex, health-oriented society such as ours that is increasingly responsive to consumer concerns related to the cost, quality, availability, and accessibiilty of health care, it is of paramount importance to define the future direction of nursing research and establish research priorities (Hinshaw, 1988, 1990).

Nursing leaders unanimously agree that the essential priority for nursing research in the future will be promotion of excellence in nursing science (Dickenson-Hazard, 1995; Grady, 1996; Hinshaw and Heinrich, 1990; Riegal et al, 1992). This priority is linked to the efforts of the discipline's scholars to develop a knowledge base that can accurately guide nursing practice (Bavier, 1995).

Research-based practice reflects the characteristics of the research from which it is derived. The quality of research by which nursing science is generated and information is provided to guide practice will be one of the major keys to producing predictable patient outcomes and improving patient care for our own discipline (Bavier, 1995). Essential to the achievement of this goal will be the continuing development of a national and international research environment (Dickenson-Hazard, 1995; Dreher, 1995; Zanotti, 1996). Within this environment an increasing number of nurses who have significant expertise in appraising, designing, and conducting research will continue to emerge within the profession. They will provide a "critical mass" of investigators who will be at the forefront of the ongoing development and refinement of our scientific knowledge base for nursing practice.

To maximize utilization of available resources and prevent wasteful duplication, researchers must develop intradisciplinary and interdisciplinary networks in similar areas of basic and applied study across disciplines (Hinshaw and Heinrich, 1990). Clinical consortia will help delineate the common and unique aspects of patient care for the various health professions.

Cluster studies, multiple-site investigations, and programs of research will facilitate the accumulation of evidence supporting or negating an existing theory and thereby contribute to defining the base of nursing practice.

Depth in nursing science will be evident when replicated, consistent findings exist in a substantive area of inquiry. Programs of research that include a series of studies in a similar area of study, each of which builds on prior investigation, both replicating and adding to the research question being studied, will promote depth in nursing science (Beck, 1994). An example of a program of research is provided by the work of Nancy Bergstrom, the principal investigator funded by a 3-year grant from the NINR for the multisite study of the Nursing Assessment of Pressure Sore Risk. Approximately 1200 patients in a variety of health care settings were studied. The study further validated the use of the Braden scale developed by Barbara Braden for evaluating pressure sore risk. The outcome of this study leads to improved patient care and ultimately to cost savings in terms of equipment use and reduction of hospital stays caused by complications of pressure sores. Consistent and replicable findings across sites yield a body of practice-relevant, in-depth knowledge of pressure sore prevention.

The preceding example illustrates the value of replication studies that are built into programs of research. Hinshaw (1990) proposes that the adoption of research findings in practice, with their potential risks and benefits, including the cost of implementation, should be based on a series of replicated studies. As such, replication studies will have much more credibility in the future and will play a crucial role in developing depth in nursing science.

Nursing research is increasingly addressing physiological as well as psychological responses to actual and potential health problems (Sigmon, Amende and Grady, 1996). Investigations that reflect state-of-the-art science will examine the interface of the biological sciences with the evolving knowledge base of nursing. Nurse researchers will continue to have increased opportunity to participate in clinical trials. This will provide direction to improve aspects of care such as symptom assessment, management, and interventions to prevent and reduce physical distress such as pain (Hinshaw, 1991).

Nurse researchers will continue to have increased methodological expertise. They are increasingly sophisticated about the development and application of computer technology to the research process. A greater emphasis will be placed on measurement issues such as the development of tools that accurately measure clinical phenomena.

The increasing focus on the need to use multiple measures to assess clinical phenomena accurately is also apparent. Related to the need to measure clinical phenomena accurately will be the development of noninvasive methods to measure physiological parameters of interest in high-technology settings. These methods may well be another aspect of using multiple measures to assess particular clinical phenomena. The development of qualitative measures and new qualitative computer analysis packages is also expanding as the qualitative mode of inquiry is more frequently used in research.

Nurse researchers will employ new, more diverse, and advanced methods for the design of research studies and analysis of findings. For example, qualitative research methods have become increasingly respected as a mode of scientific inquiry, contributing to theory development and providing essential descriptive data that provide direction for clinical practice and future research studies. Consider the importance of the findings of Beck's qualitative studies (1992, 1993, 1995) of the Lived Experience of Postpartum Depression, which revealed that the fundamental structure of postpartum depression, as described by the study subjects, differed significantly from that assessed by the questions contained in the most frequently used depression assessment tools. Beck (1992) suggests that quantitative assessment tools should include the gamut of possible behavioral manifestations from which a mother can rate her depressive symptoms. Beck proposes that the fundamental structure of postpartum depression developed from this study can be a starting point for future methodological research focused on developing a quantitative instrument to measure postpartum depression specifically. Researchers using quantitative research methods will expand the frontiers of empirically derived knowledge through the use of advanced analytical programs related to causation.

Outcome Research Studies

Another trend is the proliferation of outcomes research that is both patient- and delivery system–focused (Bavier, 1995; Bidwell-Cerone et al, 1995). Stimulated by the need for cost-effective care that makes a difference without compromising quality, outcome studies will provide an unprecedented opportunity for nurses to pursue research that will contribute to the scientific basis of nursing practice. By verifying the relationship between nursing interventions and patient outcomes, nurse researchers will be adding to the body of nursing interventions that are scientifically sound and document the impact of nursing care. The outcome study of Brooten et al (1986) described earlier in this chapter, which tested an innovative client care delivery model for very-low-birth-weight infants, is a classic example of an outcome study that documents the impact of nursing care.

Through examination of outcomes related to organizational systems outcomes, the most cost-effective models for the delivery of high-quality collaborative care are being identified. For example, the pioneering work of Ethridge and Lamb (1989) in nursing case management illustrates a research program designed to describe the process of case management and evaluate its impact on quality and costs of care for high-risk patients. Lamb (1992) reports that a series of research studies, which have incorporated both qualitative and quantitative research designs, have convincingly demonstrated that the previously cited community-based nursing care delivery model has a positive impact on quality outcomes such as greater confidence in self-care, symptom management, and patient satisfaction and on cost-effectiveness outcomes such as hospital length of stay, hospital admissions, and emergency department visits. It is clear that nurses must capitalize on the opportunity to lead other health care providers in ensuring that outcomes are measured fully.

Programs of Research

Research training for the scientific role will increasingly become an essential component of a research career plan. Nurse researchers will be committed to developing programs of research that are supported by public and private funding sources. They will also subscribe to a lifestyle of periodic education and retraining that will be funded by awards, grants, and fellowships. For example, the NINR awards funding for predoctoral, postdoctoral, midcareer, and senior scientist programs of study. These programs facilitate growth in the depth and breadth of research expertise and recognize the need of some researchers to be retrained as they develop or shift the emphasis of their research, seek to broaden their scientific background, acquire new research capabilities, and enlarge their command of an allied research field.

Nurses who are prepared to direct the conduct of research will head an expanding number of nursing research departments in clinical settings. Currently there are more than 100 clinical research centers in as many as 32 states. Nurse researchers who head these centers will involve the nursing staff in generating and conducting research projects and critically evaluating existing research data before using it to guide changes in clinical practice. An expanded number of centers for nursing research will be established in university settings as faculty members become qualified to direct them.

An International Perspective

With the discipline's emphasis on cultural aspects of nursing care and the influence of such factors on practice, increasing international research is a natural futuristic trend. Access to multiple populations as a function of globalization allows the generation and testing of nursing science from many different perspectives. Interaction with colleagues from other countries provides a rich context for the generation and dissemination of research issues (Bower, 1995; Zanotti, 1996).

Alliances with international organizations committed to the goal of health for all will create natural research partnerships. For example, the World Health Organization (WHO), through the Pan-American Health Organization, has designated that four WHO Collaborating Centers for Research and Clinical Training in Nursing be located in American schools and colleges of nursing. These centers will provide research and clinical training in nursing to colleagues worldwide. The International Council of Nurses (ICN) and the ANA Council of Nursing Research conferences are examples of international nursing research forums designed to inform nurses of the global breadth of health problems. Such forums for dissemination of research will continue to increase, challenging nurse researchers in various regions of the world to form collaborative research relationships in which they share research expertise, educational opportunities, and the ability to conduct research projects of mutual interest and, perhaps, ultimately create an international research agenda (Shaver, 1991; School of Nursing, University of California at San Francisco, 1992).

Future Research Priorities

In 1996 the U.S. Department of Health and Human Services published the revised summary report, "Healthy People 2000 Review 1994." The original document, published in 1992, was a product of 22 expert working groups and nearly 300 national organizations, including nursing bodies, and contained 22 priority areas geared to the improvement of the health of the nation. The current document reaffirms these priority areas. The National Research Agenda identifies priorities that are consistent with the goals of this national health agenda. By the year 2000 and into the twenty-first century, a cost-effective, community-based health care delivery system that emphasizes primary care and promotes prevention in partnership with members of a culturally diverse society will actualize a high-quality health care vision. One of the objectives, for example, is "to reduce physical abuse directed at women by male partners to no more than 27 instances per 1000 couples" (U.S. Department of Health and Human Services, 1992, 1996). Several nurse researchers, such as Campbell (1989); Campbell et al (1992); McFarlane (1992); McFarlane, Parker, and Soeken (1996a, 1996b); Parker et al (1993); and

Sampselle (1992), have been conducting research, developing theoretical perspectives, and conducting synthesis conferences in the area of abuse of women. In at least one case a study conducted by Campbell and Alford (1989) was used to assist in legislative change.

Concern about vulnerable populations will be integral with shaping the focus of a nursing research agenda. By the year 2000 the population will include a higher proportion of children and elderly adults who are chronically ill or disabled. The health problems of mothers and infants will continue to spur concern for dealing effectively with the rising maternal-infant mortality rate. Individuals who have sustained life-threatening illnesses will live by means of new life-sustaining technology that will create new demands for self-care and family support. Cancer, heart disease, arthritis, chronic pulmonary disease, diabetes, and Alzheimer's disease are prevalent during middle and later life and will command large proportions of the available health care resources. Mental health problems will result from rapid technological and social change; understanding of mental disorders will expand as a result of the psychobiological knowledge explosion and research initiatives. Alcohol and drug abuse will continue to be responsible for significant health care expense. The impact of human immunodeficiency virus (HIV) on individuals, families, and communities dealing with the crisis of acquired immunodeficiency syndrome (AIDS) will have a major effect on the health care delivery system. Increasingly, the settings where care is provided will be homes, schools, workplaces, and primary care centers. Over the next 10 years many hard questions of cost containment and access to care will be addressed through an interdisciplinary approach and which will need to address the related ethical dilemmas.

The emphasis of research studies will be related to clinical and systems issues and problems. The preeminent goal of scientific inquiry by nurses will be the ongoing development of knowledge for use in the practice of nursing. This refers to an action agenda that establishes how the quality of patient care is connected to nursing practice and how the interventions of nurses are related to patient satisfaction and important clinical outcomes. It also refers to patient care initiatives related to the organization and delivery of nursing care. This type of research, sometimes referred to as *health services research,* would include studies that predict the future supply and demand for nursing care (Kovner and Jonas [in press]). Consequently, priority will be given to nursing research that generates knowledge to guide practice in the areas listed in Box 1-2.

In light of the priority given to clinical research issues, the funding of investigations will increasingly emphasize clinical research projects in relation to populations of interest. For example, the historical exclusion of women from clinical research is now well documented. Men have been the subjects in the major contemporary research studies related to adult health. The findings of such studies have been generalized from men to all adults, despite the lack of female representation (Larson, 1994). The Baltimore Longitudinal Study on Aging began in 1958 but did not include women as subjects until 1978. Although women now make up about 60% of those in the United States who are 65 or older, the study's well-respected 1984 report, "Normal Human Aging," contained no data specific to women. Women of color have been even more likely to be excluded from research studies; as a result, research data on women of color are extremely scarce. Funding for research related to women's health issues and problems such as infertility, menopause, breast and ovarian cancer, and osteoporosis has been less than equitable. Given the indisputable nature of this research bias, the Office of Research on Women's Health has been established at the NIH to redress historical inequities in research

Box 1-2	Extramural Priority Areas for Nursing Research

Integrating biological and behavioral research is a major program priority. Three dimensions—promoting health and preventing disease, managing the symptoms and disability of illness, and improving the environments in which care is delivered—cut across the following six broad science areas:

1. Research in *chronic conditions,* including arthritis, diabetes, and urinary incontinence, as well as in long-term care and care giving
2. Research in *health and risk behaviors,* including studies of women's health, developmental transitions such as adolescence and menopause, and health and behavior research such as studies of smoking cessation
3. Research in *cardiopulmonary health,* including prevention and care of individuals with cardiac or respiratory conditions; this area also includes research in critical care, trauma, wound healing, and organ transplants
4. Research in *neurofunction and brain disorders,* including pain management, sleep disorders, symptom management in persons with brain disorders such as Alzheimer's disease, and rehabilitation after brain and spinal cord injury; this area also includes research on patient care in acute settings
5. Research in *immune and neoplastic diseases,* including symptoms primarily associated with cancer and AIDS (e.g., fatigue, nausea and vomiting, and cachexia); prevention research on specific risk factors is included
6. Research in *reproductive and infant health,* including prevention of premature labor, reduction of health-risk factors during pregnancy, delivery of prenatal care, care of neonates, infant growth and development, and fertility issues

From NINR: *National Institute of Nursing Research fact sheet,* Washington, DC, 1996, NIH.

design and allocation of federal resources. Research on women's health is likely to be a major funding focus in the future.

Areas of special research interest delineated by the NINR for 1995 to 1999 (NINR, 1996) include the following:

- Developing and testing community-based nursing models designed to promote access to, utilization of, and quality of health services by rural, minority, and other underserved populations
- Assessing the effectiveness of biobehavioral nursing interventions to foster health-promoting behaviors of individuals at risk for HIV and AIDS and the effectiveness of biobehavioral interventions to ameliorate the effects of illness in individuals who are already infected. The focus is on persons of different cultural backgrounds—especially women. The need to incorporate biobehavioral markers is noted
- Development and testing of biobehavioral and environmental approaches to remediating cognitive impairment and to examine prevention strategies that target those at risk
- Testing interventions that increase individual and family adaptation to chronic illness
- Identifying biobehavioral factors and test interventions to promote immunocompetence

Other types of research investigations such as those using historical, feminist, or case study methods embody the rich diversity of extant nursing research methods. Brink (1990) states that the enormous, exponential growth in nursing research since the early 1950s seems attributable to the diversity of methodological approaches that have been used to answer the profession's research questions. The nursing profession must continue to value and promote creativity and diversity in research endeavors at all educational levels as a way of empowering nursing practice for the future. As opportunities are recognized and gaps in science are observed, nurses will engage in the conduct, critique, and utilization of nursing research in ways that give voice to how nursing care makes a difference.

Nurse researchers will have an increasingly strong voice in shaping public policy. Hinshaw (1992) states that disciplines such as nursing, which focus on treatment of chronic illness, health promotion, independence in health, and the care of the acutely ill, are going to be central to shaping health care policy, because these are heavily emphasized values for the future. Research data providing evidence that supports or refutes the merit of health care needs and programs focusing on these issues will be timely and relevant. Thus nursing and its science base will be strategically placed to shape health policy decisions (DeBack, 1991; Rains, 1995).

Because we will continue to live in the "information age," dissemination of nursing research will become increasingly important in professional and public arenas. Research findings will continue to be disseminated in professional arenas such as international, national, regional, and local publications and conferences, as well as in consultations and staff development programs. However, dissemination of research findings in the public sector is an exciting future trend that has already begun. Nurse researchers are increasingly asked to present testimony at governmental hearings and to serve on commissions and task forces related to health care. Traditionally nurses have rarely been quoted in the media when health care topics are addressed, but this has and will continue to change significantly. Today nurses and nurse researchers are participating in teleconferences, developing their own home pages for the World Wide Web, starring in videos, and appearing in interviews on television and radio and in printed and electronic media such as the Internet, newspapers, and lay magazines. Nurses have their own radio shows and are beginning to have their own television shows. Dissemination of research through the public media provides excellent exposure to thousands of potential viewers, listeners, and readers (Rockwell, 1992). Practicing nurses are using technological innovations such as computerized documentation systems and electronic access to databases and literature searches, interactive telecommunication educational offerings, on-line journals, and research-based practice guidelines to make the information revolution come of age in research-related clinical practice activities (Goldsmith, 1996; Penney and Gibbons, 1996).

It is apparent from the previous discussion that nursing has a research heritage to be proud of and a challenging and exciting future direction. Both consumers and producers of research will engage in a united effort to give voice to research findings that make a difference in the care that is provided and the lives that are touched by our commitment to research-based nursing practice.

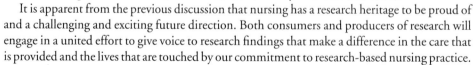

KEY POINTS

- Nursing research provides the basis for expanding the unique body of scientific knowledge that forms the foundation of nursing practice. Research links education, theory, and practice.

- Nurses become knowledgeable consumers of research through educational processes and practical experience. As consumers of research, nurses must have a basic understanding of the research process and critical appraisal skills that provide a standard for evaluating the strengths and weaknesses of research studies before applying them in clinical practice.
- In the first half of the twentieth century, nursing research focused mainly on studies related to nursing education, although some clinical studies related to nursing care were evident.
- Nursing research blossomed in the second half of the twentieth century; graduate programs in nursing expanded, research journals began to emerge, the ANA formed a research committee, and funding for graduate education and nursing research increased dramatically.
- Nurses at all levels of educational preparation have a responsibility to participate in the research process.
- The role of the baccalaureate graduate is to be a knowledgeable consumer of research. Nurses prepared at the master's and doctoral levels must be sophisticated consumers, as well as producers of research studies.
- A collaborative research relationship within the nursing profession will extend and refine the scientific body of knowledge that provides the grounding for theory-based practice.
- The future of nursing research will continue to be the extension of the scientific knowledge base for nursing expertise in appraising, designing, and conducting research and will provide leadership in both academic and clinical settings. Collaborative research relationships between education and service will multiply. Cluster research studies and replication of studies will have increased value.
- Research studies will emphasize clinical issues, problems, and outcomes. Priority will be given to research studies that focus on promoting health, diminishing the negative impact of health problems, ensuring care for the health needs of vulnerable groups, and developing cost-effective health care systems.
- Both consumers and producers of research will engage in a collaborative effort to further the growth of nursing research and accomplish the research objectives of the profession.

CRITICAL THINKING CHALLENGES

Barbara Krainovich-Miller

- How will expanding your computer technology "comfort zone" to generate nursing research data impact on health care of the future?
- What is the assumption underlying ANA's (1989) recommendation that the role of the baccalaureate graduate in the research process is primarily that of a knowledgeable consumer?
- What effects will patient outcomes studies have on the practice of nursing?
- Discuss which type of research, basic or applied, will contribute to the development of intradisciplinary and interdisciplinary networks.

REFERENCES

American Nurses Association: *Facts about nursing,* New York, 1960, ANA.

American Nurses Association: *Code for nurses with interpretive statements,* Kansas City, Mo, 1985, ANA.

American Nurses Association: *Commission on nursing research: education for preparation in nursing research,* Kansas City, Mo, 1989, ANA.

American Nurses Association: *Nursing report card for acute care settings: a tool for protecting our patients,* Washington, DC, 1994, ANA.

Barrett EAM: A nursing theory of power for nursing practice: deprivation from Rogers' paradigm. In Riehl J, ed: *Conceptual models for nursing practice,* ed 3, Norwalk, Conn, 1989, Appleton & Lange.

Barrett EAM: Rogers' science-based nursing practice. In Barrett EAM, ed: *Visions of Rogers' science-based nursing,* New York, 1990, National League for Nursing.

Batey MV: Research: a component of undergraduate education. In *Evaluating research preparation in baccalaureate nursing education: national conference for nurse educators,* published proceedings, Ames, 1982, University of Iowa College of Nursing.

Bavier AR: Where research and practice meet, *Nurs Policy Forum* 1(4):20-27, 1995.

Beck CT: The lived experience of postpartum depression: a phenomenological study, *Nurs Res* 41(3):166-170, 1992.

Beck CT: Teetering on the edge: a substantive theory of postpartum depression, *Nurs Res* 42(1):42-48, 1993.

Beck CT: Replication strategies for nursing research, *Image* 26(3):191-194, 1994.

Beck CT: Effects of postpartum depression on maternal-infant interaction: a meta-analysis, *Nurs Res* 44(5):298-305, 1995.

Beyea S, Farley JK, Williams-Burgess C: Teaching baccalaureate students to use research, *West J Nurs Res* 18(2):213-218, 1996.

Bidwell-Cerone S et al: Nursing research and patient outcomes: tools for managing the transformation of the health care delivery system, *J N Y State Nurs Assoc* 26(3):12-17, 1995.

Bower FL: Nursing research shapes global health, *Reflections* Fall:4, 1995.

Brink P: Learning how to do research requires a mentor, *West J Nurs Res* 17(4):351-352, 1995.

Brink PJ: The discipline is the method, *West J Nurs Res* 22(3):432, 1990.

Broadhurst J et al: Hand brush suggestions for visiting nurses, *Public Health Nurs* 19:487-489, 1927.

Brooten D et al: A randomized clinical trial of early hospital discharge and home follow-up of very-low-birth-weight infants, *N Engl J Med* 315(8):934-939, 1986.

Brooten D et al: Quality-cost model of early hospital discharge and nurse specialist transitional follow-up care, *Image* 20(2):64-68, 1988.

Brooten D et al: Development of a program grant using the quality-cost model of early discharge and nurse specialist transitional follow-up care, *Nurs Health Care* 10(6):315-318, 1989.

Brown EL: *Nursing for the future,* New York, 1948, Russell Sage Foundation.

Buckwalter KC: Research utilization awards, utilization versus dissemination? *Reflections* 18(3):8, 1992.

Buerhaus PI: The value of consumer and nurse partnerships, *Nurs Policy Forum* 2(2):13-20, 1996.

Campbell JC: A test of two explanatory models of women's responses to battering, *Nurs Res* 38:18-24, 1989.

Campbell JC, Alford P: The effects of marital rape on women's health, *Am J Nurs* 89:946-949, 1989.

Campbell JC et al: Correlates of battering during pregnancy, *Res Nurs Health* 15(3):219-226, 1992.

Carnegie E: *Historical perspectives of nursing research,* Boston, 1976, Boston University, Nursing Archive, Special Collections.

Clayton SL: Standardizing nursing techniques: its advantages and disadvantages, *Am J Nurs* 27:939-943, 1927.

Cohen S, Hollingsworth A, Rubin M: Another look at psychologic complications of hysterectomy, *Image* 21(1):51-54, 1989.

Committee on Nursing and Nursing Education in the United States, Josephine Goldmark, secretary, New York, 1923, Macmillan.

DeBack V: Nursing needs health policy leaders, *J Prof Nurs* 6(2):69-74, 1991.

Dickenson-Hazard N: Advancing science, *Reflections* Fall:2, 1995.

Diers D, Leonard RC: Interaction analysis in nursing research, *Nurs Res* 15:225-228, 1966.

Dock LL: What we may expect from the law, *Am J Nurs* 1:8-12, 1900.

Donaldson SK, Crowley DM: The discipline of nursing, *Nurs Outlook* 26:113-120, 1978.

Donnell H, Glick SJ: The nurse and the unwed mother, *Nurs Outlook* 2:249-251, 1954.

Downs F: Informing the media, *Nurs Res* 40(4):195, 1991.

Draucker CB, Petrovic K: Male survivors of childhood sexual abuse, *Image* 28(4):325-330, 1996.

Dreher MC: Clinical scholarship worldwide, *Reflections* Winter:6-7, 1995.

Duffy ME: The research process in baccalaureate nursing education: a ten-year review, *Image* 19:87-91, 1987.

Dumas RG, Leonard RC: The effect of nursing on the incidence of postoperative vomiting, *Nurs Res* 12:12-15, 1963.

Ethridge P, Lamb G: Professional nursing case management improves quality, access and cost, *Nurs Manage* 20(1):30-37, 1989.

Fawcett J: Hallmarks of success in nursing research, *Adv Nurs Sci* 1:1-11, 1984.

Glaser BG, Strauss AL: *Awareness of dying,* Observations series, Chicago, 1965, Aldine.

Goldsmith J: Computers and nurses changing hospital care, *Reflections* Second Quarter:8-10, 1996.

Goodrich A: *The social and ethical significance of nursing: a series of addresses,* New York, 1932, Macmillan.

Gortner SR, Nahm H: An overview of nursing research in the United States, *Nurs Res* 26:10-33, 1977.

Grady PA: Tenth anniversary speech, http://www.nih.gov/ninr, 1996.

Graff B et al: Development of a postoperative self-assessment form, *Clin Nurs Spec* 6(1):47-50, 1992.

Greenblatt M et al: *From custodial to therapeutic patient care in mental hospitals,* New York, 1955, Russell Sage Foundation.

Hall LE: A center for nursing, *Nurs Outlook* 11:805-806, 1963.

Henderson V: Research in nursing practice: when, *Nurs Res* 4:99, 1956 (editorial).

Henderson V: We've "come a long way," but what of the direction? *Nurs Res* 26:163-164, 1977 (guest editorial).

Hinshaw AS: The new National Center for Nursing Research: patient care research program, *Appl Nurs Res* 1:2-4, 1988.

Hinshaw AS: National center for nursing research: a commitment to excellence in science. In McCloskey JC, Grace HK, eds: *Current issues in nursing,* St Louis, 1990, Mosby.

Hinshaw AS: Interfacing nursing and biologic science, *J Prof Nurs* 7(5):264, 1991.

Hinshaw AS: The impact of nursing science on health policy. Silver threads: 25 years of nursing excellence, *Comm Nurs Res* 25:15-26, 1992.

Hinshaw AS, Heinrich J: New initiatives in nursing research: a national perspective. In Bergman R, ed: *Nursing research for nursing practice: an international perspective,* London, 1990, Chapman.

Joint Commission on Accreditation of Healthcare Organizations: *Accreditation manual for hospitals,* Oakbrook Terrace, Ill, 1995, JCAHO.

Keith JM: Florence Nightingale: statistician and consultant epidemiologist, *Int Nurs Rev* 35(5):147-149, 1988.

Kovner AR, Jonas S, eds: *Jonas and Kovner's health care delivery in the United States,* ed 6, New York, Springer (in press).

Lamb GS: Conceptual and methodological issues in nurse case management research, *Adv Nurs Sci* 15(2):16-24, 1992.

Larson E: Exclusion of certain groups from clinical research, *Image* 26(3):185-190, 1994.

McBride AB: Making research an activity for all nurses, *Reflections* 14:2, 1988.

McFarlane J: Battering in pregnancy. In Sampselle CM, ed: *Violence against women,* New York, 1992, Hemisphere.

McFarlane J, Parker B, Socken K: Abuse during pregnancy: associations with maternal health and infant birth weight, *Nurs Res* 45(1):37-42, 1996a.

McFarlane J, Parker B, Soeken K: Physical abuse, smoking, and substance abuse during pregnancy: prevalence, interrelationships, and effects on birth weight, *J Obstet Gynecol Neonatal Nurs* 25(4):313-320, 1996b.

NINR: *National Institute of Nursing Research fact sheet,* Washington, DC, 1996, NIH.

Nightingale, F: *Notes on hospitals,* London, 1863, Longman Group.

Nutting MA: *Educational status of nursing* (Bull No 7), Washington, DC, 1912, US Bureau of Education.

Nutting MA: *A second economic basis for schools of nursing and other addresses,* New York, 1926, GP Putnam's Sons.

Nutting MA, Dock LL: *A history of nursing* (4 vols), New York, 1907-1912, GP Putnam's Sons.

Orlando IJ: *The dynamic nurse-patient relationship,* New York, 1961, GP Putnam's Sons.

Palmer I: Florence Nightingale: reformer, reactionary, researcher, *Nurs Res* 26:84-89, 1977.

Parker B et al: Physical and emotional abuse in pregnancy: a comparison of adult and teenage women, *Nurs Res* 42(3):173-178, 1993.

Pender NJ: Environmental compatibility: accepting the challenge, *Nurs Outlook* 40(5):200-201, 1992.

Penney N, Gibbons B: Rural nurses retool for expanding health needs, *Reflections* Second Quarter:14-15, 1996.

Peplau HE: *Interpersonal relations in nursing: a conceptual frame of reference for psychodynamic nursing,* New York, 1952, GP Putnam's Sons.

Rains JW: Policy-relevant research on infant mortality: rhetorical criticism of mass media, *Nurs Outlook* 43(4):158-163, 1995.

Riegel B et al: Moving beyond: a generative philosophy of science, *Image* 24(2):115-120, 1992.

Robb IH: *Nursing: its principles and practice for hospitals and private use,* ed 3, Cleveland, 1906, EC Koeckert.

Roberts MM: *American nursing: history and interpretation,* New York, 1954, Macmillan.

Rockwell T: Emerging role for nurses in health communication, *Reflections* 18(4):4-5, 1992.

Rudy EB et al: Patient outcomes for the chronically critically ill: special care unit versus intensive care unit, *Nurs Res* 44(6):324-331, 1995.

Ryan V, Miller VB: Disinfection of clinical thermometers: bacteriological study and estimated costs, *Am J Nurs* 32:197-206, 1932.

Sampselle CM: *Violence against women,* New York, 1992, Hemisphere.

School of Nursing, University of California at San Francisco: Nursing research on an international level, *Sci Caring* 3(2):2-6, 1992.

See EM: The ANA and research in nursing, *Nurs Res* 26:165-176, 1977.

Shaver J: Global perspectives: the ANA and CNR international nursing research conference, *Council Nurs Res Newsletter* 18(3):1-6, 1991.

Sigma Theta Tau International: Nursing doctoral programs throughout the world, *Reflections* Fall:20-21, 1995a.

Sigma Theta Tau International: United States nursing doctoral programs, *Reflections* Fall:18-19, 1995b.

Sigmon HD, Amende LM, Grady PA: Development of biological studies to support biobehavioral research at the National Institute of Nursing Research, *Image* 28(2):88, 1996.

Silva MC: Research testing nursing theory: state of the art, *Adv Nurs Sci* 9:1-11, 1986.

Simmons LW, Henderson V: *Nursing research: a survey and assessment,* New York, 1964, Appleton-Century-Crofts.

Stanton AH, Schwartz MA: *The mental hospital: a study of institutional participation in psychiatric illness and treatment,* New York, 1954, Basic Books.

Titler MG et al: Infusing research into practice to promote quality care, *Nurs Res* 43(5):307-313, 1994.

US Department of Health and Human Services: *Healthy people 2000: summary report* (Pub No PH591-50213), Boston, 1992, Jones & Bartlett.

US Department of Health and Human Services: *Healthy people 2000: review 1994* (DHHS Pub No [PH5]95-1256-1), Washington, DC, 1996, USDHHS.

Wald LD: *House on Henry Street,* New York, 1915, Henry Holt & Co.

Ward SE, Berry PE, Misiewicz H: Concerns about analgesics among patients and family caregivers in a hospice setting, *Res Nurs Health* 19:205-211, 1996.

Wheeler K, Fasano N, Burr L: Strategies for teaching research: a survey of baccalaureate programs, *J Prof Nurs* 11(4):233-238, 1995.

Wiedenbach E: *Clinical nursing: a helping art,* New York, 1964, Springer.

Zanotti R: Overcoming national and cultural differences within collaborative international nursing research, *West J Nurs Res* 18(1):6-11, 1996.

ADDITIONAL READINGS

Abdellah FG: Overview of nursing research 1955-1968, Part I, *Nurs Res* 19:6-17, 1970a.

Abdellah FG: Overview of nursing research 1955-1968, Part II, *Nurs Res* 19:151-162, 1970b.

Abdellah FG: Overview of nursing research 1955-1968, Part III, *Nurs Res* 19:239-252, 1970c.

Acute Pain Managament Guideline Panel: *Acute pain mangement: operative or medical procedures and trauma. Clinical practice guideline* (AHCPR Pub No 92-0032), Rockville, Md, 1992, US Public Health Service, Agency for Health Care Policy and Research.

American Nurses Association: *Guidelines for the investigative function of nurses*, Kansas City, Mo, 1981, ANA.

Cowan MJ et al: Integration of biological and nursing sciences: a 10-year plan to enhance research and training, *Res Nurs Health* 16(1):3-9, 1993.

Dickoff J, James P: A theory of theories: a position paper, *Nurs Res* 17:197-203, 1968.

Dickoff J, James P, Wiedenbach E: Theory in a practice discipline, Part I. Practice oriented theory, *Nurs Res* 17:415-435, 1968a.

Dickoff J, James P, Wiedenbach E: Theory in a practice discipline, Part II. Practice oriented research, *Nurs Res* 17:545-554, 1968b.

Grey M, Cameron ME, Thurber FW: Coping and adaption in children with diabetes, *Nurs Res* 40(3):145-149, 1991.

Haber J et al: Shaping nursing practice through research-based protocols, *J NY State Nurs Assoc* 25(3):4-12, 1994.

Haller K, Reynolds M, Horsley J: Developing research-based innovative protocols: process, criteria and issues, *Res Nurs Health* 2:45, 1979.

Johnson TL: Health research that excludes women is bad science, *Chron Higher Educ* October 14, 1992.

Larson E: Nursing research outside academia: a panel presentation, *Image* 13:75-77, 1981.

Lindemann C: Dissemination of nursing research, *Image* 16:57-58, 1984.

McCormick K: Areas of outcome research for nursing, *J Prof Nurs* 8:71, 1992.

Mercer RT: Nursing research: the bridge to excellence in practice, *Image* 16:47-50, 1984.

National Commission for the Study of Nursing and Nursing Education: *An abstract for action*, New York, 1970, McGraw-Hill.

National Nursing Research Agenda: CNR invites your input, *Comm Nurs Res* 18(3):3, 1991.

NCNR: Priorities resulting from Second Conference on Research Priorities in Nursing Practice, March 1993, NCNR.

Nursing doctoral programs in the United States, *Reflections* 18:14-15, 1992.

Panel for the Prediction and Prevention of Pressure Ulcers In Adults: *Pressure ulcers in adults: prediction and prevention. Clinical practice guideline* (AHCPR Pub No 92-0047), Rockville, Md, 1992, Public Health Service, Agency for Health Care Policy and Research.

Phillips JR: The reality of nursing research, *Nurs Sci Q* 1:48-49, 1988.

Pollock S: Top-ranked schools of nursing: network of scholars, *Image* 18:58-60, 1986.

Rogers M: Nursing science and the space age, *Nurs Sci Q* 5(1):27-34, 1992.

Shugars DA, O'Neil EH, Bader JD, eds: *Healthy America: practitioners for 2005: an agenda for action for US health professional schools*, Durham, NC, 1991, The Pew Health Professions Commission.

Stetler CB, Marram G: Evaluating research findings for applicability in practice, *Nurs Outlook* 24:559-563, 1976.

Taylor N et al: Comparison of normal versus heparinized saline for flushing infusion devices, *J Nurs Qual Assur* 3(4):49-55, 1989.

Urinary Incontinence Guideline Panel: *Urinary incontinence in adults. Clinical practice guideline* (AHCPR Pub No 92-0038), Rockville, Md, 1992, Public Health Service, Agency for Health Care Policy and Research.

Research Process

Research Vignette
**Importance of Research
to Nursing Practice**

Chapter 2
**Overview of the Research
Process**

Chapter 3
**Research Problems and
Hypotheses**

Chapter 4
Literature Review

Chapter 5
Theoretical Framework

Chapter 6
Introduction to Design

Chapter 7
**Experimental and
Quasiexperimental
Designs**

Chapter 8
Nonexperimental Designs

Chapter 9
**Qualitative Approaches
to Research**

Chapter 10
Sampling

Chapter 11
Legal and Ethical Issues

Chapter 12
Data Collection Methods

Chapter 13
Reliability and Validity

Chapter 14
Descriptive Data Analysis

Chapter 15
Inferential Data Analysis

Chapter 16
Analysis of the Findings

Research Vignette

IMPORTANCE OF RESEARCH TO NURSING PRACTICE

Nursing research begins with nursing practice and feeds back into nursing practice. The most exciting and clinically relevant research problems that nurse researchers investigate come directly from their nursing practice. That was the case with my own research program. All my clinical practice as an RN and certified nurse-midwife have been in obstetrical nursing. Back in the late 1970s and early 1980s while I was providing nursing care to mothers and their babies during their first 6 weeks postpartum, a disturbing pattern become apparent to me. It was not so much what I had observed in the mothers that concerned me, but instead what the women painfully shared with me. The following quotes are just a couple of examples:

I was extremely insecure. I cried all the time. I didn't know what was happening to me. It was a living nightmare.

I felt like the worst mother in the world. I couldn't understand why I wasn't enjoying holding my baby or taking care of him.

When I referred back to my obstetrical nursing textbooks for guidance, much to my dismay they provided little direction. When I looked up postpartum psychological disorders in these textbooks, only a few sentences were devoted to describing postpartum depression. The books revealed only a skeleton of facts that provided little direction for nursing practice. So began the start of my research program devoted to postpartum depression. Over the past 15 years my research program has consisted of a series of quantitive and qualitative studies. Both types of research methodologies were needed to research such a complex phenomenon as postpartum depression. When I reviewed the literature before starting my research program, only quantitative studies had been conducted. These studies used Likert-type questionnaires asking women to rate the severity of different symptoms related to the depression that they were experiencing. In my own clinical experience with mothers suffering from postpartum depression I knew that these quantitative studies were only revealing the tip of the iceberg.

Based on the state of knowledge about postpartum depression at that time, I decided to conduct a phenomenological study to answer the research question: What is the meaning of mothers' experiences living through postpartum depression? (Beck, 1992). Emerging from this study were 11 themes that vividly described the complexity of this devastating syndrome. An example of one such theme was: Mothers envisioned themselves as robots stripped of all positive feelings, just going through the motions.

The next step in my research program was another qualitative study, but this time grounded theory was the method chosen to identify the basic social psychological problem women experienced in postpartum depression and what process they used to resolve this fundamental problem. Loss of control was the basic problem, and the process mothers used to cope with loss of control I called "teetering on the edge," which refers to walking the fine line between sanity and insanity (Beck, 1993). Teetering on the edge was a four-stage process that included (1) encountering terror, (2) dying of self, (3) struggling to survive, and (4) regaining control. Each of these four stages is filled with rich insights for nurses and provides clear direction for nursing practice.

In my research program I have also conducted a series of metaanalyses to help summarize the state of quantitative research surrounding postpartum depression. Topics of my different metaanalyses were the effect of postpartum depression on maternal-infant interaction (Beck, 1995), the relationship of postpartum depression and infant temperament (Beck, 1996b), and predictors of postpartum depression (Beck, 1996a). My purpose in conducting these meta-analyses was to provide direction for nursing practice and also for future nursing research. For example, one metaanalysis revealed that postpartum depression had a moderate to large adverse effect on maternal-infant interaction. Because this metaanalysis revealed a potentially serious problem in mother-infant dyads, I decided to conduct a phenomenological study (Beck, 1996c) to complement and enrich the quantitative findings. Armed with the rich description of the essence of postpartum depressed mothers' experiences interacting with their infants, nurses can design specifically tailored nursing interventions to help these troubled dyads during the first year after delivery.

The following poignant quote from one mother gives the flavor for the valuable insights into the living nightmare of postpartum depressed mothers that qualitative research can reveal (Beck, 1996c).

My husband and son got back from the store. I think my 3-year-old son wanted to tell me about something that had happened. It was physically so hard to listen that I really remember just trying to put up some kind of wall so that I wouldn't be battered to death. At this point I was really sitting on the couch trying to figure out whether I could ever move again, and I started to cry. My son started hitting me with his fists, and he said, "Where are you, Mom?" It was really painful because I didn't have a clue as to where I was either. He was really trying to wake something up, but it was just too far gone. There was no way that I could retrieve the mom that he remembered and hoped he would find, let alone the mother I wanted to be for my new baby.

Nursing research, both qualitative and quantitative, is the key for opening up opportunities to improve nursing practice. For nursing care to be effective, it must be based on specific research findings.

It is so rewarding for me, as a researcher who has devoted the last 15 years to investigating postpartum depression, to open up obstetrical nursing textbooks and see my research findings now providing the central focus of the content on postpartum depression that nursing students are learning. For this is the ultimate purpose of nursing research—to filter the findings back to practicing nurses who can incorporate this new knowledge into their delivery of care.

REFERENCES

Beck CT: The lived experience of postpartum depression: a phenomenological study, *Nurs Res* 41:166-170, 1992.

Beck CT: Teetering on the edge: a substantive theory of postpartum depression, *Nurs Res* 42:42-48, 1993.

Beck CT: The effect of postpartum depression on maternal-infant interaction: a meta-analysis, *Nurs Res* 44:398-304, 1995.

Beck CT: A meta-analysis of predictors of postpartum depression, *Nurs Res* 45:297-303, 1996a.

Beck CT: A meta-analysis of the relationship between postpartum depression and infant temperament, *Nurs Res* 45:225-230, 1996b.

Beck CT: Postpartum depressed mothers' experiences interacting with their children, *Nurs Res* 45:98-104, 1996c.

Cheryl Tatano Beck, DNSc, CNM, FAAN
Professor
University of Connecticut
School of Nursing
Storrs, Connecticut

Overview of the Research Process

Geri LoBiondo-Wood ■ Judith Haber ■ Barbara Krainovich-Miller

Chapter
TWO

Key Terms

abstract
critical reading
critical thinking
critique
critiquing criteria

Learning Outcomes

After reading this chapter the student should be able to do the following:

- Identify the importance of critical thinking and critical reading for the reading of research articles.
- Identify the steps of critical reading.
- Use the steps of critical reading for reviewing research articles.
- Use identified strategies for critically reading research articles.
- Identify the format and style of research articles.

As you venture through this text you will see the steps of the research process unfold. The steps are systematic and orderly and relate to both nursing theory and nursing practice. Understanding the step-by-step process that researchers use will assist in judging the soundness of research studies. Throughout the chapters, research terminology pertinent to each step is identified and illustrated with many examples from the research literature. Four published research studies are found in the appendixes and are used as examples to illustrate significant points in each chapter. The steps of the process generally proceed in the order outlined in Table 2-1 (pp. 50-51) but may vary depending on the nature of the research problem. It is important to remember that a researcher may vary the steps slightly, but the steps must still be addressed systematically. This chapter provides an overview of critical thinking, critical reading, and critiquing skills. It introduces the overall format of a research article and provides an overview of the subsequent chapters in the book. These topics are designed to help you read research articles more effectively and with greater understanding, thereby making this book more "user-friendly" for you as you learn about the research process.

CRITICAL THINKING AND CRITICAL READING SKILLS

As you read a research article for the first time you may be struck by the difference in style or format between a research article and a theoretical article. The terms are new, and the focus of the content is different. You may be wondering, "How will I possibly learn to evaluate all the steps of a research study, as well as all the terminology? I'm only on Chapter 2; this is not so easy." The answer, which may seem trivial, is that learning occurs with time and help. At first, reading research articles is difficult and frustrating. However, the best way to become an intelligent consumer of research is to use critical thinking and reading skills to read research articles. Students are not expected to understand a research article or critique it perfectly the first time. Nor are they expected to develop this skill on their own. An essential objective of this book is to help you acquire these critical thinking and reading skills so you can reach this goal. Remember that critical thinking and reading, like learning the steps of the research process, are learning processes that take time.

Critical thinking is the rational examination of ideas, inferences, assumptions, principles, arguments, conclusions, issues, statements, beliefs, and actions (Bandman and Bandman, 1988). This means that you are engaging in the following:

- The art of thinking *about* your thinking to make your thinking clearer, more accurate, or more defensible (Paul, 1995)
- The art of constructive skepticism
- The art of identifying and removing bias, prejudice, and one-sidedness of thought
- The art of clarifying what you do understand and what you don't know

In other words, you are consciously thinking about your own thoughts and what you say, write, read, or do, as well as what others say, write, or do. While thinking about all of this, you are questioning the appropriateness of the content, applying standards or criteria, and seeing how things measure up. Or you are thinking about alternative ways of handling the same situation. Although this is considered a highly rational process, it is a highly emotional and at times anxiety-producing one (Brookfield, 1991).

Developing the ability to evaluate research critically requires not only critical thinking skills but also critical reading skills. Paul (1995), a noted theorist on critical thinking, defines **critical reading** as:

an active, intellectually engaging process in which the reader participates in an inner dialogue with the writer. Most people read uncritically and so miss some part of what is expressed while distorting other parts. . . . [It] means entering into a point of view other than our own, the point of view of the writer. A critical reader actively looks for assumptions, key concepts and ideas, reasons and justifications, supporting examples, parallel experiences, implications and consequences and any other structural features of the written text, to interpret and assess it accurately and fairly.

This means that the reader actively looks for assumptions—those supposedly true or accepted statements that are actually unsupported. It is perhaps easier to understand how you do this by thinking about one of the early assumptions of nursing education and practice. In the late 1950s and early 1960s the nursing process was presented as "the" framework for practice. The formulation of a nursing diagnosis was viewed as an essential step of this process. Initially there was no scientific evidence to support this assumption. Yet schools of nursing began to teach these concepts and nurses began to use them in their practice. Eventually, nursing process became a part of the American Nurses Association's (ANA, 1995) social policy statement's definition of the practice of nursing.

At the same time these assumptions were introduced, nurse researchers questioned them and devised studies to examine the concepts in relation to nursing process. The results of these studies provided data to support or refute the assumptions. Numerous studies conducted over the years offer evidence that these concepts are more than assumptions.

Currently students are formally introduced to critical thinking skills through the nursing process (Miller and Babcock, 1996). Critical thinking and critical reading skills are further developed through learning the research process. You will find that beginning critical thinking and reading skills used in activating the nursing process can easily be transferred to understanding the research process and reading research articles. Gradually you will be able to read an entire article and reflect on it by identifying and challenging assumptions, identifying key concepts, questioning rationales, and determining whether supporting evidence exists and finally be able to reread it to "assess it accurately and fairly" (Paul, 1995).

PROCESS OF CRITICAL READING

To accomplish the purpose of critically reading a research study, the reader must have skilled reading, writing, and reasoning abilities. It is quite common for a research study to require several readings. A minimum of three or four readings or even as many as six readings, with your research textbook at your side, facilitates and is necessary to do the following:

- Identify concepts
- Clarify unfamiliar concepts or terms
- Question assumptions and rationale
- Determine supporting evidence

Critical reading can be viewed as a process that involves various levels or stages of understanding, including the following:

- Preliminary understanding
- Comprehensive understanding
- Analysis understanding
- Synthesis understanding

Preliminary Understanding: Familiarity

Preliminary understanding is gained by quickly or lightly reading an article to familiarize yourself with its content or to get a general sense of the material. During the preliminary reading the title and abstract are read closely, but the content is skimmed. The **abstract,** a brief overview of a study, keys the reader to the main components of the study. The title keys the reader to the main variables of the study. "Skimming" includes reading the introduction, major headings, one or two sentences under a heading, and the summary or conclusion of the study. The preliminary reading includes use of the following strategies:

- Highlighting or underlining the main steps of the research process
- Making notes on the photocopied article
- Writing key variables at the top of the photocopied article
- Highlighting or underlining on the photocopy new and unfamiliar terms and significant sentences
- Looking up the definitions of new terms and writing them in the margins of the photocopy
- Reviewing old and new terms before the next reading
- Writing comments, questions, and notes on the photocopy
- Keeping a research text and a dictionary by your side

Using these strategies enables the reader to identify the main theme or idea of the article and bring this knowledge to the second comprehensive reading. An illustration of how to use a number of these strategies is provided by the example in Box 2-1, which contains an excerpt from the introduction and literature review section of the study by Rudy et al (1995) (see Appendix C).

Comprehensive Understanding: Content in Relation to Context

Gagne (1985) refers to this level as *skilled reading.* The purpose of comprehensive understanding is to understand the article—to see the terms in relation to the context or the parts of the study in relation to the whole article. For example, when reading Draucker and Petrovic's (1996) study (see Appendix B) for comprehension, it is essential to understand that the purpose of a grounded theory study is to develop a theory about basic social processes. To simply recall that the major variable of the study was sexual abuse would be inadequate. At the comprehension level reading, you would be able to discuss the core variable that emerged: "Escaping the dungeon: The journey to freedom" and explain the metaphor of "dungeon."

Box 2-1   Example of Skimming Strategies

The original purpose of intensive care units (ICUs) was to locate groups of patients together who had similar needs for specialized monitoring and care so that
highly trained health care personnel would be available to meet these specialized
needs. As the success of ICUs has grown and expanded, the assumption that a
typical ICU patient will require only a short length of stay in the unit during the
most acute phase of an illness has given way to the recognition that stays of more
than 1 month are not uncommon (Berenson, 1984; Daly et al, 1991).

conceptual definition

These long-stay ICU patients represent a challenge to the current system, not
only because of costs but also because of concern for patient outcomes. These
patients are often elderly, have underlying chronic conditions that complicate or
exacerbate their acute illness, and often require sustained ventilatory and
nutritional support. A prime example of these types of patients are those referred
to as "ventilator dependent," found to varying degrees in nearly every ICU in the
country (American Association for Respiratory Care, 1991).

significance of problem

The term "chronically critically ill" has been previously used (Daly et al, 1991)
to describe patients who have extended stays in the ICU. Those patients have
become most burdensome to nurses and physicians who see their progress as slow
and frustrating, to hospital administrators because of extended bed occupancy in
times of high demand, and to hospital financial officers because of costs that
usually exceed the diagnosis-related group (DRG) cost allocation. Patients who
have ICU stays greater than 21 days account for approximately 3% of the total
number of patients admitted to the ICUs, yet they account for approximately
25% to 38% of the patient days (Daly et al, 1991).

previous conceptual definition

more significance

impact on resources

While ample evidence confirms that this subpopulation of ICU patients
represents a drain on hospital resources, few studies have attempted to evaluate
the effects of a delivery system outside the ICU setting on patient outcomes, cost,
and nurse outcomes. The majority of studies that have examined ICU patient

gap in the literature

Continued

Box 2-1   Example of Skimming Strategies—cont'd

outcomes have been limited primarily to mortality and length of stay (Berenson, 1984; Borlase et al, 1991; Madoff et al, 1985). More recently, attention has been given to cost in terms of risk-adjusted ICU lengths of stay, cost, utility of diagnostic and laboratory tests, and time on mechanical ventilation (Gundlach and Faulkner, 1991; Kappstein et al, 1992; Roberts et al, 1993; Schapira et al, 1993; Zimmerman et al, 1993).

previous designs and variables

In studies limited to mechanically ventilated patients, comparisons on length of stay and costs have been examined in "a before-and-after" design following initiation of a ventilatory management team (Cohen et al, 1991), on overall costs for mechanically ventilated patients cared for in an ICU versus a noninvasive respiratory care unit (Elpern et al, 1991), and on hospital charges and life expectancy for elderly mechanically ventilated ICU patients (Cohen, Lambrinos, and Fein, 1993).

gap in literature

The lack of randomized trials comparing care delivery systems for these high-cost patients is noteworthy, as are the limitations of outcome measurements to mortality and cost.

2 types of treatments = independent variables

The (purpose) of the current study was to compare the effects of a low-technology environment of care based on a nurse-managed care delivery system (special care unit [SCU] environment) with the traditional high-technology ICU environment based on a primary nursing care delivery system.

outcome variables = dependent variables

The two groups were compared on the outcomes of length of stay, mortality, readmission to the hospital, complications, patient and family satisfaction, and cost.

definitions

The complications were defined as number and types of infections, number and types of respiratory complications, and number and type of life-threatening complications.

Text from Rudy E et al: Patient outcomes for the chronically ill: special care unit versus intensive care unit, *Nurs Res* 44:324-331, 1995.

When reading for comprehension keep your research text and dictionary nearby. Although during the preliminary reading some terms may have seemed clear, on the second reading they may be unclear. Do not hesitate to write cues or key relationship words on the photocopy. If after this reading the article still does not make sense, ask for assistance before reading it again. One suggestion is to make another copy and ask your professor to read it. Indicate on the copy the unclear areas and write out your specific questions. Often what is or is not highlighted or the comments on the copy help the faculty person to understand your difficulty. The problem may be that further reading on the topic is necessary to comprehend the article. For example, if a student is unfamiliar with Rogers' Science of Unitary Human Beings (Rogers, 1990), reading a study testing a proposition of this model may be difficult unless Rogers' model is read.

Comprehensive understanding is facilitated by the following strategies:

- Reviewing all unfamiliar terms before reading for the second time
- Clarifying any additional unclear terms
- Reading additional sources as necessary
- Writing cues, relationships of concepts, and questions on the photocopy
- Making another copy of your annotated article and requesting that your faculty member read it
- Stating the main idea or theme of the article, in your own words, in one or two sentences on an index card or on the photocopy

Comprehensive understanding is necessary to analyze and synthesize the material. Understanding the author's perspective for the study reflects critical thinking (Paul, 1995) and facilitates the analysis of the study according to established criteria. The next reading or two allows for analysis and synthesis of the study.

Analysis Understanding: Breaking Into Parts

The purpose of reading for analysis is to break the content into parts to understand each aspect of the study. Some of the questions that you can ask yourself as you begin to analyze the research article are as follows:

- Did I capture the main idea or theme of this article in one or two sentences?
- How are the major parts of this article organized in relation to the research process?
- What is the purpose of this article?
- How was this study carried out? Can I explain it step by step?
- What are the author's(s') main conclusions?
- Can I say that I understand the parts of this article and summarize each section in my own words?

In a sense you are determining how the steps of the research process are presented or organized in the article and what the content related to each step is all about. This is also the time that you begin to answer the questions in the critiquing sections of each chapter. You are beginning the critiquing process that will help determine the study's merit.

The **critique** is the process of objectively and critically evaluating a research report's content for scientific merit and application to practice, theory, and education. It requires some knowledge of the subject matter and knowledge of how to critically read and how to use critiquing criteria. An in-depth exploration of the criteria for analysis required in quantitative research critiques is given in Chapters 3 through 8 and 10 through 16 and summarized in Chapter 17; the criteria for qualitative research critiques are covered in Chapter 9 and summarized in Chapter 18.

Critiquing criteria are the measures, standards, evaluation guides, or questions used to judge (critique) a product or behavior. The reader, in analyzing the research report, must evaluate each step of the research process. The reader must ask questions about whether each explanation of a step of the process meets or does not meet these criteria. For instance, Chapter 4 states that one of the objectives of a literature review is to determine gaps and consistencies and inconsistencies in the literature about a subject, concept, or problem. One critiquing guide question in Table 17-1 (see pp. 409 to 412) is "What gaps in knowledge about the problem are identified, and how does this study intend to fill those gaps?" In this example the purpose of the objective of the literature review is the evaluation question or criterion for critiquing the review of the literature.

The review of the literature section of a study by Erickson, Meyer, and Woo (1996) entitled "Accuracy of Chemical Dot Thermometers in Critically Ill Adults and Young Children" reflects the way the researchers addressed that criterion. In this section the authors review many studies; in the summary of the literature review, which appears before the purpose statement, the authors highlight the inconsistency and lack of clarity related to findings of previous research studies:

In summary, although chemical dot thermometers are widely used, their clinical accuracy is not well documented in either adults or children and the findings of available studies are inconsistent or unclear.

This statement implies that reading for analysis took place. Understanding gained by reading for analysis is facilitated by the following critiquing strategies:

- Being familiar with critiquing criteria
- Reaching the comprehensive reading stage before applying critiquing criteria; rereading if necessary
- Applying the critiquing criteria to each step of the research process in the article
- Asking whether the content meets the criteria for each step of the research process
- Asking fellow students to analyze the same study with the same criteria and comparing results
- Writing notes on the copy about how each step of the research process measures up against the established criteria

Synthesis Understanding: Putting Together

Synthesis is the "combination or putting together; combining of parts into a whole" (New Webster's Dictionary and Thesaurus, 1991). The purpose of reading for synthesis is to pull all the information together to form a new whole (Kerlinger, 1986); to make sense of it; to explain relationships. Although the process of synthesizing the material may be taking place as the reader is analyzing the article, a fourth reading is recommended. It is during the synthesis reading that the understanding and critique of the whole study are put together. During this final step you decide how well the study meets the critiquing criteria (see Chapter 17) and how useful it is to practice (see Chapter 18). It is the point at which the reader decides how well each step of the research process relates to the previous step. Synthesis can be thought of as looking at a jigsaw puzzle once it is completed. Does it form a comprehensive picture, or is there a piece out of place? In the case of reviewing or reading for synthesis of several studies, the interrelationship of the studies is assessed. Reading for high-level synthesis is essential in critiquing research studies. The previous example of Erickson, Myer, and Woo's (1996) summary statement of their review of the literature also reflects synthesis reading.

Reading for synthesis is faciliated by the following strategies:

1. Reviewing your notes on the article on how each step of the research process measured up against the established criteria
2. Briefly summarizing the study in your own words, including in your summary:
   a. The components of the study
   b. The study's overall strengths and weaknesses
3. Following the suggested format of:
   a. Limiting the summary to one page, computer-typed or handwritten on a 5 × 8 index card
   b. Including the citation at the top of the page in the specified reference style
   c. Stapling the summary to the top of the photocopied article

This type of summary is viewed as the first draft of a final written critique. It teaches brevity, facilitates easy retrieval of data to support your critiquing evaluation, and increases your ability to write a scholarly report. In addition, the ability to synthesize one study prepares you for the task of critiquing several studies on a similar topic and comparing and contrasting their findings (see Chapter 4).

PERCEIVED DIFFICULTIES AND STRATEGIES FOR CRITIQUING RESEARCH

Critiquing research articles is difficult for the beginning consumer of research and is somewhat frustrating at first. However, the best way to become an intelligent consumer of research is to use critical thinking and reading skills to read articles. Box 2-2 presents some highlighted strategies for reading and evaluating a research report. As mentioned, a helpful strategy when reading research articles for the first few times is to keep your text nearby so that unfamiliar or unclear terms can be looked up and if necessary each step of the research process can be reviewed as you read. No matter how difficult it may seem, read the entire article and reflect on it. Critically read for the levels of understanding described in this chapter. Most important, draw on previous knowledge, common sense, and the critical thinking skills you already possess.

Another important overall strategy is to ask questions; remember that questioning is essential to developing critical thinking. Asking faculty questions and sharing your concerns about what you are reading or their own published work is an effective way of developing your reading skills. Do not hesitate to write or to call a researcher if you have a question about his or her work. You will be pleasantly surprised by how willing researchers are to discuss your questions.

Throughout the chapters of this text, you will find special new features that also will assist you in refining the critical thinking and critical reading skills essential to developing your competence as a research consumer. A *Critical Thinking Decision Path* related to each step of the research process will sharpen your decision-making skills as you critique research articles.

> **Box 2-2**   Highlights of Critical Thinking and Reading Strategies
>
> - Read primary source data-based articles from referred journals (see Table 4-7, p. 109).
> - Read secondary source data-based critique/response/commentary articles from referred journals (see Table 4-7, p. 109).
> - Photocopy primary and secondary source articles; make notations directly on the copy
> - While reading data-based articles:
>   - Keep a research text and a dictionary by your side
>   - Review the chapters in a research text on various steps of the research process, critiquing criteria, unfamiliar terms, and so on
>   - List key variables at the top of photocopy
>   - Highlight or underline on photocopy new terms, unfamiliar vocabulary, and significant sentences
>   - Look up the definitions of new terms and write them on the photocopy
>   - Review old and new terms before subsequent readings
>   - Highlight or underline identified steps of the research process
>   - Identify the main idea or theme of the article; state it in your own words in one or two sentences
>   - Continue to clarify terms that may be unclear on subsequent readings
>   - Make sure you understand the main points of each reported step of the research process you identified before critiquing the article
> - Determine how well the study meets the critiquing criteria
>   - Ask fellow students to analyze the same study using the same criteria and compare results
>   - Consult faculty members about your evaluation of the study
> - Type a one-page summary and critique of each reviewed study
>   - Cite references at the top according to APA or another reference style
>   - Briefly summarize each reported research step in your own words
>   - Briefly describe strengths and weaknesses in your own words

Look for *Technology* icons in each chapter that will highlight computer resources that will enhance research consumer activities. *Critical Thinking Challenges,* which appear at the end of each chapter, are designed to reinforce your critical thinking and critical reading skills in relation to each step of the research process. *Helpful Hints* designed to reinforce your understanding and critical thinking appear at various points throughout the chapters.

RESEARCH ARTICLES: FORMAT AND STYLE

Before one considers the reading of research articles, it is important to have a sense of their organization and format. Many journals publish research, either as the sole type of article in the journal or in addition to clinical or theoretical articles. Although many journals have some common features, they also have unique characteristics. All journals have guidelines for manuscript preparation and submission, which generally are published in each journal. A review of these guides will give you an idea of the format of articles that appear in specific journals. It is important to remember that even though each step of the research process is discussed at length in this text, you may find only a short paragraph or a sentence in the research article giving the details of the step in a specific study. Because of the journal's space limitations or other publishing guidelines, the published study that one reads in a journal is a shortened version of the total work done by the researcher(s). Readers will find also that some researchers devote more space in an article to the results, whereas others present a longer discussion of the methods and procedures. In recent years most authors give more emphasis to the method, results, and discussion of implications than to details of assumptions, hypotheses, or definitions of terms. Decisions about the amount to present on each step of the research process within an article are bound by the following:

- A journal's space limitations
- A journal's author guidelines
- The type or nature of the study
- An individual researcher's evaluation of what is the most important component of the study

The following discussion provides a brief overview of each step of the research process and how it might appear in an article. Table 2-1 indicates where the step usually can be located in a journal article and where it is discussed in this text. It also is important to remember that a published article about a quantitative study will differ from one about a qualitative study. The primary difference is that a qualitative study does not test a hypothesis but may generate hypotheses based on the results. Another difference is the manner in which literature reviews are conducted and used in the study (see Chapters 5, 9, and 17).

Abstract

An abstract is a short comprehensive synopsis or summary of a study at the beginning of an article. An abstract quickly focuses the reader on the main points of a study. A well-presented abstract is accurate, self-contained, concise, specific, nonevaluative, coherent, and readable (American Psychological Association, 1994). Abstracts vary in length from 50 to 250 words. The length of an abstract is dictated by the journal's editor. An example of a succinct abstract can be found at the beginning of the study by Wikblad and Anderson (1995) (see Appendix A). It partially reads as follows:

Two hundred fifty patients undergoing heart surgery were randomized in a prospective comparative study of a semiocclusive hydroactive wound dressing, an occlusive hydrocolloid dressing, and a convential absorbent dressing. The wounds were evaluated during the 4 weeks after surgery. Color photographs were used for a blind evaluation of wound healing . . .

Within the first sentence of this example, the authors provide a view of the following information: sample (adult heart surgery patients), sample size (250), type of sampling method (probability), design (experimental), and type of procedure (group comparison of intervention effectiveness). The remainder of the abstract provides a synopsis of the variables measured and the results.

The studies in Appendixes A, B, C, and D all have abstracts.

Table 2-1

Steps of the Research Process and Journal Format

RESEARCH PROCESS STEPS AND/OR FORMAT ISSUE	USUAL LOCATION IN A JOURNAL HEADING OR SUBHEADING	TEXT CHAPTER
Research problem	Abstract and/or in the Introduction (not labeled) or in a separate labeled heading: Problem	3
Purpose	Abstract and/or in the Introduction or at the end of the literature review, theoretical framework section, or labeled as a separate heading: Purpose	3
Literature review	At the end of the heading Introduction but not labeled as such, or labeled as a separate heading: Literature Review, Review of the Literature, or Related Literature; or not labeled but the variables reviewed appear as headings or subheadings	4
Theoretical framework (TF) and/or conceptual framework (CF)	Combined with Literature Review or found in a separate heading as TF or CF; or each concept or definition used in the TF or CF may appear as a separate heading or subheading	5
Hypothesis/research questions	Stated or implied near the end of the introductory section, which may or may not be labeled or found in a separate heading or subheading: Hypothesis or Research Questions; or reported for the first time in the Results section	3
Research design	Stated or implied in the Abstract or in the Introduction or under the heading: Methods	6, 7, 8, 9,
Sample: type and size	"Size" may be stated in the Abstract, in the Methods section, or as a separate subheading under Methods section as Sample, Sample/Subjects or Subjects, or Participants	10
	"Type" may be implied or stated in any of previous headings described under size	

	Table 2-1—cont'd	
Steps of the Research Process and Journal Format		
RESEARCH PROCESS STEPS AND/OR FORMAT ISSUE	USUAL LOCATION IN A JOURNAL HEADING OR SUBHEADING	TEXT CHAPTER
Legal-ethical issues	Stated or implied in labeled headings: Methods, Procedures, Sample, or Subjects	11
Instruments (measurement tools)	Found in Headings labeled Methods, Instruments, or Measures	12, 13
Validity and reliability	Specifically stated or implied in headings labeled Methods, Instruments, Measures, or Procedures	13
Data collection procedure	Stated in Methods section under subheading Procedure or Data Collection, or as a separate heading: Procedure	12
Data analysis	Stated in Methods section under subheading Procedure or Data Analysis	14, 15
Results	Stated in separate heading: Results	15, 16
Discussion of findings and new findings	Combined with Results or as separate heading: Discussion	16
Implications, limitations, and recommendations	Combined in Discussion or presented as separate or combined major headings	16
References	At the end of the article	2, 4
Communicating research results	Research articles, poster and paper presentations	1, 2, 17, 18, 19

HELPFUL HINT

A journal abstract usually is a single paragraph that provides a general reference to the research purpose, research questions, and/or hypotheses and highlights the methodology and results.

Identification of a Research Problem

Early in a research article, in a section that may or may not be labeled *Introduction,* the researcher presents a picture of the area researched. This is the presentation of the research problem (see Chapter 3). Reading the study by Rudy et al (1995) (see Appendix C), the reader can find the research problem early in the report:

While ample evidence confirms that this subpopulation of ICU patients represents a drain on hospital resources, few studies have attempted to evaluate the effects of a care delivery system outside the ICU setting on patient outcomes, costs, and nurse outcomes.

Definition of the Purpose

The purpose of the study is defined either at the end of the researcher's initial introduction or at the end of the literature review or conceptual framework section. These components of the research process may or may not be labeled as such (see Chapters 4, 5, and 6). Following along in the study by Rudy et al (1995) (see Appendix C), in the paragraph before the *Method* section the purpose is clearly stated:

The purpose of the current study was to compare the effects of a low-technology environment of care based on a nurse-managed care delivery system (special care unit [SCU] environment) with the traditional high-technology ICU environment based on a primary nursing care delivery system.

In the study by Wikblad and Anderson (1995) (see Appendix A), the reader will find the purpose stated clearly, though positioned differently than in the previous example, in the middle of the second paragraph of the report and before the section *Related Literature:*

The objective of the present study was to assess clinical aspects of a semiocclusive hydroactive dressing and an occlusive hydrocolloid dressing in comparison with a conventional absorbent nonocclusive wound dressing.

Literature Review and Theoretical Framework

Authors of studies and journal articles present the literature review and theoretical framework in different ways. Many research articles merge the literature review and theoretical framework. The section heading may include the main concepts investigated; may be called *Review of the Literature, Literature Review, Theoretical Framework, Related Literature,* or *Conceptual Framework;* or may not be labeled at all (see Chapters 4 and 5). By reviewing Appendixes A and C, the reader will find the heading *Related Literature* (Wikblad and Anderson, 1995) and no heading (Rudy et al, 1995). These sections contain both the literature review and the theoretical frameworks of the studies. One style is not better than another; all the studies in the appendixes contain all the critical elements but present them differently.

Hypothesis/Research Question

A study's research question and hypotheses can also be presented in different ways (see Chapter 3). Quite often research reports in journals do not separate headings for reporting the *Hypotheses* or *Research Questions.* Often they are embedded in the *Introduction/Background* section or not labeled at all as in the studies in the appendixes. If a study uses hypotheses the researcher may report whether the hypotheses were or were not supported toward the end of the article in the *Results/Findings* section.

Research Design

The type of research design can be found in the abstract, within the purpose statement, in the introduction to the procedures or methods section, or not stated at all (see Chapters 6, 7, 8, and 9). For example, of the four studies in the appendixes, only two identified the type of study design used; Wikblad and Anderson (1995) (see Appendix A) identified their study as one using a prospective comparative study, and Draucker and Petrovic (1996) identified their study as one using a grounded theory method.

One of the first objectives is to determine whether the study is qualitative or quantitative. This is important because the critiquing criteria differ for qualitative and quantitative studies. In quantitative studies in particular, the way the steps of the research process are used provides clues to determine a study's design.

Do not get discouraged if you cannot easily determine the design. Unfortunately, as stated, more times than not the specific quantitative design is not stated, or if an advanced design is used the details are not spelled out. One of the best strategies is to review the chapters in this text that address quantitative designs (Chapters 6, 7, 8, and 9) and to ask your professors for assistance after you have read the chapters. Determining designs is not an easy process. The following are a few tips to help you determine whether the study you are reading uses a quantitative design:

- Hypotheses are stated or implied (see Chapter 3)
- The terms *control* and *treatment group* appear (see Chapter 7)
- The term *survey, correlational,* or *ex post facto* is used (see Chapter 8)
- The term *random* or *convenience* is mentioned in relation to the sample (see Chapter 10)
- Variables are measured by instruments or tools (see Chapter 12)
- Reliability and validity of instruments are discussed (see Chapter 13)
- Statistical analyses are used (see Chapters 15 and 16)

In contrast, generally qualitative studies do not deal with "numbers." However, some qualitative studies use standard quantitative terms, such as *subjects,* rather than the qualitative term for a phenomenological study, *informants;* they may or may not mention the number of informants used in the study (see Chapter 18). It can be confusing, so one of the best strategies is to review this text's chapter on qualitative design (Chapter 9), as well as critiquing qualitative studies (see Chapter 18). Do not hesitate to ask faculty members for assistance after you have read the chapters.

Sampling

The population from which the sample was drawn is discussed in the methods section entitled *Methods* or *Methodology* under the subheadings of *Subjects* or *Sample* (see Chapter 10). For example, both Wikblad and Anderson's (1995) (see Appendix A) and Rudy et al's (1995) (see Appendix C) studies discuss their respective samples of their quantitative studies under the heading *Method.* Both studies discuss their sample in great detail so that the reader is quite clear who the subjects were and how they were selected. Both studies state that random assignment was used.

In contrast, the qualitative grounded method study by Draucker and Petrovic (1996) (see Appendix B) drew some of its sample from area professionals in their area who worked with male survivors of sexual abuse and the remainder from survivors who had identified themselves as such. Although the type of sampling was not indicated, it can be inferred that it was a nonprobability sampling method (see Chapter 10).

Instruments: Reliability and Validity

The discussion related to method used to measure the variables of a study is usually included in a *Methods* section under the subheading of *Instruments* or *Measures* (see Chapter 12). The researcher usually describes the particular measure (instrument or tool) used by discussing its reliability and validity (see Chapter 13). Rudy et al (1995) discuss the measures used in their *Methods* section under the subheading *Instruments*. Multiple instruments were used, plus their method for measuring cost. Various validity and reliability measures are discussed.

In some cases researchers do not use space in an article to report on commonly used valid and reliable instruments such as the state-trait anxiety inventory (STAI) (Spielberger et al, 1983). Seek assistance from your instructor if you are in doubt about the validity or reliability of a study's instruments.

Procedures and Data Collection Methods

The procedures used to collect data or the step-by-step way that the researcher(s) used the measures (instruments or tools) is generally headed *Procedures* (see Chapter 12). In the study by Wikblad and Anderson (1995) (see Appendix A), the researchers indicate how they conducted the study in great detail under the subheading *Procedure*. They discuss how they took photographs and standardized both the taking of the pictures and the observations of the wounds.

Data Analysis

The data analysis procedures, that is, the statistical tests used in quantitative studies and the results of descriptive and/or inferential tests applied, are presented in the section labeled *Results* or *Findings* (see Chapters 14 and 15). Although qualitative studies do not use statistical tests, the procedures for analyzing the themes, concepts, and/or observational or print data are usually described in the *Method* or *Data Collection* section and reported in a section labeled *Results* or *Findings* (see Chapters 9 and 18).

When researchers do not indicate in a separate section what statistical test they used, it is presented in the *Results* section. For example, in the studies by Rudy et al (1995) and Ward, Berry, and Misiewicz (1996) (see Appendix D), the inferential statistical tests used are reported with the results under the heading *Results* (see Chapter 15). Draucker and Petrovic (1996) (see Appendix B) report the results of their qualitative study, which used the analysis method of grounded theory method, in the section headed *Methods*.

Results/Discussion

The last section of a research study is the *Results* or *Discussion* section. As you will find when you read Chapter 16, the researcher in this section ties together all the pieces of the study and gives a picture of the study as a whole. Researchers report the results and discussion either in one section (Wikblad and Anderson, 1995; Rudy et al, 1995) or report the results and the discussion in a separate section (Ward, Berry, and Misiewicz, 1996). One way is no better than the other. Journal and space limitations determine how these sections will be handled. Any new findings or unexpected findings are usually described in the *Discussion* section.

Recommendations and Implications

In some cases the researcher reports the implications, based on the findings, for practice and education and recommends future studies in a separate section; in other cases they appear at the end of the *Discussion* section (see quantitative studies in Appendixes A, C, and D). In contrast, the qualitative study found in Appendix B includes the recommendations based on the findings under the heading *Summary and Conclusions.* Again, one is no better than the other—only different.

References

Included at the end of a research article, or any scholarly article, are all references cited in the article. The main purpose of the reference list is to support the material presented by identifying the sources in a manner that allows easy retrieval by the reader (APA, 1994).

Communicating Results

Communicating the results of a study can take the form of a research article, a poster, or a paper presentation (see Chapter 19). All are valid ways of providing nursing with the data and the ability to provide high-quality patient care based on research findings. Research-based nursing care plans and patient protocols are outcome measures that indicate effectively communicated research.

As you develop critical thinking and reading skills by using the strategies presented in this chapter, you will become more familiar with the research and critiquing processes. Gradually your ability to read and critique research articles will improve. You will be well on your way to becoming a knowledgeable consumer of research from nursing and other scientific disciplines.

KEY POINTS

- The best way to become an intelligent consumer of research is to use critical thinking and reading skills to read research articles.
- Critical thinking is the rational examination of ideas, inferences, principles, and conclusions.
- Critical thinking enables you to question the appropriateness of the content of a research article, apply standards or criteria to assess the study's scientific merit, or consider alternative ways of handling the same topic.
- Critical reading involves active interpretation and objective assessment of an article, looking for key concepts, ideas, and justifications.
- Critical reading requires four stages of understanding: preliminary, comprehensive, analysis, and synthesis. Each stage includes strategies to increase your critical reading skills.
- Preliminary understanding is gained by quickly and lightly reading an article to familiarize yourself with its content or to get a general sense of the material.
- Comprehensive understanding is skilled reading designed to increase understanding of the terms in relation to the context or the parts of the study in relation to the whole article.

- Analysis understanding is designed to break the content into parts so that each part of the study is understood; the critiquing process begins at this stage.
- The goal of synthesis understanding is to combine the parts of a research study into a whole. During this final stage the reader determines how each step relates to all the steps of the research, how well the study meets the critiquing criteria, and the usefulness of the study for practice.
- Critiquing is the process of objectively and critically evaluating a research article for scientific merit and application to practice, theory, or education.
- Critiquing criteria are the measures, standards, evaluation guides, or questions used to judge the worth of a research study.
- Research articles have different formats and styles depending on journal manuscript requirements and whether they are quantitative or qualitative studies.
- Basic steps of the research process are presented in journal articles in various ways. Detailed examples of such variations can be found in chapters throughout this text.

CRITICAL THINKING CHALLENGES

Barbara Krainovich-Miller

? It is claimed that the critical reading of research articles may require a minimum of three or four readings. Is this always the case? What assumptions underlie this claim?

? To synthesize a research article, what questions must you be able to answer first?

? Margaret is a part-time baccalaureate nursing student, works full time as an RN in an acute care ICU setting, and is a full-time mother of two children under the age of 4. Discuss both the disadvantages and the advantages of Margaret using the critical thinking and reading strategies found in Box 2-1.

? If nurses with a baccalaureate degree are not expected to conduct research, what sense does it make to expect baccalaureate nursing students to be able to critique each step of the research process? Support either a pro or con position.

REFERENCES

American Nurses Association: *A social policy statement,* ed 2, Washington, DC, 1995, American Nurses Publishing.

American Psychological Association: *Publication manual of the American Psychological Association,* ed 4, Washington, DC, 1994, APA.

Bandman EL, Bandman B: *Critical thinking in nursing,* Norwalk, Conn, 1988, Appleton & Lange.

Brookfield SD: *Developing critical thinkers,* San Francisco, 1991, Jossey-Bass.

Draucker CD, Petrovic K: Healing of adult survivors of childhood sexual abuse, *Image* 28:325-330, 1996.

Erickson RS, Meyer LT, Woo TM: Accuracy of chemical dot thermometers in critically ill adults and young children, *Image J Nurs Sch* 28:23-28, 1996.

Gagne ED: *The cognitive psychology of school learning,* Boston, 1985, Little, Brown.

Kerlinger FN: *Foundations of behavioral research,* ed 3, New York, 1986, Holt, Rinehart & Winston.

Miller MA, Babcock DE: *Critical thinking applied to nursing,* St Louis, 1996, Mosby.

New Webster's dictionary and thesaurus, New York, 1991, Book Essentials.

Paul RW: *Critical thinking: how to prepare students for a rapidly changing world,* Santa Rosa, Calif, 1995, Foundation of Critical Thinking.

Rogers ME: Nursing: science of unitary, irreducible, human beings: update 1990. In Barrett EAN, ed: *Visions of Rogers' science-based nursing,* New York, 1990, National League for Nursing.

Rudy E et al: Patient outcomes for the chronically ill: special care unit versus intensive care unit, *Nurs Res* 44:324-331, 1995.

Spielberger CD et al: *Manual for the state-trait anxiety inventory,* Palo Alto, Calif, 1983, Consulting Psychologists Press.

Ward SE, Berry PE, Misiewicz H: Concerns about analgesics among patients and family caregivers in a hospice setting, *Res Nurs Health* 19:205-211, 1996.

Wikblad K, Anderson B: A comparison of three wound dressings in patients undergoing heart surgery, *Nurs Res* 44:312-317, 1995.

ADDITIONAL READINGS

Brooks KL, Shepherd JM: The relationship between clinical decision-making skills in nursing and general critical thinking abilities of senior nursing students in four types of nursing programs, *J Nurs Educ* 29(9):391-399, 1990.

Conger MM, Mezza I: Fostering critical thinking in nursing students in the clinical setting, *Nurs Educ* 21:11-15, 1996.

Cross KP: *Adults as learners,* San Francisco, 1987, Jossey-Bass.

Facione NC, Facione PA: Externalizing the critical thinking in knowledge development and clinical judgment, *Nurs Outlook* 44:129-135, 1996.

Miller MA, Malcolm NS: Critical thinking in the nursing curriculum, *Nurs Health Care* 11(2):67-73, 1990.

Radwin LE: Research on diagnostic reasoning in nursing, *Nurs Diagn* 1(2):70-77, 1990.

Research Problems and Hypotheses

Judith Haber

Chapter
THREE

Key Terms

conceptual definitions
dependent variable
directional hypothesis
hypothesis
independent variable
nondirectional hypothesis
operational definitions
population

problem statement
research hypothesis
research problem
statistical hypothesis
testable
theory
variable

Learning Outcomes

After reading this chapter the student should be able to do the following:

- Describe the relationship of the problem statement and hypothesis to the other components of the research process.
- Describe the process of identifying and refining a research problem.
- Identify the criteria for determining the significance of a research problem.
- Identify the characteristics of research problems and hypotheses.
- Describe the advantages and disadvantages of directional and nondirectional hypotheses.
- Compare and contrast the use of statistical versus research hypotheses.
- Discuss the appropriate use of research questions versus hypotheses in a research study.
- Identify the criteria used for critiquing a research problem and hypothesis.
- Apply the critiquing criteria to the evaluation of a problem statement and hypothesis in a research report.

Formulation of the research problem and developing hypotheses are key preliminary steps in the research process. The **research problem,** often called a ***problem statement,*** presents the question that is to be asked in the study. The hypothesis attempts to answer the question posed by the research problem.

The first step and one of the most important requirements of the research process is to be able to clearly delineate the study area and state the research problem concisely. Before the study is designed and the hypotheses are formulated, the researcher spends much time narrowing down the broad problem area to a concise and feasible research problem, which provides direction for the study.

Hypotheses can be considered intelligent hunches, guesses, or predictions that assist the researcher in seeking the solution or answer to the research question. Hypotheses are a vehicle for testing the validity of the theoretical framework assumptions and provide a bridge between theory and the real world. In the scientific world, researchers derive hypotheses from theories and subject them to empirical testing. A theory's validity is not directly examined. Instead, it is through the hypotheses that the merit of a theory can be evaluated.

The research consumer often does not see a formal statement of the research problem or hypothesis in a research article because of space constraints or stylistic considerations in such publications. What does appear more often in published articles is a statement of the aims, purpose, or goals of the research study. Nevertheless, it is equally important for both the consumer and producer of research to understand the importance of the problem statement and hypothesis as foundational elements of the research study: elements that set the stage for the development of the research study. This chapter provides a working knowledge of quantitative research problems and hypotheses, the standards for writing them, and a set of criteria for their evaluation.

DEVELOPING AND REFINING A RESEARCH PROBLEM

A researcher spends a great deal of time refining a research idea into a testable research problem. Unfortunately, the evaluator of a research study is not privy to this creative process, because it occurred during the study's conceptualization. And often, the final problem statement does not appear in the research article unless the study is qualitative rather than quantitative in nature (see Chapter 9). Although this section will not teach you how to formulate a research problem, it is important to provide a glimpse of what the process of developing a research problem may be like for a researcher.

As illustrated in Table 3-1, research problems or topics are not pulled from thin air. Research problems should indicate that practical experience, a critical appraisal of the scientific literature, or interest in untested **theory** has provided the basis for the generation of a research idea. The problem statement should reflect a refinement of the researcher's initial thinking. The evaluator of a research study should be able to discern that the researcher has done the following:

1. Defined a specific problem area
2. Reviewed the relevant scientific literature
3. Examined the problem's potential significance to nursing
4. Pragmatically examined the feasibility of studying the research problem

Table 3-1

How Practical Experience, Scientific Literature, and Untested Theory Influence the Development of a Research Idea

AREA	INFLUENCE	EXAMPLE
Practical experience	Clinical practice provides a wealth of experience from which research problems can be derived. The nurse may observe the occurrence of a particular event or pattern and become curious about why it occurs, as well as its relationship to other factors in the patient's environment.	A nurse working with patients who have chronic obstructive pulmonary disease (COPD) observes that certain patients have more dyspnea than others whose pulmonary status is equally severe. The nurse knows that dyspnea is the most common reason COPD patients seek health care, yet few obtain relief. She also observes that anxiety appears to be closely related to severity of dyspnea in certain patients. Noting the difference in the two groups of dyspneic COPD patients, those who are also anxious and those who are not, the nurse speculates about the effect of progressive muscle relaxation exercises on anxiety, dyspnea, and airway obstruction (Gift, Moore, and Soeken, 1992).
Critical appraisal of the scientific literature	The critical appraisal of research studies that appear in journals may indirectly suggest a problem area by stimulating the reader's thinking. The nurse may observe a conflict or inconsistency in the findings of several related research studies and wonder which findings are most valid.	At a staff meeting where cost-effectiveness was being discussed, a nurse reported that she had read an article indicating that saline flushes were more cost-effective than heparin flushes (saving hospitals up to $1,000,000 per year) and were equally effective in maintaining IV heparin lock patency without increasing the incidence of phlebitis. Another nurse said that other articles they had on file indicated that the heparin flush, although more costly, was more effective. The group agreed that there was a conflict in the data and began a literature review to help them scientifically resolve the discrepancy in the findings and define a problem focus (Goode et al, 1991).

Continued

Table 3-1— cont'd

How Practical Experience, Scientific Literature, and Untested Theory Influence the Development of a Research Idea

AREA	INFLUENCE	EXAMPLE
Gaps in the literature	A research idea also may be suggested by a critical appraisal of the literature that identifies gaps in the literature and suggests areas for future study. Research ideas also can be generated by research reports that suggest the value of replicating a particular study to extend or refine the existing scientific knowledge base.	A nurse who had just begun working on an oncology unit observed that the concerns and well-being of partners of patients with breast cancer were not a focus of attention after diagnosis and during treatment of their wife's breast cancer. He wondered whether the partners' emotional and physical concerns and feelings of well-being as predictors of adjustment had even been examined. Where the literature is reviewed relative to this topic, no research studies are identified that would provide a scientific basis for determining factors related to adjustment of breast cancer patients and their partners (Hoskins, 1996).
Interest in untested theory	Verification of an untested nursing theory provides a relatively uncharted territory from which research problems can be derived. Inasmuch as theories themselves are not tested, a researcher may think about investigating a particular concept or set of concepts related to a particular nursing theory. The deductive process would be used to generate the research problem. The researcher would pose questions such as, "If this theory is correct, what kind of behavior would I expect to observe in particular patients and under which conditions?" *or* "If this theory is valid, what kind of supporting evidence would I find?"	Development of theoretical models that are derived from nursing and related literature are conducted to provide empirical support for the accuracy of a specific theoretical model that examines the fit between the hypothesized model and the data. A nurse researcher sought to explain adaptation to the uncertainty of multiple sclerosis (MS) in women. A causal model, developed from the literature and from interviews with four women with MS, was tested. Successful adaptation was measured by self-esteem and mastery. The negative impact of uncertainty was found to be significantly reduced by the womens' spiritual and social relationships (Crigger, 1996).

Defining the Problem Area

Researchers generally begin with an interest in some broad topic area, such as pain management, family communication patterns, self-care patterns of elders, or management of urinary incontinence. When nurses ask such questions as "Why are things done this way?" "I wonder what would happen if . . . ?" or "What characteristics are associated with . . . ?" they are often well on their way to developing a researchable problem.

Usually the research focuses on the **dependent variable** of the study, the variable that will be predicted or explained through its relationship to the independent variable. Brainstorming with teachers, advisors, or colleagues may provide valuable feedback that helps the researcher focus on a specific problem area. Let us consider an example. Suppose a researcher told a faculty advisor that the area of interest was coping processes of children faced with stressful experiences. The advisor may have said, "What is it about the topic that specifically interests you?" Such a conversation may have initiated a chain of thought that resulted in a decision to explore coping processes of children faced with stressful hospital experiences such as surgery. Figure 3-1 illustrates how a broad area of interest (coping processes of children faced with stressful experiences) was narrowed to a specific research topic (coping processes of children faced with stressful hospital experiences such as surgery).

Beginning the Literature Review

The literature review should reveal that the literature relevant to the problem area has been critically examined. Often concluding sections on recommendations and implications for practice identify remaining gaps in the literature, the need for replication, or the need for extension of the knowledge base about a particular research focus (see Chapter 4). In the previous example about the effect of children's preoperative coping on postoperative anxiety and return to normal activity, the researcher may have conducted a preliminary review of books and journals for theories and research studies regarding factors apparently critical to how coping affects children facing stressful hospital experiences. These factors should be potentially relevant, of interest, and measurable. Possible relevant factors mentioned in the literature include stress, coping, and coping modes. Other variables, such as demographic characteristics of children and their parents, locus of control, child and parent anxiety and parent-doctor information programs that are predicted to have a direct effect on the outcome variables, postoperative anxiety, and return to normal activity, also are suggested as essential to consider. This information can then be used by the researcher to further define the research problem. At this point the researcher could write the following tentative problem statement: *What is the effect of children's preoperative coping on postoperative anxiety and return to normal activity?* Although the problem statement is not yet in its final form, the reader can envision the interrelatedness of the initial definition of the problem area, the literature review, and the refined problem statement. The person reading a research report examines the end product of this formulation process and thus should have an appreciation of this time-consuming effort.

HELPFUL HINT

Reading the literature review or theoretical framework section of a research article helps you trace the development of the implied problem statement and/or hypothesis.

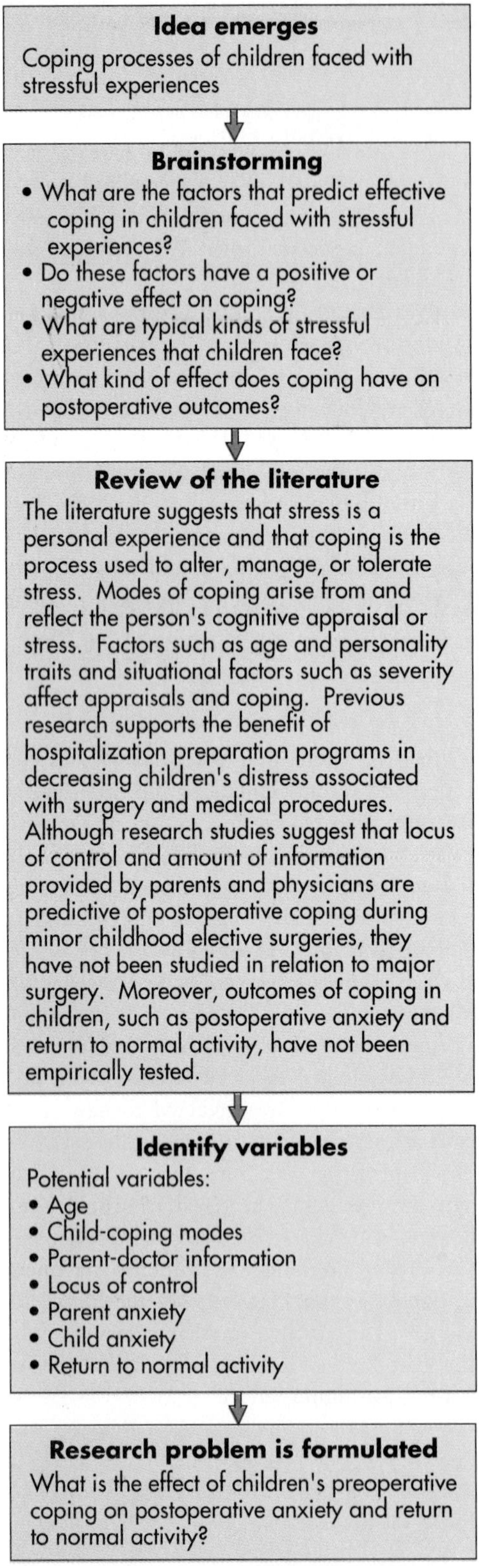

Idea emerges

Coping processes of children faced with stressful experiences

Brainstorming

- What are the factors that predict effective coping in children faced with stressful experiences?
- Do these factors have a positive or negative effect on coping?
- What are typical kinds of stressful experiences that children face?
- What kind of effect does coping have on postoperative outcomes?

Review of the literature

The literature suggests that stress is a personal experience and that coping is the process used to alter, manage, or tolerate stress. Modes of coping arise from and reflect the person's cognitive appraisal or stress. Factors such as age and personality traits and situational factors such as severity affect appraisals and coping. Previous research supports the benefit of hospitalization preparation programs in decreasing children's distress associated with surgery and medical procedures. Although research studies suggest that locus of control and amount of information provided by parents and physicians are predictive of postoperative coping during minor childhood elective surgeries, they have not been studied in relation to major surgery. Moreover, outcomes of coping in children, such as postoperative anxiety and return to normal activity, have not been empirically tested.

Identify variables

Potential variables:
- Age
- Child-coping modes
- Parent-doctor information
- Locus of control
- Parent anxiety
- Child anxiety
- Return to normal activity

Research problem is formulated

What is the effect of children's preoperative coping on postoperative anxiety and return to normal activity?

Figure 3-1 Formulation of a research problem: a process.

Significance

Before proceeding to a final formulation of the problem statement, it is crucial for the researcher to have examined the problem's potential significance to nursing. The research problem should have the potential for contributing to and extending the scientific body of nursing knowledge. The problem does not have to be of prize-winning caliber to be significant. However, it should meet the following criteria:

- Patients, nurses, the medical community in general, and society will potentially benefit from the knowledge derived from the study.

- The results will be applicable for nursing practice, education, or administration.

- The results will be theoretically relevant.

- The findings will lend support to untested theoretical assumptions, extend or challenge an existing theory, or clarify a conflict in the literature.
- The findings will potentially formulate or alter nursing practices or policies.

If the research problem has not met any of these criteria, it is wise to extensively revise the problem or discard it. For example, in the previously cited problem statement the significance of the problem includes the following facts:

- Major surgical procedures are stressful for children and/or their families.
- As health care delivery is restructured, parents play an increasingly important informational role in preparing children for hospitalization and participating in the achievement of optimal postoperative outcomes.
- The coping process may be of prime importance as it works to facilitate or impair adaptational outcomes.
- This study sought to replicate previous studies related to children's coping processes when faced with stressful experiences such as hospitalization and thereby extend the knowledge base about this phenomenon and increase generalizability of previous findings.
- This study sought to fill a gap in the literature by testing a coping model that relates coping to two untested outcomes, postoperative anxiety and return to normal activity.

Feasibility

The feasibility of a research problem needs to be pragmatically examined. Regardless of how significant or researchable a problem may be, pragmatic considerations such as time; availability of subjects, facilities, equipment, and money; experience of the researcher; and any ethical considerations may cause the researcher to decide that the problem is inappropriate because it lacks feasibility (see Chapters 6 and 11).

FINAL PROBLEM STATEMENT

A problem may be written in declarative form as illustrated in Table 3-2 or in interrogative form as illustrated in Table 3-3. Both are acceptable formats. The style chosen is largely a

Table 3-2

Problem Statements in Declarative Form

RESEARCH FOCUS	PROBLEM STATEMENT
Influence of stress management training on HIV disease	This study investigates the influence of a cognitive-behavioral stress management intervention on stress, coping patterns, quality of life, psychological distress, uncertainty, and CD4 T-lymphocyte levels in persons with HIV disease (McCain et al, 1996).
Determining the clinical accuracy of chemical dot thermometers	Clinical accuracy of chemical dot thermometers has not been well documented (Erickson, Meyer, and Woo, 1996).
Comparison of the effects of differing environments of care and nurse delivery systems on the outcomes of chronically, critically ill patients	The study examines the effect of a low-technology environment of care and a nurse case management delivery system with the traditional high-technology environment and primary nursing care delivery system on the patient outcomes of length of stay, mortality, readmission, complications, satisfaction, and cost (Rudy et al, 1995)

Table 3-3

Problem Statements in Interrogative Form

RESEARCH FOCUS	PROBLEM STATEMENT
Factors that influence adaptation of preadolescents and adolescents with diabetes	What are the influences of age, coping behavior, and self-care of psychological, social, and physiological adaptation in preadolescents and adolescents with insulin-dependent diabetes mellitus (Grey, Cameron, and Thurber, 1992)?
Comparisons of concerns about reporting pain and using analgesics in hospice patients and their family caregivers	What is the effect of patient and family caregiver concerns on reporting pain and using analgesics in a hospice patient context (Ward, Berry, and Misiewicz, 1996)?
Differences in the use of outpatient mental health services by the elderly	What are the intragroup differences in the use of mental health services by patients age 65 and older in hospital outpatient departments and emergency rooms (Blixen, 1994)?

function of the researcher's preference. A good problem statement exhibits the following three characteristics:

- It clearly identifies the variables under consideration.
- It specifies the population being studied.
- It implies the possibility of empirical testing.

Because each of these elements is crucial to the formulation of a satisfactory problem statement, the criteria will be discussed in greater detail.

Variables

Researchers call the properties that they study *variables.* Such properties take on different values. Thus a **variable** is, as the name suggests, something that varies. Properties that differ from each other, such as age, weight, height, religion, and ethnicity, are examples of variables. Researchers attempt to understand how and why differences in one variable are related to differences in another variable. For example, a researcher may be concerned about the variable of pain in postoperative patients. It is a variable because not all postoperative patients have pain or the same amount of pain. A researcher may also be interested in what other factors can be linked to postoperative pain. It has been discovered that anxiety is associated with pain. Thus anxiety is also a variable, because not all postoperative patients have anxiety or the same amount of anxiety.

When speaking of variables, the researcher is essentially asking, "Is X related to Y? What is the effect of X on Y? How are X_1 and X_2 related to Y?" The researcher is asking a question about the relationship between one or more independent variables and a dependent variable.*

An **independent variable,** usually symbolized by X, is the variable that has the presumed effect on the dependent variable. In experimental research studies the independent variable is manipulated by the researcher. For example, a nurse may study how different intramuscular injection sites affect the patient's perception of pain. The researcher may manipulate the independent variable—intramuscular injection sites—by using different injection sites (see Chapter 7). In nonexperimental research the independent variable is not manipulated and is assumed to have occurred naturally before or during the study. For example, the researcher may be studying the relationship between the level of anxiety and the perception of pain. The independent variable—the level of anxiety—is not manipulated; it is just presumed to occur and is observed and measured as it naturally happens (see Chapter 8).

The dependent variable, represented by Y, is often referred to as the *consequence* or the presumed effect that varies with a change in the independent variable. The dependent variable is not manipulated. It is observed and assumed to vary with changes in the independent variable. Predictions are made from the independent variable to the dependent variable. It is the dependent variable that the researcher is interested in understanding, explaining, or predicting. For example, it might be assumed that the perception of pain—the dependent variable—will vary with changes in the level of anxiety—the independent variable. In this case we are trying to explain the perception of pain in relation to the level of anxiety.

---

*In cases in which multiple independent or dependent variables are present, subscripts are used to indicate the number of variables under consideration.

Although variability in the dependent variable is assumed to depend on changes in the independent variable, that does not imply that there is a causal relationship between X and Y or that changes in variable X cause variable Y to change. Let us look at an example in which nurses' attitudes toward patients with acquired immunodeficiency syndrome (AIDS) were studied. The researcher discovered that older nurses had a more negative attitude about patients with AIDS than had younger nurses. The researcher did not conclude that the nurses' negative attitudes toward patients with AIDS were caused by their age, but at the same time it is apparent that there is a directional relationship between age and negative attitudes about patients with AIDS. That is, as the nurses' age increases, their attitudes about patients with AIDS become more negative. This example highlights the fact that causal relationships are not necessarily implied by the independent and dependent variables; rather, only a relational statement with possible directionality is proposed.

Although one independent and one dependent variable are used in the examples just given, there is no restriction on the number of variables that can be included in a problem statement. However, remember that problems should not be unnecessarily complex or unwieldly, particularly in beginning research efforts. Problem statements that include more than one independent or dependent variable may be broken down into subproblems that are more concise.

Finally, it should be noted that variables are not inherently independent or dependent. A variable that is classified as independent in one study may be considered dependent in another study. For example, a nurse may review an article about personality factors that are predictive of alcoholism. In this case alcoholism is the dependent variable. When another article about the relationship between alcoholism and marital conflict is reviewed, alcoholism is the independent variable. Whether a variable is independent or dependent is a function of the role it plays in a particular study.

Population

The **population** being studied needs to be specified in the problem statement. If the scope of the problem has been narrowed to a specific focus and the variables have been clearly identified, the nature of the population will be evident to the reader of a research report. For example, a problem statement that poses the question "Is there a relationship between rooming-in by mothers and preschool childrens' adjustment to hospitalization?" suggests that the population under consideration includes mothers and their hospitalized preschool children. It is also implied that some of the mothers will have had rooming-in, in contrast to other mothers who have not. The researcher or the reader will have an initial idea of the composition of the study population from the outset (see Chapter 10).

Testability

The statement of the research problem must imply that the problem is **testable;** that is, measurable by either qualitative or quantitative methods. For example, the problem statement "Should postoperative patients control how much pain medication they receive?" is incorrectly stated for a variety of reasons; one reason is that it is not testable. It represents a value statement rather than a relational problem statement. A scientific or relational problem must propose a relationship between an independent and a dependent variable and do this in such a way that it indicates that the variables of the relationship can somehow be measured. Many interesting and important questions are not valid research problems, because they are not amenable to testing.

The question "Should postoperative patients control how much pain medication they receive?" could be revised from a philosophical question to a research question that implies testability. Two examples of the revised problem statement might be the following:

- Is there a relationship between patient-controlled analgesia (PCA) versus nurse-administered analgesia and perception of postoperative pain?
- What is the effect of patient-controlled analgesia (PCA) on pain ratings by postoperative patients?

These examples illustrate the relationship between the variables, identify the independent and dependent variables, and imply the testability of the research problem.

Now that the elements of the formal problem statement have been presented in greater detail, this information can be integrating by formulating a formal problem statement about coping processes of children faced with stressful hospital experiences such as surgery. Earlier in this chapter the following unrefined problem statement was formulated: *What is the effect of children's preoperative coping on postoperative anxiety and return to normal activity?* This problem statement was originally derived from a general area of interest—coping processes of children faced with stressful experiences. The topic was more specifically defined by delineating a particular problem area—coping processes of children faced with stressful hospital experiences such as major surgery. The problem crystallized still further after a preliminary literature review and emerged in the unrefined form just given. With the four criteria inherent in a satisfactory problem statement, it is now possible to propose a refined or formal problem statement; that is, one that specifically states the problem in question form and specifies the relationship of the key variables in the study, the population being studied, and the empirical testability of the problem. Congruent with these four criteria, the following problem statement can then be formulated: *What is the effect of children's preoperative coping on postoperative anxiety and return to normal activity?* (LaMontagne et al, 1996). Table 3-4 identifies the components of this problem statement as they relate to and are congruent with the four problem statement criteria. Table 3-5 provides additional examples of unrefined problem statements. As the first column in Table 3-5 is reviewed, the reader will notice that the problem statements

Table 3-4

Components of the Problem Statement and Related Criteria

VARIABLES	POPULATION	TESTABILITY
Independent variable: preoperative coping	Children faced with hospitalization and major surgery	Differential effect of preoperative coping on postoperative anxiety and return to normal activity
Dependent variable: postoperative anxiety and return to normal activity		

Table 3-5

Examples of Unrefined and Refined Problem Statements

TYPE OF DESIGN SUGGESTED	UNREFINED PROBLEM STATEMENT	CRITIQUE OF PROBLEM STATEMENT	REFINED PROBLEM STATEMENT
Nonexperimental	Do nurses' attitudes toward patients with AIDS affect the emotional state of the patient?	Not a concise relational statement Testability is not implied	Is there a relationship between the nurse's attitude toward AIDS and the emotional status of the AIDS patient?
Experimental	How does patient teaching influence maternal anxiety in primiparas after discharge?	Not a concise relational statement Testability is not implied Variables are not clear	The relationship between the amount of patient teaching and the level of anxiety in primparas after discharge is unknown.
Experimental	To measure the effectiveness of health teaching for hospitalized patients with heart disease in a group setting.	Population is not specific	Research has not demonstrated the effect of postcardiac group health teaching on health behaviors of patients after an initial myocardial infarction.
Experimental	Does positioning have an effect on the occurrence of contractures in unconscious patients?	Variables are not clear	What is the difference in the incidence of contractures in comatose patients in relation to frequency of repositioning?
Experimental	How do nurse-run patient education classes impact on the housebound elderly?	Not a relational statement Population is not defined adequately Variables are not clearly defined Testability is not implied	The effect of nurse-administered educational rehabilitation programs on independent behavior of chronically ill housebound elderly patients has not been determined.

Table 3-5—cont'd

Examples of Unrefined and Refined Problem Statements

TYPE OF DESIGN SUGGESTED	UNREFINED PROBLEM STATEMENT	CRITIQUE OF PROBLEM STATEMENT	REFINED PROBLEM STATEMENT
Nonexperimental	How does the mother's feeling of well-being during pregnancy affect how the mother attaches to her baby?	Not a concise relational statement Variables are not clearly defined	Is there a relationship between the physical symptoms of pregnancy and maternal-fetal attachment in primigravidas?
Experimental	Do patients need sexual counseling after hysterectomies?	Not a relational statement Variables are not clearly specified Testability is not implied	Research has not demonstrated the relationship between sexual counseling and the postoperative adjustment of patients after hysterectomy.
Nonexperimental	How does assertiveness relate to feelings of power in depressed women?	Not a clear relational statement Variables are not clearly specified	Is there a relationship between assertive behavior and the perception of power in depressed women?

suggest the use of different types of research designs; that is, experimental, quasiexperimental, or nonexperimental (see Chapters 7 and 8). It is important to note that the process of moving from the general topic area to the unrefined problem and finally to the refined, formal problem statement often includes several intermediate steps.

STATEMENT OF THE PROBLEM IN PUBLISHED RESEARCH

A formal problem statement is not included in most current research articles. They are, however, used in developing grant proposals, theses, and dissertations when greater detail is required. Used more commonly in articles is a statement of purpose, usually stated in the introductory paragraph or at the beginning or end of the literature review section. As such, it is important for the research consumer to be clear about the difference between these two components of the research process.

As stated earlier, a research problem is a question for which an answer is to be described, explained, or predicted. It is a brief statement of relationships among variables. Downs (1993) highlights the importance of including a statement of the relationships the researcher hopes to establish. Presenting this information early in the article facilitates getting to the point of the study by allowing the researcher, now an author, to produce a diagram of the points that need to be addressed in the article.

HELPFUL HINT
Remember that problem statements are often not explicitly stated. The reader has to infer the problem statement from the title of the report, the abstract, the introduction, or the purpose.

PURPOSE STATEMENT

The purpose of the study encompasses the aims or goals the investigator hopes to achieve with the research, not the problem to be solved. For example, a nurse working with rehabilitation patients with bladder dysfunction may be disturbed by the high incidence of urinary tract infections. The nurse may propose the following research question: "What is the optimum frequency of changing urinary drainage bags in patients with bladder dysfunction to reduce the incidence of urinary tract infection?" If this nurse were to design a study, its purpose might be to determine the differential effect of a 1-week and 4-week urinary drainage bag change schedule on the incidence of urinary tract infections in patients with bladder dysfunction. The purpose communicates more than just the nature of the problem. Through the researcher's selection of verbs, the purpose statement suggests the manner in which the researcher sought to study the problem. Verbs like *discover, explore,* or *describe* suggest an investigation of a little researched topic that might appropriately be guided by research questions rather than hypotheses. In contrast, verb statements indicating that the purpose is to test the effectiveness of an intervention or compare two alternative nursing strategies suggest a study with a better established knowledge base that is hypothesis testing in nature. Other examples of purpose statements are illustrated in Box 3-1.

Box 3-1   Examples of Purpose Statements

- The purpose of this study was to measure sleep patterns in a sample of women during recovery from CABG surgery (Redeker et al, 1996).
- The current study was conducted to investigate the effectiveness of retention control training (RCT) in increasing bladder capacity and elimination enuresis, while controlling for frequency and type of enuresis (Ronen and Abraham, 1996).
- The primary purpose of the present study was to determine the effects of patient education and psychosocial support on physiological well-being, psychological well-being, adherence to therapeutic regimens, and knowledge about their condition among adults with hypertension (Devine and Reifschneider, 1995).
- The objective of the present study was to assess clinical aspects of a semiocclusive hydroactive dressing and an occlusive hydrocolloid dressing in comparison with a conventional absorbent nonocclusive wound dressing (Wikblad and Anderson, 1995).
- The purpose of this study was to increase the understanding of factors that influence nurses' adoption of the patient-controlled analgesia (PCA) approach (Fulton, 1996).

DEVELOPING THE RESEARCH HYPOTHESES

Like the problem statement, hypotheses are often not stated explicitly in a research article. The evaluator often will find that the hypotheses are embedded in the data analysis, results, or discussion section of the research report. It is then up to the reader to discern the nature of the hypotheses being tested. In light of that stylistic reality, it is important to be acquainted with the components of hypotheses, how they are developed, and the standards for writing and evaluating them.

Hypotheses flow from the problem statement, literature review, and theoretical framework. Figure 3-2 illustrates this flow. A **hypothesis** is an assumptive statement about the relationship between two or more variables that suggests an answer to the research question. A hypothesis converts the question posed by the research problem into a declarative statement that predicts an expected outcome.

Each hypothesis represents a unit or subset of the research problem. For example, a research problem might pose the question "Is there a relationship between nurse-expressed empathy, patient-perceived empathy, and patient distress?" (Olson, 1995). This problem can be broken down into the following two subproblems:

1. Is there a relationship between nurse-expressed empathy and patient distress?
2. Is there a relationship between patient-perceived empathy and patient distress?

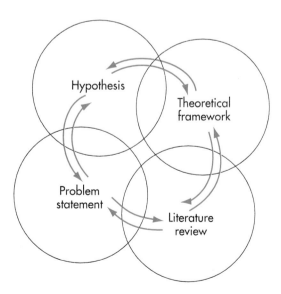

Figure 3-2   Interrelationships of problem statement, literature review, theoretical framework, and hypothesis.

A hypothesis can then be generated for each unit of the research problem—the subproblems. The hypotheses of the research problem already mentioned might be stated in the following way:

> Hypothesis 1: There will be a negative relationship between measures of nurse-expressed empathy and patient distress.
> Hypothesis 2: There will be a negative relationship between patient-perceived measures of empathy and patient distress.
> Hypothesis 3: There will be a positive relationship between nurse-expressed empathy and patient-perceived empathy.

The critiquer of a research report will want to evaluate whether the hypotheses of the study represent subsets of the main research problem as illustrated by the examples just given.

Hypotheses are formulated before the study is actually conducted, because they provide direction for the collection, analysis, and interpretation of data. Hypotheses have the following three purposes:

1. To provide a bridge between theory and reality, and in this sense they unify the two domains.
2. To be powerful tools for the advancement of knowledge, because they enable the researcher to objectively enter new areas of discovery.
3. To provide direction for any research endeavor by tentatively identifying the anticipated outcome.

HELPFUL HINT

When hypotheses are not explicitly stated by the author at the end of the introduction section or just before the methods section, they will be embedded or implied in the results or discussion sections of a research article.

Characteristics

Nurses who are conducting research or nurses critiquing published research studies must have a working knowledge about what constitutes a "good" hypothesis. Such knowledge will enable them to have a standard for evaluating their own work or the work of others. The following discussion about the characteristics of hypotheses will present criteria to be used when formulating or evaluating a hypothesis.

Relationship Statement

The first characteristic of a hypothesis is that it is a declarative statement that identifies the predicted relationship between two or more variables. This implies that there is a systematic relationship between an independent variable and a dependent variable. The direction of the predicted relationship is also specified in this statement. Phrases such as *greater than; less than; positively, negatively,* or *curvilinearly* related (∪- or ∩-shaped); and *difference in* connote the directionality that is proposed in the hypothesis. In the following example of a directional hypothesis, "Asthmatic children who receive postural drainage treatments (independent variable) will have less bronchial congestion (dependent variable) than have children with no postural drainage," the two variables are explicitly identified, and the relational aspect of the prediction is contained in the phrase *less than.*

The nature of the relationship, either causal or associative, is also implied by the hypothesis. A causal relationship is one in which the researcher is able to predict that the independent variable (X) causes a change in the dependent variable (Y). It is rare in research that one is in a firm enough position to take a definitive stand about a cause-and-effect relationship. For example, a researcher might hypothesize that relaxation training would have a significant effect on the physical and psychological health status of patients who have suffered myocardial infarction. However, it would be difficult for a researcher to predict a strong cause-and-effect relationship because of the multiple intervening variables, such as age, medication, and life-style changes, that might also influence the subject's health status. Variables are more commonly related in noncausal ways; that is, the variables are systematically related but in an associative way. This means that there is a systematic movement in the associated values of the two phenomena. For example, there is strong evidence that asbestos exposure is related to lung cancer. It is tempting to state that there is a causal relationship between asbestos exposure and lung cancer. However, do not overlook the fact that not all of those exposed to asbestos will have lung cancer and not all of those who have lung cancer have had asbestos exposure. Consequently, it would be scientifically unsound to take a position advocating the presence of a causal relationship between these two variables. Rather, one can say only that there is an associative relationship between the variables of asbestos exposure and lung cancer, a relationship in which there is a strong systematic association between the two phenomena.

Testability

The second characteristic of a hypothesis is its testability. This means that the variables of the study must lend themselves to observation, measurement, and analysis. The hypothesis is either supported or not supported after the data have been collected and analyzed. The predicted outcome proposed by the hypothesis will or will not be congruent with the actual outcome when the hypothesis is tested. Hypotheses advance scientific knowledge by confirming or refuting theories.

Hypotheses may fail to meet the criteria of testability because the researcher has not made a prediction about the anticipated outcome, the variables are not observable or measurable, or the hypothesis is couched in terms that are value laden. Table 3-6 illustrates each of these points and provides a remedy for each problem.

 HELPFUL HINT
When a hypothesis is complex, that is, it contains more than one independent or dependent variable, it is difficult for the findings to indicate unequivocally that the hypothesis is supported or not supported. In such cases the reader needs to infer from the findings or discussion section which relationships are significant in the predicted direction.

Theory Base

A sound hypothesis is consistent with an existing body of theory and research findings. Regardless of whether a hypothesis is arrived at inductively or deductively (see Chapter 5), it

Table 3-6		
Hypotheses That Fail to Meet the Criteria of Testability		
PROBLEMATIC HYPOTHESIS	PROBLEMATIC ISSUE	REVISED HYPOTHESIS
Anxiety related to learning.	No predictive statement about the relationship is made; therefore the relationship is not verifiable.	Anxiety is curvilinearly (∩-shaped) related to problem-solving behavior.
Patients who receive pre-operative instruction have less postoperative stress than have patients who do not.	The "postoperative stress" variable must be specifically defined so that it is observable or measurable, or the relationship is not testable.	Patients who attend preoperative education classes have less postoperative emotional stress than have patients who do not.
Small-group teaching will be better than individual-ized teaching for dietary compliance in diabetic patients.	"Better than" is a value-laden phrase that is not objective. Moral and ethical questions containing words such as *should, ought, better than,* and *bad for* are not scientifically testable.	Dietary compliance will be greater in diabetic patients receiving diet instruction in small groups than in diabetic patients receiving individualized diet instruction.
Widowhood causes psychosocial health dysfunction.	Causal relationships are proposed without sufficient evidence. The "widowhood" variable must be specifically defined or the relationship is not testable.	Widowed persons with greater resource strength will have less psychosocial health dysfunction than those with lower resource strength.

must be based on a sound scientific rationale. The reader of a research report should be able to identify the flow of ideas from the problem statement to the literature review, to the theoretical framework, and through the hypotheses (see Chapters 4 and 5). Table 3-7 illustrates this process in relation to the problem statement "What is the effect of children's preoperative coping on postoperative anxiety and return to normal activity?" (LaMontagne et al, 1996). In this example it is clear that there is an explicitly developed, relevant body of scientific data that provides the theoretical grounding for the study. The hypotheses, as stated in Table 3-7, are logically derived from the theoretical framework. However, the research consumer should be cautioned about assuming that the theory-hypothesis link will always be present.

Table 3-8

Examples of How Hypotheses Are Worded

HYPOTHESIS	VARIABLES*	TYPE OF HYPOTHESIS	TYPE OF DESIGN SUGGESTED
1. There will be a relationship between self-concept and suicidal behavior.	*IV:* Self-concept *DV:* Suicidal behavior	Nondirectional research	Nonexperimental
2. Synchrony of maternal and newborn sleep rhythms will be negatively related to post-partum blues.	*IV:* Synchrony of maternal and new-born sleep rhythms *DV:* Postpartum blues	Directional research	Nonexperimental
3. Structured preoperative education is more effective than struc-tured postoperative edu-cation in reducing the patient's perception of pain.	*IV:* Preoperative education *IV:* Postoperative education *DV:* Perception of pain	Directional research	Experimental
4. The incidence and de-gree of severity of subject discomfort will be less af-ter administration of medications by the Z-track intramuscular injec-tion technique than after administration of med-ications by the standard intramuscular injection technique.	*IV:* Z-track intramuscular injection technique *IV:* Standard intra-muscular injection technique *DV:* Subject discom-fort	Directional research	Experimental
5. Progressive relaxation will be more effective in reducing indices of physiological arousal than hypnotic relaxation or self-relaxation in patients undergoing cardiac rehabilitation.	*IV:* Progressive relax-ation *IV:* Hypnotic relax-ation *IV:* Self-relaxation *DV:* Physiological arousal indices	Directional research	Experimental

*IV, Independent variable; DV, dependent variable.

Continued

		TYPE OF	TYPE OF DESIGN
Table 3-8—cont'd			
Examples of How Hypotheses Are Worded			
HYPOTHESIS	VARIABLES*	TYPE OF HYPOTHESIS	TYPE OF DESIGN SUGGESTED
6. There will be a relationship between years of nursing experience and attitude toward patients with human immunodeficiency virus (HIV) disease.	*IV:* Years of experience *DV:* Attitude toward HIV patients	Nondirectional research	Nonexperimental
7. There will be a positive relationship between trust and self-disclosure in marital relationships.	*IV:* Trust *DV:* Self-disclosure	Directional research	Nonexperimental
8. There will be a greater decrease in posttest state anxiety scores in subjects treated with noncontact therapeutic touch than in subjects treated with contact therapeutic touch.	*IV:* Noncontact therapeutic touch *IV:* Contact therapeutic touch *DV:* State anxiety	Directional research	Experimental

*_IV,_ Independent variable; _DV,_ dependent variable.

ture of many studies utilizing nondirectional hypotheses, the theory base may be less well developed.

- They provide the reader with a specific theoretical frame of reference within which the study is being conducted.
- They suggest to the reader that the researcher is not sitting on a theoretical fence, and as a result, the analyses of data can be accomplished in a statistically more sensitive way.

The important point for the critiquer to keep in mind regarding directionality of the hypotheses is whether there is a sound rationale for the choice the researcher has proposed regarding directionality.

Statistical Versus Research Hypotheses

Readers of research reports may observe that a hypothesis is further categorized as either a research or a statistical hypothesis. A **research hypothesis,** also known as a _scientific hypothesis,_ consists of a statement about the expected relationship between the variables. A research hypothesis indicates what the outcome of the study is expected to be. A research hypothesis is also either directional or nondirectional. If the researcher obtains statistically significant find-

		TYPE OF	TYPE OF DESIGN
HYPOTHESIS	VARIABLES*	HYPOTHESIS	SUGGESTED

Table 3-9

Examples of Statistical Hypotheses

HYPOTHESIS	VARIABLES*	TYPE OF HYPOTHESIS	TYPE OF DESIGN SUGGESTED
Oxygen inhalation by nasal cannula of up to 6 L/min does not affect oral temperature measurement taken with an electronic thermometer.	*IV:* Oxygen inhalation by nasal cannula *DV:* Oral temperature	Statistical	Experimental
The incidence of pregnancy in adolescent girls attending birth control education classes will not differ from that of girls who do not attend birth control education classes.	*IV:* Birth control education classes *DV:* Adolescent pregnancy	Statistical	Experimental

*IV, Independent variable; *DV,* dependent variable.

ings for a research hypothesis, the hypothesis is supported. For example, in a study exploring the relative effectiveness of one intervention, the side-lying position during breastfeeding, to minimize fatigue, Milligan, Flenniken, and Pugh (1996) hypothesized that "postpartum women [who] delivered vaginally and who breastfed in the side-lying position would report less fatigue symptoms than women who breastfed in the sitting position." The authors reported a statistically significant difference in the average number of fatigue symptoms between the two breastfeeding positions in subjects who had vaginal deliveries. As such, the hypothesis is supported; that is, the predicted outcome was supported by the study findings. The examples in Table 3-8 represent research hypotheses.

A **statistical hypothesis,** also known as a *null hypothesis,* states that there is no relationship between the independent and dependent variables. The examples in Table 3-9 illustrate statistical hypotheses. If in the data analysis a statistically significant relationship emerges between the variables at a specified level of significance, the null hypothesis is rejected. Rejection of the statistical hypothesis is equivalent to acceptance of the research hypothesis. For example, in the study by Rudy et al (1995) that compared the effects of a low-technology environment of care and a nurse case management delivery system (special care unit [SCU]) with the traditional high-technology environment (intensive care unit [ICU]) and a primary nursing care delivery system, null or statistical hypotheses were implied. One example of an implied null hypothesis is "there is no difference in mortality, length of stay, infections, respiratory complications, or life-threatening complications for chronically critically ill patients receiving care in the SCU versus the ICU environment." Rudy et al (1995) reported that there were no significant differences in patient outcomes in relation to these variables. Because the difference in outcomes was not greater than expected by chance, the null hypothesis was accepted (see Chapter 15).

Some researchers refer to the null hypothesis as a statistical contrivance that obscures a straightforward prediction of the outcome. Others state that it is more exact and conservative statistically, and that failure to reject the null hypothesis implies that there is insufficient evidence to support the idea of a real difference. Readers of research reports will note that, in general, when hypotheses are stated, research hypotheses are more commonly used than statistical hypotheses. It is more desirable to state the researcher's expectation. The reader then has a more precise idea of the proposed outcome. In any study that involves statistical analysis, the underlying null hypothesis is usually assumed without being explicitly stated.

RELATIONSHIP BETWEEN THE HYPOTHESIS AND THE RESEARCH DESIGN

Regardless of whether the researcher uses a statistical or a research hypothesis, there is a suggested relationship between the hypothesis and the research design of the study. The type of design, experimental or nonexperimental (see Chapters 7 and 8), will influence the wording of the hypothesis. For example, when an experimental design is utilized, the research consumer would expect to see hypotheses that reflect relationship statements, such as the following:

- X_1 is more effective than X_2 on Y.
- The effect of X_1 on Y is greater than that of X_2 on Y.
- The incidence of Y will not differ in subjects receiving X_1 and X_2 treatments.
- The incidence of Y will be greater in subjects after X_1 than after X_2.

Such hypotheses indicate that an experimental treatment will be used and that two groups of subjects, experimental and control groups, are being used to test whether the difference predicted by the hypothesis actually exists.

In contrast, hypotheses related to nonexperimental designs reflect associative relationship statements, such as the following:

- X will be negatively related to Y.
- There will be a positive relationship between X and Y.

Additional examples of this concept are illustrated in Table 3-8. The Critical Thinking Decision Path will help you determine the type of hypothesis presented in a study, as well as the study's readiness for a hypothesis-testing design.

RESEARCH QUESTIONS

Research studies do not always contain hypotheses. As you become more familiar with the scientific literature, you will notice that exploratory studies usually do not have hypotheses. This is particularly common where there is a dearth of literature or related research studies in a particular area that is of interest to the researcher. The researcher, interested in finding out more about a particular phenomenon, may engage in a fact-finding or relationship-finding mission guided only by research questions. The outcome of the exploratory study may be that data about the phenomenon are amassed and the researcher is then able to formulate hypotheses for a future study. This is sometimes called a *hypothesis-generating study.*

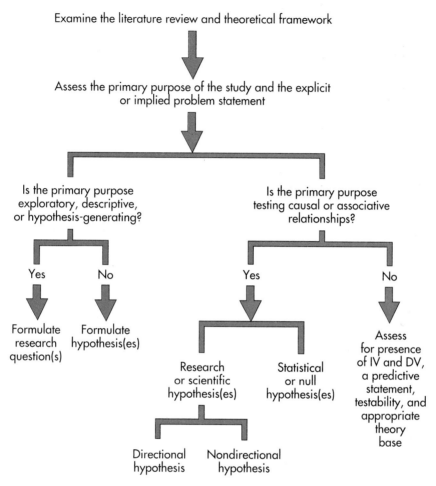

Examine the literature review and theoretical framework

Assess the primary purpose of the study and the explicit or implied problem statement

Is the primary purpose exploratory, descriptive, or hypothesis-generating?

Is the primary purpose testing causal or associative relationships?

Yes   No

Yes   No

Formulate research question(s)

Formulate hypothesis(es)

Research or scientific hypothesis(es)

Statistical or null hypothesis(es)

Assess for presence of IV and DV, a predictive statement, testability, and appropriate theory base

Directional hypothesis   Nondirectional hypothesis

Critical Thinking Decision Path   Determining the type of hypothesis or readiness for hypothesis testing.

A study by Failla et al (1996) examining the influence of psychosocial variables, uncertainty, health-related hardiness, hopelessness, and social support in women with systemic lupus erythematosus (SLE) illustrates how an investigation designed to generate relationships and fill a gap in the literature was guided by research questions. Research questions included the following:

- What relationships exist among the variables of uncertainty, health-related hardiness, hopelessness, social support, and adjustment in women with SLE?
- What demographic and psychosocial variables predict adjustment in women with SLE?

Because there has been little research on SLE, research questions rather than hypotheses are appropriate for this baseline phase of a study. The findings of the study highlighted the importance of hope as a significant predictor of adjustment and the need for future hypothesis-

﹔studies to identify nursing interventions that will be instrumental in instilling and sus-
﹒g hope in women with SLE.

꜄ualitative research studies also are guided by research questions rather than hypotheses. The descriptive findings of qualitative studies also can provide the basis for future hypothesis-testing studies. "What is the meaning of postpartum depressed mothers' experiences during interactions with their infants and older children?" is an example of a research question, from a qualitative study by Beck (1996) that sought to enrich understanding about the adverse effects of postpartum depression on maternal-child interactions.

As you can see, research questions tend to be more general than the research problems discussed in the problem statement section of this chapter. However, the more specific they are, the more they provide direction for the study.

In other studies, research questions are formulated in addition to hypotheses to answer questions related to ancillary data. Such questions do not directly pertain to the proposed outcomes of the hypotheses. Rather, they may provide additional and sometimes serendipitous findings that are enriching to the study and valuable in providing direction for further study. Sometimes they are the kernels of new or future hypotheses. The evaluator of a research study needs to determine whether it was appropriate to formulate a research question rather than a hypothesis, given the nature and context of the study.

HELPFUL HINT

Remember that research questions are most often used in exploratory or hypothesis-generating studies.

CRITIQUING THE RESEARCH PROBLEM AND HYPOTHESES

The care that a researcher takes when developing the problem statement and hypotheses is often representative of the overall conceptualization and design of the study. A methodically formulated research problem provides the basis for hypothesis development. In an empirical research study, the remainder of a study revolves around testing the hypotheses or, in some cases, the research questions. This may be a time-consuming, sometimes frustrating endeavor for the researcher. But in the final analysis, the product, as evaluated by the consumer, most often has been worth the struggle. Because this text focuses on the nurse as a critical consumer of research, the following sections will pertain primarily to the evaluation of research problems and hypotheses in research reports.

Critiquing the Problem Statement

The Critiquing Criteria box provides several criteria for evaluating this initial phase of the research process—the problem statement. Because the problem statement represents the basis for the study, it is usually introduced at the beginning of the research report. This will indicate the focus and direction of the study to the readers, who will then be in a position to evaluate whether the rest of the study logically flows from its base. Often the author will begin by identifying the general problem area that originally represented some vague discontent or question regarding an unsolved problem. The experimental and scientific background that led to the specific problem is briefly summarized, and the purpose, aim, or goal of the study is identified. Finally, the problem statement and any related subproblems are proposed in those instances that they are used in an article.

The purpose of the introductory summary of the experimental and scientific background is to provide the reader with a glimpse of how the author critically thought about the research problem's development. The introduction to the research problem places the study within an appropriate conceptual framework and sets the stage for the unfolding of the study. This introductory section should also include the significance of the study; that is, why the investigator is doing the study. For example, the significance may be to solve a problem encountered in the clinical area and thereby improve patient care, to resolve a conflict in the literature regarding a clinical issue, or to provide data supporting an innovative form of nursing intervention that is cost effective.

 ## CRITIQUING CRITERIA

THE PROBLEM STATEMENT

1. Was the problem statement introduced promptly?
2. Is the problem stated clearly and unambiguously in declarative or question form?
3. Does the problem statement express a relationship between two or more variables or at least between an independent and a dependent variable, implying empirical testability?
4. Does the problem statement specify the nature of the population being studied?
5. Has the problem been substantiated with adequate experiential and scientific background material?
6. Has the problem been placed within the context of an appropriate theoretical framework?
7. Has the significance of the problem been identified?
8. Have pragmatic issues, such as feasibility, been addressed?
9. Have the purpose, aims, or goals of the study been identified?

THE HYPOTHESES

1. Does the hypothesis directly relate to the research problem?
2. Is the hypothesis concisely stated in a declarative form?
3. Are the independent and dependent variables identified in the statement of the hypothesis?
4. Are the variables measurable or potentially measurable?
5. Is each of the hypotheses specific to one relationship so that each hypothesis can be either supported or not supported?
6. Is the hypothesis stated in such a way that it is testable?
7. Is the hypothesis stated objectively, without value-laden words?
8. Is the direction of the relationship in each hypothesis clearly stated?
9. Is each hypothesis consistent with the literature review?
10. Is the theoretical rationale for the hypothesis explicit?
11. Are research questions appropriately used (i.e., exploratory or qualitative study or in relation to ancillary data analyses)?

In reality, the reader often will find that the research problem is not clearly stated at the conclusion of this section. In fact, in some cases it is only hinted at, and the reader is challenged to identify the problem under consideration. In other cases the problem statement is embedded in the introductory text or purpose statement. To some extent, this will depend on the style of the particular journal. Nevertheless the evaluator must remember that the main problem statement should be clearly delineated in the introductory section even if the subproblems are not.

The reader looks for the presence of four key elements that are described and illustrated in an earlier section of this chapter. They are the following:

- Is the problem stated clearly and unambiguously?
- Does the problem statement express a relationship between two or more variables, or at least between an independent and dependent variable?
- Does the problem statement specify the nature of the population being studied?
- Does the problem statement imply the possibility of empirical testing?

The reader will use these four elements as criteria for judging the soundness of a stated research problem. It is likely that if the problem is unclear in terms of the variables, the population, and the implications for testability, the remainder of the study is going to falter. For example, a research study contained introductory material on anxiety in general, anxiety as it relates to the perioperative period, and the potentially beneficial influence of nursing care in relation to anxiety reduction. The author concluded that the purpose of the study was to determine whether selected measures of patient anxiety could be shown to differ when different approaches to nursing care were used during the perioperative period. The author did not go on to state the research problems. A restatement of the problem in question form might be the following:

$$(Y_1) \qquad\qquad (X_1, X_2, X_3)$$
What is the difference in patient anxiety level in relation to different approaches to nursing care during the perioperative period?

If this process is clarified at the outset of a research study, all that follows in terms of the design can be logically developed. The reader will have a clear idea of what the report should convey and can evaluate knowledgeably the material that follows.

Critiquing the Hypothesis

As illustrated in the Critiquing Criteria box, several criteria for critiquing the hypotheses should be used as a standard for evaluating the strengths and weaknesses of the hypotheses in a research report.

1. When reading a research study the research consumer may find the hypotheses clearly delineated in a separate hypothesis section of the research article, after the literature review or theoretical framework section(s). In many cases the hypotheses are not explicitly stated and are only implied in the *Results* or *Discussion* section of the article. As such, they must be inferred by the critiquer from the purpose statement and the type of analysis used. The reader must be cognizant of this variation and not think that because hypotheses do not appear at the beginning of the article, they do not exist in the particular study. Even when hypotheses are

stated at the beginning of an article, they are reexamined in the *Results* or *Discussion* section as the findings are presented and discussed. However, the critiquer should expect hypotheses to be appropriately reflected depending on the purpose of the study and format of the article.

2. The hypothesis should directly answer the research problem that was posed at the beginning of the report. Its placement in the research report logically follows the the problem statement, the literature review, and the theoretical framework, because the hypothesis should reflect the culmination and expression of this conceptual process. It should be consistent with both the literature review and the theoretical framework. The flow of this process, as depicted in Table 3-8, should be explicit and apparent to the reader. If this criterion is met, the reader feels reasonably assured that the basis for the hypothesis is theoretically sound.

3. As the reader examines the actual hypothesis, several aspects of the statement should be critically appraised. First, the hypothesis should consist of a declarative statement that objectively and succinctly expresses the relationship between an independent and a dependent variable. In wording a complex versus a simple hypothesis, there may be more than one independent and dependent variable.

Second, the reader can expect that there may be more than one hypothesis, particularly if there is more than one independent and dependent variable. This will be a function of the type of study being conducted.

Third, the variables of the hypothesis should be understandable to the reader. Often in the interest of formulating a succinct hypothesis statement, the complete meaning of the variables is not apparent. The critiquer must realize that sometimes a researcher is caught between the "devil and the deep blue sea" on that issue. It may be a choice between having a complete but verbose hypothesis paragraph, or a less complete but concise hypothesis. The solution to this dilemma is for the researcher to have a definition section in the research report. The inclusion of **conceptual definitions** and **operational definitions** (see Chapter 5) provides the complete explication of the variables. The critiquer is then able to examine the hypothesis side by side with the definitions and determine the exact nature of the variables under consideration. An excellent example of this process appears in a research article by Woods, Haberman, and Packard (1993), who hypothesized that

> women reporting more direct disease effect demands will report poorer individual adaptation to the illness
>
> and
>
> women reporting more personal disruption demands will report poorer individual adaptation to the illness.

These are appropriately worded hypotheses. However, it is not completely clear what the variables "direct disease effect demands" and "personal disruption demands" imply. It is only when one examines the definitions of these variables, which are included in the literature review section, that the exact nature of the variables becomes clear to the reader:

- Direct disease effect demands: "the physical and psychosocial experiences that people attribute directly to the disease with which they live . . . and may include such symptoms as nausea, fatigue, pain, dyspnea, and weakness"
- Personal disruption demands: "represent challenges to one's sense of integrity, continuity, and normalcy"

The context of the variables is now revealed to the evaluator.

Fourth, although a hypothesis can legitimately be nondirectional, it is preferable to indicate the direction of the relationship between the variables in the hypothesis. The reader will find that when there is a dearth of data available for the literature review—that is, the researcher has chosen to study a relatively undefined area of interest—the nondirectional hypothesis may be appropriate. There simply may not be enough information available to make a sound judgment about the direction of the proposed relationship. All that could be proposed is that there will be a relationship between two variables. Essentially, the critiquer wants to determine the appropriateness of the researcher's choice regarding directionality of the hypothesis.

4. The notion of testability is central to the soundness of a hypothesis. One criterion related to testability is that the hypothesis should be stated in such a way that it can be clearly supported or not supported. Whereas the previous statement is very important to keep in mind, the reader should also understand that ultimately neither theories nor hypotheses are ever proven beyond the shadow of a doubt through hypothesis testing. Researchers who claim that their data have "proven" the validity of their hypothesis should be regarded with grave reservation. The reader should realize that, at best, findings that support a hypothesis are considered tentative. If repeated replication of a study yields the same results, greater confidence can be placed in the conclusions advanced by the researchers. An important thing to remember about testability is that although hypotheses are more likely to be accepted with increasing evidence, they are never ultimately proven.

Another point about testability for the consumer to consider is that the hypothesis should be objectively stated and devoid of any value-laden words. Value-laden hypotheses are not empirically testable. Quantifiable words such as *greater than; less than; decrease; increase;* and *positively, negatively,* and *curvilinearly related* convey the idea of objectivity and testability. The reader should be immediately suspicious of hypothesis that are not stated objectively.

5. The evaluator of a research study should be cognizant of the fact that the way that the proposed relationship of the hypothesis is phrased suggests the type of research design that will be appropriate for the study. For example, if a hypothesis proposes that treatment X_1 will have a greater effect on Y than treatment X_2, an experimental or quasiexperimental design is suggested (see Chapter 7). If a hypothesis proposes that there will be a positive relationship between variables X and Y, a nonexperimental design is suggested (see Chapter 8). A review of Table 3-6 provides you with additional examples of hypotheses and the type of research design that is suggested by each hypothesis. The reader of a research report should evaluate whether the selected research design is congruent with the hypothesis. This factor has important implications for the remainder of the study in terms of the appropriateness of sample selection, data collection, data analysis, interpretation of findings, and ultimately the conclusions advanced by the researcher.

6. If the research report contains research questions rather than hypotheses, the reader will want to evaluate whether this is appropriate to the study. The criterion for making this decision, as presented earlier in this chapter, is whether the study is of an exploratory or qualitative nature. If it is, then it is appropriate to have research questions rather than hypotheses. Ancillary research questions should be evaluated as to whether they answer additional questions secondary to the hypotheses. Sometimes the substance of an additional research question is more appropriately posed as another hypothesis in that it relates in a major way to the original research problem.

KEY POINTS

- Formulation of the research problem and stating the hypothesis are key preliminary steps in the research process. The care with which they are developed is often representative of the overall conceptualization and design of the study.
- The research problem is refined through a process that proceeds from the identification of a general idea of interest to the definition of a more specific and circumscribed topic.
- A preliminary literature review reveals related factors that appear critical to the research topic of interest and aids in further definition of the research problem.
- The significance of the research problem must be identified in terms of its potential contribution to patients, nurses, the medical community in general, and society. Applicability of the problem for nursing practice, as well as its theoretical relevance, must be established. The findings should also have the potential for formulating or altering nursing practices or policies.
- The feasibility of a research problem must be examined in light of pragmatic considerations such as time; availability of subjects, money, facilities, and equipment; experience of the researcher; and ethical issues.
- The final problem statement consists of a statement about the relationship between two or more variables. It clearly identifies the relationship between the independent and dependent variables; it specifies the nature of the population being studied; and it implies the possibility of empirical testing.
- A hypothesis attempts to answer the question posed by the research problem. When testing the validity of the theoretical framework's assumptions, the hypothesis bridges the theoretical and real worlds.
- A hypothesis is a declarative statement about the relationship between two or more variables that predicts an expected outcome. Characteristics of a hypothesis include a relationship statement, implications regarding testability, and consistency with a defined theory base.
- Hypotheses can be formulated in a directional or a nondirectional manner. Hypotheses can be further categorized as either research or statistical hypotheses.
- Research questions may be used instead of hypotheses in exploratory or qualitative research studies. Research questions may also be formulated in addition to hypotheses to answer questions related to ancillary data.
- The critiquing criteria provide a set of guidelines for evaluating the strengths and weaknesses of the problem statement and hypotheses as they appear in a research report.
- The critiquer assesses the clarity of the problem statement, as well as the related subproblems, the specificity of the population, and the implications for testability.
- The interrelatedness of the problem statement, the literature review, the theoretical framework, and the hypotheses should be apparent.
- The appropriateness of the research design suggested by the problem statement is also evaluated.
- The purpose of the study (i.e., why the researcher is doing the study) should be differentiated from the problem statement or the research question to be answered.
- The reader evaluates the wording of the hypothesis in terms of the clarity of the relational statement, the implications for testability, and its congruence with a theory base. The appropriateness of the hypothesis in relation to the type of research design suggested by the

design also is examined. The appropriate use of research questions is also evaluated in relation to the type of study conducted.

CRITICAL THINKING CHALLENGES
Barbara Krainovich-Miller

❓ Do you think the problem statements found in Tables 3-2 and 3-3 equally meet the three characteristics of a good problem statement listed on p. 67? Justify your answer.

❓ You are listening to two of your classmates from your nursing research class argue over whether a variable is independent or dependent. Joseph states that in the study they reviewed in class, anxiety was the dependent variable. Therefore anxiety is the dependent variable in the current study on the clinical validation of the nursing diagnosis preop anxiety they are reviewing for assignment one. Do you think Joseph is correct? What explanations would you offer him?

❓ Is it always the case that hypotheses are explicitly stated for experimental studies? What evidence do you have to support your answer?

❓ Table 3-7 lists three hypotheses for the stated problem statement. Do you agree that these hypotheses meet the characteristics of hypotheses, including a relationship between variables that predict an expected outcome, implications regarding testability, and consistency with a defined theory base? Discuss your conclusion for each of these hypotheses and your reasons for your decision.

REFERENCES

Beck CT: Postpartum depressed mothers' experiences interacting with their children, *Nurs Res* 45(2):98-104, 1996.

Blixen CE: Differences in the use of hospital-based outpatient mental health services by the elderly, *Image* 26(3):195-200, 1994.

Crigger NJ: Testing an uncertainty model for women with multiple sclerosis, *Adv Nurs Sci* 18(3):37-47, 1996.

Devine EC, Reifschneider E: A meta-analysis of the effects of psychoeducational care in adults with hypertension, *Nurs Res* 44(4):237-245, 1995.

Downs F: How to get to the point, *Nurs Res* 42(1):3, 1993.

Erickson RS, Meyer LT, Woo TM: Chemical dot thermometers, *Image* 28(1):23-28, 1996.

Failla S et al: Adjustment of women with systemic lupus erythematosus, *Appl Nurs Res* 9(2):87-92, 1996.

Fulton TR: Nurses' adoption of a patient-controlled analgesia approach, *West J Nurs Res* 18(4):383-396, 1996.

Gift AG, Moore T, Soeken K: Relaxation to reduce dyspnea and anxiety in COPD patients, *Nurs Res* 41(4):242-246, 1992.

Goode CJ et al: A meta-analysis of effects of heparin flush and saline flush: quality and cost implications, *Nurs Res* 40(6):324-330, 1991.

Grey M, Cameron ME, Thurber FW: Coping and adaptation in children with diabetes, *Nurs Res* 40(3):144-149, 1991.

Hoskins C et al: Social support and patterns of adjustment to breast cancer, *Sch Inq Nurs Pract* 10(2):99-123, 1996.

LaMontagne LL et al: Children's preoperative coping and its effect on postoperative anxiety and return to normal activity, *Nurs Res* 45(3):141-147, 1996.

McCain NL et al: The influence of stress management training in HIV disease, *Nurs Res* 45(4):246-253, 1996.

Milligan RA, Flenniken PA, Pugh LC: Positioning intervention to minimize fatigue in breast-feeding women, *Appl Nurs Res* 9(2):67-70, 1996.

Olson JK: Relationships between nurse-expressed empathy, patient-perceived empathy and patient distress, *Image* 27(4):317-322, 1995.

Redeker NS et al: Sleep patterns in women after coronary artery bypass surgery, *Appl Nurs Res* 9(3):115-122, 1996.

Ronen T, Abraham Y: Retention control training in the treatment of younger versus older enuretic children, *Nurs Res* 45(2):78-82, 1996.

Rudy EB et al: Patient outcomes for the chronically critically ill: special care unit versus intensive care unit, *Nurs Res* 44(6):324-331, 1995.

Ward SE, Berry PE, Misiewicz H: Concerns about analgesics among patients and family caregivers in a hospice setting, *Res Nurs Health* 19:205-211, 1996.

Wikblad K, Anderson B: A comparison of three wound dressings in patients undergoing heart surgery, *Nurs Res* 44(5):312-316, 1995.

Woods NF, Haberman MR, Packard NJ: Demands of illness and individual, dyadic, and family adaptation in chronic illness, *Nurs Res* 15(1):10-25, 1993.

ADDITIONAL READINGS

Campbell DT, Stanley JC: *Experimental and quasi-experimental designs for research,* Chicago, 1963, Rand McNally.

Downs FS, Newman MA: *A source book of nursing research,* Philadelphia, 1977, FA Davis.

Kerlinger FN: *Foundations of behavioral research,* New York, 1986, Holt, Rinehart & Winston.

Newman MA: *Theory development in nursing,* Philadelphia, 1979, FA Davis.

Van Dalen DB: *Understanding educational research,* New York, 1979, McGraw-Hill.

Literature Review

Barbara Krainovich-Miller

Key Terms

CD-ROM
computer database
conceptual
    literature
Cumulative Index
    to Nursing and
    Allied Health
    Literature
    (CINAHL)

data-based
    literature
empirical literature
Internet
on-line
primary source
print databases
refereed or
    peer-reviewed
    journals

research literature
review of the
    literature
scholarly literature
scientific literature
secondary source
theoretical
    literature
Web browser
World Wide
    Web (WWW)

Learning Outcomes

After reading this chapter the student should be able to do the following:

- Discuss the relationship of the review of the literature to nursing theory, research, education, and practice.
- Discuss the purposes of the literature review for research and consumer research activities.
- Discuss the use of the review of the literature for quantitative designs and qualitative approaches.
- Differentiate between conceptual and data-based literature.
- Differentiate between primary and secondary sources.
- Compare the advantages and disadvantages of the most commonly used computer CD-ROM and on-line Internet databases and traditional print database sources for conducting a relevant review of the literature.
- Identify the characteristics of a relevant literature review.
- Critically read (summarize and critique), at a beginning consumer of research level, conceptual and data-based resources.
- Apply critiquing criteria to the evaluation of literature reviews in selected research studies.

Y ou may wonder why an entire chapter of a research text is devoted to the review of the literature. The main reason is because the literature review is not only a key step in the research process but also is used in all steps of the process. A more personal question you might ask yourself is, "Will knowing more about the literature review really help me in my student role or later in my research consumer role as a practicing professional nurse?" The answer is that it most certainly will. The ability to review the literature is a skill essential to your role as a student and your future nursing role as a research consumer (ANA, 1993).

The **review of the literature** is traditionally considered a systematic and critical review of the most important published scholarly literature on a particular topic (Carroll-Johnson, 1992). The term *scholarly literature* can refer to published and unpublished data-based (research) literature, as well as conceptual literature materials found in print and nonprint forms. *Data-based literature* are reports of completed research. **Conceptual literature** can be reports of theories, some of which underlie reported research, as well as other consumer research material. For example, an article that discusses a particular theory or reviews the research and nonresearch literature related to a concept such as anxiety is considered conceptual rather than data-based or research literature.

As illustrated in Figure 4-1, this chapter introduces the review of the literature as a concept essential to the growth of nursing theory, research, education, and practice. In turn, knowledge, generated from theorists, researchers, educators, and practitioners, builds the literature through scholarly publications and presentations. In relation to these four concepts, a critical review of the literature does the following:

- Uncovers conceptual and data-based knowledge in relation to a particular subject/concept/problem.
- Uncovers new knowledge that can lead to the development, validation, or refinement of theories.
- Reveals appropriate research questions for the discipline.
- Provides the latest knowledge for education.
- Uncovers research findings that can lead to changes in clinical practice, especially for the development of research-based nursing interventions/practice protocols.

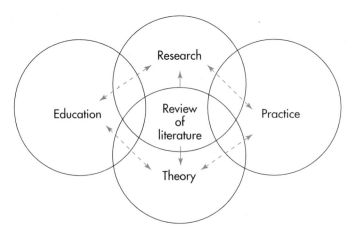

Figure 4-1   Relationship of the review of the literature to theory, research, education, and practice.

The purpose of this chapter is to introduce you to the use of the review of the literature in quantitative research and other scholarly consumer activities. The primary focus of the discussion is the perspective of the consumer of research rather than the "conductor of research."

REVIEW OF THE LITERATURE: PURPOSES

Overall Purpose: Knowledge

The overall purpose of a review of the literature is to develop a strong knowledge base to carry out research and other consumer research scholarly activities in the educational and clinical practice settings (Feldman et al, 1993; Glass, 1991). The objectives listed in Box 4-1 relate to research and consumer of research purposes. The knowledge uncovered from a critical review of the literature contributes to the development, implementation, and results of both quantitative and qualitative studies. Such knowledge enhances the writing of scholarly papers. In the clinical practice arena, the knowledge from a critical literature review contributes to the implementation of research-based practice interventions, protocols, and evaluation programs that improve the quality of patient care (see Chapter 19).

Research Purpose of the Literature Review

All 10 objectives listed in Box 4-1 can reflect the use of a literature review for the conduct of quantitative research. Critically reading the literature is essential to meeting these objectives. The main goal of a literature review is to develop the foundation of a sound study. Table 4-1

Box 4-1	Overall Purposes of a Review of Literature

Major goal: To develop a strong knowledge base to carry out research and other scholarly educational and clinical practice setting activities

Objectives: A review of the literature does the following:

1. Determines what is known and not known about a subject, concept, or problem
2. Determines gaps, consistencies, and inconsistencies in the literature about a subject, concept, or problem
3. Discovers unanswered questions about a subject, concept, or problem
4. Discovers conceptual traditions used to examine problems
5. Uncovers a new practice intervention(s), or gains support for current practice intervention(s)
6. Promotes development of new or revising practice protocols, policies, and projects/activities related to nursing practice and the discipline
7. Generates useful research questions and hypotheses for the discipline
8. Describes the strengths and weaknesses of designs/methods of inquiry and instruments used in earlier works
9. Determines an appropriate research design/method (instruments, data collection, and analysis methods) for answering the research question(s)
10. Determines the need for replication of a well-designed study or refinement of a study

Table 4-1	
Examples of the Uses of Review of Literature for Research Process: Quantitative and Qualitative	
QUANTITATIVE DESIGNS AND STEPS	QUALITATIVE PROCESS
The review of the literature is used for all designs/levels: experimental, quasiexperimental, and nonexperimental	The use of the literature review depends on the selected designs/types and phases; usually an extensive database is not available, conceptual data are somewhat limited, and for this reason a qualitative design is being used.
The review of the literature is usually defined as a step of the research process. When a research study is written as a proposal or is published, the literature review often is written as a separate aspect of the study. However, the actual review of the literature (i.e., the results of the review) is used in developing all steps of the process.	The following examples highlight the predominant use of the literature review for the particular qualitative approach: Phenomenological—compare findings with information from the review of the literature (Moore, 1997)
The review of the literature is essential to the following steps of the research process (see Appendix A; Wikblad and Anderson, 1995): Problem Need/significance Question/hypothesis(es) Theoretical/conceptual framework Design/methodology Specific instruments (validity and reliability) Data collection method Type of analysis Findings (interpretation) Implications of the findings Recommendations based on the findings	Grounded theory—constantly compare literature with data being generated (Draucker and Petrovic, 1996; see Appendix B) Ethnographic—more conceptual than data based; provides framework for study (Russell, 1996) Historical—review of literature is source of data (Roberts, 1996)

summarizes the main focus of the literature review for use in the steps of the research process for quantitative and qualitative designs. Box 4-2 lists the characteristics of a literature review that meet critiquing criteria; these characteristics are discussed throughout the chapter.

Consumer of Research Purposes of the Literature Review

The major consumer of research focus of the literature review is uncovering knowledge for use in educational and clinical practice settings. Objectives 1 through 6 in Box 4-1 address the

> **Box 4-2   Characteristics of a Written "Relevant" Review of Literature**
>
> Each reviewed source of information reflects critical thinking and scholarly writing, is relevant to the study/topic/project, and the content satisfies the following criteria:
> - Purposes of a literature review were met.
> - Summary is succinct and adequately represents the reviewed source.
> - Critiquing (objective critical evaluation) reflects analysis and synthesis of material.
> - Application of accepted "critiquing criteria" to analyze for strengths, weaknesses, or limitations and conflicts or gaps in information as it relates directly and indirectly to the area of interest.
> - Evidence of synthesis of the critiques of each source of information. Putting the parts (i.e., each critique) together to form a new whole (Kerlinger, 1986) or connecting link for what is to be studied, replicated, developed, or implemented.
> - Review consists of mainly primary sources.
> - Sufficient number of sources are used, especially data-based sources.
> - Summarizes/paraphrases material rather than continually quoting content.
> - Summaries/critiques of studies are presented in a logical flow ending with a conclusion or synthesis of the reviewed material that reflects why the study, project, or conceptual stand should be taken.

consumer of research purposes. Critically reading the literature generates useful projects for these settings. Table 4-1 indicates the ways the review of the literature is used for research purposes. Table 4-2 illustrates a few examples of consumer of research scholarly activities.

From a student perspective, a critical review of the literature is essential to acquiring knowledge for the development of scholarly papers, presentations, and debates. Faculty usually require that students use data-based and conceptual literature resources to support their rationale for each nursing intervention written for a particular nursing diagnosis. For example, a student assignment might involve retrieving and critically reviewing the primary sources (i.e., data-based references) listed for a particular practice protocol to determine the degree of support found for the interventions in the protocol. A **primary source** is one that is written by a person(s) who actually conducted the research or developed the theory. This will be discussed in more depth later in the chapter.

Differences Between Research Conduct and Consumer of Research Purposes

How does the literature review differ when it is used for research versus consumer of research purposes? Traditionally for research, the literature review is used in the development of a sound research proposal. It includes a critical evaluation of both conceptual and data-based literature related to the proposed study, as well as a summary of the overall strengths or weakness of the reviewed studies' conflicts and gaps in the literature; it concludes with a statement relating the proposed study to the reviewed research. It is not a rehash or simple paraphrasing of what each article stated.

Table 4-2

Examples of the Uses of the Literature for Research Consumer Purposes:
Educational and Practice Settings

EDUCATIONAL SETTING	CLINICAL/PROFESSIONAL SETTING
Undergraduate students	**Nurses in the clinical setting**
Develop academic scholarly papers (i.e., researching a topic, problem, or issue)	Implement research-based nursing interventions
Prepare oral presentations or debates of a topic, problem, or issue; clinical projects	Develop hospital-specific nursing protocols or policies related to patient care
	Develop, implement, and evaluate hospital-specific QA, CQI, or TQM projects or protocols related to patient outcome data
Graduate students (master's and doctoral)	**Professional nursing organizations/governmental agencies**
Develop research proposals	Develop ANA's major documents (e.g., Social Policy Statement, 1995; Nursing Care
Develop research-based practice protocols and other scholarly projects	Report Card for Acute Care, 1995;
Faculty	Women's Primary Health Care: Protocols for Practice, 1995; Standards of Clinical
Develop and revise curricula	Practice, 1991 [in revision]; Annotated Bibliography for Ethical Guidelines, 1995).
Develop theoretical papers for presentations and/or publication	Develop AHCPR's practice guidelines (e.g., Acute Pain Management, 1992).
Develop research proposals	

QA, quality assurance; *CQI,* continuous quality improvement; *TQM,* total quality management.

Should a literature review for consumer of research purposes be any different? Absolutely not; both reviews should be critical, framed in the context of previous data-based and conceptual literature, and pertinent to the objectives presented in Box 4-1. A critical review of the literature is essential to meeting ANA's Practice Standard VII (ANA, 1991) related to consumer of research implementation activities of the baccalaureate prepared nurse. Table 4-2 lists a number of consumer of research projects conducted in the educational and clinical/professional settings.

A critical literature review is central to developing and implementing these consumer of research activities. A practice protocol or nursing interventions implemented in a health care setting should be based on nurses' "critical" review of data-based (research) literature. For example, since 1992 the federal government's interdisciplinary Agency for Health Care Policy and Research (AHCPR) has published 18 guidelines for frequently occurring health problems. AHCPR's *Acute Pain Management Guideline* (1992) was one of the first guidelines; a later Guideline was *Evaluation and Management of Early HIV Infection* (1994). An extensive literature review was conducted for the development of these practice guidelines rather than as a step in the research process to develop and implement a research study. Stetler (1994) incorporates an extensive review of all types of research studies in her nursing model for research utilization (see Chapter 19).

REVIEW OF THE LITERATURE FOR QUANTITATIVE STUDIES: CONDUCTOR OF RESEARCH PERSPECTIVE

The literature review is considered essential to all steps of the quantitative research process. From this perspective the review is broad and systematic, as well as in-depth but not usually exhaustive; it is a critical collection and evaluation of the important published scholarly literature (conceptual and data-based) in journals, monographs, books, and/or book chapters, as well as unpublished scholarly (data-based) print and computer accessed materials (e.g., doctoral dissertations and master's theses), audiovisual materials (e.g., audiotapes and videotapes), and personal communications (e.g., conference presentations and one-to-one interviews).

From the perspective of a producer of research, objectives 1 through 5 and 7 through 10 of Box 4-1 represent different ways of thinking about the literature; these objectives direct the questions the researcher asks while reading the literature to determine a useful research question(s) and an appropriate design and method and/or the need for replication or refinement of a particular study.

As a consumer of research the following brief overview of the use of the literature review in relation to the steps of the quantitative research process will help you to understand the researcher's focus. (For an in-depth presentation in relation to qualitative research, see Chapter 9.) A critical reading of relevant literature is done in the following quantitative steps of the research process.

- *Theoretical or conceptual framework:* A critical literature review reveals conceptual traditions, concepts, and/or theories or conceptual models from nursing and other related fields that can be used to examine problems; it presents the context for studying the problem and can be viewed as a map for understanding the relationships between or among the variables in quantitative studies. The literature review provides rationale for the variables and explicates propositions in relation to the individual variables for the theoretical framework of the study.
- *Problem statement and hypothesis:* The literature review helps to determine what is known and not known; to uncover gaps, consistencies, or inconsistencies; and/or to reveal unanswered questions in the literature about a subject, concept, theory, or problem. The review allows for refinement of research problems and questions and/or hypotheses.
- *Design and method:* The literature review reveals the strengths and weaknesses of designs and methods of previous research studies. The review is crucial to choosing an appropriate design, data collection method, sample size, valid and reliable instruments, and effective data analysis method(s), as well as assisting in the development of an appropriate consent form that addresses ethical concerns. A critical literature review reveals the appropriateness of a study's design and can help the researcher determine whether a previous study should be replicated and/or refined. It also can uncover instruments that lack validity and reliability and thus identify the need for instrument refinement or development through testing.
- *Outcome of the analysis (findings, discussion, implications, and recommendations):* The literature review is used to accurately interpret and discuss the results/findings of a study. The researcher returns to the literature and uses conceptual and data-based literature to accomplish this goal. For instance, findings from a study on the clinical validation of the nursing diagnosis of anxiety may indicate that the most common indicator used to diagnose anxiety is the patient's subjective expression, "I'm anxious." The research would then indicate in this section of the journal article/report that this particular

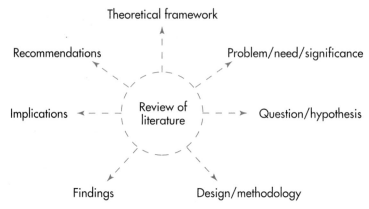

Figure 4-2   Relationship of the review of the literature to the steps of the quantitative research process.

finding was supported in the literature review. The literature review also helps to develop the implications of the findings for practice, education, and further research.

Figure 4-2 relates the literature review to all aspects of the quantitative research process. The literature review is essential to all aspects of conducting and/or writing the results of quantitative studies.

REVIEW OF THE LITERATURE: CONSUMER OF RESEARCH PERSPECTIVE

As a consumer of research you are not expected to write a complete scholarly review of the literature on your own, but you are expected to know how to conduct a literature review and critically evaluate it (ANA, 1993). Understanding the purpose(s) of a review of the literature for research and consumer of research purposes will enable you to meet this outcome (see Box 4-1). Embedded in the purposes is the ability to do the following:

- Efficiently retrieve an adequate amount of scholarly literature using computer **CD-ROM** (computer capability to use compact disk-read only memory) or **on-line** (accessing via Internet, which is a world-wide computer communication capability) programs such as **Cumulative Index to Nursing and Allied Health Literature (CINAHL),** as well as traditional print resources for material not entered into the common databases. CINAHL is a database of nursing and allied health literature.
- Critically evaluate data-based and conceptual material based on accepted literature review critiquing criteria for the respective literature.
- Synthesize the critically evaluated literature (e.g., the entire compilation of conceptual and data-based literature about patient-controlled analgesia [PCA]).

The objectives in Box 4-1 reflect both academic and professional expectations for a beginning consumer of research (see Chapter 1). Table 4-3 presents an overview of the steps for con-

Table 4-3

Steps and Strategies for Searching the Literature

STEPS OF LITERATURE REVIEW	STRATEGY
Step I: Determine concept/issue/topic/ problem	Keep focused on the types of patients/clients you deal with in your work setting. You know what works and doesn't work in the delivery of nursing care.
Step II: Identify variables/terms	Ask your reference librarian for help and read the data-based guide books usually found near the computers used for student searches; include "research" as one of your variables.
Step III: Conduct computer search	Do it yourself with the help of your librarian; it is essential for nurses to use CINAHL's database; prior to 1982 requires the use of print indexes.
Step IV: Weed out irrelevant sources before printing	Scan through your search, read the *abstracts* provided, and highlight or otherwise mark only those that fit your topic; ask your librarian how to include "references" (RF) in your print field for your search.
Step V: Organize sources from printout for retrieval	Organize by journal type and year, and reread abstracts to determine if the articles chosen are relevant.
Step VI: Retrieve relevant sources	Scan each article to determine if it is worth your time and money to retrieve it.
Step VII: Copy articles	Save yourself time and money; ahead of time buy a library copying card or bring plenty of change, so that you avoid wasting time midway to secure change. Copy the *entire* article including the references, making sure that you can clearly read the name of the journal, year, volume number, and pages; this can save you an immense amount of time when you are word processing your paper.
Step VIII: Conduct preliminary reading and weed out irrelevant sources	Review critical reading strategies (see Chapter 2) (e.g., read the abstract at the beginning of the article; see example in this chapter).
Step IX: Critically read each source (summarize and critique each source)	Use the critical reading strategies from Chapter 2; take the time to word process each summary, no more than 1 page long, include reference in APA style at the top or bottom of each, and staple copied article to back of summary.
Step X: Synthesize critical summaries of each article	Decide how you will present your synthesis of the reviewed articles (e.g., chronologically, according to type—conceptual or data-based), and word process the synthesized material and a reference list.

ducting a literature search. In the right-hand column you will find some useful tips/strategies or rationales for successfully and efficiently completing these steps. This process is the same whether the purpose is critiquing or writing a literature review; it reflects the cognitive processes and manual techniques of retrieving and critically reviewing sources from the literature. The remainder of this chapter presents the essential material for accomplishing these goals.

SCHOLARLY LITERATURE
Conceptual and Data-Based Literature: Synonyms and Sources

Synonyms for conceptual and data-based scholarly literature are presented in Table 4-4. Often these terms are used interchangeably. Most frequently the term *theoretical literature* is interchanged with conceptual literature; the terms *empirical literature, scientific literature,* or *research literature* are interchanged with *data-based literature.* Definitions and general examples of conceptual and data-based literature are presented in Table 4-5. For example, if you were interested in the topic "Critical Thinking and Nursing" you would use these variables in your search request.

The common sources of both conceptual and data-based literature are books, chapters of books, journal articles, abstracts, critique reviews, abstracts published in conference proceedings, professional and governmental reports, and unpublished doctoral dissertations. *Abstracts* are concisely written summaries of the main aspects of a research study or conceptual paper (see Chapter 2). Many published data-based and conceptual articles have a very brief summary or abstract on the first page, set off from the beginning of the article. Most computer searches have the feature of including the abstract for the reference, as well as all of the references used in the article. Another important source for abstracts is the *Annual Review of Nursing Research* (Fitzpatrick and Norbeck, 1996).

Less common and less used sources of scholarly material are audiotapes, videotapes, personal communications (letters or telephone or in-person interviews), unpublished doctoral dissertations, and master's theses. Also, there is a growing number of data-based and concep-

Table 4-4

Literature Review Synonyms

CONCEPTUAL LITERATURE	DATA-BASED LITERATURE
Theoretical literature	Empirical literature
Scholarly nonresearch literature	Scientific literature
Scholarly literature	Research literature
Soft- versus hard-science	Scholarly research literature
Literature review article	Research study
Analysis article	Concept analysis (as methodology)
Integrative review	Study

tual articles and abstracts available through electronic Internet sources. The **Internet** is not really a place; it is an international network of networks, which allows one computer to communicate with another, regardless of where it is located in the world (Prohaska and Chang, 1996). You may be most familiar with the Internet through hearing about or using the **World Wide Web (WWW).** The WWW is a part of the Internet that combines text and graphic materials and makes this information available through files, Web pages, or electronic mail (e-mail) (Kaufeld and Kaufeld, 1996).

Examples of Theoretical Material

Some conceptual or theoretical articles are an extensive literature review of conceptual and data-based articles on a particular concept or are a report about research that has been conducted on a particular phenomenon. These articles are often published in a journal that mainly publishes data-based articles. For example, *IMAGE* also includes theoretical papers. *IMAGE* published Larrabee's (1996) conceptual article entitled *Emerging Model of Quality.* The following abstract from Larrabee's article demonstrates the nature of a theoretical article:

A theoretical model of quality, based on an organismic worldview, provides a framework for understanding health care quality. This retroductively developed model incorporates ethical and economic concepts: value, beneficence, prudence, and justice. The model supports viewing patients and families as equal partners with providers in defining, evaluating, and achieving health care quality. Further model development can generate mid-range theories useful for improving quality in an ethical and economic manner.

Table 4-5

Types of Information Sources for a Review of Literature*

CONCEPTUAL LITERATURE	DATA-BASED LITERATURE
Published articles, documents, chapters in books, or books discussing theories, conceptual frameworks, and/or conceptual models, concept(s), constructs, theorems.	Published quantitative and qualitative studies, including concept analysis and/or methodology studies on a concept. Such material is found in journals, monographs, or books that are directly related to or indirectly related to the problem of interest.
Literature reviews of a concept that include both conceptual and data-based critiques.	Unpublished studies: master's theses and doctoral dissertations.
Proceedings and audiotapes and videotapes from scholarly conferences containing abstracts of a conceptual paper or the entire conceptual presentation.	Unpublished research abstracts or entire studies from print, audio, on-line: proceedings of conferences, compendiums, professional organizations' home page, or listservs (see library/computer activities section in text).

*Many of the examples given are or will be available by Internet services.

Larrabee performed an extensive review of the theoretical literature on the concepts related to quality and ethical philosophy as well as empirical studies that examined quality as a variable in developing a theoretical model of quality for use by health professionals.

Another excellent example of a conceptual article is Reed's (1996) analysis of the works of Peplau and the relevance of her theory for today's practice. The author critiqued both Peplau's theoretical works and studies that used Peplau's theory. Hays et al's (1994) article on *Informatics Issues for Nursing's Future* examined conceptual and data-based publications, as well as the reality issues surrounding the development of clinical databases to improve nursing practice. Their abstract clearly indicates (as noted by the bolded words) that its purpose was a theoretical paper rather than a research report. Hays et al stated:

Automated clinical databases are crucial to the future of nursing but presently are not meeting the needs of clinicians, administrators, educators, or researchers. **This article examines theoretical, empirical, and practical issues relating to the development of automated nursing clinical databases that will foster safe, effective practice and further nursing's knowledge base.** A series of key questions are identified relevant to each issue. These issues must be resolved if nurses are to take full advantage of the possibilities inherent in the evolving information technology. Key words: computers, informatics, information management, nomenclature, secondary data analysis.

Another related example of a conceptual article was published 2 years later. Turley (1996) proposed a new model for the further development of informatics for nursing based on a critical review of historical precedents in the field.

Sometimes the title of a scholarly article can help you determine if it is a conceptual rather than a research article. For example, the title of Bowles and Naylor's (1996) article is *Nursing Intervention Classification Systems.* The title suggests that the manuscript is conceptual in nature rather than a research study. If the title had been "A Study of Nursing's Intervention Classification Systems," then you might think it was a data-based (noted bolded words) article. Furthermore, do not assume because an article's abstract uses terms such as *purpose, organizing framework, conclusions,* and *implications* that it is a research study. Bowles and Naylor's abstract used these terms; however, it is clear from reading the entire article that these authors conducted a critical review of the unique components of the three ANA (1993) approved nursing intervention classification systems or taxonomies: Omaha Classification System (OCS), the IOWA Nursing Intervention Classification (NIC), and the Home Health Care Classification (HHC). Although the North American Nursing Diagnosis Association's (NANDA) taxonomy is the other ANA approved taxonomy, it was not critiqued in this analysis because it is a labeling rather than an intervention taxonomy (McCormick et al, 1994).

Other examples of theoretical literature are Maas, Johnson, and Moorhead's (1996) report of the research conducted on *Classifying Nursing-Sensitive Patient Outcomes* and Rafael's (1996) dialectical analysis between the concepts of power and caring. The reference list at the end of Rafael's article indicated that 50 conceptual and data-based resources, published between 1968 and 1995, were used in the manuscript. It is interesting to note that Hawks' (1991) concept analysis of power, published in the *Journal of Advanced Nursing,* was not included in Rafael's literature review. Another example of a conceptual article is Tiesinga, Dassen, and Halfens' (1996) *Fatigue: A Summary of the Definitions, Dimensions, and Indicators.* These authors reviewed 98 conceptual and data-based articles and books on the concept of fatigue;

however, they did not use concept analysis methodology and their research is therefore not considered a data-based article.

Data-Based Material

Nursing does have an ever-growing body of this type of scholarly literature that focuses on the use of specific nursing theories or models, as well as a variety of variables related to the nature and practice of nursing. For example, there are studies that tested various propositions of Rogers' model of Unitary Human Being (1970, 1980, 1990), such as the work of Barrett (1984, 1986) and Malinski (1981).

There are studies that examine multiple variables in relation to a cadre of patient-focused clinical problems, such as Wikblad and Anderson's 1995 study that compared three types of wound dressing that would be more effective with heart surgery patients (see Appendix A). Other studies examine a particular type of nursing care delivery system in relation to patient outcomes such as Rudy et al's (1995) study that compared the effects of a special care unit versus intensive care unit with chronically critically ill patients (see Appendix C). There are qualitative studies that generate a framework for practice such as Draucker and Petrovic's (1996) healing framework for survivors of sexual abuse (see Appendix B).

As discussed with conceptual-based or theoretical articles, most data-based articles indicate in their title that a study was conducted. For example, the title of Wikblad and Anderson's (1995) quantitative study is *A Comparison of Three Wound Dressings in Patients Undergoing Heart Surgery* (see Appendix A). Data-based articles that are published in a scholarly professional journal usually include an abstract following the title of the article. Wikblad and Anderson's abstract starts with the following: "Two hundred fifty patients undergoing heart surgery were randomized in a prospective comparative study. . . ." Reading the abstract helps the reader determine whether it is a data-based or theoretical article, and if it is data-based what type of design was used by the researcher. The complete abstract includes comments on the method, findings, conclusions, and clinical implications. This type of abstract is very helpful to the beginner consumer of research and the experienced researcher. (Specific examples of data-based and conceptual literature will be provided in the Critiquing Criteria box on p. 125.)

Refereed Journals

A major portion of most literature reviews consists of journal articles. Journals are a ready source of the latest information on almost any conceivable subject. A number of journals can be accessed through various subscription services of the Internet. Currently time and cost remain a disadvantage. Unfortunately books and texts, despite the inclusion of multiple data-based sources, take much longer to publish than journals. Therefore, journals are the preferred mode for communicating the latest theory or results of a research study. As a beginning consumer of research you should use **refereed or peer-reviewed journals** as your first source of primary scholarly literature. A refereed journal uses a panel of external and internal reviewers (peer-reviewed) or editors who review submitted manuscripts for possible publication. The external reviewers are drawn from a pool of nurse scholars who are experts in various fields. In most cases these reviews are "blind;" that is, the manuscript to be reviewed does not include the name of the author(s). The review panels use the same set of scholarly criteria to judge whether a manuscript is worthy of publication. The credibility of the reported research is enhanced through this peer review process.

PRIMARY AND SECONDARY SOURCES

A credible literature review reflects the use of mainly primary sources. Table 4-6 gives the general definition and examples of these sources. As defined earlier in the chapter, a *primary source* is written by a person(s) who developed the theory or conducted the research. Most primary sources are found in published literature. A **secondary source** is written by a person(s) other than the individual who developed the theory or conducted the research. Often a secondary source represents a response to or a summary and critique of a theorist's or researcher's work or an in-depth analysis on a topic/issue/problem/concept.

Box 4-3 illustrates journals that contain both primary and secondary data-based and conceptual articles. Table 4-6 highlights the differences between primary and secondary sources. Table 4-7 offers examples of primary and secondary print sources. For example, the first column of Table 4-7 indicates that Benner's (1984) book, *From Novice to Expert,* is a primary source of her theory for practices; it is a primary source because Benner is the originator of this theory and also the author of this publication (i.e., you would be reading first-hand information). The second column of Table 4-7 represents secondary sources. For instance, *Theoretical Perspectives in Nursing* (Nicoll, 1996) has many chapters that are conceptual secondary sources that represent critiques on nursing theory, nursing research, and their application to education and practice. In most cases the original paper usually discusses the work of another nurse author. These authors write about another nurse's theory or research by summarizing, responding to, or critiquing it in relation to implications for theory verification, practice, education, and/or development of nursing science. This is considered "second-hand" information—hence the term *secondary source.* However, it should be noted that it also includes a number of primary source conceptual articles.

There are two general reasons for using secondary sources. One reason is that a primary source is literally unavailable. This is rarely the case in this age of computer searches and interlibrary loan of books and the ability of libraries to copy an article and send or fax it to the person requesting the information. Of course there is usually a charge for this service. Another reason, which is more common, is that a secondary source can provide different ways of looking at an issue or problem. Secondary sources can help students develop the ability to see things from another person's point of view, which is an essential aspect of critical reading (Paul, 1995). However, secondary sources should not be overused, especially for literature reviews, although they can have tremendous value for the beginning consumer of research.

Table 4-6

Primary and Secondary Sources

PRIMARY: ESSENTIAL	SECONDARY: USEFUL
The person who conducted the study, developed the theory (model), or prepared the scholarly discussion on a concept, topic, or issue of interest (i.e., the original author).	Someone other than the original author (i.e., the person who conducted the original work—whether data-based or conceptual) writes or presents the author's original work. These are usually in the form of a summary and critiques (analysis and synthesis) of someone else's scholarly work.
Primary sources can be published or unpublished.	Secondary sources can be published or unpublished.
Data-based examples: An investigator's report of his or her research study (question/hypothesis[es], design/method, sample/setting, findings, results; e.g., articles in Appendixes A, B, C, and D) is a primary source of data-based reports; McCloskey and Bulechek's (1996) book on NIC is also a primary source for this data-based nursing intervention classification system.	Response/commentary/critique articles of a research study, a theory/model, or a professional view of an issue; review of literature article published in a refereed scholarly journal; abstracts of a published work written by someone other than the original author; a doctoral dissertation's review of the literature.
Conceptual or theoretical example: A theorist's work reported in the literature by the author in an article, chapter of a book, or a book (Rogers, 1990).	Bowles and Naylor's (1996) review of the three ANA approved taxonomies—NIC, OCS, HHC—is a secondary source of these taxonomies.
HINT: Critical evaluation of mainly primary sources is essential to a thorough and relevant review of the literature.	HINT: Use secondary sources sparingly; however, secondary sources, especially of studies that include a critique by a seasoned researcher, are a valuable learning tool for a beginning consumer of research.

Secondary sources that are published in referred journals are generally written by experienced nursing scholars. Such articles usually provide a critical evaluation of or a response to a theory or research study. They usually include implications for practice and/or contributions of the work to the development of the science of nursing. Occasionally the *Western Journal of Nursing Research* includes a critique entitled "Commentary." Mosby published a variety of research critiques from 1992 to 1996 under the journal title *Capsules and Comments*. However, as stressed earlier, to develop the competency of critiquing research, the consumer of research must read primary sources and use standardized critiquing criteria. Consulting faculty, advisors, or librarians about secondary sources is an effective way to secure an appropriate resource.

Box 4-3   Examples of Nursing Journals for Literature Reviews*

Advances in Nursing Science
American Journal of Critical Care
AORN
Applied Nursing Research
Archives of Psychiatric Nursing
Clinical Nursing Research
Computers in Nursing
Dimensions of Critical Nursing
Heart & Lung
Holistic Nursing Practice
Image: Journal of Nursing Scholarship
International Journal of Nursing Studies
Issues in Mental Health Nursing
Journal of the American Psychiatric Nurses Association
Journal of Advanced Nursing
Journal of Clinical Nursing
Journal of Neonatal Nursing
Journal of Nursing Administration
Journal of Nursing Education
Journal of Nursing Management
Journal of Nursing Scholarship
Journal of Obstetric, Gynecologic and Neonatal Nursing
Journal of Professional Nursing
Journal of Qualitative Research
Journal of Nursing Scholarship
Journal of Professional Nursing
Journal of Qualitative Research
NACOG
Nursing Clinics of North America
Nurse Educator
Nursing Diagnosis
Nursing & Health Care
Nursing Management
Nursing Outlook
Nursing Research
Nursing Science Quarterly
Research in Nursing & Health
Scholarly Inquiry for Nursing Practice
Western Journal of Nursing Research

*Main focus: Primary sources of research studies and conceptual articles; sources of some secondary sources, such as extensive reviews of literature on a particular concept, issues, and responses or critiques of data-based and conceptual articles; most are refereed journals; all can be searched through CINAHL print and computer CD-ROM and on-line.
NB: Dissertation Abstracts International is not a journal but a source of data-based studies.

Table 4-7

Conceptual and Data-Based Examples of Primary and Secondary Journal Articles, Books, Chapters in Books, or Documents

PRIMARY	SECONDARY
Journal article Wikblad K, Anderson B: A comparison of three wound dressings in patients undergoing heart surgery, *Nurs Res* 44(5):312-316, 1995.	**Journal commentary** Koop PM: Commentary: a family's coming to terms with Alzheimer's disease, *West J Nurs Res* 18(1):22-23, 1996.
Book Benner P: *From novice to expert: excellence and power in clinical nursing practice,* Menlo Park, Calif, 1984, Addison-Wesley.	**Book** Nicoll LH: *Perspectives on nursing theory,* ed 3, Philadelphia, 1996, Lippincott.
Chapter in a book McEvoy MD: The relationships among the experience of dying, the experience of paranormal events, and creativity in adults. In Barrett EAM, ed: *Visions of Rogers' science-based nursing,* New York, 1990, NLN.	**Chapter in a book** Belcher JR, Fish LJB: Hildegard E Peplau. In George JB, ed: *Nursing theories: the base for profession nursing practice,* ed 4, Norwalk, Conn, 1995, Appleton & Lange.
Doctoral dissertation Campagna A: The lived experience of step-families, doctoral dissertation, Dissertation Abstracts International, 8824404, New York, 1995, Columbia University Teachers College.	**Documents** Rantz MF: *Nursing quality measurement: a review of nursing studies,* Washington, DC, 1995, ANA.
Document American Nurses Association: *Nursing's social policy statement,* Washington, DC, 1995, ANA.	Early HIV Infection Guideline Panel: *Evaluation and management of early HIV infection,* AHCPR Pub No 94-0572, Rockville, Md, 1994, Agency for Health Care Policy and Research, Public Health Service, US Department of Health and Human Services.

HELPFUL HINT

- Remember that a secondary source of a theory or data-based study usually does not include all of the theory's concepts or aspects of a study, and/or definitions may not be fully presented.
- If concepts or variables are included, the definitions may be collapsed or paraphrased to such a degree that it no longer represents the theorist's actual work.
- Perhaps the critique (whether positive or negative) is based on the condensed summary or abstract; as such it would be less useful to the consumer.
- Read a primary data-based study, as well as a secondary source critique on the same study; compare your critique with the critique of the secondary source.

CONDUCTING A SEARCH AS A CONSUMER OF RESEARCH

Most students who are preparing an academic paper read the required course materials, as well as additional library materials. Students often state that they are researching a topic or writing a research paper. However, in this situation it would be more accurate to state that the student is "searching" the literature to uncover knowledge to prepare an academic term paper on a certain topic rather than to uncover knowledge on a specific topic to carry out a research project. Reviewing the literature for research and consumer of research activities requires the same critical thinking and reading skills. This point is discussed at the beginning of the chapter. From an academic standpoint, the level, type of course, and objective of the assignment determines whether a student's literature search needs to be minor, selected, cursory, major, in-depth, extensive, or exhaustive. Regardless, discovering knowledge is the goal of any "search;" therefore a consumer of research needs to know how to search the literature. Box 4-2 summarizes the important characteristics of a relevant review of the literature.

Becoming a competent consumer of research requires knowing the way to search the literature *quickly* and *efficiently*. Reference librarians are excellent people to ask about various sources of scholarly literature. If you are unfamiliar with the process of conducting a scholarly computer search, your reference librarian can certainly help.

TYPES OF RESOURCES

Print Databases

Before the 1980s, usually a search was done by hand using print index databases. This was a tedious and time-consuming process. **Print databases** consist mainly of indexes, card catalogues, and abstract reviews; they are useful for finding sources that have not been entered into electronic databases. Print indexes are used to find journal sources (periodicals) of data-based and conceptual articles on a variety of topics, as well as publications of professional organizations and various governmental agencies. Card catalogues are used to secure books, monographs, conference proceedings, master's theses, and doctoral dissertations. Abstract reviews contain summaries of data-based articles and prepared bibliographies. Box 4-4 lists examples of the more commonly used print indexes that are still published. Most CD-ROM and on-line databases include sources from their particular form's publication date or a few years before that date; for example, CINAHL's **computer database** sources are from 1982 to the present, whereas the print index covers 1956 to the present. The most *relevant* and frequently used print source for nursing literature remains the CINAHL, also known as the "Red Books." CINAHL covers all nursing and related literature from 1956 to the present. Print resources are still relied on if a search requires materials not entered into an electronic database before a certain year (e.g., CINAHL on CD-ROM or on-line database cover literature from 1982 to the present) or if a library is not equipped for electronic computer CD-ROM and on-line databases.

Almost all print databases are now available through some type of computer/electronic means. The nineteenth edition of the *Interagency Council on Information Resources for Nursing* published its biennial list of essential references (ICIRN et al, 1996); 26 computerized databases were listed.

During the 1980s almost all libraries of larger universities and health care agencies and those near metropolitan areas provided students and health care workers with direct access to computer searches. Currently, in most areas of the country, students are able to access a com-

---

Box 4-4   Common Print Databases

Indexes

Cumulative Index to Nursing and Allied Health Literature (CINAHL)—initially called Cumulative Index to Nursing Literature, published in 1956; print version known as the "Red Books"

Index Medicus (IM)—oldest health-related index, first published in 1879; medicine, allied health, biophysical sciences, humanities, veterinary medicine, and nursing

International Nursing Index (INI)—quarterly publication by American Journal of Nursing Company in cooperation with National Library of Medicine, started in 1966; over 200 journals, all languages; includes nursing publications in nonnursing journals

Nursing Studies Index—developed by Virginia Henderson; publishes nursing literature 1900 to 1959, as well as from other disciplines (see INI above)

Hospital and Health Administration Index (HHAI), formerly known as Hospital Literature Index (HLI)—published in 1945 by American Hospital Association in cooperation with National Library of Medicine (NLM); included over 700 journals and related ones from IM; main focus: hospital administration and delivery of care

Current Index to Journals in Education (CIJE)—first published in 1969 in cooperation with Educational Resources Information Center (ERIC)

Card Catalogues

Lists books, monographs, theses, dissertations, audiovisuals, and conference proceedings

Abstract Reviews

Dissertation Abstracts International, Master's Abstracts Nursing Abstracts, Psychological Abstracts, Sociological Abstracts

---

puter search from their computer center, library, classrooms, or even from on-campus dorms; faculty have access from their office or even from home; some health care workers have access from their work stations.

 ## Internet: On-Line Databases

The Internet is a global resource, a rather broad term that describes an international network that links a cadre of participating networks (e.g., commercial, educational, and governmental agencies). These resources share computer power, software, and information. There are multiple uses for the Internet that are beyond the objectives of this chapter. However, the Internet's main objective of communication is in concert with the objectives of this chapter. Other Internet objectives are to share ideas, provide selected information, and to provide entertainment (Hutchinson, 1997; Kaufeld and Kaufeld, 1996; Nicoll and Ouellette, 1997). Tables 4-8 and 4-9 present various capabilities of the Internet and their usefulness for conducting a literature review.

Internet services, such as e-mail and the WWW, are part of the Internet (Hutchinson, 1997; Kaufeld and Kaufeld, 1996; Nicoll and Ouellette, 1997). E-mail and the WWW are important to learn but have varying levels of usefulness for the consumer of research. Although

Table 4-8

Examples of Internet Services

INTERNET CAPABILITIES	EXAMPLES OF SERVICES	COST	OUTCOMES FOR LITERATURE REVIEW BY UNDERGRADUATE STUDENT (ESSENTIAL POSSIBILITIES, NOT RECOMMENDED AT THIS TIME)
Gopher (protocol and software)—a menu-driven browser; text-based; supports FTP for downloading; user friendly; WWW page sites have replaced its use for many, especially nursing home page sites and chat rooms	Access Gopherspace: search, display, and retrieve documents (e.g., reports, books out of print) from remote sites on Internet; can do broad Gopherspace search using *Veronica*, or confined search using *Jughead*	?	Not recommended as first-line scholarly search: some possibilities for doctoral students; can access Library and Information Science Internet Resources, Library of Congress, Reference Desk, and U.S. National Library of Medicine
ListServ (list server) lists—software program that supports e-mail lists or electronic discussion; lists are special interest groups; over 300 health-related lists software application; if you have e-mail capabilities you can subscribe	Helpful but very time consuming without a very fast computer; one can keep abreast of various topics; NURSERES—nursing research—to join e-mail: listserv@kentvm.kent.edu	Costly on own unless using the services at an academic or health care agency; if join service you pay for connection charges; may be costly because you can receive multiple messages/day	Not recommended at this time: possibilities for doctoral students; can discover latest on a particular topic; theoretically can ask a particular research-related question (e.g., to NURSERES) and receive 50 replies from various colleagues who subscribe
Remote login 1. Telenet—various interactive login to remote host (protocol and program); check at your institution,	No library card: browse the library but usually no file transfer; protocols for login are site specific; check library's catalog for holdings;	Need an account for just Telenet?	Not recommended as a first-line search

or follow directions if you download this program via your AOL or NET-SERV communication service	may be possible to download search results and send yourself search via e-mail For journals would need to log on to following:	
	MEDLINE or CINAHL Direct (see text discussion under CINAHL)	Need an account for CINAHL Direct, etc.	CINAHL and MEDLINE are recommended as first-line search: usually both are available at library via CD-ROM; if you have Telenet you may not be able to log on unless you set up an account directly or via library, because of license agreements
	CARL (Colorado Alliance of Research Libraries)	CARL: no charge	Possibilities: can access book reviews and reference sources; CINAHL still first choice
2. FTP (file transfer protocol)—transfer text and nontext (binary) files; two types: personal and anonymous (public); check with librarian for FTP to protocol; need FTP to download a file you find on the Internet	Library card: browse via computer and access public files; personal (must be able to log on to another's account—need password) and over 700 anonymous open sites	Anonymous FTP-free open sites only need Internet access; personal—requires some cost	Not recommended as first-line search, but capabilities in the future

Data from Corel, 1996; CINAHL, 1996; Kaufeld and Kaufeld, 1996; Kay, 1995; Nicoll and Ouellette, 1997; Prohaska and Chang, 1996; Weinberg, 1996.

Table 4-9

Selected Examples of WWW/Chat Sites

NURSING WEB SITES/CHAT ROOMS AND ADDRESSES	SOURCES	OUTCOME FOR LITERATURE REVIEW
AJN Company Online Services http://www.ajn.org:80/	Subscription required, journals: AJN, Nursing Research, MCN; books, videos, and so on	Interesting way of keeping up with latest issues; same sources can be accessed via CINAHL CD-ROM or on-line at academic or health care agency library without a fee
AORN (Association of Operating Room Nurses, Inc.) Online Service http://www.aorn.org/	General information about AORN activities, membership, research projects	Interesting way to keep up with a speciality; able to discuss research projects AORN is currently involved in; if published, this research would be in CINAHL database
CINAHL Information Systems http://cinahl.com/	Offers general information regarding search capabilities in various print, CD-ROM, and on-line services; CINAHLdirect on-line requires a membership fee	If you can afford this go for it; otherwise use CINAHL CD-ROM at your academic or health care agency library
Journal of Nursing Jocularity http://www.jocularity.com/toc.html Contact: Laffin RN@neta.com	On-line journal: articles and cartoons on the humor in the nursing profession	Sometimes you need a break—just seeing if you were awake!
Judy Norris' Home Page http://www.oise.on.ca/~jnorris/welcom.html Contact: Judy Norris: jnorris@oise.utoronto.ca	Website of J. Norris; QualPage—resource of qualitative research; Parse Page—Parse's theory; NURSENET Page—resources for NURSENET listserv subscribers	More helpful for doctoral students conducting qualitative studies
Midwest Nursing Research Society (MNRS) http://www.umich.edu/~nursing/mnrs/	MNRS goals are developing and using nursing research; website provides information on nursing research, funding,	Depending on where you live, this might be an interesting organization to learn about; not specific to literature search

	publication, and membership	
Contact: mnrs@amctec.com National Institute of Nursing Research (NINR) http://www.nih.gov/ninr/	NINR: promote science for nursing practice; supports interdisciplinary research; linked to nurse scientist training program	Not particularly useful for your level literature search; doctoral and postdoctoral students may find this an interesting resource
NURSERES: listserv@kentvm.kent.edu Subscribe NURSERES Firstname Lastname	Provides a discussion list on nursing research and related health and professional issues	May lead to some new sources; not an expectation for the beginning consumer of research for a literature search
Sigma Theta Tau International Nursing Honor Society http://stti-web.iupui.edu/	Can visit and be updated on the news and activities of the society; subscription fee required to access the *Online Journal of Knowledge Synthesis for Nursing* and the *Virginia Henderson International Nursing Library*; link to chapter websites	Great possibilities; may have some unpublished research in abstract form not found on CINAHL; check if your library subscribes—try it out; also don't miss the opportunity to see if you are eligible for STTI at your school of nursing or join as a community member

Data from Corel, 1996; CINAHL, 1996; Nicoll and Ouellette, 1997; Prohaska and Chang, 1996; STTI, 1996; Weinberg, 1996.

only a modem and a basic communication software package are needed for e-mail, accessing the WWW requires an additional commercial communication on-line service. Basically this communication service allows computers to talk to each other. In the case of the WWW, because it is a hypertext interface, in addition to text capabilities it also has video, audio, and nontext capabilities.

Table 4-8 presents examples of the other sophisticated services of the Internet; a number require the downloading of additional software to use a particular service, such as Telenet and file transfer protocol (FTP) (see "Remote Login" in Table 4-9). As noted in Table 4-9, Sigma Theta Tau International's (STTI) *Registry of Nursing Research* and the *Online Journal of Knowledge Synthesis for Nursing* are available on-line; however, in addition to the cost of subscribing, it will require that your computer has the software program called Adobe or that it be downloaded to use it.

Most Internet communication providers include a **Web browser,** such as America On-Line (AOL), or another popular browser called *Netscape Navigator.* Internet providers are developing new versions every month. It is suggested that you check with your local academic computer center for individual or group classes and/or visit your local computer store regarding accessing such services from your home and the availability of classes and up-to-date handbook guides on the subject. The suggested reading list at the end of the chapter indicates a few help guides for surfing or browsing the Net (Internet).

HELPFUL HINT
- Find someone who is experienced with using the Internet (e.g., e-mail, AOL, or WWW browser). Watch what they do. Make sure you find time to learn it and do it.
- Make sure you have enough hard drive space to accommodate new software browser programs (e.g., Netscape Navigator, Telenet, or Adobe) and that your CD-ROM has at least 32-bit drivers.

Table 4-9 lists selected examples of the hundreds of nursing sites, Web home pages, and chat rooms of mainly the WWW. It includes their Internet addresses, main services, and if they are presently considered a primary source of information for a literature review by a beginning consumer of research. Many college and university schools of nursing and individual nurses and nursing organizations have Web sites; they are too numerous to list in this chapter. See Nicoll and Ouellette's (1997) book on the Internet for a complete list (see reference list at the end of the chapter). More and more nursing site chat rooms are available every day. However, in general these chat rooms do not provide literature search and retrieval capabilities anywhere similar to that of CINAHL; a number require a subscription fee for access, as well as the need for additional software programs. Although you may find that some of these sites provide interesting information, it can be a very time-consuming process. In managing your time for doing a literature search, you must consider whether you can afford to spend the time getting on-line, as well as browsing the various chat rooms. Unless Internet services can be accessed through your academic setting, this can also be very costly to access through your personal computer (PC). You need to ask yourself if your outcome from searching the Internet provided essential primary data needed for meeting the objectives of a literature review. If not, continue reading the remainder of the chapter on searching databases on-line or on CD-ROM for scholarly material.

On-Line Database: CINAHLdirect

CINAHL Information Systems introduced their new on-line service (via Internet and WWW) at the end of 1995, called *CINAHLdirect*. This new service is aimed at professionals and students and has a number of services in addition to its journal database; for information call toll-free 1-800-959-7167. If you wish to secure their services, fees are based on the number of hours purchased in a block; there is a discount for students with identification. If you do not have access to CINAHL CD-ROM (see discussion below) and you can afford the subscription and have access to a PC with the following capabilities: a high-speed modem to connect to the Internet directly or via an on-line service through WWW, with Internet software with Telenet capability, you are set to access your scholarly searches on-line from your home or worksite. You can then think of yourself as riding or surfing the wave of the future. While you are on the Web, browse CINAHL's Information Systems Website; it is a key access point to multidisciplinary professional literature (Nicoll and Ouellette, 1997).

Box 4-5 lists a number of databases available on-line or on CD-ROM. Box 4-6 lists the advantages of using CINAHL's database. As indicated, CINAHLdirect offers the user the capability of acquiring an article. There is a charge for this service that compensates the server and the publisher in keeping with copyright laws.

CD-ROM Databases

CD-ROM refers to the capability of the computer to use compact disk (CD) information in a read only memory (ROM) format. Currently this remains the most useful database to use, especially in your consumer of research role as a student or practicing nurse. Typically, CINAHL CD-ROM is available via software programs, such as Silver Platter (1996), Ovid, or PaperChase. These software programs are referred to as major vendors of CD-ROM and on-line databases. This program enables CINAHL to be accessed in a quick and efficient manner. Box 4-5 indicates a few of the print databases that are available on CD-ROM or on-line; they are numbered in order of importance and usefulness to nursing. In addition to those listed in Box 4-5, there are approximately 20 other discipline-specific CD-ROM or on-line databases (ICIRN, 1996). MEDLINE uses medical model terminology rather than nursing

---

Box 4-5 CD-ROM and On-Line Databases*

1. CINAHL (Cumulative Index to Nursing and Allied Health Literature)†
2. MEDLINE (Medical Literature analysis and retrieval system on-line)
3. AIDSLINE (AIDS literature on-line)
4. CancerLit (Cancer literature)
5. HealthSTAR (Merged: AHA, Health Planning and Administration [HEALTH], and Health Services/Technology Assessment Research [HSTAR])
6. PsycLIT (Psychology Literature; on-line PsycINFO—APA)
7. ERIC (Educational Resources Information Center)

*Listed in order of importance and usefulness to nursing.
†Most important database for the nurse consumer of research.

Box 4-6   Advantages of CINAHL CD-ROM and On-Line for Nurse Consumer of Research*

1. Quick (CD-ROM) or instant (on-line) access to more than 240,000 records from 1982 to present (e.g., journals, books, chapters in books, abstracts, software, audiovisual)
2. Contains author abstracts for more than 922 journal titles, dissertations, educational software, and audiovisuals including nursing and 17 allied health disciplines, biomedicine, consumer health, and health sciences librarianship
3. Includes thousands of abstracts for more than 275 journal titles, dissertations, educational software, and audiovisuals; book and audiovisual reviews; reading level for patient education teaching materials; cited references for the articles indexed in health sciences librarianship journals
4. Provides access to the full text from selected nursing standards of practice, nurse practice acts, STTI nursing journals, and even critical paths
5. Uses major nursing and allied health fields: 8100 plus subject headings (over 2500 unique to CINAHL over MEDLINE)
6. Uses ANA's (McCormick et al, 1994) four approved taxonomies terms (NANDA, NIC, OMAHA, and HHC)
7. Access to methodologies, conceptual frameworks, variables, and identifies all research instruments
8. Monthly updates
9. Provides author's professional affiliations for increased networking
10. Document retrieval and delivery via fax or mail for CINAHLdirect

Modified from CINAHL: *CINAHLnews,* Glendale, Calif, 1997, CINAHL Information Systems.
*Access time and all features not available with PRINT Index

---

terminology. MEDLINE does not cover all the nursing literature. In fact, CINAHL reported that there are many nursing citations not reported in MEDLINE. Examples are *AORN Journal, AIDS Patient Care, American Journal of Health Promotion,* and *Harvard Health Letter.* SilverPlatter introduced a product in 1995, called RNDEX, which is comprised of 100 nursing journals. Box 4-6 lists a number of the advantages of using CINALH's database.

CINAHL CD-ROM

As indicated, for more than 40 years CINAHL has been the best choice for most searches in nursing—at first by using the red print books and now by accessing it through a computer via CD-ROM or on-line. According to librarians familiar with nursing literature searches, CINAHL's database is excellent for searches by nursing students from associate degree, baccalaureate, master's, and doctoral programs, as well as practicing nurses and faculty members. It contains the most comprehensive nursing information as compared to any other databases via CD-ROM or on-line for the purposes of a review of the literature for research and consumer of research purposes. Box 4-6 lists many of the advantages of CINAHL over the other databases.

CINAHL CD-ROM is the most frequently used program for searches by nursing students and nurses. In most institutions both students and faculty are able to conduct their own searches, print the results on site, and/or download the results on their own 3.5" microdisk, without any additional charge. CINAHL CD-ROM is a very cost-effective and fast data-based program to use for your searches. As indicated in Box 4-6 CINAHL uses major subject headings specific to nursing (e.g., nursing process terms, nursing taxonomies such as NANDA diagnoses, major nursing models and theories), which is crucial for your search. CINAHL provides easy access to research literature. Subject headings are established for many specific types of research variables (e.g., designs, conceptual frameworks, data collection methods, and statistical methods of data analysis). In addition, CINAHL provides an instrumentation field that lists all the instruments used in a study (CINAHL, 1996).

Most college, university, and health care agency libraries are set up for staff and students to conduct their own computer searches; most subscribe to CINAHL and other databases. Designated computers are CD-ROM–ready and have menu driven "user-friendly" databases. For instance, the computer's menu usually lists the various databases available (e.g., CINAHL, MEDLINE); in your case your first choice should be CINAHL—select it and follow the prompts on the screen. Step-by-step printed guides for the search, as well as search guides for each database, are usually available. These guides provide information about variables/terms, broadening or narrowing a search, marking or eliminating unwanted records, and printing the citations (i.e., references found at the end of an article).

PERFORMING A COMPUTER SEARCH

Why a Computer Search?

Perhaps you are still not convinced that computer searches are the best way to acquire information for a review of the literature. Then think about it once again from another perspective. If you use CINAHL's print indexes (the red book), you will have to write out each relevant reference you find, unless of course you have access to a copier, in which case you could copy each page an entry is on. However, this can be a very time-consuming and costly proposition—but at least you would have all the necessary information for retrieving the articles. Then again, as you demonstrated your critical thinking abilities in your previous analysis of why Rafael did not include Hawks' article as a reference, it is conceivable that you could miss an important entry because you must read through all possible entries of the subject heading you are reviewing. Furthermore, if you cannot photocopy each page you need from the CINAHL print index, then you will need to transcribe each entry by hand. Find out the protocol your library uses (i.e., what type of call slip used) and write your information from the print index directly on the call slip. If you at least try to do a CINAHL computer search even once, you will see how easy it is to do, and you will feel confident that you did a thorough search; in addition, you will have avoided the pitfalls previously discussed (Holmes, 1996). The critical thinking decision path illustrates the way to conduct a research consumer focused computer literature search.

HELPFUL HINT
Think of a CINAHL computer search first. It can facilitate all steps of critically reviewing the literature, especially Steps III, IV, and V.

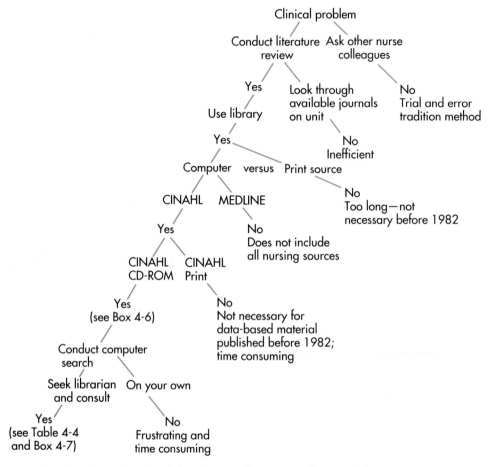

Critical Thinking Decision Path   Consumer of research literature review.

How Far Back Must the Search Go?

Questions frequently asked by students are "How many articles do I need?" "How much is enough?" "How far back in the literature do I need to go?" Often a computer search done on CINAHL will recover information from 1982 until the time of your search; it will yield more than enough materials to complete the purpose of your search.

A general time line for conceptual academic or clinical practice papers/projects is to go back in the literature at least 3 but preferably 5 years; a research project may warrant 10 years or more. Another cue is if you come across an extensive literature review on a particular topic or a concept clarification methodology study. This usually means you can begin your search at the date of their last reviewed citation or at least a year or two before that time. An example is the AHCPR *Guideline on Evaluation and Management of Early HIV Infection.* It was published in 1994. In their literature review it indicated that a search between 1981 and 1992 revealed 36,000 abstracts; a first review reduced references to 2831, which were put through a rigorous review process, during which time additional citations were added through August of 1993. Therefore, if you were searching this topic you could use their review and conduct your search from January 1993 to the present.

The pitfalls to avoid with print indexes were discussed earlier in this chapter. With experience you will know when enough is enough. As noted, each computer database has its own time limitations. Another consideration is the cost of your search. Many academic institutions include the use of the computer for searches and word processing in students' tuition fees. Sometimes an academic institution limits the number of citations that can be printed at any one time. Check with your reference librarian regarding this issue and whether you can instead download your search to a 3.5" microdisk and print it off on your own PC. Make sure you find out this information before printing your search.

What Do I Need to Know?

Each database usually has a specific search guide that provides information on the organization of the entries and the terminology used. For instance, CINAHL uses nursing-specific terms. Finding the right variables/concepts/terms to "plug in" for a computer search is an important aspect of conducting a search. CINAHL is very user friendly in regard to this aspect of your search; it has an explode feature, which means you can search multiple headings with a single command. Another feature is the mapping capability of this program. If the term you use is not exactly the same as is in the database, the program maps or connects you to a term nearest to what you typed in (CINAHL, 1996). If you are still having difficulty, of course do not hesitate to ask your reference librarian.

Box 4-7 offers a quick overview of how user friendly the CINAHL database is; it provides a number of helpful hints that literally walk you through the steps of a search. This particular protocol is based on CINAHL through SilverPlatter. SilverPlatter (1996) is a vendor, or company, that develops a program so that multiple CD-ROM databases can be accessed in a similar manner. As indicated in Box 4-8, an entry usually consists of the author, title, source (e.g., book or journal), and type (e.g., data-based or conceptual) and may include an abstract. CINAHL uses the following abbreviations for the terms: title (TI), author (AU), source (SO), abstract (AB) if available, document type (DT), and references (RF). This is a typical CINAHL computer search entry through SilverPlatter. The main focus of this search was on retrieving nursing research related to the treatment of adults with depression. This entry's TI, SO, AB, DE, and RF indicate its usefulness for this purpose. As indicated, the first set was too broad—3365 articles. Using the Boolean connector "and" with nursing interventions resulted in 133 entries (see explanation of *Boolean* and connector "*and*" in Box 4-7). This was a manageable number to review on screen by quickly reading over the abstracts and marking those for print retrieval. Before printing your search, remember to check and see if your fields indicate that references (RF) for each entry will be printed; this was a new feature added in 1996. If not, follow the directions provided in Box 4-7, or ask the reference librarian for assistance. Because it makes the printout considerably longer, many libraries make it an optional field for printing. One advantage of using this option is that you will frequently come across some classic document or one that was not entered in the computer database because it was published before 1982. If you intend to download your search to a 3.5" microdisk, make sure you include this option. When you

Box 4-7   Helpful Hints: Using CINAHL CD-ROM

- Choose (i.e., highlight) "CINAHL" on the computer search menu; hit [Enter].
- Once CINAHL is loaded look for the Find prompt at the bottom of the screen.
- Type in your search words (e.g., nursing intervention); do not use complete sentences (if a manual is not handy press [F9] for Thesaurus); reenter search words if necessary.
- Press [Enter].
- Each word is searched separately and "hits" or a set of items is created for each word.
- Final set combines your search words:
    1. 68978 nursing
    2. 45892 intervention
    3. 2986 nursing intervention
- 2986 is too many "hits" to scroll or browse through.
- Add additional variables to narrow search (e.g., if interested in); but first type in at the Find prompt: nursing in SB [Enter].
    4. SB = Nursing
  Then type in at the Find prompt: research in DT
    5. DT = Research
- When you do your next Find type in the Boolean connector "and" between each of the above numbers you wish to use plus additional variables; if you wanted nursing intervention and nursing research you would at the Find prompt type in: 3 and 4 and 5 and psychiatric [Enter].
    6. 102 (= psychiatric nursing intervention nursing research)
- The Boolean "or" broadens your search.
- Booleans save time because you don't have to retype each search word.
- Press [F4] to view your search; the first entry will be marked 1 of 102.
- To browse through, use down arrow key or [Ctrl] and [Page Down]; do the reverse for paging up.
- To mark the entry or record you want to print at the end press [M] or [Enter]; the [Enter] key will also unmark, as will the [U] key.
- Print by pressing [P] and [Enter]; start print will be highlighted; a menu will be shown that indicates the various fields for printing; if the first field does not end with RF, look at the bottom of your screen and you can change options by using the [Tab] key to highlight "Change." Highlight "Change" and press [Enter]. This will bring you to the first field, which will indicate that it will print TI, AU, etc. Press the [End] key, which will bring you to the end of this first field; type in RF and Press [P] or [Enter] key. Your search will print all the references used in the preparation of each of the articles/documents you marked.
- If you wish to download to a disk and print your search at home, then insert a 3.5" diskette in drive available (usually A or B); press [D] for download.
- Advantage of downloading: can print as many citations as you wish and when you load the search into your computer you can edit the search document by cutting and pasting each entry and create an instant reference list for your paper.

Modified from Rosedale, 1997; Weinberg, 1996.

Box 4-8   Example of CINAHL on SilverPlatter Retrieved Entry

SilverPlatter 3.11: CINAHL ® 1982-8/96

No.	Records	Request
1.	3275	depression
2.	38462	research
3.	3365	depression research
4.	133	3 and nursing intervention and adult

1 of 133

TI	TITLE:
AU	AUTHOR(S):
SO	SOURCE (BIBLIOGRAPHIC CITATION):
SI	
AB	ABSTRACT:

upload it on your PC you will be able to retrieve all your references, as well as the references of each entry, into your word processing program. Think how much time you will save! Your reference list will be typed and you will only have to do some editing to put it into the style required by your instructor.

If, as suggested, you did your preliminary reading of available abstracts as you marked an entry before printing your search you should be ready to photocopy each article. Having a copy of each article will allow you to organize them for priority critical reading.

How Do I Complete the Search?

Now the truly important aspect of the search begins, your critical reading of the retrieved materials. Critically reading scholarly material, especially data-based articles, requires several readings and the use of critiquing criteria. Do not be discouraged if all the retrieved articles are not as useful as you first thought; this happens to the most experienced researcher. If most of the articles are not useful, be prepared to do another search, but discuss the variables you will use next time with your instructor and/or the reference librarian. Remind yourself how quickly you will be able to do it, now that you are experienced. It is also a good idea to review the references of your articles; if any seem relevant, you can retrieve them.

LITERATURE REVIEW FORMAT: WHAT TO EXPECT

Becoming familiar with the format of the literature review assists the research consumer in the task of using critiquing criteria to evaluate the review. To decide which style you will use so that your review is presented in a logical and organized manner, you need to consider the following:

- The research question/topic
- The number of retrieved sources reviewed
- The number and type of data-based versus conceptual materials

Some reviews are written according to the variables being studied and presented chronologically under each variable. Others present the material chronologically with subcategories or variables discussed within each period; still others present the variables and include subcategories related to the study's types or designs or related subvariables.

An example of a literature review that is logically presented according to the variables under study is Appendix C (Rudy et al, 1995). The researchers state that "the purpose of the current study was to compare the effects of a low-technology environment of care based on a nurse-managed care delivery system (special care unit [SCU] environment) with the traditional high-technology ICU environment based on a primary nursing care delivery system." The authors did not label the first five introductory paragraphs as a *review of the literature* or provide subheadings for the variables. However, it was evident by this review that studies discussed the following variables: length of stay (LOS) of a typical intensive care unit (ICU) patient, the concerns of cost and patient outcomes in ICU patients, definition of the term *chronically critically ill*, the negative impact of ICU patients on hospital resources, and LOS and costs with ICU ventilated patients using other than randomized trial designs. The last paragraph concluded with the support for their chosen methodology, followed by a last paragraph of this introductory section that introduced the purpose of the study, as previously stated.

In contrast to the styles of the previous quantitative studies, the literature reviews' of qualitative studies are much shorter. This is because little is known about the topic under study, or the very nature of the qualitative design dictates that a review of the literature be conducted after the study is completed and then the researchers compare the literature review with their findings. For example, Draucker and Petrovic's grounded theory study was to generate a framework or a theory of healing by male survivors of childhood sexual abuse (see Appendix B). There are a few overview paragraphs on sexual abuse survivors, but the researchers conclude that little is known from the survivor's perspective. Thus the rationale for using a grounded theory methodology is supported (see Chapter 9).

CRITIQUING CRITERIA FOR A REVIEW OF THE LITERATURE

As you analyze (critique) a scholarly report you must use appropriate criteria. If you are reading a research study, it must be evaluated in terms of each step of the research process. The characteristics of a relevant review of the literature (see Box 4-3) and the purposes of the review of the literature (see Box 4-1) provided the framework for the development of literature review evaluation criteria. Difficulties that the consumer of research might have regarding this task and related strategies are presented after a discussion of the critiquing criteria.

Critiquing the literature review of data-based or conceptual reports is a challenging task for the consumer of research. Critiquing criteria have been developed for all aspects of the quantitative research process, for various quantitative designs and qualitative approaches, and for consumer of research projects for the educational and clinical settings. Critiquing criteria for the review of the literature are usually presented from the quantitative research process perspective. Because the focus of this book is on the baccalaureate nurse in the research consumer role, the critiquing criteria for the literature review incorporates this frame of reference. However, Chapter 17 presents an overview of evaluating quantitative research studies. The processes used in qualitative studies are specifically presented in Chapter 9, and a qualitative study is evaluated in Chapter 18.

The important issue is for the reader to determine the overall value of the data-based or conceptual report. Does the review of the literature permeate the report? Does the review of the literature contribute to the significance of the report in relation to nursing theory, research, education, or practice (see Figure 4-1)? The overall question to be answered is, "Does the review of the literature uncover knowledge?" This question is based on the overall purpose of a review of the literature, which is to uncover knowledge (see Box 4-1). The major goal turns into the question, "Did the review of the literature provide a strong knowledge base to carry out the reported research or scholarly educational or clinical practice setting project?" The Critiquing Criteria box provides questions for the consumer of research to ask about literature review.

Questions related to the logical presentation of the reviewed articles are somewhat more challenging for the beginning consumer of research. The more you read scholarly articles, the easier this question is to answer. At times the type of question being asked in relation to the particular concept lends itself to presenting the reviewed studies chronologically (i.e., perhaps beginning with early or landmark data-based or conceptual literature).

Questions must be asked about whether each explanation of a step of the research process met or did not meet these guidelines (criteria). For instance, Box 4-1 illustrates the overall purposes of a review of the literature. The second objective listed states that the review of the literature is to determine gaps, consistencies, and inconsistencies in the literature about a subject,

CRITIQUING CRITERIA

IMPORTANT QUESTIONS TO ASK ABOUT LITERATURE REVIEW

1. Does the literature review uncover gaps or inconsistencies in knowledge?
2. How does the review reflect critical thinking?
3. Are all the relevant concepts and variables included in the review?
4. Does the summary of each reviewed study reflect the essential components of the study design (e.g., in a quantitative design: type and size of sample, instruments' validity and reliability; in a qualitative design: does it indicate the type, such as phenomenological)?
5. Does the critique of each reviewed study include strengths, weaknesses, or limitations of the design; conflicts; and gaps or inconsistencies in information in relation to the area of interest?
6. Are both conceptual and data-based literature included?
7. Are primary sources mainly used?
8. Is there a written summary synthesis of the reviewed scholarly literature?
9. Does the synthesis summary follow a logical sequence that leads the reader to why there is the need for the particular research or nonresearch project?
10. Does the organization of the reviewed studies (e.g., chronologically, according to concepts/variables, or by type/design/level of study) flow logically, enhancing the ability of the reader to evaluate the need for the particular research or nonresearch project?
11. Does the literature review follow the purpose(s) of the study or nonresearch project?

concept, or problem. The guide question in Table 17-1 (see Chapter 17) is, "What gaps or conflicts in knowledge about the problem are identified? How does this study intend to fill those gaps or resolve those conflicts?" In this example, the purpose or objective of the literature review became the evaluation question or criterion for critiquing the review of the literature.

Two other important questions to ask are, "Were both conceptual and data-based literature included?" and "Does the review consist of mainly primary sources?" Other sets of critiquing criteria may phrase these questions differently or more broadly. For instance, the question may be, "Does the literature search seem adequate?" or "Does the report demonstrate scholarly writing?" These may seem to be difficult questions for you to answer; however, one place to begin is by determining whether the source is a refereed journal (see Box 4-3). It is fairly reasonable to assume that a scholarly refereed journal publishes manuscripts that are adequately searched, use mainly primary sources, and are written in a scholarly manner. However, this does not mean that every study reported in a refereed journal will meet all the criteria in an equal manner. You still must answer the critiquing questions by what is stated rather than by what you think the researchers meant. Consultation with a faculty advisor may be necessary to develop skill in answering this question.

Other questions that should be asked are, "Is there a written summary of each reviewed source?" and "Does the summary of the study include a critique?" These questions seem as if they would be easily answered by reading what is reported in the literature review. However, because of style differences and space constraints, each citation summarized is usually very brief and often lacks a critique. Other possible reasons for critiques not being written are discussed earlier in the chapter.

More typically an entire study is summarized in one or two sentences. For example, Ward, Berry, and Misiewicz's (1996) study illustrates this point (see Appendix D). They report the following:

In a study of 40 patient-spouse dyads Dar et al found that 43% of the spouses believed that the patient . . . should not take narcotic medication on a regular basis, but only when the pain is extreme (Dar et al, 1992).

A critique was not apparent in this written report; perhaps their evaluation did not seem essential to the review, or page constraints prevented its inclusion.

In addition to a summary and critique of each source, a literature review requires a complete summary or a synthesis of all reviewed sources. The relationship between and among these studies must be explained. The summary should reflect the putting together of the main points or value of all the sources in relation to the research question. A synthesis of a written review of the literature usually appears at the end of the review section before the research question or hypothesis reporting section. If not labeled as such, it is usually evident in the last paragraph. A relevant literature review demonstrates synthesis of the reviewed sources (see Box 4-2). Therefore, demonstrating synthesis becomes an essential critiquing criterion for the review of the literature.

Wikblad and Anderson (1995) end their literature review (see Appendix A) with the following:

However, the results from controlled studies on wound dressings in postoperative settings are inconsistent, and further controlled clinical studies are required to resolve the ambiguities.

The preceding summary synthesis meets the objective of uncovering knowledge, determining what is known and not known, and finding gaps and inconsistencies in the literature. Their synthesis was brief, yet it provided enough data to conclude that their literature review reflected critical thinking and scholarly writing, and it provided the bridge or reason for carrying out the study. This example specifically addresses a number of the questions found in the Critiquing Criteria box. Another example is Rudy et al's (1995) concluding statement found at the end of their review, which states that the lack of randomized trials comparing care delivery systems for these high-cost patients is noteworthy, as well as the limitation of outcome measurements to mortality and cost (see Appendix C). Their summary (synthesis) statement, also brief, demonstrates that their randomized study comparing the relationship between these two variables was needed.

Critiquing a review of the literature is an acquired skill. Continue reading and rereading, as well as seeking advice from faculty and seasoned researchers. Think about using the literature review as your essential key to implementing a research-based practice.

KEY POINTS

- The role of the consumer of research for critiquing a literature review is based on ANA's *Educational Guidelines for Research Activities* (1993), ANA's *Standards of Clinical Practice* (1991), and ANA's *Social Policy Statement* (1995).
- The review of the literature is defined as a broad, comprehensive, in-depth, systematic, and critical review of scholarly publications, unpublished scholarly print materials, audiovisual materials, and personal communications.
- The review of the literature is for research and consumer of research activities. The main objectives for the consumer of research in relation to the literature review are to acquire the ability to do the following: (1) conduct a computer data-based search, (2) efficiently retrieve a sufficient amount of scholarly materials for a literature review, (3) critically evaluate data-based and conceptual material based on accepted reviewing criteria, and (4) critically evaluate a review of the literature based on accepted reviewing criteria.
- Primary resources are essential for literature reviews.
- Secondary sources, from peer reviewed journals, are part of a learning strategy for developing critical evaluation skills.
- There are many advantages for using computer databases rather than print databases for retrieving scholarly material.
- Strategies for efficiently retrieving scholarly literature include consulting the reference librarian and using computer CINAHL CD-ROM database.
- Literature reviews are organized according to variables, as well as chronologically.
- Critiquing criteria for scholarly literature reflect the purposes and characteristics of a relevant literature review and are presented in the form of questions.
- The ability to critically review data-based literature is necessary for implementing a research-based practice in nursing.

CRITICAL THINKING CHALLENGES
Barbara Krainovich-Miller

? How is it possible that the review of the literature can be both an individual step of the research process and a research component used in each of the steps of the process? Support your answer with specific examples.

❓ How does a researcher justify using both conceptual and data-based literature in a literature review; and would you for research consumer purposes, such as developing an academic scholarly paper, use the same types of literature?

❓ A classmate in your research class tells you that she has access to the Internet and can do all her searches from home. What essential questions do you need to ask her to determine if database sources can be accessed?

❓ An acute care agency's nursing research committee is developing a research-based practice protocol for patient-controlled analgesia (PCA). One suggestions is to use AHCPR's *Pain Guideline* (1992), and another is to conduct a review of the literature from the past 6 years on pain control. How would you settle the question—which one is these suggestions will contribute most effectively to the goal of a research-based protocol?

REFERENCES

Acute Pain Management Guideline Panel: *Acute pain management: operative or medical procedures and trauma practice guideline,* AHCPR Pub No 92-0023, Rockville, Md, 1992, Agency for Health Care Policy and Research, Public Health Service, US Department of Health and Human Services.

American Nurses Association: *Education for participation in nursing* research, Washington, DC, 1993, ANA.

American Nurses Association: *Nursing's social policy statement,* Washington, DC, 1995, ANA.

American Nurses Association: *Standards of clinical nursing practice,* Kansas City, Mo, 1991, ANA (in revision).

Barrett EAM: An empirical investigation of Martha E Rogers' principle of helicy: the relationship of human field motion and power, *Dissert Abstr Int* 45:615A, 1984 (University Microfilms No 8406278).

Barrett EAM: Investigation of the principle of helicy: the relationship of human field motion and power. In Malinski V, ed: *Explorations on Martha Rogers' science of unitary human beings,* Norwalk, Conn, 1986, Appleton-Century-Crofts.

Belcher JR, Fish LJB: Hidegard E Peplau. In George JB, ed: *Nursing theories: the base for profession nursing practice,* ed 4, Norwalk, Conn, 1995, Appleton & Lange.

Benner P: *From novice to expert: excellence and power in clinical nursing practice,* Menlo Park, Calif, 1984, Addison-Wesley.

Bowles KH, Naylor MD: Nursing intervention classification systems, *Image* 28(4):303-308, 1996.

Campagna A: The lived experience of step-families, doctoral dissertation, Dissertation Abstracts International, 8824404, New York, 1995, Columbia University Teacher's College.

Carroll-Johnson RM: Searching . . . one of the first steps of writing is to conduct a comprehensive literature search, *Oncol Nurs Forum* 19(5):705, 1992.

CINAHL: *CINAHLnews,* Glendale, Calif, 1997, CINAHL Information Systems.

Corel: *Corel wordperfect suite 7: quick results,* Ireland, 1996, Corel Corporation.

Draucker CB, Petrovic K: Healing of adult male survivors of childhood sexual abuse, *Image* 28(4):325-330, 1996.

Early HIV Infection Guideline Panel: *Evaluation and management of early HIV infection,* AHCPR Pub No 94-0572, Rockville, Md, 1994, Agency for Health Care Policy and Research, Public Health Service, US Department of Health and Human Services.

Feldman HR et al: Bridging the nursing research-practice gap through research utilization, *JNY State Nurs Assoc* 42(3):4-10, 1993.

Fitzpatrick JJ, Norbeck JS: *Annual review of nursing research,* Vol 14, New York, 1996, Springer.

Glass EC: Importance of research to practice. In Mateo MA, Kirchhoff KT, eds: *Conducting and using nursing research in the clinical setting,* Baltimore, 1991, Williams & Wilkins.

Hays BJ et al: Informatics issues for nursing's future, *Adv Nurs Sci* 16(4):71-81, 1994.

Hawks JH: Power: a concept analysis, *J Adv Nurs* 16:754-762, 1991.

Holmes S: Systematic search offers a sound evidence base, *Nurs Times* 92(4):37-39, 1996.

Hutchinson D: A nurse's guide to the Internet, *RN* 60(1):46-51, 1997.

Interagency Council on Information Resources for Nursing (ICIRN) et al: Essential nursing references, *Nurs Health Care Perspect Comm* 17(5):255-259, 1996.

Kaufeld J, Kaufeld J: *America On-Line for dummies,* Foster City, Calif, 1996, IDG Books Worldwide.

Kay CL: Introduction to the Internet, Unpublished guide, Garden City, NY, 1995, Adelphi University.

Kerlinger FN: *Foundations of behavioral research,* ed 3, New York, 1986, Holt, Rinehart & Winston.

Koop PM: Commentary: a family's coming to terms with Alzheimer's disease, *West J Nurs Res* 18(1):22-23, 1996.

Larrabee JH: Emerging model of quality, *Image* 28(4):353-358, 1996.

Malinski V: The relationship between hyperactivity in children and perception of short wavelength light: an investigation into the conceptual system proposed by Martha E Rogers, *Dissert Abstr Int* 41:4459B, 1981 (University Microfilms No 8110669).

Maas ML, Johnson M, Moorhead S: Classifying nursing-sensitive patient outcomes, *Image* 28(4):295-301, 1996.

McCloskey JC, Bulechek GM, eds: *Iowa intervention project: nursing interventions classification (NIC),* ed 2, St Louis, 1996, Mosby.

McCormick KA et al: Toward standard classification schemes for nursing language: recommendations of the American Nurses Association Steering Committee on databases to support clinical nursing practice, *J Am Med Informatics Assoc (JAMIA)* 1(6):421-427, 1994.

McEvoy MD: The relationships among the experience of dying, the experience of paranormal events, and creativity in adults. In Barrett EAM, ed: *Visions of Rogers' science-based nursing,* New York, 1990, NLN.

Moore SL: A phenomenological study of meaning in life in suicidal older adults, *Arch Psychiatr Nurs* 11(1):29-36, 1997.

Nicoll LH: *Perspectives on nursing theory,* ed 3, New York, 1996, Lippincott.

Nicoll LH, Ouellette TH: *Nurses' guide to the Internet: computers in nursing,* Philadelphia, 1997, Lippincott.

Paul RW: *Critical thinking: how to prepare students for a rapidly changing world,* Rohnert Park, Calif, 1995, Center for Critical Thinking & Moral Critique.

Prohaska, JL, Chang BL: Computer use and nursing research: using the Internet to enhance nursing knowledge and practice, *West J Nurs Res* 18(3):365-370, 1996.

Rafael ARF: Power and caring: a dialectic in nursing, *Adv Nurs Sci* 19 (1):3-17, 1996.

Rantz MF: *Nursing quality measurement: a review of nursing studies,* Washington, DC, 1995, ANA.

Reed PG: Transforming practice knowledge into nursing knowledge: a revisionist analysis of Peplau, *Image* 28(1):29-33, 1996.

Roberts J: British nurses at war 1914-1918: ancillary personnel and the battle for registration, *Nurs Res* 45(3):167-172, 1996.

Rogers ME: *An introduction to the theoretical basis of nursing,* Philadelphia, 1970, FA Davis.

Rogers ME: Nursing: a science of unitary man. In Riehl JP, Roy C, eds: *Conceptual models for nursing practice,* ed 2, New York, 1980, Appleton-Century-Crofts.

Rogers ME: Nursing: science of unitary, irreducible, human beings: update 1990. In Barrett EAM, ed: *Visions of Rogers' science-based nursing,* New York, 1990, NLN.

Rosedale J: Personal communication, January 6, 1997.

Rudy EB et al: Patient outcomes for the chronically critically ill: special care unit versus intensive care unit, *Nurs Res* 44:324-331, 1995.

Russell CK: Elder care recipients' care-seeking process, *West J Nurs Res* 18:43-62, 1996.

SilverPlatter Information: *1996 directory of CD-ROM databases,* Norwood, Ma, 1996, Silver-Platter Information.

Stetler CB: Refinement of the Stetler/Marram model for application of research findings to practice, *Nurs Outlook* 42(1):15-25, 1994.

Sigma Theta Tau International (STTI): *The online journal of knowledge synthesis for nursing,* Indianapolis, 1996, STTI.

Tiesinga LJ, Dassen TWN, Halfens RJG: Fatigue: a summary of the definitions, dimensions, and indicators, *Nurs Diagn* 7(2):51-62, 1996.

Turley JP: Toward a model for nursing informatics, *Image* 28(4):309-314, 1996.

Ward SE, Berry PE, Misiewicz H: Concerns about analgesics among patients and family caregivers in a hospice setting, *Res Nurs Health* 19:205-211, 1996.

Weinberg L: How to use CINAHL, Unpublished guide, Garden City, NY, 1996, Adelphi University.

Wikblad K, Anderson B: A comparison of three wound dressings in patients undergoing heart surgery, *Nurs Res* 44(5):312-316, 1995.

ADDITIONAL READINGS

American Nurses Association: *The scope of practice for nursing informatics,* Washington, DC, 1994, ANA.

American Psychological Association: *Publication manual of the American Psychological Association,* ed 4, Washington, DC, 1994, APA.

Heddle NM, Gagliardi K, Flemming T: Searching the scientific literature, *Can J Med Tech* 53(4):210-213, 1991.

Hinzmann C: Educational innovations. BSN students present research findings on complex health problems in poster session format, *J Nurs Educ* 35(4):177-178, 1996.

Hutchinson D, Hogarth M: *An Internet guide for the health professional,* ed 2, Sacramento, Calif, 1996, New Wind.

Larson E, Satterthwaite R: Searching the literature: a professional imperative, *Am J Infect Control* 17(6):359-364, 1989.

Malinski V: The meaning of a progressive world view in nursing: Rogers' science of unitary human beings. In Chaska NL, ed: *The nursing profession: turning points,* St Louis, 1990, Mosby.

McCain NL, Lynn MR: Meta-analysis of a narrative review: studies evaluating patient teaching, *West J Nurs Res* 12(3):347-58, 1990.

Nicoll LH, Ouellette TH: *Nurses' guide to the Internet: computers in nursing,* Philadelphia, 1997, Lippincott.

Silverstein JL: Strengthening the links between health sciences information users and providers, *Bull Med Libr Assoc* 83(4):407-417, 1995.

Strunk W, White EB: *The elements of style,* ed 3, New York, 1979, Macmillan.

Tornquist EM: From proposal to publication: an informal guide to writing about nursing research, Menlo Park, Calif, 1986, Addison-Wesley.

Westra BL, Rodgers BL: The concept of integration: a foundation for evaluating outcomes of nursing care, *J Prof Nurs* 7(5):277-282, 1991.

Theoretical Framework

Harriet R. Feldman

Key Terms

concept
conceptual definition
conceptual model
deductive reasoning
hypothesis
inductive reasoning

operational definition
propositions
theoretical framework
theories
variable

Learning Outcomes

After reading this chapter the student should be able to do the following:

- Identify the major sources of human knowledge.
- Contrast the strengths and weaknesses of the major sources of human knowledge.
- Compare the inductive and deductive modes of inquiry.
- Differentiate between theory, conceptual model, and theoretical framework.
- Identify the purpose and nature of a theoretical framework.
- Describe how a theoretical framework guides research.
- Differentiate between conceptual and operational definitions.
- Describe the relationship between theory and research.
- Differentiate among grand, middle range, and practice theories in nursing.
- Describe the points of critical appraisal used to evaluate the appropriateness, cohesiveness, and consistency of a theoretical framework.

"**K**nowledge is the awareness or perception of reality acquired through insight, learning, or investigation and expressed in a form that can be shared" (Chinn and Kramer, 1995). Knowledge is developed within the context of a belief system cherished by a particular discipline. Nursing knowledge comes from a variety of sources including intuition, tradition and authority, trial and error, and research. The quality of nursing practice depends on the quality of knowledge learned. Think about the quality and validity of new information that you read and learn. For example, were the nursing interventions you were taught based on research evidence or tradition? How many research-based interventions that you learned about need further study to determine their effectiveness? Research is an important source of knowledge for the nursing profession, because it promotes development of the scientific base for nursing practice. This chapter examines the sources of human knowledge and the components of theory, as well as approaches to developing theory and the relationship between theory and research. The nature, purpose, and critique of a theoretical framework in a research study are discussed.

WAYS OF KNOWING—SOURCES OF KNOWLEDGE

Ideas are generated in many ways. Some sources of knowledge are highly structured and are generally bound by defined rules of process or method; other sources are less structured and have few defined rules. Examples of sources of knowledge include research, critical thinking, logical reasoning, intuition, trial-and-error experience, and tradition and authority. These approaches are summarized in Box 5-1.

Sources of Knowledge

Intuition
Intuition or innate knowledge is a frequently used method of problem solving. It can operate either as a form of inference, in which intuition closely resembles sensory perception, or as an extrasensory experience independent of sensory input. Intuition depends on some familiarity with a subject area. Intuitive leaps in science and the arts, made by such people as Einstein and Beethoven, have led to great contributions.

Minick (1995) conducted a study of the processes that critical care nurses used in the early recognition of patient problems. She said that "intuitive early recognition of patient problems may be a key aspect in the identification of complications and thus in reducing mortality among critically ill patients." Based on her interviews of critical care nurses she concluded that "decision-making that is based on the immediate recognition of patient problems with-

Box 5-1	Approaches to Generating Knowledge
Less Structured	**Structured**
Intuition	Induction
Trial and error	Deduction
Tradition	Nursing process
Authority	Science/research

out objective data has traditionally been viewed as less important, yet clinicians in this study suggest that it is extremely important. Nurses need to be alert to and act on this embodied knowledge."

Intuition also plays a role in research. Although intuition is not a sufficient means to approach information in a research context, it can serve as a guiding and creative adjunct. Often it is an initial "hunch" or inference that leads investigators to examine anticipated relationships or a later hunch that opens new avenues for understanding research findings.

> **HELPFUL HINT**
> Regarding the use of intuition in the research process, authors do not always include information about how they arrived at the problem studied, nor do they necessarily document insights that arose along the way.

Trial-and-Error Experience

One approach to solving problems is by the process of trial and error. When a problem is identified, a solution is attempted. Depending on whether or not the solution works, the nurse either adopts the trial solution or tries another one. When the second trial solution fails, the nurse keeps trying, eliminating one possible solution after another until the problem is actually solved. For example, a nurse may try several interventions in an attempt to promote healing of a decubitus ulcer before finding the one solution that works for a particular patient. For a second patient with a similar problem the solution found for the first patient may not work, so other trials are implemented until a successful method for groups of similar patients is discovered. This method of problem solving can be inefficient in terms of both time and energy, because it may take a long time to find a successful solution and the solution that is found may not be effective for more than one patient. In addition, a solution with broader applicability may have already been determined by someone else. A more structured approach would save time, money, and inconvenience to patients.

Tradition and Authority

Often people believe that something is right or acceptable because it is backed by tradition and authority. When trial-and-error experiences lead to problem resolution, a ready source of known solutions becomes available and this forms the basis for tradition. As individuals become more invested in those traditional solutions, the solutions take on an air of authority. In nursing the temperature-taking ritual is an example of this problem solving evolution from trial and error to authority. In many instances nurses have come to accept that individuals require temperature readings every 4 hours, simply because they are admitted to an acute care facility. The initial rationale for this procedure has been long forgotten, and more current investigations have refuted this practice. In fact some hospitals have discontinued this temperature-taking routine on the basis of their own research.

Although it is important to be aware of what has existed for a long time and listen to what those in authority are saying, knowledge derived from tradition and authority must be critically evaluated in light of other available data, for example, related literature and experts in the field. Research consumers can assess the accuracy of knowledge by questioning, identifying, and synthesizing all available data sources and noting the ones that clearly and logically support valid solutions.

The study by Rudy et al (1995; see Appendix C) exemplifies a challenge to what has become the traditional practice of long-stay intensive care units (ICUs), despite the fact that when ICUs were originally created it was assumed that "a typical ICU patient will require only a short length of stay in the unit during the most acute phase of illness." These investigators found that there was a lower readmission rate after discharge in patients cared for in a special care unit (SCU), which was a low-technology environment with a nurse case management case delivery system, versus those cared for in the ICU; they also found a lower mortality rate in SCU versus ICU patients.

Science/Research

Science/research is a systematic planned method or process of inquiry conducted to develop knowledge (Chinn and Kramer, 1995; Kerlinger, 1986). As a body of knowledge, science is concerned with interrelated principles, laws, and theories rather than with random or unrelated data. Science becomes the medium for systematically collecting, analyzing, and evaluating data.

The scientific approach or research process involves the processes of logical reasoning concerning the phenomena about which more information, or new knowledge, is sought through a systematically planned investigation. The two major approaches to research are termed *inductive* and *deductive,* as reflected in their respective approaches to inquiry, that is, the *qualitative* and *quantitative* approaches. As nurses tackle daily problems, they often use these approaches or mental operations without realizing it. **Inductive reasoning** involves the observation of a particular set of instances that belong to and can be identified as part of a larger set. This reasoning moves from the particular to the general and underlies qualitative approaches to inquiry (see Chapter 9). On the other hand, **deductive reasoning** uses two or more variables or related statements that, when combined, form the basis for a concluding assertion of a relationship between the variables, called *relational statements.* This reasoning moves from the general to the particular and is typically applied through quantitative inquiry approaches (see Chapters 7 and 8). The two approaches are compared in Box 5-2.

Box 5-2	Differences in the Research Process When Using Inductive and Deductive Reasoning
Inductive/Qualitative	**Deductive/Quantitative**
State problem	State problem
Review literature	Review literature
Select method	Identify theoretical framework
Collect data	State hypothesis
Analyze data	Select method
Interpret results	Collect data
Develop concepts	Analyze data
Draw conclusions	Accept/reject hypothesis
Examine universality	Interpret results
Create hypotheses	Examine generalizability
Communicate results	Communicate results

Inductive reasoning. Logical reasoning about abstract concepts and empirical observations permits the researcher to consider how best to formulate a research study. As stated previously, inductive reasoning moves from the particular to the general. Conclusions are developed from specific observations. For example, a nurse may notice that more and more newborns in the nursery are developing rashes on their backs. The nurse may inductively reason that a problem exists with the method of laundering the sheets on which the newborns lie. Based on this information alone, however, it is not reasonable to conclude that the laundromat is using harsh detergents on all the sheets. The problem may well be caused by an inadequate amount of rinse water. The nurse can attribute the problem to the method of laundering but has insufficient information to conclude that the detergent is the culprit and is causing skin rashes in the nursery.

Inductive reasoning is exemplified in the qualitative study conducted by Draucker and Petrovic (1996; see Appendix B), who interviewed men living in the community who had experienced some healing from childhood sexual abuse. The purpose of the study was to generate a framework of healing by male survivors of childhood sexual abuse and to identify some problems that male sexual abuse survivors experience that might be important for clinicians to consider. In another example, Fisher (1995) noted that "requiring that staff act quickly to predict and control potential violence remains a significant component of contemporary nursing work in psychiatric emergency and inpatient settings." This observation led to her qualitative study of "ethical problems encountered in the day-to-day practices of psychiatric nurses, as they cared for and managed the dangerous mentally ill." The inductive approach, then, begins with an observation or some other way of obtaining information and leads to a conclusion.

HELPFUL HINT

Investigators may not state explicitly what observation(s) led them to their conclusion(s); their reason for using an inductive approach may, instead, be implicit.

Deductive reasoning. Deductive reasoning moves from the general to the particular. A specific **hypothesis** (prediction) or research question can be deduced or drawn from a theory or an organizing statement about abstract concepts that serves as a more general statement or network of interrelated concepts (see Chapter 3). As a result of deduction, observations can be made and predictions tested through quantitative research approaches. Rather than generating or discovering sources of new information, deductive reasoning can serve as an approach to confirming existing relationships. For example, if it is known that theory X has been substantiated, the nurse researcher could anticipate what outcomes and behaviors are logically expected. The three examples in Box 5-3 show how a nurse uses deductive reasoning.

Shaio et al (1995) conducted a quasiexperimental (quantitative) clinical study (see Chapter 7) that evolved through deductive reasoning. The following statements show how deduction was used to develop their study of nasogastric tube placement in very-low-birth-weight (VLBW) infants:

1. A nasogastric (NG) tube is commonly used during the initial hospitalization of preterm infants. During the transitional period from tube feedings to oral feedings, the nursery staff may place the NG tube only for tube feedings or keep it in place continuously between and during tube and oral feedings.

Box 5-3   Examples of Deductive Reasoning

It is known that certain physiological changes take place in bedridden clients as a result of continuous or uneven pressure to bony prominences. A nurse could deduce that pressure-relieving methods will decrease the incidence and intensity of decubitus ulcer development. In research-based practice the nurse would apply this knowledge of specific relationships to the prevention of decubiti by relieving pressure on a client's bony prominences.

The gate control theory of pain identifies the interaction of motivational, affective, and sensory processing that modulates the perception of and response to pain. According to that theory, such variables as anxiety, attention, age, culture, meaning of the present pain experience, and pathophysiological findings are associated with the pain experience. Because anxiety and the pain sensation tend to reinforce each other, thereby increasing the intensity of the pain experience, the nurse could deduce that anxiety-reducing measures such as empathic interaction, a back rub, an explanation to the patient, and prompt administration of pain medication would result in decreased pain. If the nurse wanted to know which of these methods worked best to relieve distress in patients with certain painful conditions, a research study could be designed to test which of the hypothesized or predicted relationships between pain relief method and relief would be confirmed.

Social support helps an individual to see an event as less stressful so that the person can cope with it more effectively. One stressful situation that affects the health of an individual is breast cancer. On the basis of what is known about social support and its effects on stress and health, a researcher studying the adjustment of women to mastectomy might deduce that breast cancer patients who receive social support after mastectomy would have fewer adjustment problems than those who do not receive social support.

2. NG tube insertion involves laryngeal stimulation, which is associated with apnea and bradycardia. The continuous presence of an NG tube may be an additional stimulus to laryngeal chemoreceptors during and between oral feedings.
3. Continuous tube placement can affect distribution of ventilation.
4. VLBW infants are unable to compensate for nasal occlusion by converting to oral breathing; partial blocking of one naris by an NG tube would probably be a significant problem for VLBW infants.
5. Using NG tubes continuously has been found to be an important contributor to a less successful transition to oral feeding.

On the basis of their observations and documented research findings, the researchers deduced that "because an NG tube may affect the functions of both breathing and sucking, it is important to examine the tube'e effect on development of coordinated breathing and sucking." Information about appropriate tube placement could significantly improve such outcomes as respiratory status, feeding status, weight gain, and length of hospital stay.

As with inductive reasoning, there may be inherent problems in using the deductive approach. First, not all deductions can be verified, particularly when the measurement methods are poor or undeveloped. Second, a deduction that is based on a tentative premise may result in a conclusion that is logically valid, yet unsound. Third, an unsound conclusion may be assumed sound, especially if it seems reasonable. If a systematic, scientific approach, that is, quantitative design, is used to test a prediction deduced from a theory, the conclusion is more likely to be sound and to be useful to the discipline.

HELPFUL HINT

When an investigator has used a deductive approach, the theoretical framework should be described to substantiate how the conclusion (e.g., hypothesis or research question) was determined.

Concepts, Propositions, and Hypotheses

A **concept** is an image or symbolic representation of an abstract idea. It is formed by generalizing from particular characteristics. To illustrate, health is a concept formed by generalizing from particular behaviors, for example, being mobile and being free of infection. Other concepts include pain, weight, grieving, and self-concept. Some concepts are directly observable, such as a chair or rain, and others are indirectly observable, for example, anxiety or intelligence.

Because concepts are the basis for refining ideas and developing theory, it is important that a researcher selects those concepts that clearly reflect the subject matter. In evaluating a piece of research, research consumers must consider whether the concepts as defined are examined both in general and specifically in the context of the problem under investigation (see Chapters 3 and 12). Furthermore, one must consider whether they are being measured with the appropriate instruments (see Chapters 12 and 13).

In the process of examining the concepts or variables that guide the research effort, relationships emerge. For example, from a review of the literature in a particular area such as stress, information about related variables can be found (e.g., onset of illness, certain physiological responses, and learning ability). Relationships can also be identified through systematic observation and experience. A relationship may be invariable, tentative, or inconclusive. One type of invariable relationship is a scientific law, for example, Newton's three laws of motion. In this case, no known contradiction has been observed. A tentative or inconclusive relationship is a hypothesis, which expresses a relationship between two or more variables and does not convey truth or falsity. Both laws and hypotheses are types of **propositions,** which are statements that link concepts and lay a foundation for the development of methods that test relationships. The Critical Thinking Decision Path identifies the linkages among concepts, propositions, and hypotheses.

HELPFUL HINT

For a quantitative study, the literature review is the part of the research report that generally includes discussion of the theoretical basis for formulating hypotheses (which is the researcher's prediction about the outcome of the study). It should also explicitly identify propositions in relation to the individual variables described. The hypotheses should express relationships between variables in an unambiguous, precise manner, and they should be based on the propositions that evolved from the theoretical framework.

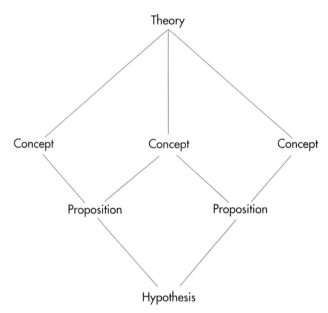

Theory

Concept   Concept   Concept

Proposition   Proposition

Hypothesis

Critical Thinking Decision Path   The development of a hypothesis.

Conceptual Models, Theories, and Theoretical Frameworks

Various terms are used to describe the conceptual background for a research study. The terms *conceptual framework, theory,* and *theoretical framework* are used independently of each other but as used by others can have some similarities. The contrasts presented here are not universal but do provide a clarification of the terms.

A **conceptual model** is analogous to an architectural blueprint for a house. It is a group of interrelated concepts that fit together because of their relevance to a common theme or matrix, for example, a blueprint that provides a rational scheme or design for the architect's vision. "It reflects the philosophical stance, cognitive orientation, and research tradition of a group of scholars, rather than the beliefs, values, thoughts, and research methods of all members of a discipline" (Fawcett and Downs, 1986).

Theories serve the function of describing, explaining, and making predictions about phenomena particular to the conceptual model, for example, the arrangement of materials to build the heating system of a house that is appropriate to the architect's blueprint. Theory is defined as a set of interrelated concepts, definitions, and propositions that present a systematic view of phenomena for the purpose of explaining and predicting phenomena (Chinn and Kramer, 1995; Kerlinger, 1986). Theories are linked to the real world through definitions that specify how concepts will be observed and measured.

As discussed earlier in this chapter, theories are *generated* by using inductive processes, which lead to predictions about observed phenomena. A deductive approach, however, is used to evaluate and modify existing theory by *testing* predictions about relationships between observed phenomena. As current research findings are reported in the literature, a body of knowledge about a phenomenon accumulates. Theories are always evolving as new information is discovered or verified about particular concepts through both inductive and deductive research approaches.

A **theoretical framework** is like the frame of a house. Just as the foundation supports a house, a theoretical framework provides a rationale for predictions about the relationships among variables of a research study. A theoretical framework specifies the relationship between the concepts in a study. It provides a context for examining a problem, that is, the theoretical rationale for developing hypotheses, just as a direction indicator (N-S-E-W) provides a context for using a road map.

The theoretical framework is a frame of reference that is a basis for observations, definitions of concepts, research designs, interpretations, and generalizations, much as the frame that rests on a foundation defines the overall design of a house. For example, Cole and Slocumb (1995), in their study of factors influencing safer sexual behaviors in heterosexual late adolescent and young adult collegiate males, used the PRECEDE model of health behavior as a basis for their research. This model, used for educational diagnosis and evaluation, contains three factors that precede and influence health behavior, namely, predisposing, enabling, and reinforcing factors. Cole and Slocumb studied the predisposing factors. Based on their review of the literature, they identified the following predisposing factors: self-esteem, acquired immunodeficiency syndrome (AIDS) knowledge, internal health locus of control, chance health locus of control, powerful other health locus of control, perceived susceptibility, and attitudes toward condoms, thereby defining the concept of predisposing factors. They selected a quantitative research design and a number of instruments to measure these factors, such as the AIDS-HIV Knowledge Scale developed by Thomas, Gilliam, and Iwrey (1989) and a visual analog scale (VAS) to measure perceived susceptibility to AIDS. Their discussion of findings related to the PRECEDE model, as indicated by the following: "The results of this study lend support to the use of the predisposing factors of the PRECEDE model for examining variables that affect the practice of safer sexual behaviors. Continued use of the model, adding variables to measure enabling and reinforcing factors, is recommended and will fully operationalize the model."

Why is a theoretical framework necessary for a research study? Why can't a researcher just match any two variables that make sense and look at their relationship? As an analogy, consider the first time you traveled by car to an unfamiliar place. How did you get to your destination? Did you use a map? Did you follow someone's directions? Did you stick to the prescribed route, or did you try a shortcut? Did you turn left instead of right because it seemed logical, or did you use known information to make that decision? The map served as a guide to your destination, and when conducting research, a theoretical framework serves as a guide or map to systematically identifying a logical, precisely defined relationship between variables.

An investigator who reports research is obliged to state clearly the theoretical basis for hypothesis formulation, study findings, and outcome interpretations. As in the analogy presented earlier, each piece of lumber that the frame of the house comprises must be connected to another piece, as in the relationship between two or more variables. The frame must rest squarely on a solid foundation, just as the relationship between two variables rests firmly on a theoretical framework. The "fit" must be precise, or the house will fall; similarly, the theoretical fit must be precise or the prediction made about the relationship of the variables will in all likelihood not be supported through testing of the hypothesis.

Defining Concepts

To develop a theoretical framework that can generate and test hypotheses, concepts must be clearly defined. In thinking back to the earlier illustration about traveling to an unfamiliar place, how do you think you would have arrived if the directions simply read, "First you take one road, then turn at another, and proceed to three more roads"? Without a clear conception of which road, what direction to turn, and how far to proceed, you probably would get lost. The same process applies to any concept. For example, how would you define pain, anxiety, or intelligence? In addition to knowing the names of the roads to travel, other specifics are clearly needed, such as what type of vehicle you will use, what town you will travel through, how you will know when you have arrived, and how far you will travel. These parameters delineate the procedure to follow by identifying what operations must occur to make the trip. When defining concepts for the purpose of testing, researchers must include both conceptual and operational information.

Conceptual Definitions

Concepts, no matter what their level of abstraction, must be defined as unambiguously as possible, so that they can be easily communicated to others. Even the word *can* is open to various interpretations, for example, a container, being able to, or a commode. A **conceptual definition** conveys the general meaning of the concept, as does a dictionary definition. It reflects the theory used in the study of that concept. Box 5-4 provides several examples of conceptual definitions. Because these are general definitions, they do not include an indication of how the concepts will be measured.

Operational Definitions

Operationalization delineates the procedures or operations required to measure the concept. It supplies the information needed to collect data on the problem being studied. Some concepts are easily defined in operational terms; for example, pulse can be measured numerically

---

Box 5-4   Examples of Conceptual Definitions

Motivation—"the inner urge that moves or prompts a person to action" (Resnick, 1996)

Coaching—"an ongoing, face-to-face process of influencing behavior by which the manager (superior, supervisor) and employee collaborate to achieve increased job knowledge, improved skills in carrying out job responsibilities, a stronger and more positive working relationship, and opportunities for personal as well as professional growth of the protege" (Yoder, 1995)

Postoperative pain—discomfort an individual experiences after a surgical procedure

Weaning—"gradual reduction . . . in mechanical ventilation support" (Hanneman, 1994.)

Metamemory—"knowledge, perceptions, and beliefs about the functioning, development, and capacities of one's own memory and the human memory system" (McDougall, 1995)

Maternal identity—"maternal cognitions and affect with regard to the maternal-infant relational system" (Walker and Montgomery, 1994)

after finding the radial pulse and counting the number of beats or pulsations for a minute. Other concepts are more difficult to define operationally, such as coping, leaving it up to the investigator to locate and select an instrument that bests measures the concept as defined. Box 5-5 provides several examples of operational definitions.

Each of these examples has a conceptual definition and at least one index of measurement that makes it operational. To summarize, an **operational definition** provides specificity and direction for constructs to guide the development of the research study. Once a construct is operationalized (made measurable), it is termed a **variable,** and at that point it begins to play a significant role in formulating the theoretical rationale. The research consumer is responsible for evaluating whether variables are clearly defined, both conceptually and operationally. If the meaning of the variable is vague or if the measurement used does not reflect the same meaning as the variable, comparisons of the research with the other investigations will not be valid and the research will be impossible to replicate (see Chapter 3).

 HELPFUL HINT

Some research reports present conceptual definitions followed by a description of measurement in another section, such as methodology or instrumentation. Other reports present operational definitions; still others may present no definitions, leaving interpretations about the meaning of the variables to the reader. Of course, in the latter instance, it is easy to get lost en route.

Box 5-5   Examples of Operational Definitions

Obesity—"defined on the basis of two indices of body mass, the Quetelet Index (weight in kilograms/height in meters-squared) and the Rohrer Index (weight in kilograms/height in meters-cubed) and by triceps skinfold thickness [measured with Lange skin-fold calipers]" (Hayman et al, 1995)

Preschool mental health—"children's social competence and the presence/absence of behavior problems" (Gross et al, 1995), measured by the Kohn Social Competence Scale and Kohn Symptom Checklist

Imitating/animating—"the movement cycle that begins within 5 seconds of a child's initiation (e.g., child utters a vocalization, jumps up and down) wherein the parent imitates the child's behavior in an animated manner (e.g., with exaggerated affect, lively movement)" (Elder, 1995)

Perceived role attainment—"a sense of confidence and comfort in the maternal role, as measured by the Pharis Self-Confidence Scale" (Walker and Montgomery, 1994)

Barriers to reporting pain—"fear of addiction to analgesics, fatalism about the possibility of achieving pain control, concern about drug tolerance, belief that 'good' patients do not complain, belief that side effects from analgesics are even more bothersome than pain, fear of injections, fear of distracting a physician from treating one's disease, and belief that increased pain signifies disease progression" (Ward, Berry, and Misiewicz, 1996), measured by the Barriers Questionnaire (BQ)

RELATIONSHIP BETWEEN THEORY AND RESEARCH

Theory is tested through research, and research contributes to theory development and clinical practice. Chinn and Kramer (1995) view the interaction between theory and research as a spiral (Figure 5-1). "If you begin with theory, research derived from the theory is used to clarify and extend the theory. If you begin with research, theory that is formed from the findings can be subsequently used to direct research." The examples that follow clarify how theory guides the research process.

Suppose a nurse researcher were interested in alternatives to medication for the treatment of postoperative pain. An examination of the literature might lead to the identification of relaxation training as an intervention. The following questions might be posed:

- On what basis has a linkage between pain and relaxation been established?
- What is the nature of the linkage?
- How can this linkage or relationship be tested?
- What methods can be used for the purpose of testing?

To answer these questions, the researcher must begin by exploring a theoretical framework that is suitable for pursuing the research problem. Figure 5-2 illustrates this linkage between the independent variable (relaxation) and dependent variable (pain) of this study, showing that by influencing certain psychological and physiological components of the pain experience, that experience can be altered. Taking this rationale a step further, the following hypotheses can be generated:

- Individuals who practice a relaxation technique will experience reduced intensity of postoperative pain as compared with those who do not practice a relaxation technique.

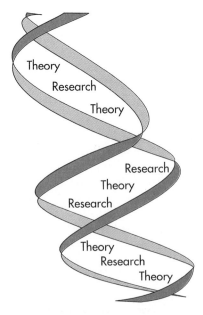

Figure 5-1   Interaction between theory and research as a spiral. (Redrawn from Chinn PL, Kramer MK: *Theory and nursing: a systematic approach,* ed 4, St Louis, 1995, Mosby.)

- Individuals who practice a relaxation technique will experience reduced postoperative pain distress as compared with those who do not practice a relaxation technique.

The first hypothesis evolved from the theoretical linkage between relaxation and physiological factors associated with pain, and the second hypothesis evolved from theoretically based psychological factors associated with pain.

A theory that comprises abstract concepts provides a framework for the deductive approach to research by guiding the selection of research variables. Variable selection in the quantitative study of nurses' attitudes toward caring for patients with AIDS (Baylor and McDaniel, 1996), for example, was directed by the Ajzen-Fishbein Theory of Reasoned Action (Ajzen and Fishbein, 1980) and past research, and particular attention was paid to substantiating empirically that an individual's intention to act influences the actual behavior. Attitude toward caring for AIDS patients was "assessed using a scale modified from an original instrument by Scherer, Haughey, and Wu (1989)," along five dimensions: "1) fears and concerns relating to caring for AIDS patients, 2) attitudes toward health care utilization by AIDS patients, 3) attitudes toward caring for terminally ill patients, 4) attitudes toward homosexuality, and 5) attitudes of significant others toward AIDS patients." These dimensions were deemed important to establishing therapeutic relationships with AIDS patients.

Theory also guides decision making with regard to subsequent interpretation of research results. In a qualitative study by Badger (1996), her review of the literature provided descrip-

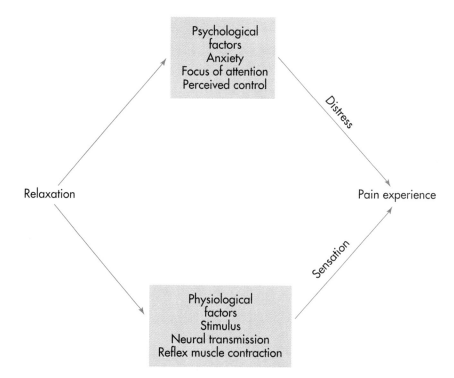

Figure 5-2 Inventory of relationship between relaxation and pain.

tions of the concept of depression as developed and researched by others, as well as research pertaining to family functioning. Through extensive interviews with family members and a data analysis method that identified, refined, and merged categories that formed patterns, she found that "a central or core category that best explained the process of living with a person with depression was . . . family transformations." This inductive clustering of data uncovered a social psychological process whereby "family members move through the three stages of family transformations, all family members are transformed, and family functioning is changed." It also expanded knowledge about depression.

The theoretical framework plays an important role in guiding the entire process of the research study. If the framework is logically sound and substantiated by previous research studies, there is a strong possibility that the predictions or hypotheses evolving from that framework will be supported; however, if hypotheses are not based firmly on a theoretical rationale, there can be no confidence in the findings. Research consumers must be able to evaluate whether the theoretical framework is consistent with the concepts, definitions, and hypotheses stated by the investigator.

HELPFUL HINT

As a research consumer, you might ask the following questions: Is the theoretical rationale explicitly stated? Are the hypotheses explicitly substantiated, that is, are they grounded in the theory? Are the concepts defined and measured in a manner consistent with the theory?

RELATIONSHIP BETWEEN THEORY AND METHOD

Theory also guides the methods used to conduct research. When little is known about a phenomenon, research is usually conducted for the purpose of discovery and exploration of the phenomenon as it occurs in the natural world. At this level of inquiry the researcher may use either inductive or deductive methods to organize the study.

When an investigation is undertaken from the inductive (qualitative) perspective, the relationship between theory and methods proceeds from data collection and content analysis to the discovery of abstract concepts that best capture both the objective and subjective aspects of the phenomenon. As in deductive (quantitative) studies, systematic procedures for data collection and analysis are followed. When the findings are discrepant with what is already known, the investigator reviews the original design and methods for limitations, such as misclassification of the data or other limitations related to the occurrence of the phenomenon.

An example of how the conceptual and research processes of an inductive study reveal the fit between theory and method is demonstrated in the study by Badger (1996). To understand the experiences of individuals who were living with family members who were depressed, the investigator used her experience and current literature to ask the following: "Tell me what it has been like living with your [husband, wife, child] who [is/was] depressed." From these interviews, she developed, then refined "categories into smaller sets of higher level concepts to fit the emerging theory" of family transformations. The theory emerged using grounded theory methodology (see Chapter 9). The exploratory study by Baylor and McDaniel (1996) exemplifies the fit between theory and method using a deductive approach. A review of literature revealed factors that were found to contribute to nurses' attitudes toward caring for patients with AIDS, for example, social stigma, fear of contracting AIDS, and negative attitudes toward homosexual patients. The Ajzen-Fishbein Theory of Reasoned Action (1980) was the basis for understanding these attitudes in relation to behavioral intentions and behavior. If, indeed, attitudes predict behavior, then knowing the attitudes of nurses toward AIDS patients "is essential before developing interventions to affect these attitudes and enhance care" (Baylor and McDaniel, 1996). The survey instrument was used to explore nurses' attitudes in relation to selected demographic characteristics of the nurses and their experience in caring for patients with AIDS. Theory guided instrument modifications and overall methods for data collection.

> **HELPFUL HINT**
> When links between theory and method are made explicit in a research report, it is easier for the research consumer to examine the study for definitional consistency and congruency of the concepts in the theoretical framework with their application or derivation through data collection, analysis, and interpretation of the results.

THEORY—WHAT AND WHOSE

The theoretical frameworks for nursing research studies either come from knowledge developed primarily in other disciplines such as sociology or psychology and borrowed for the purpose of answering nursing questions or are derived from nursing theories. For example, a study by LoBiondo-Wood et al (1997) explored quality of life in liver transplant recipients before and after transplant using a sociological theory of quality of life. The questions asked in the study focused on nursing issues, and the framework was borrowed from another discipline. The contributions made by using borrowed theories are most appropriate when data are specifically made relevant to nursing. Theories unique to nursing help nursing define how it is different from other disciplines. Nursing theories reflect particular views of the person, health, and other concepts that contribute to the development of a body of knowledge specific to nursing's concerns.

Fawcett (1989) defines nursing theory as "a relatively specific and concrete set of concepts and propositions that purports to account for or characterize phenomena of interest to the discipline of nursing." The central phenomena of interest (concern) to nursing are persons, their environment, their health, and nursing itself. Therefore theories that deal with these phenomena are termed *nursing theories*. These phenomena, as stated, are not conceptualized or operationalized.

There are several well-known nursing theorists whose conceptual models have served as a basis for theory development. Among these models are Rogers' (1986) life process interactive person–environment model; King's (1981) model of personal, interpersonal, and social systems; Orem's (1991) model of self-care; Neuman's health care systems model (1988); Johnson's behavioral system model (1980); King's open systems model (1983); and Roy's (1984) adaptation model. Each of these theorists addresses the four phenomena of concern to nursing from a different perspective. For example, Rogers views the person and the environment as energy fields coextensive with the universe, where person-environment interactions are mutual and simultaneous. King, however, views the person and the environment as separate, and interactions as cause and effect processes.

---

x 5-6   Examples of Grand, Middle-Range, and Practice Theories

Grand
Health belief model (Becker, 1974)
Transactional model of stress and coping (Lazarus and Folkman, 1984)
Life process interactive person–environment model (Rogers, 1986)
Roy's adaptation model (Roy, 1984)
Interacting systems conceptual framework (King, 1981)
Self-care conceptual framework (Orem, 1991)

Middle-Range
Theory of self-care deficit (Orem, 1991)
Theory of health promotion (Pender, 1987)
Theory of self-regulation (Leventhal and Johnson, 1983)
Theory of uncertainty in illness (Mishel, 1988)
Theory of acute pain management (Good and Moore, 1996)
Theory of families, children, and chronic illness (Frey, 1993)

Practice
Theory of interpersonal relations (Peplau, 1992)
Theory of representativeness heuristic (Tversky and Kahneman, 1982)
Theory of communicative action (Habermas, 1984)
Theory of clinical reasoning in nursing practice (Tanner et al, 1987)
Theory of end-of-life decision making (Stewart, 1994)

Fawcett and Downs (1986) state that "theories with high precision tend to be narrow in scope; and those with high explanatory power, broad in scope." Broad nursing theories are known as *grand theory* and may be so abstract that they tend to explain everything while at the same time explain nothing. An example of a grand theory is a conceptual model. Theories must therefore be somewhat general and complex, yet encompass a small number of well-defined concepts. These are referred to as "theories of the middle range." It has been suggested by Suppe (1993) that middle-range theory becomes more important than grand theory as a discipline matures, because it is through middle-range theories that substantive knowledge develops to guide practice (Good and Moore, 1996). Examples of grand and middle-range theories appear in Box 5-6. Another type of theory, practice theory, is important to developing a science of nursing practice (Kim, 1994). "A science of nursing practice is, therefore, aimed at providing knowledge about what nurses do in their practice, how they get to do what they do in practice, and what is affected [client outcomes] by what nurses do in their practice" (Kim, 1994). Practice theories can be derived from both nursing and nonnursing middle-range theories. Examples of practice theories appear in Box 5-6.

CRITIQUING THE THEORETICAL FRAMEWORK

The theoretical framework provides the context that clarifies and specifies problems, develops and tests hypotheses, evaluates research findings, and makes generalizations. As research consumers, nurses need to know how to critically appraise the theoretical bases for research (Critiquing Criteria box). The following discussion is intended to assist in this process.

Initially, the research consumer focuses on the concepts being studied. Concepts should clearly reflect the area of investigation; for example, using the general concept of stress when anxiety is more appropriate to the research focus creates difficulties in defining variables and delineating hypotheses. Next, the consumer must evaluate the completeness and appropriateness of the operational definitions of each concept. Once they are defined, it is important to consider whether the variables are examined in general and specifically in the context of the problem under investigation. The literature review is the source of this kind of discussion. Finally, it is important to appraise the instruments used to measure the variables in terms of appropriateness; for example, does the instrument measure the variables as defined and is the instrument consistent with the theoretical framework? How do they hold up when compared with other instruments? Are all of the subparts consistently measuring the same characteristics? Are the instruments maintaining their stability when repeatedly used over time (see Chapter 12)?

A second aspect of appraising the theoretical rationale relates to the interrelationships among concepts (hypotheses). Briefly stated, hypotheses should express precisely and unambiguously the relationships between variables. They should be based on the propositions that arise from the theoretical framework and directly answer the research problem identified early in the report. A more detailed discussion of critiquing hypotheses appears in Chapter 3.

When evaluating the theoretical rationale itself, it is important to examine both the depth and breadth of the literature review. Has the investigator included sufficient information to substantiate the problem and hypothesis, considering a broad range of possibilities? Is there consistency throughout in terms of the philosophical view of phenomena? Are previous studies sufficiently described so that their validity can be determined? Is there a firm basis for linking the variables and determining the direction of the hypotheses? Can the theory be empirically tested? Does the research contribute to the understanding of the phenomena of interest? Are the findings discussed in relation to the theoretical framework? In summary, the research consumer must evaluate whether the theoretical framework or the map led the researcher to the expected findings or destination in a logical and systematic way.

KEY POINTS

- It has been demonstrated that knowledge generated through structured approaches is more likely to be valid than that which is arrived at through intuition, authority, or trial and error.
- The scientific approaches used to generate nursing knowledge reflect both inductive and deductive conceptualizations of phenomena.
- Theories help to organize the discipline, both in practice and in research endeavors, by providing explanations and making predictive statements about concepts.
- The use of theory is important as a guide to systematically identifying and studying the logical, precise relationships between variables.
- Concept formulation and concept testing are two purposes of nursing research.
- Consistency and congruency in the development and use of nursing concepts and their validation through credible research will contribute to the quality of nursing's scientific base and to the acceptance of new knowledge within the discipline and by other scientists.
- A construct is an image or symbolic representation of an abstract idea that is adapted for a scientific purpose. Constructs help us refine the ideas that form the basis for developing theory.
- To facilitate the process of refinement, constructs must be clearly defined. In addition, operationalization of the definitions serves to delineate the procedures or operations required to measure the construct.
- A theoretical rationale provides a road map or context for examining problems and generating and testing hypotheses. It gives meaning to the problem and study findings by summarizing existing knowledge in the field of inquiry and identifying linkages among concepts.
- Nursing conceptual models provide a context for constructing theories that deal with the central phenomena of concern to nursing, that is, the person, the environment, health, and nursing.
- In developing a theoretical framework for nursing, knowledge may be acquired from other disciplines or directly from nursing. In either case, that knowledge is used to answer specific nursing questions.
- Of significance to the research consumer is the evaluation or critique of the theoretical rationale of a research study. It is important to consider not only the clarity and logic of the theoretical rationale itself but also whether the operational definitions, measurement instruments, and methods of carrying out collection of data about the variables, hypotheses, and findings are consistent with the theory.

CRITICAL THINKING CHALLENGES

Barbara Krainovich-Miller

? You are taking an elective course in advanced pathophysiology. The professor is comparing the knowledge of various disciplines and states that nursing is an example of a nonscientific discipline. She supports this assertion by citing that nursing's knowledge has been generated with unstructured methods such as intuition, trial and error, tradition, and authority. What assumptions have been made by this professor? Would you defend or support her position?

❔ Nurse researchers claim that a theoretical framework is essential for systematically identifying the relationship between the chosen variables. If this is true, why don't nonnursing research studies identify theoretical frameworks?

❔ How would you as a consumer of research use computer databases to verify tools for measuring operational definitions?

❔ How would you argue against the following statement: "As a beginning consumer of research it is ridiculous to expect me to determine if a researcher's study has an appropriate theoretical framework; I only had Nursing Theory 101."

REFERENCES

Ajzen I, Fishbein M: *Understanding attitudes and predicting social behavior,* Englewood Cliffs, NJ, 1980, Prentice Hall.

Badger TA: Family members' experience living with member with depression, *West J Nurs Res* 18:140-171, 1996.

Baylor RA, McDaniel AM: Nurses' attitudes toward caring for patients with acquired immunodeficiency syndrome, *J Prof Nurs* 12:99-105, 1996.

Becker MH: The health belief model and personal health behavior, *Health Educ Monogr* 2:324-473, 1974.

Chinn PL, Kramer MK: *Theory and nursing: a systematic approach,* ed 4, St Louis, 1995, Mosby.

Cole FL, Slocumb EM: Factors influencing safer sexual behaviors in heterosexual late adolescent and young adult collegiate males, *Image J Nurs Sch* 27:217-223, 1995.

Draucker CB, Petrovic K: Healing of adult male survivors of childhood sexual abuse, *Image* 28:325-330, 1996.

Elder JH: In-home communication intervention training for parents of multiply handicapped children, *Sch Inq Nurs Pract* 9:71-92, 1995.

Fawcett J: The "what" of theory development. In *Theory development: what, why, how?* New York, 1989, National League for Nursing.

Fawcett J, Downs FS: *The relationship of theory and research,* Norwalk, Conn, 1986, Appleton-Century-Crofts.

Fisher A: The ethical problems encountered in psychiatric nursing practice with dangerous mentally ill persons, *Sch Inq Nurs Pract* 9:193-208, 1995.

Frey MA: A theoretical perspective of family and child health derived from King's conceptual framework for nursing: a deductive approach to theory building. In Feetham SL et al, eds: *The nursing of families,* Newbury Park, Calif, 1993, Sage.

Good M, Moore SM: Clinical practice guidelines as a new source of middle-range theory: focus on acute pain, *Nurs Outlook* 44:74-79, 1996.

Gross D et al: A longitudinal study of maternal depression and preschool children's mental health, *Nurs Res* 44: 96-101, 1995.

Habermas J: *The theory of communicative action. Volume One: Reason and the rationalization of society,* Boston, 1984, Beacon Press (Translated by T McCarthy).

Hanneman SKG: Multidimensional predictors of success or failure with early weaning from mechanical ventilation after cardiac surgery, *Nurs Res* 43:4-10, 1994.

Hayman LL et al: Nongenetic influences of obesity on risk factors for cardiovascular disease during two phases of development, *Nurs Res* 95 44:277-283, 1995.

Johnson DE: The behavioral system model for nursing. In Riehl JP, Roy C, eds: *Conceptual models for nursing practice,* ed 2, New York, 1980, Appleton-Century-Crofts.

Kerlinger F: *Foundations of behavioral research,* ed 2, New York, 1986, Holt, Rinehart & Winston.

Kim HS: Practice theories in nursing and a science of nursing practice, *Sch Inq Nurs Pract* 8:145-158, 1994.

King IM: King's theory of nursing. In Clements IW, Roberts FB, eds: *Family health: a theoretical approach to nursing,* New York, 1983, John Wiley & Sons.

King T: *A theory for nursing: systems, concepts, process,* New York, 1981, John Wiley & Sons.

Lazarus RS, Folkman S: *Stress, appraisal and coping,* New York, 1984, Springer.

Leventhal H, Johnson JE: Laboratory and field experimentation: development of a theory of self-regulation. In Schmitt M, Skipper J, Leonard R, eds: *Behavioral science and nursing theory,* St Louis, 1983, Mosby.

LoBiondo-Wood G et al: The impact of transplantation on quality of life: a longitudinal perspective, *Appl Nurs Res* 10:27-32, 1997.

McDougall GJ: Metamemory and depression in cognitively impaired elders, *Nurs Res* 44:306-311, 1995.

Minick P: The power of human caring: early recognition of patient problems, *Sch Inq Nurs Pract* 9:303-317, 1995.

Mishel MH: Uncertainty in illness, *Image J Nurs Sch* 20:225-232, 1988.

Neuman BM: The Betty Neuman health care systems model: a total person approach to patient problems. In Riehl JP, Roy C, eds: *Conceptual models of nursing practice,* ed 3, New York, 1988, Appleton-Century-Crofts.

Orem D: *Nursing: concepts of practice,* ed 4, St Louis, 1991, Mosby.

Pender N: *Health promotion in nursing,* ed 2, Norwalk, Conn, 1987, Appleton & Lange.

Peplau HE: Interpersonal relations: a theoretical framework for application in nursing practice, *Nurs Sci Q* 5:13-18, 1992.

Resnick B: Motivation in geriatric rehabilitation, *Image* 28:41-45, 1996.

Rogers ME: Science of unitary human beings. In Malinski VM, ed: *Explorations on Martha E Rogers' science of unitary human beings,* Norwalk, Conn, 1986, Appleton-Century-Crofts.

Roy C: *Introduction to nursing: an adaptation model,* ed 2, Englewood Cliffs, NJ, 1984, Prentice-Hall.

Rudy EB et al: Patient outcomes for the chronically critically ill: special care unit versus intensive care unit, *Nurs Res* 44:324-331, 1995.

Scherer YK, Haughey BP, Wu YB: AIDS: what are nurses' concerns? *Clin Nurs Spec* 3(1):48-54, 1989.

Shiao SPK et al: Nasogastric tube placement: effects on breathing and sucking in very-low-birth-weight infants, *Nurs Res* 44:82-88, 1995.

Stewart BM: End-of-life family decision-making from disclosure of HIV through bereavement, *Sch Inq Nurs Pract* 8:321-352, 1994.

Suppe F: Middle range theories: what they are and why nursing science needs them. Paper presented at the 1982 American Nurses Association/Council of Nurse Researchers Symposium, Washington, 1993.

Tanner C et al: Diagnostic reasoning strategies of nurses and nursing students, *Nurs Res* 36:359-363, 1987.

Taversky A, Kahneman D: Judgements of and by representativeness. In Kahneman D, Slovic P, Tversky A, eds: *Judgement under uncertainty: heuristics and biases,* Cambridge, 1982, Cambridge University Press.

Thomas SB, Gilliam AG, Iwrey CG: Knowledge about AIDS and reported risk behaviors among Black college students, *J Am Coll Health* 38:61-66, 1989.

Walker LO, Montgomery E: Maternal identity and role attainment: long-term relations to children's development, *Nurs Res* 43:105-110, 1994.

Ward SE, Berry PE, Misiewicz H: Concerns about analgesics among patients and family caregivers in a hospice setting, *Res Nurs Health* 19:205-211, 1996.

Yoder LH: Staff nurses' career development relationships and self-reports of professionalism, job satisfaction, and intent to stay, *Nurs Res* 44:290-297, 1995.

ADDITIONAL READINGS

Agor WH: *The logic of intuitive decision making,* New York, 1986, Quorum Books.

Cody WK, Mitchell GJ: Parse's theory as a model for practice: the cutting edge, *Adv Nurs Sci* 15(2):52-65, 1992.

Fawcett J: *Analysis and evaluation of conceptual models of nursing,* ed 2, Philadelphia, 1989, FA Davis.

Gortner SR: Nursing values and science: toward a science philosophy, *Image J Nurs Sch* 22:101-105, 1990.

Johnson D: Development of theory: a requisite for nursing as a primary health profession, *Nurs Res* 23:372-377, 1974.

Nicoll L, ed: *Perspectives on nursing theory,* ed 3, Philadelphia, 1996, JB Lippincott.

Phillips LR: *A clinician's guide to the critique and utilization of nursing research,* Norwalk, Conn, 1986, Appleton & Lange.

Rogers ME: Nursing science and the space age, *Nurs Sci Q* 5:1:27-34, 1992.

Silva M: Philosophy, science, theory: interrelationships and implications for nursing research, *Image J Nurs Sch* 9:59-63, 1977.

Silva MC, Rothbart D: An analysis of changing trends in philosophies of science on nursing theory development and testing, *Adv Nurs Sci* 6(2):1-13, 1984.

Strauss A, Corbin J: *Basics of qualitative research: grounded theory, procedures, and techniques,* Newbury Park, Calif, 1990, Sage.

Watson J: *Nursing: human science and human care,* Norwalk, Conn, 1985, Appleton-Century-Crofts.

Introduction to Design

Geri LoBiondo-Wood

Key Terms

constancy
control
control group
experimental group
external validity
extraneous or mediating
  variable
history

homogeneity
instrumentation
internal validity
maturation
mortality
randomization
reactivity
selection bias
testing

Learning Outcomes

After reading this chapter the student should be able to do the following:

- Define research design.
- Identify the purpose of the research design.
- Define control as it affects the research design.
- Compare and contrast the elements that affect control.
- Begin to evaluate what degree of control should be exercised in the design.
- Define internal validity.
- Identify the threats to internal validity.
- Define external validity.
- Identify the conditions that affect external validity.
- Evaluate the design using the critiquing questions.

The word *design* implies the organization of elements into a masterful work of art. In the world of art and fashion, design conjures up images of processes and techniques that are used to express a total concept. When an individual creates, process and form are employed. The form, process, and degree of adherence to structure depend on the aims of the creator. The same can be said of the research process. The research process does not need to be a sterile procedure but one where the researcher develops a masterful work within the limits of a problem and the related theoretical basis. The framework that the researcher creates is the design. When reading a study, the research consumer should be able to recognize that the problem statement, purpose, literature review, theoretical framework, and hypothesis all interrelate with, complement, and assist in the operationalization of the design (Figure 6-1).

Nursing is concerned with a variety of structures that require varying degrees of process and form, such as the provision of quality, cost-effective patient care, staff organization, and student education. When patient care is administered, the nursing process is used. Previous chapters stress the importance of theory and subject matter knowledge. How a researcher structures, implements, or designs a study affects the results of a research project.

For the consumer to understand the implications and the use of research, the central issues in the design of a research project should be understood. This chapter provides an overview of the meaning, purpose, and issues related to quantitative research design, and Chapters 7 and 8 present specific types of designs. Chapter 9 focuses the consumer on the meaning, purpose, issues, and specific types of designs in qualitative research.

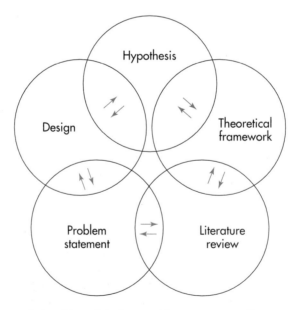

Figure 6-1   Interrelationships of design, problem statement, literature review, theoretical framework, and hypothesis.

PURPOSE OF RESEARCH DESIGN

The purpose of the research design is to provide the plan for answering research problems. The design in quantitative research then becomes the vehicle for hypothesis testing or answering research questions. The design involves a plan, structure, and strategy. These three design concepts guide a researcher in writing the hypothesis or research questions, during the operationalization or the conduct of the project, and in the analysis and evaluation of the data. The overall purpose of the research design is twofold: to aid in the solution of research problems and to maintain control. All research attempts to solve problems. The design coupled with the methods and procedures are the mechanisms for finding solutions to research problems. *Control* is defined as the measures that the researcher uses to hold the conditions of the study uniform and avoid possible impingement of bias on the dependent variable or outcome.

A research example that demonstrates how the design can aid in the solution of a research question and maintain control is the study by Rudy et al (1995; see Appendix C). The purpose of the study was to compare the effects of a low-technology care environment and a nurse case management case delivery system (special care unit [SCU]) with a traditional high-technology environment (intensive care unit [ICU]) and primary nursing care delivery system on patient outcomes such as length of stay, mortality, readmission, complications, satisfaction, and cost. To maintain control the investigators randomly assigned chronically critically ill patients to either the SCU or the ICU. To further maintain control and be eligible for the study, potential subjects had to meet the eligibility criteria, which included a length of stay (LOS) in the ICU of greater than 5 days, not currently receiving intravenous (IV) vasopressors, no pulmonary artery monitor in place, no acute event in the past 3 days, APACHE II 18 or less, TISS class II or III, and unable to be cared for on a general unit. By establishing the specific sample criteria of randomization, subject eligibility, and the use of a control group, the researchers were able to say which care environment would benefit patients the most and could extend this outcome study with further research in this and other clinical areas. A variety of considerations, including the type of design chosen, affect the accomplishment of the study. These considerations include objectivity in the conceptualization of the problem, accuracy, feasibility, control of the experiment, internal validity, and external validity. There are statistical principles behind the many forms of control, but a clear conceptual understanding is of greater importance for the research consumer.

OBJECTIVITY IN THE PROBLEM CONCEPTUALIZATION

Objectivity in the conceptualization of the problem is derived from a review of the literature and development of a theoretical framework (see Figure 6-1). Using the literature the researcher assesses the depth and breadth of available knowledge concerning the problem. The literature review and theoretical framework should demonstrate to the reader that the researcher reviewed the literature with a critical and objective eye (see Chapters 4 and 5), because this affects the type of design chosen. For example, a question regarding the relationship of the length of a breastfeeding teaching program may suggest either a correlational or an experimental design (see Chapters 7 and 8), whereas a question regarding the physical changes in a woman's body during pregnancy and maternal perception of the unborn child may suggest a survey or case study (see Chapters 8 and 9). Therefore the literature review should reflect the following:

- When the problem was studied
- What aspects of the problem were studied
- Where it was investigated
- By whom it was investigated
- The gaps or inconsistencies in the literature

HELPFUL HINT

A review that incorporates the above aspects allows the consumer to judge the objectivity of the problem area and therefore whether the design chosen matches the problem.

ACCURACY

Accuracy in determining the appropriate design is also accomplished through the theoretical framework and review of the literature (see Chapters 4 and 5). Accuracy means that all aspects of a study systematically and logically follow from the problem statement. The beginning researcher is wise to answer a question involving few variables that will not require the use of sophisticated designs. The simplicity of a research project does not render it useless or of a lesser value for practice. Although the project is simple, the researcher should not forego accuracy. The consumer should feel that the investigator used the appropriate type of design to answer the research question with a minimum of contamination. The issues of contamination or control are discussed later in this chapter. Also, many clinical problems have not yet been researched. Therefore, a preliminary or pilot study would be a wise approach. The key is the accuracy, validity, and objectivity used by the researcher in attempting to answer the question. Accordingly, the researcher should read various levels of studies and assess how and if the criteria for each step of the research process were followed. Research consumers will find that many nursing journals publish not only sophisticated clinical research projects but also smaller clinical studies that can be applied to practice.

An example of a preliminary study that investigated a clinical problem was conducted by Hill et al (1996). This study was done to generate hypotheses for future research about the relationship between end stage renal disease (ESRD) and foot complications in people with long-term diabetes. The idea for the study grew from clinical observations about the increasing and pressing nursing needs of ESRD patients with diabetic foot complications. The researchers felt that if a relationship were found between foot complications and ESRD then nursing and medical interventions to decrease the incidence and negative consequences would be important for improving the quality of care provided. Diabetic foot disease and ESRD are two very important comorbid conditions associated with long-term and potentially costly complications. The researchers acknowledge the limitations of the study and the need for future research. Although this study does not give nurses all the data to decide whether these variables are related, it does provide a beginning outcome study of the question and suggests avenues of future inquiry for nursing research and utilization in nursing practice.

FEASIBILITY

When critiquing the research design the evaluator also needs to be aware of the pragmatic consideration of feasibility. Sometimes the reality of this does not truly sink in until one does research. It is important to consider feasibility when reviewing a study, including availability of the subjects, timing of the research, time required for the subjects to participate, costs, and analysis of the data (Table 6-1). These pragmatic considerations are not presented as a step in the research process as are the theoretical framework or methods, but they do affect every step of the process. As such, the reader of a study should consider these when assessing a study. The student researcher may or may not have monies or accessible services. When critiquing a study, note the credentials of the author and whether the investigation was part of a student project or part of a fully funded grant project. If the project was a student project, the standards of critiquing are applied more liberally than for a doctorally prepared, experienced researcher or clinician. Finally, the pragmatic issues raised affect the scope and breadth of an investigation and therefore its generalizability.

CONTROL

A researcher attempts to use a design to maximize the degree of control over the tested variables. Control involves holding the conditions of the study constant and establishing specific sampling criteria as described by Rudy et al (1995). An efficient design can maximize results, decrease errors, and control preexisting conditions that may affect outcome. To accomplish these tasks the research design and methods should demonstrate the researcher's efforts at control.

For example, in a study by Frey (1996) the researcher attempted to examine the relationships between and among general health behavior, illness management behavior, indicators of health, and indicators of illness among several groups of chronically ill youth. The research questions were the following:

- Is general health behavior related to illness management behavior?
- Is general health behavior related to illness outcome?
- Is illness management behavior related to health status?
- Is health status related to illness outcome?

To test these questions and apply control the investigator included in the study children between the ages of 9 and 16 years of age with no major health problems other than insulin-dependent diabetes mellitus (IDDM) or asthma, appropriate grade in school for age, and diagnosed for more than 6 months. This study illustrates how the investigator in one study planned the design to apply controls. Control is important in all designs. When various research designs are critiqued, the issue of control is always raised but with varying levels of flexibility. The issues discussed here will become clearer as you review the various types of designs discussed in later chapters (see Chapters 7 to 9). Control is accomplished by ruling out extraneous or mediating variables that compete with the independent variables as an explanation for a study's outcome. An **extraneous or mediating variable** is one that interferes with the operations of the phenomena being studied, such as age and gender, or as in the previous example of chronically ill youth. Means of controlling extraneous variables include the following:

- Use of a homogeneous sample

Table 6-1

Pragmatic Considerations in Determining Feasibility of a Research Problem

FACTOR	PRAGMATIC CONSIDERATION
Time	The research problem must be one that can be studied within a realistic period of time. All researchers have deadlines for completion of a project. It is essential that the scope of the problem be circumscribed enough to provide ample time for the completion of the entire project. Research studies generally take longer than anticipated to complete.
Subject availability	The researcher needs to determine whether a sufficient number of eligible subjects will be available and willing to participate in the study. If one has a captive audience, like students in a classroom, it may be relatively easy to enlist their cooperation. When a study involves the subjects' independent time and effort, they may be unwilling to participate when there is no apparent reward for doing so. Other potential subjects may have fears about harm or confidentiality and may be suspicious of the research process in general. Subjects with unusual characteristics are often difficult to locate. In general, people are fairly cooperative about participating, but a researcher must consider needing a larger subject pool than will actually participate. At times, when reading a research report the researcher may note how the procedures were liberalized or the number of subjects was altered. This was probably a result of some unforeseen pragmatic consideration.
Facility and equipment availability	All research projects require some kind of equipment. The equipment may be questionnaires, telephones, stationery, stamps, technical equipment, or other apparatus. Most research projects require the availability of some kind of facility. The facility may be a hospital site for data collection or laboratory space or a computer center for data analyses.
Money	Research projects require some expenditure of money. Before embarking on a study the researcher probably itemized the expenses and projected the total cost of the project. This provides a clear picture of the budgetary needs for items like books, stationery, postage, printing, technical equipment, telephone and computer charges, and salaries. These expenses can range from about $100 for a small-scale student project to hundreds of thousands of dollars for a large-scale federally funded project.
Researcher experience	The selection of the research problem should be based on the nurse's realm of experience and interest. It is much easier to develop a research study related to a topic that is either theoretically or experientially familiar. Selecting a problem that is of interest to the researcher is essential for maintaining enthusiasm when the project has its inevitable ups and downs.
Ethics	Research problems that place unethical demands on subjects may not be feasible for study. Researchers must take ethical considerations seriously. The consideration of ethics may affect the choice between an experimental design and a nonexperimental design.

- Use of consistent data collection procedures
- Manipulation of the independent variable
- Randomization

The following example illustrates and defines these concepts:

An investigator might be interested in how a new stop-smoking program (independent variable) affects smoking behavior (dependent variable). The independent variable is assumed to affect the outcome or dependent variable. But the investigator needs to be relatively sure that the decrease in smoking is truly related to the stop-smoking program rather than to some other variable, such as motivation. The design of the research study alone does not inherently provide control. But an appropriately designed study with the necessary controls built in can increase the researcher's ability to answer this research question.

Homogeneous Sampling

In the stop-smoking study, extraneous variables may affect the dependent variable. The characteristics of a study's subjects are common extraneous variables. Age, gender, and even smoking rules may affect the outcome in the stop-smoking example. These variables may therefore affect the outcome, even though they are extraneous or outside of the study's design. As a control for these and other similar problems, the researcher's subjects should demonstrate **homogeneity** or similarity with respect to the extraneous variables relevant to the particular study (see Chapter 10). Extraneous variables are not fixed but need to be reviewed and decided on, based on the study's purpose and theoretical base. By using a sample of homogeneous subjects, the researcher has used a straightforward step of control.

For example, in the study described earlier by Frey (1996), the researcher ensured homogeneity of the sample. The sample was homogenous based on disease states and demographics. This control step limits the generalizability or the application of the outcomes to other populations when analyzing and discussing the outcomes (see Chapter 16). Results can then be generalized only to a similar population of individuals. You may say that this is limiting. This is not necessarily so because no treatment or program may be applicable to all populations and the consumer of research findings needs to take the differences in populations into consideration. In the case of Frey's study (1996) the findings provided information for nursing practice and raised several important questions for specialty practice areas and future research.

 HELPFUL HINT

When reviewing studies remember that it is better to have a "clean" study that can be used to make generalizations about a specific population than a "messy" one that can generalize little or nothing.

If the researcher feels that one of the extraneous variables is important, it may be included in the design. In the smoking example, if individuals are working in an area where smoking is not allowed and this is considered to be important, the researcher could build it into the design and set up a control for it. This can be done by comparing two different work areas—one where smoking is allowed and one where it is not. The important idea to keep in mind is that before the data are collected, the researcher should have identified, planned for, or controlled the important extraneous variables.

Constancy in Data Collection

Another basic, yet critical, component of control is **constancy** in data collection procedures. Constancy refers to the notion that the data collection procedures should reflect to the consumer a cookbooklike recipe of how the researcher controlled the conditions of the study. This means that environmental conditions, timing of data collection, data collection instruments, and data collection procedures used to gain the data are the same for each subject (see Chapters 10 and 12). An example of a well-controlled clinical study was done by Wikblad and Anderson (1995; see Appendix A). The objective of this study was to assess clinical aspects of a semiocclusive hydroactive dressing and an occlusive hydrocolloid dressing in comparison with a conventional absorbent nonocclusive wound dressing in patients undergoing heart surgery. To control conditions, the nurses who made the wound observations were trained to apply and examine the dressings in the same way, wound cultures were obtained on the same postoperative day for all patients, and a color photograph was taken on the same postoperative day and rated by two trained independent raters who were unaware of the experimental conditions. A review of this study shows that data were collected from each subject in the same manner and under the same conditions. This type of control aided the researcher's ability to draw conclusions, discuss, and cite the need for further research in this area. For the consumer it demonstrates a clear, consistent, and specific means of data collection. Another method of ensuring constancy of data collection methods in a study that uses equipment would be to test the equipment for accuracy before and during data collection.

Manipulation of Independent Variable

A third means of control is manipulation of the independent variable. This refers to administration of a program, treatment, or intervention to only one group within the study but not to the other subjects in the study. The first group is known as the **experimental group**, and the other group is known as the **control group.** In a control group the variables under study are held at a constant or comparison level. For example, suppose a researcher wants to study the level of infection rates between a new type of surgical dressing and an old type as in the Wikblad and Anderson's (1995) study. The usual method represents the control group and the new method the experimental groups. Experimental designs use manipulation. Nonexperimental designs do not manipulate the independent variable. This does not decrease the usefulness of a nonexperimental design, but the use of a control group in an experimental design is related to the level of the problem and, again, its theoretical framework.

HELPFUL HINT

Be aware that the lack of manipulation of the independent variable does not mean a weaker study. The level of the problem, the amount of theoretical work, and the research that has preceded a project all affect the researcher's choice of a design. If the problem is amenable to a design that manipulates the independent variable, it increases the power of a researcher to draw conclusions; that is, if all of the considerations of control are equally addressed.

Randomization

Researchers may also choose other forms of control, such as randomization. **Randomization** is used when the required number of subjects from the population is obtained in such a manner that each subject in a population has an equal chance of being selected. Randomization eliminates bias, aids in the attainment of a representative sample, and can be used in various designs (see Chapters 7 and 10). Rudy et al (1995; see Appendix C) used one method of randomization when assigning chronically critically ill patients to type of hospital unit.

Randomization can also be done with paper-and-pencil type instruments. By randomly ordering items on the instruments the investigator can assess if there is a difference in responses that can be related to the order of the items. This may be especially important in longitudinal studies where bias from giving the same instrument to the same subjects on a number of occasions can be a problem (see Chapters 8 and 13).

QUANTITATIVE CONTROL AND FLEXIBILITY

The same level of control cannot be exercised in all types of designs. At times, when a researcher wants to explore an area in which little or no literature on the concept exists, the researcher will probably use an exploratory design. In this type of study the researcher is interested in describing or categorizing a phenomenon in a group of individuals. Rubin's (1967a, 1967b) early work on the development of maternal tasks during pregnancy is an example of exploratory research. In this research she attempted to categorize conceptually the various maternal tasks of pregnancy. Rubin interviewed women throughout their pregnancies and from these extensive interviews developed a framework of the maternal tasks of pregnancy. In critiquing this type of study the issue of control should be applied in a highly flexible manner because of the preliminary nature of the work.

If it is determined from a review of a study that the researcher intended to conduct a correlational study, or a study that looks at the relationship between or among the variables, then the issue of control takes on more importance (see Chapter 8). Control needs to be strictly exercised as much as possible. At this intermediate level of design it should be clear to the reviewer that the researcher considered the extraneous variables that may affect the outcomes.

All aspects of control are strictly applied to studies that use an experimental design (see Chapter 8). The reviewer should be able to locate in the research report how the researcher met the following criteria: the conditions of the research were constant throughout the study, assignment of subjects was random, and an experimental group and control group were utilized. The Wikblad and Anderson study (1995) is an example in which the aspects of control were addressed. Because of the control exercised in the study the reviewer can see that issues related to control were considered and that extraneous variables were addressed.

INTERNAL AND EXTERNAL VALIDITY

When reading research one needs to feel that the results of a study are valid, based on precision, and faithful to what the researcher wanted to measure. For a study to form the basis of further research, practice, and theory development, it must be believable and dependable. There are two important criteria for evaluating the credibility and dependability of the results: internal validity and external validity. Threats to validity are listed in Box 6-1, and discussion follows.

Box 6-1   Threats to Validity

Internal Validity	External Validity
History	Effects of selection
Maturation	Reactive effects
Testing	Effects of testing
Instrumentation	
Mortality	
Selection bias	

Internal Validity

Internal validity asks whether the independent variable really made the difference. This requires the researcher to rule out other factors or threats as rival explanations of the relationship between the variables. There are a number of threats to internal validity, and six of the major threats to internal validity are defined by Campbell and Stanley (1966). These should be considered by the researcher in planning the design and by the consumer before implementing results in practice. The consumer of research should note that the threats to internal validity are most clearly applicable to experimental designs, but attention to those factors that can compromise outcomes should be considered to some degree in all quantitative designs. If these threats are not considered, they could negate the results of the research. How these threats may affect specific designs are addressed in Chapters 7 and 8. Threats to internal validity include history, maturation, testing, instrumentation, mortality, and selection bias.

History

In addition to the independent variable, another specific event that may have an effect on the dependent variable may occur either inside or outside the experimental setting; this is referred to as **history**. For example, in a study of the effects of a breastfeeding teaching program on the length of time of breastfeeding, an event such as government-sponsored advertisements on the importance of breastfeeding featured on television and newspapers may be a threat of history.

Another example may be that of an investigator testing the effects of a breast self-examination teaching program on the incidence of monthly breast self-examination. Concurrently, a famous movie star or news correspondent is diagnosed as having breast cancer. The occurrence of this diagnosis in a public figure engenders a great deal of media and press attention. In the course of the media attention medical experts are interviewed widely and the importance of a breast self-examination is supported. If the researcher finds that breast self-examination behavior is improved, the researcher may not be able to conclude that the change in behavior is the result of the teaching program; it may be the result of the diagnosis given the known figure and the resultant media coverage.

Maturation

Maturation refers to the developmental, biological, or psychological processes that operate within an individual as a function of time and are external to the events of the investigation. For example, suppose one wishes to evaluate the effect of a specific teaching method on baccalaureate students' achievements on a skills test. The investigator would record the students' abilities before and after the teaching method. Between the pretest and posttest the students have grown older and wiser. This growth or change is unrelated to the investigation and may explain differences between the two testing periods rather than the experimental treatment.

The Wikblad and Anderson study (1995; see Appendix A) is an example of how investigators controlled for the possibility of maturation, which in this case would be the processes of normal wound healing. Normal wound healing could have been a factor had the investigators not controlled the conditions of the study as they did (see procedures found in Appendix A, p. 502). Maturation could also occur in a study focused on investigating the relationship between two methods of teaching on children's knowledge of self-care measures. Posttests of student learning would need to be conducted in a relatively short time period after the teaching sessions were completed. A relatively short interval would allow the investigator to conclude that the results were the result of the design of the study and not maturation in a population of children who are learning new skills rapidly.

Testing

Testing is defined as the effect of taking a pretest on the score of a posttest. The effect of taking a pretest may sensitize an individual and improve the score of the posttest. Individuals generally score higher when they take a test a second time regardless of the treatment. The differences between posttest and pretest scores may not be a result of the independent variable but rather of the experience gained through testing.

An example in which testing might have affected the results was in a study conducted by Keefe et al (1996). The purpose of this study was to explore the differences in behavior and mother-infant interaction in infants with irritability or colic and nonirritable infants. The researchers followed a group of mothers and infants over 4 months. The findings revealed differences between the groups. The researchers in their discussion note that "relying on the mothers to provide sufficient and consistent data over time was a challenge." The researchers noted in discussing the results that the bias of repeated measures of pain during labor may have primed the postpartum responses and that the practice of reporting pain repeatedly on the same instrument during labor and memory may have influenced the results.

Instrumentation

Instrumentation threats are changes in the measurement of the variables or observational techniques that may account for changes in the obtained measurement. Flo and Brown (1995) used various types of thermometers (tympanic, oral Diatek, oral mercury-in-glass) to compare accuracy of the tympanic to the other temperature-taking methods. To prevent instrumentation the researchers checked calibration of the thermometers according to the manufacturer's specifications before and after data collection.

Another example that fits into this area is related to techniques of observation. If an investigator has several raters collecting observational data, all must be trained in a similar manner. If they are not similarly trained, a lack of consistency may occur in their ratings and therefore a major threat to internal validity will occur. The study by Wikblad and Anderson (1995; see Appendix A) is an example of a study that trained observers to use the same methods of dressing application, observation, and recording of data for each subject, thereby reducing the risk of instrumentation. At times, even though the researcher takes steps to prevent problems of instrumentation, this threat may still occur. In a study by Lipson (1992) that was designed to explore the health and adjustment processes of Iranian immigrants, the investigator in English and two highly qualified research assistants who were Iranian and therefore spoke Persian conducted semistructured interviews with the study's subjects. The researcher notes that when the interviewer was an Iranian, the subjects described the political nature of their immigration responses to the Iranian interviewers, but when the interviewer was an American, they did not. This is a problem that would be difficult to prevent because of the delicate political circumstances of the immigrants. When a critiquer finds such a threat, it needs to be evaluated within the total context of the study, as, in fact, the researcher did in this study.

Mortality

Mortality is the loss of study subjects from the first data collection point (pretest) to the second data collection point (posttest). If the subjects who remain in the study are not similar to those who dropped out, the results could be affected. In a study of the ways a media campaign affects the incidence of breastfeeding, if most dropouts were nonbreastfeeding women, the perception given could be that exposure to the media campaign increased the number of breastfeeding women, whereas it was the effect of experimental mortality that led to the observed results. A study in which mortality may have influenced the results was conducted by Ziemer, Cooper, and Pigeon (1995). The study evaluated a dressing to reduce nipple pain and improve skin condition in breastfeeding women. The investigators noted a high dropout rate in the study and noted several reasons for the problem such as timing of data collection (all were new mothers) and discomfort of the dressing (discomfort of dressing removal). Even though the dropout rate was high as noted by the researchers the results do provide valuable information on the problem area, the possible use of the dressing and the continued need for more research in the area.

Selection Bias

If the precautions are not used to gain a representative sample, a bias of subjects could result from the way the subjects were chosen. Selection effects are a problem in studies in which the individuals themselves decide whether to participate in a study. Suppose an investigator wishes to assess if a new breastfeeding program contributes to the incidence and length of time of breastfeeding. If the new program is offered to all, chances are that women who are more motivated to learn about breastfeeding will take part in the program. Assessment of the effectiveness of the program is problematic, because the investigator cannot be sure if the new program increased the number of women who breastfed their newborns or if only highly motivated individuals joined the program. The way to avoid **selection bias** in this case is to randomly assign the women to either the new teaching method group or a control group that receives a different type of instruction. In the study by Rudy et al (1995) the researchers controlled for selection bias by establishing selection criteria and by randomly assigning subjects to one of the study groups.

HELPFUL HINT

The list of internal validity threats is not exhaustive. More than one threat can be found in a study depending on the type of study design. Finding a threat to internal validity in a study does not invalidate the results and is usually acknowledged by the investigator in the results or discussion section of the study.

External Validity

External validity deals with possible problems of generalizability of the investigation's findings to additional populations and to other environmental conditions. External validity questions under what conditions and with what types of subjects the same results can be expected to occur. The goal of the researcher is to select a design that maximizes both internal and external validity. This is not always possible; if this is the case, the researcher needs to establish a minimum requirement of meeting the criteria of external validity.

The factors that may affect external validity are related to selection of subjects, study conditions, and type of observations. These factors are termed *effects of selection, reactive effects,* and *effects of testing.* The reader will notice the similarity in names of the factors of selection and testing and those of threats to internal validity. When considering them as internal threats the consumer assesses them as they relate to the independent and dependent variables within the study, and when assessing them as external threats the consumer considers them in terms of the generalizability or use outside the study to other populations and settings. The Critical Thinking Decision Path for threats to validity displays the way threats to internal and external validity can interact with each other. It is important to remember that this path is not exhaustive of the type of threats and their interaction. Problems of internal validity are generally easier to control. Generalizability issues are more difficult to deal with, because it means that the researcher is assuming that other populations are similar to the one being tested. External validity factors include effect of selection, reactivity effects, and effect of testing.

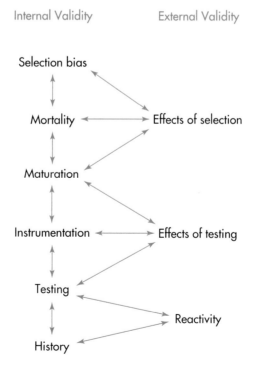

Internal Validity   External Validity

Selection bias

Mortality ←——→ Effects of selection

Maturation

Instrumentation ←——→ Effects of testing

Testing

Reactivity

History

Critical Thinking Decision Path   Threats to study's validity.

Effect of Selection

Selection refers to the generalizability of the results to other populations. An example of the effects of selection occurs when the researcher is not able to attain the ideal sample population. At times, numbers of available subjects may be low or not accessible to the researcher; the researcher may then need to choose a nonprobability method of sampling over a probability method (see Chapter 10). Therefore the type of sampling method utilized and how subjects are assigned to research conditions affect the generalizability to other groups or the external validity.

An example of the effect of selection is depicted with the following example. Koniak-Griffin and Brecht (1995) studied the relationship of sexual risk taking to substance use and acquired immunodeficiency syndrome (AIDS) knowledge in pregnant adolescents and nonpregnant young mothers. The sample consisted of 58 pregnant adolescents and 93 nonpregnant young mothers. The researchers in the discussion of the findings noted the following: "The results of this study must be interpreted with considerations of the study limitations. A convenience sample of moderate size was employed. Therefore, the possibility of self-selection bias influencing the findings must be considered." The investigators also comment on the comparability of their sample to other urban samples in general and on the steps they took to ensure complete anonymity of data collection. These remarks caution the reader but also point out the usefulness of the findings for practice and future research aimed at building the data in this area.

Reactive Effects

Reactivity is defined as the subjects' responses to being studied. Subjects may respond to the investigator not because of the study procedures but merely as an independent response to being studied. This is also known as the *Hawthorne effect,* named after Western Electric Corporation's Hawthorne plant, where a study of working conditions was conducted. The researchers developed several different working conditions (i.e., turning up the lights, piping in music loudly or softly, and changing work hours). They found that no matter what was done, the workers' productivity increased. They concluded that production increased as a result of the workers' knowing that they were being studied rather than because of the experimental conditions.

A threat to internal validity can also be a threat to external validity. An example in which this can be found is the study conducted by Lipson (1992) on the Iranian immigrants. The reaction to the interviewer in this study is a threat to instrumentation and is also reactivity and therefore a threat to the generalizability of the findings. It should be noted that even though this is a problem in the study, the study is excellent because it points out the many needs of immigrants related to health care and to health care providers. Chrisman (1992), a reviewer, noted that the immigrants demonstrated concerns related to language and different ways of expression and explanation of their illnesses. Yet Chrisman notes also that more research in this area is needed so that nurses can better assess and intervene with immigrants. This study is a good example of how a researcher took an interest in a relevant nursing care issue, developed a study to explore the issue, dealt with the real problems of research in the area, and is also developing an area of specialty that will ultimately improve patient care.

Effect of Testing

Administration of a pretest in an experimental situation affects the generalizability of the findings to other populations. Just as pretesting affects the posttest results within a study, pretesting affects the posttest results and generalizability outside the study. For example, suppose a researcher wants to conduct a study with the aim of changing attitudes toward AIDS. To accomplish this an education program on the risk factors for AIDS is incorporated. To test whether the education program changes attitudes toward AIDS, tests are given before and after the teaching intervention. The pretest on attitudes allows the subjects to examine their attitudes regarding AIDS. The subjects' responses on follow-up testing may be different from those of individuals who were given the education program and who did not see the pretest. Also, the study by Keefe et al (1996) is an example of how testing can be both an internal and external validity threat. Therefore, when a study is conducted and a pretest is given, it may prime the subjects and affect their ability to generalize to other situations.

> **HELPFUL HINT**
> When reviewing a study be aware of the internal and external threats to validity. These threats do not make a study useless but actually more useful to you. Recognition of the threats allows researchers to build on data and consumers to think through what part of the study can be applied to practice. Specific threats to validity depend on the type of design and the type of generalizations the researcher hopes to make.

There are other threats to external validity that depend on the type of design and methods of sampling utilized by the researcher, but these are beyond the scope of this text. Detailed coverage of the issues related to internal and external validity is offered by Campbell and Stanley (1966).

CRITIQUING THE RESEARCH DESIGN

Critiquing the design of a study requires one to first have knowledge of the overall implications that the choice of a particular design may have for the study as a whole (Critiquing Criteria box). The concept of the research design is an all-inclusive one that parallels the concept of the theoretical framework. The research design is similar to the theoretical framework in that it deals with a piece of the research study that affects the whole. For one to knowledgeably critique the design in the light of the entire study, it is important to understand the fac-

CRITIQUING CRITERIA

1. Is the type of design employed appropriate?
2. Does the researcher use the various concepts of control that are consistent with the type of design chosen?
3. Does the design used seem to reflect the issues of economy?
4. Does the design used seem to flow from the proposed research problem, theoretical framework, literature review, and hypothesis?
5. What are the threats to internal validity?
6. What are the controls for the threats to internal validity?
7. What are the threats to external validity?
8. What are the controls for the threats to external validity?

tors that influence the choice and the implications of the design. In this chapter the meaning, purpose, and important factors of design choice, as well as the vocabulary that accompanies these factors, have been introduced.

Several criteria for evaluating the design can be drawn from this chapter. One should remember that these criteria are applied differently with various designs. Different application does not mean that the consumer will find a haphazard approach to design. It means that each design has particular criteria that allow the evaluator to classify the design as to type, such as experimental or nonexperimental. These criteria need to be met and addressed in conducting an experiment. The particulars of specific designs are addressed in Chapters 7 and 8. The following discussion pertains primarily to the overall evaluation of a research design.

The research design should reflect that an objective review of the literature and the establishment of a theoretical framework guided the choice of the design. There is no explicit statement regarding this in a research study. A consumer can evaluate this by critiquing the theoretical framework (see Chapter 5) and literature review (see Chapter 4). Is the problem new and not researched extensively? Has a great deal been done on the problem, or is it a new or different way of looking at an old problem? Depending on the level of the problem, certain choices are made by the investigators. Rice, Mullin, and Jarosz (1992) conducted a study to compare the effects of two approaches to teaching postoperative therapeutic exercise (preadmission self-instruction and postadmission instruction by a nurse) to coronary artery bypass graft (CABG) patients on postadmission indicators such as mood state, exercise performance behaviors, teaching time postadmission, analgesia needs, and length of hospitalization. They used theory, their previous research, and others' previous research to design their study and extend the research in this area as objectively and as accurately as possible. The study was intended to build on previous research and fill a gap through replication and extension and to explore the mood of patients, which had not been studied previously.

The consumer should be alert for the means used by investigators to maintain control, such as homogeneity in the sample, consistent data collection procedures, how or if the independent variable was manipulated, and whether randomization was used. As the reader can see in Chapter 7 all of these criteria must be met for an experimental design. As the reader begins to understand the types of designs and levels of research, namely, quasiexperimental and nonexperimental designs such as survey and interrelationship designs, the reader will find that these concepts are applied in varying degrees, or, as in the case of a survey study, the independent variable is not manipulated at all (see Chapter 8). The level of control and its applications presented in Chapters 7 and 8 provide the remaining knowledge to fully critique the aspects of the design in a study.

Once it has been established whether the necessary control or uniformity of conditions has been maintained, the evaluator needs to determine whether the study is believable or valid. The evaluator should ask whether the findings are the result of the variables tested and internally valid or whether there could be another explanation. To assess this aspect the threats to internal validity should be reviewed. If the investigator's study was systematic, was well grounded in theory, and followed the criteria for each of the processes, the reader will probably conclude that the study is internally valid.

In addition, the critical reader needs to know whether a study has external validity or generalizability to other populations or environmental conditions. External validity can be claimed only after internal validity has been established. If the credibility of a study (internal validity) has not been established, a study could not be generalized (external validity) to other populations. Determination of external validity goes hand in hand with the sampling frame (see Chapter 10). If the study is not representative of any one group or phenomena of interest, external validity may be limited or not present at all. The evaluator will find that establishment of internal and external validity needs not only knowledge of the threats to internal and external validity but also a knowledge of the phenomena being studied. A knowledge of the phenomena being studied allows critical judgments to be made regarding the linkage of theories and variables for testing. The critical reader should find that the design follows from the theoretical framework, literature review, problem statement, and hypotheses. The evaluator should feel, on the basis of clinical knowledge and knowledge of the research process, that the investigators in a study are not comparing apples to oranges.

KEY POINTS

- The purpose of the design is to provide the format of a masterful and creative piece of research.
- There are many types of designs. No matter which type of design the researcher uses, the purpose always remains the same.
- The consumer of research should be able to locate within the study a sense of the question that the researcher wished to answer. The question should be proposed with a plan or scheme for the accomplishment of the investigation. Depending on the question, the consumer should be able to recognize the steps taken by the investigator to ensure control.
- The choice of the specific design depends on the nature of the problem. To specify the nature of the problem requires that the design reflects the investigator's attempts to maintain objectivity, accuracy, pragmatic considerations, and, most important, control.
- Control affects not only the outcome of a study but also its future use. The design should also reflect how the investigator attempted to control threats to both internal and external validity.
- Internal validity needs to be established before external validity can be. Both are considered within the sampling structure.
- No matter which design the researcher chooses, it should be evident to the reader that the choice was based on a thorough examination of the problem within a theoretical framework.
- The design, problem statement, literature review, theoretical framework, and hypothesis should all interrelate to demonstrate a woven pattern.
- The choice of the design is affected by pragmatic issues. At times, two different designs may be equally valid for the same problem.

CRITICAL THINKING CHALLENGES
Barbara Krainovich-Miller

- Would you support or refute the following statement: "All research attempts to solve problems"?
- As a consumer of research you recognize that control is an important concept in the issue of research design. You are critiquing an assigned experimental study as part of your "open

book" midterm exam. You cannot determine from what is written how the researchers kept the conditions of the study constant. How would you use computer or other forms of technology to answer your question?

❓ Box 6-1 lists six major threats to the internal validity of an experimental study. Prioritize them and defend the one that you have made the essential or number one threat to address in a study.

❓ This is your first time as a consumer of research that you will be critiquing the research design of an assigned study. Discuss the process you will use. What must you do first?

REFERENCES

Campbell D, Stanley J: *Experimental and quasi-experimental designs for research,* Chicago, 1966, Rand McNally.

Chrisman NJ: Review of the health and adjustment of Iranian immigrants (commentary), *West J Nurs Res* 14:27-28, 1992.

Flo G, Brown M: Comparing three methods of temperature taking: oral mercury-in-glass, oral Diatek, and tympanic First Temp, *Nurs Res* 44:120-122, 1995.

Frey M: Behavioral correlates of health and illness in youths with chronic illness, *Appl Nurs Res* 9:167-176, 1996.

Hill MN et al: Risk of foot complications in long-term diabetic patients with and without ESRD: a preliminary study, *ANNA J* 23:381-388, 1996.

Keefe MR et al: A longitudinal comparison of irritable and nonirritable infants, *Nurs Res* 45:4-9, 1996.

Koniak-Griffin D, Brecht ML: Linkages between sexual risk taking, substance use and AIDS knowledge among pregnant adolescents and young mothers, *Nurs Res* 44:340-346, 1995.

Lipson JG: The health and adjustment of Iranian immigrants, *West J Nurs Res* 14:10-24, 1992.

Rice VH, Mullin MH, Jarosz P: Preadmission self-instruction effects on post-admission and post-operative indicators in CABG patients: partial replication and extension, *Res Nurs Health* 15(4):253-259, 1992.

Rubin R: Attainment of the maternal role: 1. Processes, *Nurs Res* 16:237-245, 1967a.

Rubin R: Attainment of the maternal role: 2. Models and referents, *Nurs Res* 16:342-346, 1967b.

Rudy EB et al: Patient outcomes for the chronically ill: special care unit versus intensive care unit, *Nurs Res* 44:324-331, 1995.

Wikblad K, Anderson B: Comparison of three wound dressings in patients undergoing heart surgery, *Nurs Res* 44:312-316, 1995.

Ziemer MM, Cooper DM, Pigeon JG: Evaluation of a dressing to reduce nipple pain and improve nipple skin condition in breast feeding women, *Nurs Res* 44:347-351, 1995.

ADDITIONAL READINGS

Cook TD, Campbell DT: *Quasi-experimentation: design analysis issues for field settings,* Boston, 1979, Houghton-Mifflin.

Kerlinger FN: *Foundations of behavioral research,* ed 3, New York, 1986, Holt, Rinehart & Winston.

Lipsey MW: *Design sensitivity: statistical power for experimental research,* Newbury Park, 1990, Sage.

Miller DC: *Handbook of research design and social measurement,* ed 5, Newbury Park, 1991, Sage.

Experimental and Quasiexperimental Designs

Margaret Grey

Key Terms

after-only design
after-only
    nonequivalent
    control group
    design
antecedent
    variable
control
dependent variable
design

evaluation research
experiment
experimental
    design
independent
    variable
intervening
    variable
manipulation

nonequivalent
    control group
    design
quasiexperiment
quasiexperimental
    design
randomization
Solomon four-
    group design
time series design
true experiment

Learning Outcomes

After reading this chapter the student should be able to do the following:

- List the criteria necessary for inferring cause-and-effect relationships.
- Distinguish the differences between experimental and quasiexperimental designs.
- Define internal validity problems associated with experimental and quasiexperimental designs.
- Describe the use of experimental and quasiexperimental designs for evaluation research.
- Critically evaluate the findings of selected studies that test cause-and-effect relationships.

One of the fundamental purposes of scientific research in any profession is to determine cause-and-effect relationships. In nursing, for example, we are concerned with developing effective approaches to maintaining and restoring wellness. Testing such nursing interventions to determine how well they actually work—that is, evaluating the outcomes in terms of efficacy and cost-effectiveness—is accomplished by using experimental and quasiexperimental **designs.** These designs differ from nonexperimental designs in one important way: the researcher actively seeks to bring about the desired effect and does not passively observe behaviors or actions. In other words, the researcher is interested in making something happen, not merely observing customary patient care. Experimental and quasiexperimental studies also are important to consider in relation to research utilization. It is the findings of such studies that provide the validation of clinical practice and rationale for changing specific aspects of practice (see Chapter 19).

Experimental designs are particularly suitable for testing cause-and-effect relationships because they help eliminate potential alternative explanations (threats to validity) for the findings. To infer causality requires that the following three criteria be met:

- The causal variable and effect variable must be associated with each other
- The cause must precede the effect
- The relationship must not be explainable by another variable

When the reader critiques studies that use experimental and quasiexperimental designs, the primary focus will be on the validity of the conclusion that the experimental treatment, or the **independent variable,** caused the desired effect on the outcome, or **dependent variable.** The validity of the conclusion depends on just how well the researcher has controlled the other variables that may explain the relationship studied. Thus the focus of this chapter is to explain how the various types of experimental and quasiexperimental designs control extraneous variables.

It should be made clear, however, that most research in nursing is not experimental. This is because nursing, unlike the physical sciences, is still identifying the content and theory that are the exclusive province of nursing science. In addition, an experimental design requires that all of the relevant variables have been defined so that they can be manipulated and studied. In most problem areas in nursing this requirement has not been met. Therefore nonexperimental designs used in identifying variables and determining their relationship to each other often need to be done before experimental studies are performed.

The purpose of this chapter is to acquaint you with the issues involved in interpreting studies that use **experimental design** and **quasiexperimental design.** These designs are listed in Box 7-1. The Critical Thinking Decision Path shows an algorithm that influences a researcher's choice of experimental or quasiexperimental design.

TRUE EXPERIMENTAL DESIGN

An **experiment** is a scientific investigation that makes observations and collects data according to explicit criteria. A **true experiment** has three identifying properties—randomization, control, and manipulation. These properties allow for other explanations of the phenomenon to be ruled out and thereby provide the strength of the design for testing cause-and-effect relationships.

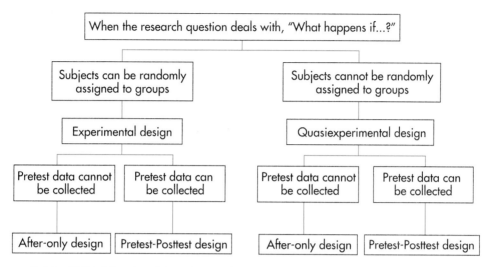

Critical Thinking Decision Path   Experimental and quasiexperimental design.

Box 7-1   Summary of Experimental and Quasiexperimental Research Designs

Experimental Designs
True experiment (pretest-posttest control group) design
Solomon four-group design
After-only design

Quasiexperimental Designs
Nonequivalent control group design
After-only nonequivalent control group design
Time series design

Randomization

Randomization, or random assignment to group, involves the distribution of subjects to either the experimental or control group on a purely random basis. That is, each subject has an equal and known probability of being assigned to any group. Random assignment may be done individually or by groups (Conlon and Anderson, 1990; Rudy et al, 1993). Random assignment to experimental or control groups allows for the elimination of any systematic bias in the groups with respect to attributes that may affect the dependent variable being studied. The procedure for randomization assumes that any important intervening variables will be equally distributed between the groups and, as discussed in Chapter 6, minimizes variance. Note that random assignment to groups is different from random sampling discussed in Chapter 10.

Control

Control means the introduction of one or more constants into the experimental situation. Control is acquired by manipulating the causal or independent variable, by randomly assigning subjects to a group, by very carefully preparing experimental protocols, and by using comparison groups. In experimental research the comparison group is the control group, or the group that receives the usual treatment, rather than the innovative experimental one.

Manipulation

As discussed previously, experimental designs are characterized by the researcher "doing something" to at least some of the involved subjects. This "something," or the independent variable, is manipulated by giving it (the experimental treatment) to some participants in the study and not to others or by giving different amounts of it to different groups. The independent variable might be a treatment, a teaching plan, or a medication. It is the effect of this **manipulation** that is measured to determine the result of the experimental treatment.

The concepts of control, randomization, and manipulation and their application to experimental design are sometimes confusing for students. To see the way these properties allow researchers to have confidence in the causal inferences they make by allowing them to rule out other potential explanations, the use of these properties is examined in one report. Rudy et al (1995) used a clinical randomized experiment to study the effects of a low-technology environment of care and a nurse case management case delivery system (special care unit) with a traditional high-technology environment and primary nursing care delivery system on patient outcomes. Chronically critically ill patients were randomly assigned to one of two groups before the patients or their guardians consented to participation in the study. This means that all of the patients who met the study criteria had an equal chance of being assigned to the control or the experimental group. The use of random assignment to groups helps ensure that the two study groups are comparable on preexisting factors that might affect the outcome of interest, such as gender, age, length of stay in the intensive care unit, and severity of illness. Note that the researchers checked statistically whether the procedure of random assignment did in fact produce groups that are similar.

The two study groups were a special care environment and the traditional intensive care environment. The special care environment was designed to decrease technology and ensure privacy, allow for more interaction with family and friends, ensure continuity of care with nurse case managers working with medical protocols, and create an opportunity for self-directed governance (Rudy et al, 1995; see Appendix C). The degree of control exerted over the experimental conditions is illustrated by the detailed description in the report of the special care program. This helps to ensure that all members of the experimental group receive similar treatment and assists the reader in understanding the nature of the experimental treatment. The control group provides a comparison against which the experimental group can be judged.

In this study, the type of care environment—routine intensive care or the special care unit—was manipulated. Patient outcomes of length of stay, mortality, readmission, complications, satisfaction, and cost were determined for all of the participants.

The use of the experimental design allowed the researchers to rule out many of the potential threats to internal validity of the findings, such as selection, history, and maturation (see

Chapter 6). By exerting clear and careful control over the experimental special care program, the investigators were able to make the assertion that the special care program was effective in decreasing costs and charges to produce a survivor with equivalent clinical outcomes.

The strength of the true experimental design lies in its ability to help the researcher and the reader to control the effects of any extraneous variables that might constitute threats to internal validity. Such extraneous variables can be either antecedent or intervening. The **antecedent variable** occurs before the study but may affect the dependent variable and confuse the results. Factors such as age, gender, socioeconomic status, and health status might be important antecedent variables in nursing research, because they may affect dependent variables such as recovery time and ability to integrate health care behaviors. Antecedent variables that might affect the dependent variables in the study by Rudy et al (1995) might include characteristics of the nursing staff, preexisting health status, and socioeconomic status. Random assignment to groups helps to ensure that groups will be similar on these variables so that differences in the dependent variable may be attributed to the experimental treatment. It should be noted, however, that the researcher should check and report how the groups actually compared on such variables. An **intervening variable** occurs during the course of the study and is not part of the study, but it affects the dependent variable. An example of an intervening variable that might affect the outcomes of this study (Rudy et al, 1995) is a change in health care financing that would lead to sicker patients being admitted to the intensive care unit. Certainly, if care provided to patients changed in any major way while the study was being implemented, the study would be affected.

Types of Experimental Designs

There are several different experimental designs (Campbell and Stanley, 1966). Each is based on the classic design called the *true experiment* diagrammed in Figure 7-1, *A.* In this figure, you will note that subjects have been assigned randomly to the experimental or the control group. The experimental treatment is given only to those in the experimental group, and the pretests and posttests are those measurements of the dependent variables that are made before and after the experimental treatment is performed. All true experimental designs have subjects randomly assigned to groups, have an experimental treatment introduced to some of the subjects, and have the effects of the treatment observed. Designs vary primarily in the number of observations that are made.

As shown, subjects are randomly assigned to the two groups, experimental and control, so that antecedent variables are controlled. Then pretest measures or observations are made so that the researcher has a baseline for determining the effect of the independent variable. The researcher then introduces the experimental variable to one of the groups and measures the dependent variable again to see whether it has changed. The control group gets no experimental treatment but is also measured later for comparison with the experimental group. The degree of difference between the two groups at the end of the study indicates the confidence the researcher has that a causal link exists between the independent and dependent variables. Because random assignment and the control inherent in this design minimize the effects of many threats to internal validity, it is a strong design for testing cause-and-effect relationships. However, the design is not perfect. Some threats cannot be controlled in true experimental studies (see Chapter 6). Mortality effects are often a problem in such studies, because people tend to

Comparison of experimental designs

A True or classic experiment

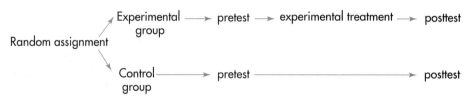

B Solomon four-group design

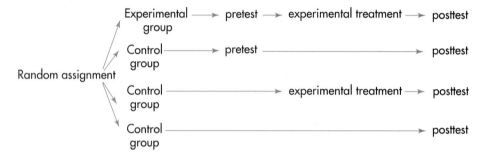

C After-only experimental design

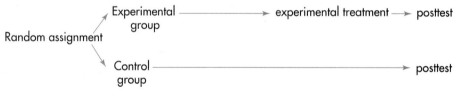

Figure 7-1   Comparison of experimental designs. **A,** True or classic experiment.
B, Solomon four-group design. **C,** After-only experimental design.

drop out of studies that require their participation over an extended period. If there is a difference in the number of people who drop out of the experimental group from that of the control group, a mortality effect might explain the findings. When reading such a work, it is important to examine the sample and the results carefully to see if deaths occurred. Testing is also
a problem in these studies, because the researcher is usually giving the same measurement
twice, and subjects tend to score better the second time just by learning the test. Researchers
can get around this problem in one of two ways: they might use different forms of the same
test for the two measurements, or they might use a more complex experimental design called
the *Solomon four-group design.*

The **Solomon four-group design**, shown in Figure 7-1, *B,* has two groups that are identical to those used in the classic experimental design, plus two additional groups, an experi-

mental after-group and a control after-group. As the diagram shows, all four groups have randomly assigned subjects as in all experimental studies. However, the addition of these last two groups helps to rule out testing threats to internal validity that the before and after groups may experience. Suppose a researcher is interested in the effects of some counseling on chronically ill patients' self-esteem, but just taking a measure of self-esteem may influence how the subjects report themselves. For example, the items might make the subjects think more about how they view themselves so that the next time they fill out the questionnaire, their self-esteem might appear to have improved. In reality, however, their self-esteem may be the same as it was before; it just looks different because they took the test before. The use of this design with the two groups that do not receive the pretest allows for evaluating the effect of the pretest on the posttest in the first two groups. Although this design helps to evaluate the effects of testing, the threat of mortality remains a problem as with the classic experimental design.

Another frequently used experimental design is the **after-only design**, shown in Figure 7-1, *C.* This design, which is sometimes called the *posttest-only control group design,* is composed of two randomly assigned groups, but unlike in the true experimental design, neither group is pretested or measured. Again, the independent variable is introduced to the experimental group and not to the control group. The process of randomly assigning the subjects to groups is assumed to be sufficient to ensure a lack of bias so that the researcher can still determine whether the treatment created significant differences between the two groups. This design is particularly useful when testing effects are expected to be a major problem and the number of available subjects is too limited to use a Solomon four-group design. O'Sullivan and Jacobson (1992) used this design in their study of the impact of a program for adolescent mothers because it was inappropriate to measure infant outcomes before the birth of the infant. They carefully examined the two groups to ensure that the groups were equivalent at baseline, so that they could be assured that random assignment had yielded equivalent groups.

Field and Laboratory Experiments

Experiments also can be classified by setting. Field experiments and laboratory experiments share the properties of control, randomization, and manipulation, and they use the same design characteristics, but they are conducted in various environments. Laboratory experiments take place in an artificial setting that is created specifically for the purpose of research. In the laboratory the researcher has almost total control over the features of the environment, such as temperature, humidity, noise level, and subject conditions. On the other hand, field experiments are exactly what the name implies—experiments that take place in some real, existing social setting such as a hospital or clinic where the phenomenon of interest usually occurs. Because most experiments in the nursing literature are field experiments and control is such an important element in the conducting of experiments, it should be obvious that studies conducted in the field are subject to treatment contamination by factors specific to the setting that the researcher cannot control. However, studies conducted in the laboratory are by nature "artificial," because the setting is created for the purpose of research. Thus laboratory experiments, although stronger in relationship in internal validity questions than field work, suffer more from problems with external validity. For example, a subject's behavior in the laboratory may be quite different from the person's behavior in the real world—a dichotomy that presents problems in generalizing findings from the laboratory to the real world. When research reports are read, then, it is important to consider the setting of the experiment and what impact it might have on the findings of the study.

Consider the study of three different wound dressings in patients undergoing heart surgery (Wikblad and Anderson, 1995). This study could have been done in a laboratory using animals, which would have allowed complete control over the external environment of the study, a variable that might be important in studying wound healing. However, there is no guarantee that the results found in a study in a laboratory would be applicable to cardiac surgery patients in hospital settings, so the study would lose some external validity.

Advantages and Disadvantages of the Experimental Design

As previously discussed, experimental designs are the most appropriate for testing cause-and-effect relationships. This is because of the design's ability to control the experimental situation. Therefore it offers better corroboration than if the independent variable is manipulated in a certain way, in which certain consequences can be expected to ensue. Such studies are important because one of nursing's major research priorities is documenting outcomes to provide a basis for changing or supporting current nursing practice (see Chapter 1). In the study by Rudy et al (1995, see Appendix C), the authors were able to conclude from their study that there were no differences in the length of stay, mortality, or complications in patients in a nurse managed special care unit compared to a traditional intensive care unit. Their study helps to support new methods of providing care to patients. Similarly, in the classic study by Brooten et al (1986), the authors were able to conclude that infants with low birth weight who were discharged early and received follow-up care from nurse specialists had outcomes that were as good as or better than those of infants who received routine care. These studies and others like them allow nurses to anticipate in a scientific manner the outcomes of their actions and provide the basis for effective high-quality care strategies.

Still, experimental designs are not the ones most commonly used. There are several reasons that most nursing research studies are not experimental. First, experimentation assumes that all of the relevant variables involved in a phenomenon have been identified. For many areas of nursing research this simply is not the case, and descriptive studies need to be completed before experimental interventions can be applied. Second, there are some significant disadvantages to these designs.

One problem with an experimental design is that many variables important in predicting outcomes of nursing care are not amenable to experimental manipulation. It is well known that health status varies with age and socioeconomic status. No matter how careful a researcher is, no one can assign subjects randomly by age or a certain level of income. In addition, some variables may be technically manipulable, but their nature may preclude actually doing so. For example, the ethics of a researcher who tried to randomly assign groups for the study of the effects of cigarette smoking and asked the experimental group to smoke two packs of cigarettes a day would be seriously questioned. It is also potentially true that such a study would not work, because nonsmokers randomly assigned to the smoking group would be unlikely to comply with the research task. Thus, sometimes, even when a researcher plans to conduct a true experiment, subjects dropping out of the study or other factors may, in effect, make the study a **quasiexperiment**. This was the case in a study by Gross, Fogg, and Tucker (1995), in which subjects were randomly assigned to either a training program for promoting positive parent child interactions or a comparison group. Because subjects dropped out of the experimental group due to the time involved, the authors treated their study as a quasiexperimental study.

Another problem with experimental designs is that they may be difficult or impractical to perform in field settings. It may be quite different to randomly assign patients on a hospital floor to different groups when they might talk to each other about the different treatments. Experimental procedures may also be disruptive to the usual routine of the setting. If several nurses are involved in administering the experimental program, it may be impossible to ensure that the program is administered in the same way to each subject.

Finally, just the act of being studied may influence the results of a study. This is called the *Hawthorne effect*. As discussed in Chapter 6, this effect means that merely because subjects know that they are subjects in a study, they may answer questions or perform differently.

HELPFUL HINT

Remember that the Hawthorne effect is nearly always a problem in research situations, simply because of the attention being paid to the subjects. The difficulty is in determining when the findings of the study may be applicable to real clinical situations.

Because of these problems in carrying out true experiments, researchers frequently turn to another type of research design to evaluate cause-and-effect relationships. Such designs, because they look like experiments but lack some of the control of the true experimental design, are called *quasiexperiments*.

QUASIEXPERIMENTAL DESIGNS

In a quasiexperimental design full experimental control is not possible. Quasiexperiments are research designs in which the researcher initiates an experimental treatment but some characteristic of a true experiment is lacking. Control may not be possible because of the nature of the independent variable or the nature of the available subjects. Usually what is lacking in a quasiexperimental design is the element of randomization. In other cases the control group may be missing. However, like experiments, quasiexperiments involve the introduction of an experimental treatment.

Compared with the true experimental design, quasiexperiments are similar in their utilization. Both types of designs are used when the researcher is interested in testing cause-and-effect relationships. However, the basic problem with the quasiexperimental approach is a weakened confidence in making causal assertions. Because of the lack of some controls in the research situation, quasiexperimental designs are subject to contamination by many, if not all, of the threats to internal validity discussed in Chapter 6.

HELPFUL HINT

Remember that researchers often make trade-offs and sometimes use a quasiexperimental design instead of an experimental design because it may be pragmatically impossible to randomly assign subjects to groups. Not using the "purest" design does not decrease the value of the study even though it may decrease the utility of the findings.

Types of Quasiexperimental Designs

There are many different quasiexperimental designs. Only the ones most commonly used in nursing research are discussed in this book. Again, the notations introduced earlier in the chapter are used. Refer back to the true experimental design shown in Figure 7-1, *A,* and compare it with the **nonequivalent control group design** shown in Figure 7-2, *A.* Note that this design looks exactly like the true experiment except that subjects are not randomly assigned to groups. Suppose a researcher is interested in the effects of a new diabetes education program on the physical and psychosocial outcome of patients newly diagnosed with diabetes. If conditions were right, the researcher might be able to randomly assign subjects to either the group receiving the new program or the group receiving the usual program, but for any number of reasons, that design might not be possible. For example, nurses on the unit where patients are admitted might be so excited about the new program that they cannot help but include the new information for all patients. So the researcher has two choices—to abandon the experiment or to conduct a quasiexperiment. To conduct a quasiexperiment the researcher might find a similar unit that has not been introduced to the new program and study the newly diagnosed diabetic patients who are admitted to that unit as a comparison group. The study would then involve this type of design.

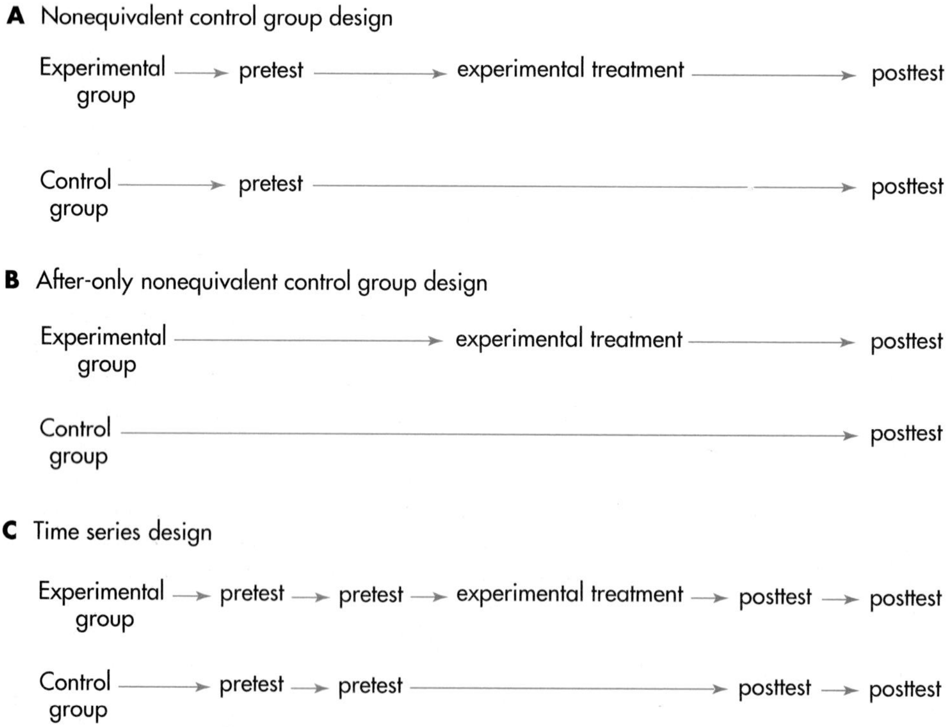

A Nonequivalent control group design

    Experimental ⟶ pretest ⟶ experimental treatment ⟶ posttest
      group

    Control ⟶ pretest ⟶ posttest
      group

B After-only nonequivalent control group design

    Experimental ⟶ experimental treatment ⟶ posttest
      group

    Control ⟶ posttest
      group

C Time series design

    Experimental ⟶ pretest ⟶ pretest ⟶ experimental treatment ⟶ posttest ⟶ posttest
      group

    Control ⟶ pretest ⟶ pretest ⟶ posttest ⟶ posttest
      group

Figure 7-2   Comparison of quasiexperimental designs. **A,** Nonequivalent control group design. **B,** After-only nonequivalent control group design. **C,** Time series design.

Gross, Fogg, and Tucker (1995) used the classic nonequivalent control group design to study the effectiveness of a parent training program for promoting positive parent-child relationships among families of 2-year-old children. Although the study was designed as experimental, a number of families dropped out of the study, so that the groups could not be considered randomly assigned. Nonetheless, the researchers collected data on parental self-efficacy, depression, stress, and perceptions of their toddlers behaviors before and after the intervention was introduced to some of the subjects. They demonstrated that their program led to significant increases in maternal self-efficacy, decreases in maternal stress, and improvements in the quality of mother-toddler interactions. In discussing their findings, the authors carefully note that the differences they found may be due to self-selection of participants in the intervention.

The nonequivalent control group design is commonly used in nursing research studies conducted in field settings. The basic problem with the design is the weakened confidence the researcher can have in assuming that the experimental and comparison groups are similar at the beginning of the study. Threats to internal validity, such as selection, maturation, testing, and mortality, are possible with this design. However, the design is relatively strong, because the gathering of the data at the time of pretest allows the researcher to compare the equivalence of the two groups on important antecedent variables before the independent variable is introduced. In the previous example the motivation of the patients to learn about their diabetes might be important in determining the effect of the new teaching program. The researcher could include in the measures taken at the outset of the study some measure of motivation to learn. Then differences between the two groups on this variable could be tested, and if significant differences existed, they could be controlled statistically in the analysis. Nonetheless the strength of the causal assertions that can be made on the basis of such designs depends on the ability of the researcher to identify and measure or control possible threats to internal validity, as was true in the study by Gross, Fogg, and Tucker (1995).

Now suppose that the researcher did not think to measure the subjects before the introduction of the new treatment (or she or he was tired after the new program began) but later decided that it would be useful to have data demonstrating the effect of the program. Perhaps, for example, a third party asks for such data to determine whether the extra cost of the new teaching program should be paid. Sometimes, the outcomes simply cannot be measured before the intervention, as with prenatal interventions that are expected to impact birth outcomes. The study that could be conducted would look like the **after-only nonequivalent control group design,** shown in Figure 7-2, *B.*

This design is similar to the after-only experimental design, but randomization is not used to assign subjects to groups. This design makes the assumption that the two groups are equivalent and comparable before the introduction of the independent variable. Thus the soundness of the design and the confidence that we can put in the findings depend on the soundness of this assumption of preintervention comparability. Often it is difficult to support the assertion that the two nonrandomly assigned groups are comparable at the outset of the study, because there is no way of assessing its validity. In the example of the teaching program for patients with newly diagnosed diabetes, measuring the subjects' motivation after the teaching program would not tell us whether their motivations differed before they received the program, and it is possible that the teaching program would motivate individuals to learn more about their health problem. Therefore the researcher's conclusion that the teaching program improved physical status and psychosocial outcome would be subject to the alternative conclusion that the results were an effect of preexisting motivations (selection effect) in combination with greater learning in those so motivated (selection-maturation interaction). Nonetheless this design is frequently used in nursing research, because there often are limited opportunities for data collection and because it is particularly useful when testing effects may be problematic. Consider again the example of the experiment conducted by Rudy et al (1995). Suppose that they had not randomly assigned the patients to the special care unit, but rather took all patients before a certain point and assigned them to the control group and then assigned all new patients to the experimental treatment setting. The study would then be an example of an after-only nonequivalent control group design. Had the authors chosen to conduct the study with this design and if they had found the same results, they would have been less confident of the results, because selection and effects may have been stronger.

A study by Archbold et al (1995) used an after-only quasiexperimental design to test the effectiveness of a system of nursing interventions designed to increase preparedness, enrichment, and predictability in families providing care to older people. Due to the nature of the clinical sample, randomization could not always be used to assign families to groups, so a quasiexperimental approach was used. Further, data could not be collected from families until after the home care intervention had begun, so an after-only design was used. The researchers were still able to demonstate that their program led to greater preparedness, enrichment, and predictability than a control group of families receiving routine home health care.

One approach that is used by researchers when only one group is available is to study that group over a longer period. This quasiexperimental design is called a *time series design,* and it is illustrated in Figure 7-2, *C.* Time series designs are useful for determining trends. Keefe et al (1996) studied the differences over time of infants who were irritable versus infants who were nonirritable. Obviously the researcher cannot make infants more or less irritable, but the unwritten hypothesis in the study is that the irritability of the infant affects the maternal-infant relationship. By showing that the trends over time were consistently different, the authors demonstrated that infant irritability affected synchrony in the maternal-child relationship. This study can be considered a quasiexperiment because the authors were interested in determining the effect of irritability on the maternal-infant relationship. However, they could not assign infants to be irritable or nonirritable, so they examined trends over time in both groups.

To rule out some alternative explanations for the findings of a one-group pretest-posttest design, researchers can measure the phenomenon of interest over a longer period and introduce the experimental treatment sometime during the course of the data collection period. Even with the absence of a control group, the broader range of data collection points helps to rule out such threats to validity as history effects. Obviously our problem related to the earlier example of teaching patients with diabetes will not lend itself to this design, because we do not have access to the patients before the diagnosis.

An example of how a time series design would strengthen causal conclusions is provided by Gardner (1991), who compared primary and team nursing by studying units using team nursing and after conversion to primary nursing. Data on quality of care, impact on nursing staff, and cost were collected once before the transition and twice after. There were no comparison units that were not changing, so that there was no control group. It is difficult to be confident that the outcomes described are the result of the change in nursing care delivery rather than the development of the profession or changes in patient mix. If the author had more data from before the transition, showing that there was not a trend, it would strengthen the conclusion that the increased quality of care and decreased cost were caused by the change in nursing delivery systems. The use of a time series design would weaken the alternative explanation that the changes occurred because of something else that happened during the study period. However, the testing threat to validity looms large in these designs, because measures are repeated so many times (see Chapters 6 and 8).

> **HELPFUL HINT**
> One of the reasons replication is so important in nursing research is that so many problems cannot be subjected to experimental methods. Therefore the consistency of findings across many populations helps support a cause-and-effect relationship even when an experiment cannot be conducted.

Advantages and Disadvantages of Quasiexperimental Designs

Given the problems inherent in interpreting the results of studies using quasiexperimental designs, you may be wondering why anyone would use them. Quasiexperimental designs are used frequently because they are practical, feasible, and generalizable. These designs are more adaptable to the real-world practice setting than the controlled experimental designs. In addition, for some hypotheses these designs may be the only way to evaluate the effect of the independent variable of interest.

The weaknesses of the quasiexperimental approach involve mainly the inability to make clear cause-and-effect statements. However, if the researcher can rule out any plausible alternative explanations for the findings, such studies can lead to furthering knowledge about causal relationships. Researchers have several options for ferreting out these alternative explanations. They may control them *a priori* by design or control them statistically, or in some cases, common sense of knowledge of the problem and the population can suggest that a particular explanation is not plausible. Nonetheless it is important to replicate such studies to support the causal assertions developed through the use of quasiexperimental designs.

The literature on cigarette smoking is an excellent example of how findings from many studies, experimental and quasiexperimental, can be linked to establish a causal relationship. A large number of well-controlled experiments with laboratory animals randomly assigned to smoking and nonsmoking conditions have documented that lung disease will develop in smoking animals. Although such evidence is suggestive of a link between smoking and lung disease in humans, it is not directly transferable because animals and humans are different. But we cannot randomly assign humans to smoking and nonsmoking groups for ethical and other reasons. So researchers interested in this problem have to use quasiexperimental data to test their hypotheses about smoking and lung disease. Several different quasiexperimental designs have been used to study this problem, and all had similar results—that there is a causal relationship between cigarette smoking and lung disease. Note that the combination of results from both experimental and quasiexperimental studies led to the conclusion that smoking causes cancer, because the studies together meet the causal criteria of relationship, timing, and lack of an alternative explanation. Nonetheless, the tobacco industry has taken the stand that because the studies on humans are not true experiments, there may be another explanation for the relationships that have been found. For example, they suggest that the tendency to smoke is linked to the tendency for lung disease to develop and smoking is merely an unimportant intervening variable. The reader needs to study the evidence from studies to determine whether the cause-and-effect relationship that is postulated is believable.

EVALUATION RESEARCH AND EXPERIMENTATION

As the science of nursing expands and the cost of health care rises, nurses and others have become increasingly concerned with the ability to document the costs and the benefits of nursing care (see Chapter 1). This is a complex process, but at its heart is the ability to evaluate or measure the outcomes of nursing care. Such studies are usually associated with quality assurance, quality improvement, and evaluation. Studies of evaluation or quality assurance do exactly what the name implies: such studies are concerned with the determination of the quality of nursing and health care and with assurance that the public is receiving high-quality care.

Quality assurance and quality improvement in nursing are in their infancy. Experimentation techniques are just beginning to be applied to the study of the delivery of nursing care. Many early quality assurance studies documented whether nursing care met predetermined standards. The goal of quality improvement studies is to evaluate the effectiveness of nursing interventions and to provide direction for further improvement in the achievement of quality clinical outcomes and cost effectiveness.

Evaluation research is the utilization of scientific research methods and procedures to evaluate a program, treatment, practice, or policy; it uses analytical means to document the worth of an activity. Such research is not a different design. Evaluation research uses both experimental and quasiexperimental designs (as well as nonexperimental) for the purpose of determining the effect or outcomes of a program. Bigman (1961) listed the following purposes and uses of evaluation research:

1. To discover whether and how well the objectives are being fulfilled
2. To determine the reasons for specific successes and failures
3. To direct the course of experiment with techniques for increasing effectiveness
4. To uncover principles underlying a successful program
5. To base further research on the reasons for the relative success of alternative techniques
6. To redefine the means to be used for attaining objectives and to redefine subgoals, in light of research findings

Evaluation studies may be either formative or summative. Formative evaluation refers to assessment of a program as it is being implemented; usually the focus is on evaluation of the process of a program rather than the outcomes. Summative evaluation refers to the assessment of the outcomes of a program that is conducted after completion of the program. An example of a study using both formative and summative evaluation with experimental design is found in the study by McCain et al (1996). The authors studied the effects of a 6-week stress management training program with standard outpatient care for 45 men with the human immunodeficiency virus (HIV) disease. In addition to the summative evaluation, they described the evaluation of the stress-management program as it developed. Data were collected before the interventions and at 6 weeks and 6 months after the intervention. The study by Rudy et al (1995) that evaluated the effectiveness of the nurse special care unit is another example of the experimental design applied to summative evaluation.

The use of experimental and quasiexperimental designs in quality assurance and evaluation studies allows for the determination of not only whether care is adequate but also which method of care is best under certain conditions. Furthermore, such studies can be used to determine whether a particular type of nursing care is cost effective; that is, that the care not only does what it is intended to do but that it also does it at less or equivalent cost. The study by Brooten et al (1986) was very important to nursing, as well as the health care in general, because the authors were able to demonstrate that the intervention was safe and efficacious and that there was a significant cost savings because of early discharge from the hospital with follow-up care by clinical nurse specialists. That model has now been expanded to other clinical areas, such as gerontological nursing (Naylor, 1990). In an era of health care reform and cost containment for health expenditures, it has become increasingly important to evaluate the relative costs and benefits of new programs of care. Relatively few studies in nursing and medicine have done so, but in terms of outcomes, nursing costs and cost savings will be important to future studies.

HELPFUL HINT

Think of quality assurance and quality improvement projects as research-related activities that enhance the ability of nurses to generate cost and quality outcome data. These outcome data contribute to documenting the way nursing practice makes a difference.

CRITIQUING EXPERIMENTAL AND QUASIEXPERIMENTAL DESIGNS

As discussed earlier in the chapter, various designs for research studies differ in the amount of control the researcher has over the antecedent and intervening variables that may impact the results of the study. True experimental designs offer the most possibility for control, and preexperimental designs offer the least. Quasiexperimental designs fall somewhere in between. Research designs must balance the needs for internal validity and external validity to produce useful results. In addition, judicious use of design requires that the chosen design be appropriate to the problem, free of bias, and capable of answering the research question.

Questions that the reader should pose when reading studies that test cause-and-effect relationships are listed in the Critiquing Criteria box. All of these questions should help the reader judge whether it can be confidently believed that a causal relationship exists.

For studies in which either experimental or quasiexperimental designs are used, first try to determine the type of design that was used. Often a statement describing the design of the study appears in the *Abstract* and in the *Methods* sections of the paper. If such a statement is not present, the reader should examine the paper for evidence of the following three characteristics: control, randomization, and manipulation. If all are discussed, the design is probably experimental. On the other hand, if the study involves the administration of an experimental treatment but does not involve the random assignment of subjects to groups, the design is quasiexperimental. Then try to identify which of the various designs within these two types of designs was used. Determining the answer to these questions gives you a head start, because each design has its inherent threats to validity and this step makes it a bit easier to critically evaluate the study. The next question to ask is whether the researcher required a solution to a

CRITIQUING CRITERIA

1. What design is used in the study?
2. Is the design experimental or quasiexperimental?
3. Is the problem one of a cause-and-effect relationship?
4. Is the method used appropriate to the problem?
5. Is the design suited to the setting of the study?

EXPERIMENTAL DESIGNS

1. What experimental design is used in the study, and is it appropriate?
2. How are randomization, control, and manipulation applied?
3. Are there any reasons to believe that there are alternative explanations for the findings?
4. Are all threats to validity, including mortality, addressed in the report?
5. Whether the experiment was conducted in the laboratory or a clinical setting, are the findings generalizable to the larger population of interest?

QUASIEXPERIMENTAL DESIGNS

1. What quasiexperimental design is used in the study, and is it appropriate?
2. What are the most common threats to the validity of the findings of this design?
3. What are the plausible alternative explanations, and have they been addressed?
4. Are the author's explanations of threats to validity acceptable?
5. What does the author say about the limitations of the study?
6. Are there other limitations related to the design that are not mentioned?

EVALUATION RESEARCH

1. Does the study identify a specific problem, practice, policy, or treatment that it will evaluate?
2. Are the outcomes to be evaluated identified?
3. Is the problem analyzed and described?
4. Is the program to be analyzed described and standardized?
5. Is measurement of the degree of change (outcome) that occurs identified?
6. Is there a determination of whether the observed outcome is related to the activity or to some other causes?

cause-and-effect problem. If so, the study is suited to these designs. Finally, think about the conduct of the study in the setting. Is it realistic to think that the study could be conducted in a clinical setting without some contamination?

The most important question to ask yourself as you read experimental studies is, "What else could have happened to explain the findings?" Thus it is important that the author provide adequate accounts of how the procedures for randomization, control, and manipulation were carried out. The paper should include a description of the procedures for random assignment to such a degree that the reader could determine just how likely it was for any one subject to be assigned to a particular group. The description of the independent variable should also be detailed. The inclusion of this information helps the reader decide if it is possible that the treatment given to some subjects in the experimental group might be different from what was given to others in the same group. In addition, threats to validity, such as testing and the occurrence of deaths, should be addressed. Otherwise there is the potential for the findings of the study to be in error and less believable to the reader.

HELPFUL HINT

Remember that mortality is a problem in most experimental studies, because data are usually collected more than once. The researcher should demonstrate that the groups are equivalent when they enter the study and at the final analysis.

This question of potential alternative explanations or threats to internal validity for the findings is even more important when critically evaluating a quasiexperimental study, because quasiexperimental designs cannot possibly control many plausible alternative explanations. A well-written report of a quasiexperimental study will systematically review potential threats to the validity of the findings. Then the reader's work is to decide if the author's explanations make sense.

When critiquing evaluation research, the reader should look for a careful description of the program, policy, procedure, or treatment being evaluated. In addition, the reader may need to determine the design used to evaluate the program and assess the appropriateness of the design for the evaluation. Once the design has been determined, the reader assesses threats to validity for the appropriate design in determining the appropriateness of the authors' conclusions related to the outcomes. As with all research, studies using these designs need to be generalizable to a larger population of people than those actually studied. Thus it is important to decide whether the experimental protocol eliminated some potential subjects and whether this affected not only internal validity but also external validity.

KEY POINTS

- Two types of design commonly used in nursing research to test hypotheses about cause-and-effect relationships are experimental and quasiexperimental designs. Both are useful for the development of nursing knowledge, because they test the effects of nursing actions and lead to the development of prescriptive theory.

- True experiments are characterized by the ability of the researcher to control extraneous variation, to manipulate the independent variable, and to randomly assign subjects to research groups.

- Experiments conducted either in clinical settings or in the laboratory provide the best evidence in support of a causal relationship because the following three criteria can be met: (1) the independent and dependent variables are related to each other, (2) the independent variable chronologically precedes the dependent variable, and (3) the relationship cannot be explained by the presence of a third variable.

- Researchers frequently turn to quasiexperimental designs to test cause-and-effect relationships, because there are many times when experimental designs are impractical or unethical.

- Quasiexperiments may lack either the randomization or comparison group characteristics of true experiments or both of these factors. Their usefulness in studying causal relationships depends on the ability of the researcher to rule out plausible threats to the validity of the findings, such as history, selection, maturation, and testing effects.

- The overall purpose of critiquing such studies is to assess the validity of the findings and to determine whether these findings are worth incorporating into the nurse's personal practice.

CRITICAL THINKING CHALLENGES

Barbara Krainovich-Miller

? Discuss the barriers to nurse researchers meeting the three criteria of a true experimental design.

? How is it possible to have a research design that includes an experimental treatment intervention and a control group yet is not considered a true experimental study?

? Argue your case for supporting or not supporting the following claim, include examples with your reasons: A study that does not use the "purest" design (i.e., true experimental design) does not decrease the value of the study even though it may decrease the utility of the findings.

? How would you use the Internet to determine if your critique of an assigned study is accurate and fair?

REFERENCES

Archbold PG et al: The PREP system of nursing interventions: a pilot test with families caring for older members, *Res Nurs Health* 18:3-18, 1995.

Bigman SK: Evaluating the effectiveness of religious programs, *Rev Relig Res* 2:99-110, 1961.

Brooten D et al: A randomized clinical trial of early hospital discharge and home follow-up of very-low-birth-weight infants, *N Engl J Med* 315:934-939, 1986.

Campbell D, Stanley J: *Experimental and quasiexperimental designs for research,* Chicago, 1966, Rand-McNally.

Conlon M, Anderson GC: Three methods of random assignment: comparison of balance achieved on potentially confounding variables, *Nurs Res* 39(6):376-378, 1990.

Gardner K: A summary of findings of a five-year comparison study of primary and team nursing, *Nurs Res* 40(2):113-117, 1991.

Gross D, Fogg L, Tucker S: The efficacy of parent training for promoting positive parent-toddler relationships, *Res Nurs Health* 18:489-499, 1995.

Keefe MR et al: A longitudinal comparison of irritable and nonirritable infants, *Nurs Res* 45: 4-9, 1996.

McCain NL et al: The influence of stress management training in HIV disease, *Nurs Res* 45:246-253, 1996.

Naylor M: Comprehensive discharge planning for hospitalized elderly: a pilot study, *Nurs Res* 39:156-161, 1990.

O'Sullivan AO, Jacobson BJ: A randomized trial of a health care program for first-time adolescent mothers and their infants, *Nurs Res* 41(4):210-215, 1992.

Rudy EB et al: Permuted block design for randomization in a clinical nursing trial, *Nurs Res* 42:287-289, 1993.

Rudy EB et al: Patient outcomes for the chronically critically ill: special care unit versus intensive care unit, *Nurs Res* 44:324-331, 1995.

Wikblad K, Anderson B: A comparison of three wound dressings in patients undergoing heart surgery, *Nurs Res* 44(5):312-316, 1995.

ADDITIONAL READINGS

Atwood JR, Taylor W: Regression discontinuity design: alternative for nursing research, *Nurs Res* 40(5):312-315, 1991.

Cook TD: The generalization of causal connections: multiple theories in search of clear practice. In Sechrest L, Perrin E, Bunker J, eds: *AHCPR conference proceedings: research methodology: strengthening causal interpretations of nonexperimental data,* Rockville, Md, 1990, Agency for Health Care Policy and Research.

Cook TD, Campbell DT: *Quasi-experimentation: design and analysis issues for field settings,* Chicago, 1979, Rand-McNally.

Given BA et al: Strategies to minimize attrition in longitudinal studies, *Nurs Res* 39(3): 184-186, 1990.

Jacobson BS, Meininger JC: Seeing the importance of blindness, *Nurs Res* 39:54-57, 1990.

Polivka BJ, Nickel JT: Case-control design: an appropriate strategy for nursing research, *Nurs Res* 41:250-253, 1992.

Weinert C, Burman M: Nurturing longitudinal samples, *West J Nurs Res* 18:360-364, 1996.

Nonexperimental Designs

Geri LoBiondo-Wood ■ Judith Haber

Key Terms

correlational study
cross-sectional studies
descriptive/exploratory
   surveys
developmental studies
ex post facto studies
interrelationship/difference
   studies
longitudinal studies

metaanalysis
methodological research
nonexperimental research
   designs
prediction studies
prospective studies
psychometrics
retrospective studies

Learning Outcomes

After reading this chapter the student should be able to do the following:

- Describe the overall purpose of nonexperimental designs.
- Describe the characteristics of descriptive/exploratory survey and interrelationship designs.
- Define the differences between descriptive/exploratory survey and interrelationship designs.
- List the advantages and disadvantages of surveys and each type of interrelationship design.
- Identify methodological and metaanalysis types of research.
- Identify the purposes of methodological and metaanalysis types of research.
- Discuss relational inferences versus causal inferences as they relate to nonexperimental designs.
- Identify the criteria used to critique nonexperimental research designs.
- Apply the critiquing criteria to the evaluation of nonexperimental research designs as they appear in research reports.

onexperimental research designs are used in studies in which the researcher wishes to construct a picture of a phenomenon or explore events, people, or situations as they naturally occur. In experimental research the independent variable is manipulated; in nonexperimental research it is not. In nonexperimental research the independent variables have already occurred, so to speak, and the investigator cannot directly control them by manipulation. Thus in an experimental design the researcher actively manipulates one or more variables, but in a nonexperimental design the researcher explores relationships or differences.

Many phenomena that are of interest and relevant to nursing do not lend themselves to an experimental design. For example, nurses studying pain may be interested in the amount of pain, variations in the amount of pain, and patient responses to postoperative pain. The investigator would not design an experimental study that would potentially intensify a patient's pain just to study the pain experience. Instead, the researcher would examine the factors that contribute to the variability in a patient's postoperative pain experience using a nonexperimental design. Nonexperimental research also requires a clear, concise problem statement that is based on a theoretical framework. Even though the researcher does not actively manipulate the variables, the concepts of control (see Chapter 6) should be considered as much as possible.

Researchers are not in agreement on how to classify nonexperimental studies. For purposes of discussion this chapter will divide nonexperimental designs into descriptive/exploratory survey studies and interrelationship/difference studies as illustrated in Box 8-1. A continuum of quantitative research design is presented in Figure 8-1. These categories are somewhat flexible, and other sources may classify nonexperimental studies in a different way. Some studies fall exclusively within one of these categories, whereas other studies have characteristics of more than one category. This chapter will introduce the various types of nonexperimental designs, the advantages and disadvantages of nonexperimental designs, the use of nonexperimental research, the issues of causality, and the critiquing process as it relates to nonexperimental research. The Critical Thinking Decision Path outlines the path to the choice of a nonexperimental design.

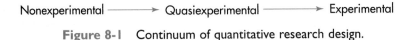

Figure 8-1 Continuum of quantitative research design.

Box 8-1   Summary of Nonexperimental Research Designs

I. Descriptive/exploratory survey studies
II. Interrelationship/difference studies
   A. Correlational studies
   B. Ex post facto studies
   C. Prediction studies
   D. Developmental studies
      1. Cross-sectional and longitudinal studies
      2. Retrospective and prospective studies

DESCRIPTIVE/EXPLORATORY SURVEY STUDIES

The broadest category of nonexperimental designs is the survey study. Survey studies are also further classified as descriptive or exploratory research designs. **Descriptive/exploratory surveys** collect detailed descriptions of existing variables and use the data to justify and assess current conditions and practices or to make more intelligent plans for improving health care practices. The reader of research will find that the terms *exploratory, descriptive,* and *survey* are used either alone, interchangeably, or together to describe the design of a study. Investigators use this design to search for accurate information about the characteristics of particular subjects, groups, institutions, or situations or about the frequency of a phenomenon's occurrence, particularly when little is known about the phenomenon. The types of variables of interest can be classified as opinions, attitudes, or facts. An example of a study whose aim was to explore an opinion or attitude variable was conducted by Grenier, Joseph, and Jaccobi (1996). The purpose of this study was to explore the perceptions and attitudes toward organ procurement in the medical community. Studies such as this provide the basis for further exploration into this area and also for the development of educational programs for nurses and physicians that will promote increased organ donation.

Facts include attributes of individuals that are a function of their membership in society, such as gender, income level, political and religious affiliations, ethnicity, occupation, and educational level. An example of a study that explored facts was conducted by Mullins (1996). The purpose of this study was to identify the nursing behaviors that are perceived as desirable

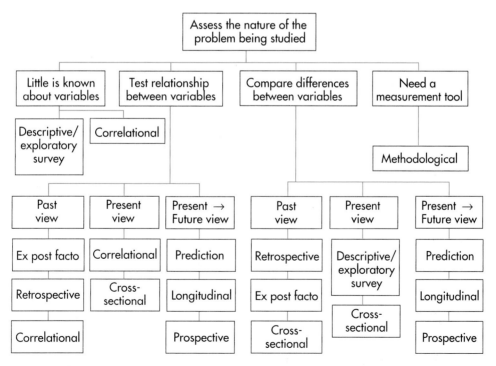

Critical Thinking Decision Path   Nonexperimental design choice.

by persons with acquired immunodeficiency syndrome (AIDS) or human immunodeficiency virus (HIV). The researcher noted that the significance of this study would be to better understand this area due to the physical, social, and economic costs related to the care of AIDS and HIV patients. The researcher conducted the study by surveying 46 subjects with AIDS or HIV from four geographical areas in the southwestern United States. The results provide useful information for nurses caring for patients with AIDS and HIV.

Descriptive/exploratory survey studies are also used to determine differences between variables. An example of a descriptive/exploratory survey that examined differences was conducted by Schneider and LoBiondo-Wood (1992). Appropriate assessment and intervention of children's responses to various health care procedures are important parts of nursing care. An exploratory study was conducted to assess whether there were differences among a group of subjects regarding children's pain perceptions. This study assessed whether children, their parents, and their nurses differ in their perception of pain associated with a health care procedure (immunization). This study, like the two previously discussed, does not manipulate variables but assesses perceptions of children's pain to provide data for future nursing intervention studies.

Data in survey research can be collected by either a questionnaire or an interview (see Chapter 12). Survey researchers study either small or large samples of subjects drawn from defined populations. The sample can be either broad or narrow and can be made up of people or institutions. For example, if a primary care rehabilitation unit based on a case management model were to be established in a hospital, a survey might be taken of the prospective applicants' attitudes with regard to case management before the staff of the unit are selected. In a broader example, if a hospital were contemplating converting all patient care units to a case management model, a survey might be conducted to determine attitudes of a representative sample of nurses in hospital X toward case management. The data might provide the basis for projecting in-service needs of nursing regarding case management. The scope and depth of a survey are a function of the nature of the problem.

In descriptive/exploratory surveys, investigators attempt only to relate one variable to another; they do not attempt to determine causation. There are both advantages and disadvantages of survey research. Two major advantages are that a great deal of information can be obtained from a large population in a fairly economical manner and that survey research information can be surprisingly accurate. If a sample is representative of the population (see Chapter 10), a relatively small number of subjects can provide an accurate picture of the population.

There are several disadvantages of descriptive/exploratory survey studies. First, the information obtained in a survey tends to be superficial. The breadth rather than the depth of the information is emphasized. Second, conducting a survey requires a great deal of expertise in a variety of research areas. The survey investigator must know sampling techniques, questionnaire construction, interviewing, and data analysis to produce a reliable and valid study. Third, large-scale surveys can be time-consuming and costly, although the use of on-site personnel can reduce costs.

HELPFUL HINT

Research consumers should recognize that a well-constructed descriptive/exploratory survey can provide a wealth of data about a particular phenomenon of interest even though relationships between variables are not being examined.

INTERRELATIONSHIP/DIFFERENCE STUDIES

In contrast to survey research, investigators also endeavor to trace the relationships or differences between variables that will provide a deeper insight into a phenomenon. These studies can be classified as **interrelationship/difference studies.** The following types of interrelationship/difference studies will be discussed: correlational studies, ex post facto studies, prediction studies, and developmental studies.

Correlational Studies

In a **correlational study** an investigator uses a correlational design to examine the relationship between two or more variables. The researcher is not testing whether one variable causes another variable or how different one variable is from another variable. The researcher is testing whether the variables covary; that is, as one variable changes, does a related change occur in the other variable? The researcher using this design is interested in quantifying the strength of the relationship between the variables. The positive or negative direction of the relationship is also a central concern (see Chapter 15 for an explanation of the correlation coefficient). For example, Ward, Berry, and Misiewicz (1996; see Appendix D) conducted a correlation study whose purpose was to explore if there was a relationship between the concerns about analgesic use between patients and caregivers in a hospice setting. The researchers noted that patients receiving curative treatment for cancer are concerned with reporting pain and using analgesics and that these concerns are associated with underutilization of analgesics. They also noted the need to extend knowledge about such concerns to the context of palliative care and explore analgesics concerns in hospice patients and their families. Each step of this study was consistent with the aims of exploring a relationship among the variables. The study's findings highlight the need for studying relationships between concerns and usage in both the patient and the caregiver, the need for patient and caregiver education about reporting pain, using analgesics, and the need to include both persons in regard to assessment and intervention.

It should be remembered that the researchers were not testing a cause-and-effect relationship. All that is known is that the researchers found a relationship and that one variable (patient's concerns) varied in a consistent way with another variable (family member's concerns) for the particular sample studied. When reviewing a correlational study remember what relationship the researcher is testing and notice whether the researcher implied a relationship that is consistent with the theoretical framework and hypotheses being tested. Correlational studies offer researchers and research consumers the following advantages:

- An increased flexibility when investigating complex relationships among variables
- An efficient and effective method of collecting a large amount of data about a problem
- A potential for practical application in clinical settings
- A potential foundation for future, experimental research studies
- A framework for exploring the relationship between variables that are inherently not manipulable

The reader will find that the correlational design has a quality of realism and is particularly appealing because it suggests the potential for practical solutions to clinical problems. The following are disadvantages of correlational studies:

- The researcher is unable to manipulate the variables of interest

- The researcher does not employ randomization in the sampling procedures because of dealing with preexisting groups, and therefore generalizability is decreased
- The researcher is unable to determine a causal relationship between the variables because of the lack of manipulation, control, and randomization

One of the most common misuses of a correlational design is the researcher's conclusion that a causal relationship exists between the variables. In the Ward, Berry, and Misiewicz (1996) study the investigators appropriately concluded that a relationship did not exist between the variables, not that patient's concerns did not cause the family member's level of concern. The investigators also appropriately concluded that the ability to generalize from this study is limited by the small homogeneous sample and the fact that a subscale of one of the instruments used did not yield reliable correlations. The study concludes with some very thoughtful recommendations for future studies in this area. This study is a good example of a clinical study that uses a correlational design well. The inability to draw causal statements should not lead the research consumer to conclude that a nonexperimental correlational study uses a weak design. It is a very useful design for clinical research studies, because many of the phenomena of clinical interest are beyond the researcher's ability to manipulate, control, and randomize. For instance, a researcher interested in studying the grief experiences of women who have recently miscarried could not randomly assign subjects to grief and nongrief groups. Also, the experience of a miscarriage is a naturally occurring process and, as such, cannot be manipulated.

Ex Post Facto Studies

When scientists wish to explain causality or the factors that determine the occurrence of events or conditions, they prefer to employ an experimental design. However, they cannot always manipulate the independent variable X or use random assignments. In cases in which experimental designs cannot be employed, **ex post facto studies** may be used. Ex post facto literally means "from after the fact." Ex post facto studies are also known as causal-comparative studies or comparative studies. As we discuss this design further, you will see that many elements of ex post facto research are similar to quasiexperimental designs because they explore differences between variables (Campbell and Stanley, 1963).

In ex post facto studies a researcher hypothesizes, for instance, that X (cigarette smoking) is related to and a determinant of Y (lung cancer), but X, the presumed cause, is not manipulated and subjects are not randomly assigned to groups. Rather, a group of subjects who have experienced X (cigarette smoking) in a normal situation is located and a control group of subjects who have not is chosen. The behavior, performance, or condition (lung tissue) of the two groups is compared to determine whether the exposure to X had the effect predicted by the hypothesis. Table 8-1 illustrates a paradigm for ex post facto design. Examination of Table 8-1 reveals that although cigarette smoking appears to be a determinant of lung cancer, the researcher is still not in a position to conclude that there is a causal relationship between the variables, because there has been no manipulation of the independent variable or random assignment of subjects to groups.

The advantages of the ex post facto design are similar to those in the correlational design. The additional benefit of the ex post facto design is that it offers a higher level of control than

Table 8-1

Paradigm for the Ex Post Facto Design

GROUPS (NOT RANDOMLY ASSIGNED)	INDEPENDENT VARIABLE (NOT MANIPULATED BY INVESTIGATOR)	DEPENDENT VARIABLE
Exposed group: Cigarette smokers	X Cigarette smoking	Y_E Lung cancer
Control group: Nonsmokers		Y_C No lung cancer

a correlational study. For example, in the cigarette smoking study a group of nonsmokers' lung tissue samples are compared with samples of smokers' lung tissue. This comparison enables the researcher to establish that there is a differential effect of cigarette smoking on lung tissue. However, the researcher remains unable to draw a causal linkage between the two variables, and this inability is the major disadvantage of the ex post facto design.

Another disadvantage of ex post facto research is the problem of an alternative hypothesis being the reason for the documented relationship. If the researcher obtains data from two existing groups of subjects, such as one that has been exposed to X and one that has not, and the data support the hypothesis that X is related to Y, the researcher cannot be sure whether X or some extraneous variable is the real cause of the occurrence of Y. Finding naturally occurring groups of subjects who are similar in all respects except for their exposure to the variable of interest is very difficult. There is always the possibility that the groups differ in some other way, such as exposure to some other lung irritants such as asbestos, which can affect the findings of the study and produce spurious results. Consequently, the critiquer of such a study needs to cautiously evaluate the conclusions drawn by the investigator.

Prediction Studies

Researchers at times want to make a forecast or prediction about how patients will respond to an intervention or a disease process or how successful individuals will be in a particular setting or field of specialty. In this case, **prediction studies** are used. For example, in a study conducted by Mills et al (1992), first-time nurse candidates from a 4-year baccalaureate nursing program were examined to identify predictors of success on NCLEX-RN examinations. Retrospective data from student records (e.g., gender, high school GPA, ACT scores, and cumulative GPA for nursing courses) and NCLEX-RN scores reported by the state board of nursing were the data sources. The researchers stated that having this information would enable faculty to recognize students at risk for NCLEX-RN failure. The goal of the study was to identify preexisting characteristics of the individual that were predictive of a relationship to the dependent variable, success on the state board examinations.

In another example, in a study conducted by Failla et al (1996), the researchers studied which demographic and psychosocial variables predicted adjustment in women with systemic lupus erythematosus (SLE). The purpose of this study was to examine the influence of psychosocial variables on the adjustment of women with SLE. The variables selected were those identified within the Adaptation to Chronic Disease Model. The researchers chose SLE because of its incidence (1 in 400 individuals) and because of the limited research on SLE. The Adaptation to Chronic Disease Model was chosen because of its use in studying other chronic diseases. To test the model the researchers used instruments that reflected the psychosocial and demographic variables consistent with the model.

The research consumer will find that prediction studies may also use retrospective data from one group to make predictions about a similar group or test a model for its usefulness. This type of design generally employs sophisticated statistical techniques (see section on "Causality in Nonexperimental Designs"; Chapter 15) when exploring relationships among variables in one group to make predictions about the behavior of another group.

The major advantage of predictive studies is that they facilitate intelligent decision making, because objective criteria are available to guide the process. This can be particularly important in situations where critical choices, such as student selection, are made. The major disadvantage or limitation of prediction studies is that the design does not imply a cause-and-effect relationship between the chosen independent predictor variables and the dependent criterion variable. In addition, if the predictor variables were not chosen with a sound rationale, a study may not be valid.

Developmental Studies

There are also classifications of nonexperimental designs that use a time perspective. Investigators who use **developmental studies** are concerned not only with the existing status and interrelationship of phenomena but also with changes that result from elapsed time. The following four types of developmental study designs will be discussed: cross-sectional, longitudinal, retrospective, and prospective.

Cross-Sectional Studies

Cross-sectional studies examine data at one point in time; that is, the data collected on only one occasion with the same subjects rather than on the same subjects at several points in time. For example, Meleis, Messias, and Arruda (1996) studied the nature of women's work environment as perceived by a group of Brazilian clerical workers. They collected data on only one occasion from a group of clerical and lower administrative position women to explore how women conceptualized their work environment, how they perceived work-related health concerns, and how they coped with the stress of their work environment.

Another cross-sectional study approach is to simultaneously collect data on the variables of interest from different cohort groups. An excellent sample of a cross-sectional study with different age cohort groups is the one conducted by Grey, Cameron, and Thurber (1991). This study focused on comparing the influence of age, coping behavior, and self-care on psychological, social, and physiological adaptation in preadolescents and adolescents with diabetes. Children with insulin-dependent diabetes mellitus between 8 and 18 years of age and their parents participated in the study and filled out several questionnaires at one point in time measuring the study's variables. Differences between preadolescent and adolescent groups were analyzed by dividing the subjects according to Tanner's stages of sexual maturation.

Longitudinal Studies

In contrast to the cross-sectional design, **longitudinal studies** collect data from the same group at different points in time. For instance, the investigator conducting the study with diabetic children could elect to use a longitudinal design. In that case the investigator could collect yearly data or follow the same children over a number of years to compare changes in the variables at different ages. By collecting data from each subject at yearly intervals, a longitudinal perspective of the diabetic process is accomplished. A study by Keefe et al (1996) is an example of a longitudinal study. In this study the researchers followed a group of infants and their mothers for the first four months of the newborn's life to explore the processes of underlying idiopathic irritability or colic and to evaluate the mother-infant interactions during that period. The data collected at the five data collection points allowed the researchers to compare two groups and explore changes in infant behavior and mother-infant interactions.

There are many advantages and disadvantages of both designs. When assessing the appropriateness of a cross-sectional study versus a longitudinal study, the research consumer should first assess what the goal of the researcher was in light of the theoretical framework. In the example of the infant colic study, the researchers were looking at a developmental process; therefore, a longitudinal design seems more appropriate. However, the disadvantages inherent in a longitudinal design must also be considered. Data collection may be of long duration because of the time it takes for the subjects to progress to each data collection point. In the infant colic study it took the researchers between 12 months and 18 months to collect the data from the total sample. Internal validity threats such as testing and mortality are also ever-present and unavoidable in a longitudinal study.

These realities make a longitudinal design costly in terms of time, effort, and money. There is also a chance of confounding variables that could affect the interpretation of the results. Subjects in such a study may respond in a socially desirable way that they believe is congruent with the investigators' expectations (see *Hawthorne Effect* in Chapter 6). However, despite the pragmatic constraints imposed by a longitudinal study, the researcher should proceed with this design if the theoretical framework supports a longitudinal developmental perspective.

The advantages of a longitudinal study are that each subject is followed separately and thereby serves as his or her own control, increased depth of responses can be obtained, and early trends in the data can be investigated. The researcher can assess changes in the variables of interest over time, and both relationships and differences can be explored between variables.

In contrast, cross-sectional studies are less time consuming, less expensive, and thus more manageable for the researcher. Because large amounts of data can be collected at one point, the results are more readily available. In addition, the confounding variable of maturation, resulting from the elapsed time, is not presented. However, the investigator's ability to establish an in-depth developmental assessment of the interrelationships of the phenomena being studied is lessened. Thus the researcher is unable to determine whether the change that occurred is related to the change that was predicted, because the same subjects were not followed over a period of time. In other words, the subjects are unable to serve as their own controls (see Chapter 6). In summary, longitudinal studies begin in the present and end in the future and cross-sectional studies look at a broader perspective of a cross section of the population at a specific point in time.

Retrospective and Prospective Studies

Retrospective studies are essentially the same as ex post facto studies. The term *retrospective* is mainly used by epidemiologists, whereas the term *ex post facto* is preferred by social scientists. In either case, the dependent variable has already been affected by the independent variable, and the investigator attempts to link present events to events that have occurred in the past. An example of a retrospective study is one in which a researcher conducted a retrospective chart review comparing patients who had received heparin with patients who had not received heparin in normal saline injection for maintenance of intermittent intravenous sites to assess efficacy of the two methods for site patency.

The investigator would begin with a theoretical framework that was derived from a systematic retrospective search to identify the factors related to the development of intermittent intravenous site maintenance. The findings of such retrospective studies can provide the basis for further investigation and require additional research information.

In another example of a retrospective study Noedel et al (1996) studied the influence of critical pathways on clinical management, length of hospitalization, and hospital charges. To conduct the study within a retrospective design, the researchers conducted a retrospective review of medical and billing records from 74 consecutive transplantation procedures within a defined time period. Patients were divided into two groups before the pathway institution and after institution. Data were collected from the hospital chart, transplantation chart, hospital billing records, and transplantation database. The parameters that were evaluated were perioperative patient data, donor information, intraoperative and postoperative data, and billing costs. The researchers found that the critical pathway provided for systematic delivery of care and decreased hospitalization stay charges without compromising safety or quality. This is an excellent example of how researchers develop and expand clinical knowledge by conducting studies that can directly contribute to patient care.

Prospective studies explore presumed causes, presumed differences, or presumed relationships and move forward in time to the presumed effect. As such, they are much like longitudinal studies; they start in the present and end in the future. For example, a researcher might want to test the incidence of alcohol consumption during pregnancy in relation to resulting low-birth-weight infants. To test this hypothesis the investigator would draw a sample of pregnant women, some who regularly consumed alcohol during their pregnancy and others who did not. The occurrence of low-birth-weight infants in both groups would then be analyzed. These data would allow the investigator to assess whether regular alcohol consumption during pregnancy was related to the birth weight of the infant.

In another situation a researcher may wish to study the development of a particular health outcome. In this type of study the investigator selects the participants from a population known to be free of the health outcome under study and classifies the participants according to whether they have one or more factors (independent variables) presumably related to the outcome. These participants, who are frequently referred to as a *cohort*, are then studied over a period, ranging from months to years, to determine who develops the health outcome. The Framingham heart study examined the effect of blood pressure, cholesterol levels, smoking, exercise, and other variables on the development of coronary artery disease in a cohort of healthy men. The subjects were studied at specified intervals over a period of years.

An example of a prospective study was conducted by McFarlane, Parker, and Soeken (1996). The aim of this study was to examine the relationship of abuse during pregnancy to acknowledged risk factors for low birth weight and their joint relationship with low birth weight. The first data collection was at the woman's first prenatal visit, and all subjects were reinterviewed during subsequent visits. Therefore, data were collected from each subject over time.

HELPFUL HINT
When reading research reports the reader will note that at times researchers classify study design with more than one design type label. This is correct, because research studies often reflect aspects of more than one design label.

Prospective studies are less common than retrospective studies. This may be explained by the fact that it can take a long time for the phenomenon of interest to become evident in a prospective study. For example, if researchers were studying pregnant women who regularly consume alcohol, it would take 9 months for the effect of low birth weight in the subjects' infants to become evident. The problems inherent in a prospective study are therefore similar to those of a longitudinal study. However, prospective studies are considered to be stronger than retrospective studies because of the degree of control that can be imposed on extraneous variables that might confound the data.

HELPFUL HINT
Remember that nonexperimental designs can test relationships, differences, comparisons, or predictions depending on the purpose of the study.

CAUSALITY IN NONEXPERIMENTAL RESEARCH

A concern of researchers and research consumers is the issue of causality. Researchers are interested in explaining cause-and-effect relationships. Historically researchers have said that only experimental research can support the concept of causality. For example, nurses are interested in discovering what causes anxiety in many settings. If we can uncover the causes, we could perhaps develop interventions that would prevent or decrease the anxiety. Causality makes it necessary to order events chronologically; that is, if we find in a randomly assigned experiment that event 1 (stress) occurs before event 2 (anxiety) and that those in the stressed group were anxious whereas those in the unstressed group were not anxious, we can say that the hypothesis of stress causing anxiety is supported by these empirical observations. If these results were found in a nonexperimental study where some subjects underwent the stress of surgery and were anxious and others did not have surgery and were not anxious, we would say that there is an association or relationship between stress (surgery) and anxiety. But on the basis of the results of a nonexperimental study we could say that the stress of surgery caused the anxiety.

There are also many variables like anxiety that nurse researchers wish to study that cannot be manipulated, nor would it be wise to try to manipulate them. Yet there is a need to have studies that can assert a causal sequence; in light of this need, many nurse researchers are using several analytical techniques that can explain the relationships among variables to establish causal links. These techniques are called *causal modeling* and *associated causal analysis techniques* (Aaronson, Frey, and Boyd, 1988; Asher, 1983; Boyd, Frey, and Aaronson, 1988; Ferketich and Verran, 1984; Verran and Ferketich, 1984). The reader of research will also find the terms *path analysis, LISREL, analysis of covariance structures,* and *structural equation mod-*

eling (SEM) used to describe these techniques (Pedhazur and Schmelkin, 1991). An example of a study that used causal modeling was conducted by Diorio, Hennessy, and Manteuffel (1996). In this study the researchers studied the role of social support, self-efficacy, outcome expectancy, and anxiety as predictors of medication management in persons with epilepsy. The researchers developed and tested a model based on social cognitive theory. To accomplish a test of the model the researchers had the subjects respond to a number of questionnaires that corresponded to the variables in the model. The study results have led to an increased understanding of the components of medication practices and will assist in the development of epilepsy self-management programs. The researchers' recommendations of further research also point to the fact that no matter which type of design or which statistical procedure is used, there is a need for future testing and refinement of the principles that guide nursing care.

A full description of the techniques and principles of causal modeling is beyond the scope of this text. A review of the additional references will provide the reader with the basic assumptions and principles of these techniques.

HELPFUL HINT

Nonexperimental clinical research studies have progressed to the point where prediction models are used to explore or test relationships between independent and dependent variables.

ADDITIONAL TYPES OF DESIGNS

Other types of designs that complement the science of research exist that use a different perspective to collect, analyze, and interpret data. These additional types of designs provide a means of viewing and interpreting phenomena that gives further breadth and knowledge to nursing science and practice. The additional types are *methodological* and *metaanalysis*. **Methodological research** is the development of data collection instruments; **metaanalysis** is the synthesis of research studies in a specific area.

Methodological Research

Methodology is a general term and has many meanings. It may mean different ways of doing research for different purposes, ways of stating hypotheses, methods of data collection and measurement, and techniques of data analysis. As you will find in succeeding chapters (see Chapters 12 and 13), methodology influences research strongly. Methodological research is the controlled investigation of the theoretical and applied aspects of mathematics, statistics, measurement, and the means of gathering and analyzing data (Kerlinger, 1986).

The most significant and critically important aspect of methodological research that is addressed in measurement and statistics is called *psychometrics.* Psychometrics deals with the theory and development of measurement instruments (such as questionnaires) or measurement techniques (such as observational tools) through the research process. Psychometrics thus deals with the measurement of a concept, such as anxiety or interpersonal conflict, with reliable and valid tools (see Chapter 13 for a discussion of reliability and validity). Psychometrics is a critical issue for nurse researchers. In the past 2 decades nurse researchers have used the principles of psychometrics to develop and test measurement instruments that focus on nursing phenomena. Nurse researchers also use instruments developed by other disciplines, such as psychology and sociology. Sound measurement tools are critical to the reliability and validity of a study. Although a study's purpose, problems, and procedures may be clear and the data analysis correct and consistent, if the measurement tool that was used by the researcher has inherent psychometric problems, the findings are rendered questionable or limited.

The main problem for nurse researchers is locating appropriate measurement tools. Many of the phenomena of interest to nursing practice and research are intangible, such as interpersonal conflict, caring, and maternal-fetal attachment. The intangible nature of various phenomena, yet the recognition of the need to measure them, places methodological research in an important position. Methodological research differs from other designs of research. First, it does not include all of the research process steps as discussed in Chapter 2. Second, to implement its techniques the researcher must have a sound knowledge of psychometrics or must consult with a researcher knowledgeable in psychometric techniques. The methodological researcher is not interested in the interrelationship of the independent variable and dependent variable or in the effect of an independent variable on a dependent variable. The methodological researcher is interested in identifying an intangible construct and making it tangible with a paper-and-pencil tool or observation protocol.

Basically a methodological study includes the following steps:

- Defining the construct or behavior to be measured
- Formulating the tool's items
- Developing instructions for users and respondents
- Testing the tool's reliability and validity

These steps require a sound, specific, and exhaustive literature review to identify the theories underlying the construct. The literature review provides the basis of item formulation. Once the items have been developed, the researcher assesses the tool's reliability and validity (see Chapter 13). Various aspects of these procedures may differ according to the tool's use, purpose, and stage of development.

An example of methodological research can be found in the study by Neelon et al (1996). In this study the researchers identified the construct of acute confusion and defined it conceptually and operationally. Common considerations that researchers incorporate into methodological research are outlined in Table 8-2. Many more examples of methodological research can be found in nursing research literature (Frank-Stromberg, 1992; Strickland and Waltz, 1988; Waltz and Strickland, 1988) and many nursing journals. Psychometric or methodological studies are found primarily in journals that report research. One journal, the *Journal of Nursing Measurement,* is devoted to the publication of information on instruments, tools, and approaches for measurement of variables. The specific procedures of methodological research are beyond the scope of this book, but the reader is urged to look closely at the tools used in studies. References of psychometric and methodological research are provided in the "Additional Readings" list in this chapter.

Metaanalysis

Metaanalysis is not a design per se but a research method that takes the results of many studies in a specific area and synthesizes their findings to draw conclusions regarding the state of

Table 8-2

Common Considerations in the Development of Measurement Tools

CONSIDERATION	EXAMPLE
The well-constructed scale, test, interview schedule, or other form of index should consist of an objective, standardized measure of samples of a behavior that has been clearly defined. Observations should be made on a small but carefully chosen sampling of the behavior of interest, thus permitting us to feel confident that the samples are representative.	In their study of acute confusion, Neelon et al (1996) based the tool on clinical bedside observations, clinical consultants, and selected factors that were assessed as being representative of "acute confusion in hospitalized older patients" as it had been defined. The tool was also based on a thorough review of previous theoretical and research literature.
The tool should be *standardized;* that is, a set of uniform items and response possibilities that are uniformly administered and scored.	In the study by Neelon et al (1996) the evaluation of the confusion scale consisted of objective assessment by research nurses in various settings. Without specific criteria and ratings for the observed behaviors, the evaluations would be based on the nurses' subjective impressions, which may have varied significantly between observers and conditions.
The items of a measurement tool should be unambiguous; they should be clear-cut, concise, exact statements with only one idea per item. Negative stems or items with negatively phrased response possibilities result in a double negative and ambiguity in meaning and scoring.	In constructing a tool to measure job satisfaction, a nurse scientist writes the following items, "I never feel that I don't have time to provide good nursing care." The response format consists of "Agree," "Undecided," and "Disagree." It is very likely that a response of "Disagree" will not reflect the respondent's true intent because of the confusion that is created by the double negatives.
The type of items used in any one test or scale should be restricted to a limited number of variations. Subjects who are expected to shift from one kind of item to another may fail to provide a true response as a result of the distraction of making such a change.	Mixing true-or-false items with questions that require a yes-or-no response and items that provide a response format of five possible answers is conducive to a high level of measurement error.
Items should not provide irrelevant clues. Unless carefully constructed, an item may furnish an indication of the expected response or answer. Furthermore the correct answer or expected response to one item should not be given by another item.	An item that provides a clue to the expected answer may contain value words that convey cultural expectations, such as, "A good wife enjoys caring for her home and family."

Table 8-2—cont'd

Common Considerations in the Development of Measurement Tools

CONSIDERATION	EXAMPLE
The items of a measurement tool should not be made difficult by requiring unnecessarily complex or exact operations. Furthermore, the difficulty of an item should be appropriate to the level of the subjects being assessed. Limiting each item to one concept or idea helps to accomplish this objective.	A test constructed to evaluate learning in an introductory course in research methods may contain an item that is inappropriate for the designated group, such as, "A nonlinear transformation of data to linear data is a useful procedure before testing a hypothesis of curvilinearity."
The diagnostic, predictive, or measurement value of a tool depends on the degree to which it serves as an indicator of a relatively broad and significant area of behavior known as the *universe of content* for the behavior. As already emphasized, a behavior must be clearly defined before it can be measured. The definition is developed from the universe of content; that is, the information and research findings that are available for the behavior of interest. The items should reflect that definition. To what extent the test items appear to accomplish this objective is an indication of the validity of the instrument.	Two nurse researchers, A and B, are studying the construct of patient satisfaction. Each has defined this construct in a different way. Consequently, the measurement tool that each nurse devises will include different questions. The questions on each tool will reflect the universe of content for patient satisfaction as defined by each researcher.
The instrument should also adequately cover the defined behavior. The primary consideration is whether the number and nature of items in the sample are adequate. If there are too few items, the accuracy or reliability of the measure must be questioned. In general, there should be a minimum of 10 items for each independent aspect of the behavior of interest.	Very few people would be satisfied with an assessment of such traits as intelligence if the scales were limited to three items.
The measure must prove its worth empirically through tests of reliability and validity.	A researcher should demonstrate to the reader that the scale is accurate and measures what it purports to measure (see Chapter 13).

the art in the area of focus. The synthesis of the data can be accomplished in several different ways (Beck, 1996a; Glass, McGaw, and Smith, 1981; Hunter and Schmidt, 1990). The consumer of research should note that a researcher who conducts a metaanalysis does not conduct the original analysis of data in the area but rather takes the data from already published studies and synthesizes the information by following a set of controlled and systematic steps. Metaanalysis can be used to synthesize both descriptive and experimental research studies (Reynolds et al, 1992). Only recently have studies of this nature become more prevalent in nursing research. An example of a nursing metaanalysis was conducted by Labyak and Metzger (1997). The researchers analyzed the data from nine studies that evaluated the efficacy of massage and its role as a nursing therapy. Labyak and Metzger chose studies in which the physiological effects of back rubs were assessed and used metaanalysis techniques to examine how the findings differed by gender and presence of cardiovascular disease.

Another example of a metaanalysis was conducted by Beck (1996b). This metaanalysis of 17 studies was conducted to determine the strength of the relationship between postpartum depression and infant temperament during the first year of life. The literature is reflecting an increased use of metaanalysis. Studies like the two examples can provide nurses with a synthesis and integration of research findings in an area and provide indicators of future research needs.

CRITIQUING NONEXPERIMENTAL DESIGNS

Criteria for critiquing nonexperimental designs are presented in the Critiquing Criteria box. When critiquing nonexperimental research designs the consumer should keep in mind that such designs offer the researcher the least amount of control. The first step in critiquing nonexperimental research is to determine which type of design was used in the study. Often a statement describing the design of the study appears in the *Abstract* and in the *Methods* section of the report. If such a statement is not present, the reader should closely examine the paper for evidence of which type of design was employed. The reader should be able to discern that either a survey or interrelationship design was used, as well as the specific subtype. For example, the reader would expect an investigation of self-concept development in children from birth to 5 years of age to be an interrelationship study using a longitudinal design.

Next, the critiquer should evaluate the theoretical framework and underpinnings of the study to determine if a nonexperimental design was the most appropriate approach to the problem. For example, many of the studies on pain discussed throughout this text are suggestive of a nonmanipulable interrelationship between pain and any of the independent variables under consideration. As such, a nonexperimental correlational, longitudinal, or cross-sectional design is suggested by these studies. Investigators will use one of these designs to examine the relationship between the variables in naturally occurring groups. Sometimes the reader may think that it would have been more appropriate if the investigators had used an experimental or quasiexperimental design. However, the reader must recognize that pragmatic or ethical considerations may also have guided the researchers in their choice of design (see Chapters 6 and 11).

Then the evaluator should assess whether the problem is at a level of experimental manipulation. Many times researchers merely wish to examine if relationships exist between variables. Therefore when one critiques such studies, the purpose of the study should be deter-

CRITIQUING CRITERIA

1. Which nonexperimental design is utilized in the study?
2. Based on the theoretical framework, is the rationale for the type of design evident?
3. How is the design congruent with the purpose of the study?
4. Is the design appropriate for the research problem?
5. Is the design suited to the data collection methods?
6. Does the researcher present the findings in a manner that is congruent with the utilized design?
7. Does the research go beyond the relational parameters of the findings and erroneously infer cause-and-effect relationships between the variables?
8. Are there any reasons to believe that there are alternative explanations for the findings?
9. Where appropriate, how does the researcher discuss the threats to internal and external validity?
10. How does the author deal with the limitations of the study?

mined. If the purpose of the study does not include describing a cause-and-effect relationship, the researcher should not be criticized for not looking for one. However, the evaluator should be wary of a nonexperimental study in which the researcher suggests a cause-and-effect relationship in the findings.

Finally, the factor(s) that actually influence changes in the dependent variable are often ambiguous in nonexperimental designs. As with all complex phenomena, multiple factors can contribute to variability in the subjects' responses. When an experimental design is not used for controlling some of these extraneous variables that can influence results, the researcher must strive to provide as much control of them as possible within the context of a nonexperimental design. For example, when it has not been possible to randomly assign subjects to treatment groups as an approach to controlling an independent variable, the researcher may use a strategy of matching subjects for identified variables. For example, in a study of infant birth weight, pregnant women could be matched on variables such as weight, height, smoking habits, drug use, and other factors that might influence birth weight. The independent variable of interest, such as the type of prenatal care, would then be the major difference in the groups. The reader would then feel more confident that the only real difference between the two groups was the differential effect of the independent variable, because the other factors in the two groups were theoretically the same. However, the consumer should remember also that there may be other influential variables that were not matched, such as income, education, and diet. Rival factors represent a major influence on the interpretation of a nonexperimental study, because they impose limitations on the generalizability of the results.

If the consumer is critiquing one of the additional types of research discussed, it is important first to identify the type of research used. Once the type of research is identified, its specific purpose and format need to be understood. The format and methods of methodological research and metaanalysis vary; knowing how they vary allows a consumer to assess whether the process was applied appropriately. Some of the basic principles of these methods were presented in this chapter. The specific criteria for evaluating these designs are beyond the scope of this text, but the references provided will assist in this process. Even though the format and methods vary, it is important to remember that all research has a central goal: to answer questions scientifically.

KEY POINTS

- Nonexperimental research designs are used in studies that construct a picture or make an account of events as they naturally occur. The major difference between nonexperimental and experimental research is that in nonexperimental designs the independent variable is not actively manipulated by the investigator.
- Nonexperimental designs can be classified as either survey studies or interrelationship studies.
- Survey studies and interrelationship studies are both descriptive and exploratory in nature.
- Survey research collects detailed descriptions of existing phenomena and uses the data either to justify current conditions and practices or to make more intelligent plans for improving them.
- Interrelationship studies endeavor to explore the interrelationships between variables that provide deeper insight into the phenomena of interest.
- Correlational, ex post facto, prediction, and developmental studies are examples of interrelationship studies. Developmental studies are further broken down into categories of cross-sectional, longitudinal, retrospective, and prospective studies.
- Methodological research and metaanalysis are examples of other means of adding to the body of nursing research. The advantages and disadvantages of each type of design must be considered by the researcher and critiquer when evaluating the merits of nonexperimental design.
- Nonexperimental research designs do not enable the investigator to establish cause-and-effect relationships between the variables. Consumers must be wary of nonexperimental studies that make causal claims about the findings unless a causal modeling technique is used.
- Nonexperimental designs also offer the researcher the least amount of control. Rival factors represent a major influence on the interpretation of a nonexperimental study because they impose limitations on the generalizability of the results and as such should be fully assessed by the critical reader.
- The critiquing process is directed toward evaluating the appropriateness of the selected non-experimental design in relation to factors such as the research problem, theoretical framework, hypothesis, methodology, and data analysis and interpretation.

CRITICAL THINKING CHALLENGES

Barbara Krainovich-Miller

? Discuss which type of nonexperimental design might help to validate the defining characteristics of a particular nursing diagnosis you use in practice. Do you think it is possible to use nurses, as well as patients/clients, as the subjects in this type of study?

? The midterm group (five students) assignment for your research class is to critique an assigned quantitative study. To proceed you must first decide its overall type. You think it is an ex post facto nonexperimental design; the others think it is an experimental design because it has several explicit hypotheses. How would you convince them that you are correct?

❓ You are beginning your senior practicum on a surgical step-down unit. The nurses completed a research-based practice protocol for PCAs, which will be implemented in the near future. What are the advantages and disadvantages to developing a research study to test the effectiveness of this protocol? Discuss whether an experimental or nonexperimental design could be used.

❓ Discuss the reasons for conducting a methodological study and how the researcher's use of the Internet might contribute to implementing such a study.

REFERENCES

Aaronson LS, Frey MA, Boyd CJ: Structural equation models and nursing research: Part II, *Nurs Res* 37:315-318, 1988.

Asher HB: *Causal modeling,* ed 2, Beverly Hills, Calif, 1983, Sage.

Beck CT: Use of a meta-analytic database management system, *Nurs Res* 45:181-184, 1996a.

Beck CT: A meta-analysis of the relationship between postpartum depression and infant temperament, *Nurs Res* 45:225-230, 1996b.

Boyd CJ, Frey MA, Aaronson LS: Structural equation models and nursing research: Part I, *Nurs Res* 37:249-251, 1988.

Campbell DT, Stanley JC: *Experimental and quasi-experimental designs for research,* Chicago, 1963, Rand McNally.

Diorio C, Hennessy M, Manteuffel B: Epilepsy self-management: a test of theoretical model, *Nurs Res* 45:211-217, 1996.

Failla S et al: Adjustment of women with systemic lupus erythematosus, *Appl Nurs Res* 9:87-92, 1996.

Ferketich SL, Verran JA: Residual analysis for causal model assumptions, *West J Nurs Res* 6(1):41-60, 1984.

Frank-Stromberg MF, ed: *Instruments for clinical nursing research,* Boston, 1992, Jones and Bartlett.

Glass G, McGaw B, Smith M: *Meta-analysis in social research,* Newbury Park, Calif, 1981, Sage.

Grenier CE, Joseph AS, Jaccobi LM: Perceptions and attitudes toward organ procurement and transplantation: a medical community survey analysis, *J Transpl Coord* 6:69-74, 1996.

Grey M, Cameron ME, Thurber FW: Coping and adaptation in children with diabetes, *Nurs Res* 40:144-149, 1991.

Hunter JE, Schmidt FL: *Methods of meta-analysis,* Newbury Park, Calif, 1990, Sage.

Keefe MR et al: A longitudinal comparison of irritable and nonirritable infants, *Nurs Res* 45:4-9, 1996.

Kerlinger FH: *Foundations of behavioral research,* ed 3, New York, 1986, Holt, Rinehart & Winston.

Labyak SE, Metzger BL: The effects of effleurage backrub on the physiological components of relaxation: a meta-analysis, *Nurs Res* 46:59-61, 1997.

McFarlane J, Parker B, Soeken K: Abuse during pregnancy: associations with maternal health and infant birth weight, *Nurs Res* 45:37-42, 1996.

Meleis AI, Messias DKH, Arruda EN: Women's work environment and health: clerical workers in Brazil, *Res Nurs Health* 19:53-62, 1996.

Mills AC et al: The odds for success on NCLEX-RN by nurse candidates from a four-year baccalaureate nursing program, *J Nurs Educ* 31(9):403-408, 1992.

Mullins IL: Nursing caring behaviors for persons with acquired immunodeficiency syndrome/human immunodeficiency virus, *Appl Nurs Res* 9:18-23, 1996.

Neelon VJ et al: The NEECHAM confusion scale: construction, validation, and clinical testing, *Nurs Res* 45:324-330, 1996.

Noedel NR et al: Critical pathways as an effective tool to reduce cardiac transplantation hospitalization and charges, *J Transpl Coord* 6:14-19, 1996.

Pedhazur EJ, Schmelkin LP: *Measurement, design, and analysis,* Hillsdale, NJ, 1991, Lawrence Erlbaum Associates.

Reynolds NR et al: Meta-analysis for descriptive research, *Res Nurs Health* 15:467-476, 1992.

Schneider EM, LoBiondo-Wood G: Perceptions of procedural pain: parents, nurses, and children, *Child Health Care* 21:157-162, 1992.

Strickland OL, Waltz CF: *Measurement of nursing outcomes: measuring client outcomes,* vol 1, New York, 1988, Springer.

Verran JA, Ferketich SL: Residual analysis for statistical assumptions of regression equations, *West J Nurs Res* 6(1):27-40, 1984.

Waltz CF, Strickland OL: *Measurement of nursing outcomes: measuring client outcomes,* vol 2, New York, 1988, Springer.

Ward S, Berry PE, Misiewicz H: Concerns about analgesics among patients and family caregivers in a hospice setting, *Res Nurs Health* 19:205-211, 1996.

ADDITIONAL READINGS

Anastasi A: *Psychological testing,* ed 6, New York, 1988, Macmillan.

Creswell JW: *Research design: qualitative & quantitative approaches,* Thousand Oaks, Calif, 1994, Sage.

Miller D: *Handbook of research design and social measurement,* ed 5, Newbury Park, Calif, 1991, Sage.

Minnick A et al: An analysis of posthospitalization telephone survey data, *Nurs Res* 44:371-375, 1995.

Waltz CF, Bausell RB: *Nursing research, design, statistics and computer analysis,* Philadelphia, 1991, FA Davis.

Qualitative Approaches to Research

Marianne Taft Marcus ■ Patricia R. Liehr

Key Terms

axial coding
bracketed
case study method
constant
  comparative
  method
data saturation
domains
emic view
ethnographic
  method

etic view
external criticism
grounded theory
  method
historical research
  method
internal criticism
key informants
life context
lived experience

phenomenological
  method
primary sources
qualitative
  research
secondary sources
symbolic
  interaction
theoretical
  sampling

Learning Outcomes

After reading this chapter the student should be able to do the following:

- Distinguish the characteristics of qualitative research from those of quantitative research.
- Recognize the uses of qualitative research for nursing.
- Identify the processes of phenomenological, grounded theory, ethnographic, and historical methods.
- Recognize nursing phenomena that lend themselves to use of case study methodology.
- Identify research methodology emerging from nursing theory.
- Discuss significant issues that arise in conducting qualitative research in relation to such topics as ethics, criteria for judging scientific rigor, combination of research methods, and use of computers to assist data management.
- Apply the critiquing criteria to evaluate a report of qualitative research.

Nursing is both a science and an art. **Qualitative research** combines the scientific and artistic natures of nursing to enhance understanding of the human health experience. It is a general term encompassing a variety of philosophical underpinnings and research methods. According to Denzin and Lincoln (1994), "qualitative researchers study things in their natural settings, attempting to make sense of, or interpret, phenomena in terms of the meanings people bring to them."

Over recent years, there has been heightened interest in qualitative research methods as recorded by an increasing number of reports of qualitative research in professional nursing journals. A review of four journals, *Advances in Nursing Science, Image, Nursing Research,* and *Research in Nursing and Health,* indicated that from 1988 until 1995, reports of qualitative research doubled. This count included only full research reports (not abstracts or briefs) that were conducted by using inductive strategies and does not conclusively reflect the total amount of qualitative research being done by nurses. It is offered merely as an example of an upward trend in established nursing publications.

This chapter focuses on four qualitative research methods most commonly used by nurses: phenomenological, grounded theory, ethnographic, and historical. Each of these methods, although distinct from the others, also shares characteristics that identify it as a method within the qualitative research approach. Some of the basic tenets distinguishing the qualitative from the quantitative approach are reviewed to establish a foundation before discussing qualitative methodologies. Use of the qualitative approach requires different beliefs, different research activities, and different questions than the use of the quantitative research approach. The Critical Thinking Decision Path diagrams an algorithm that compares the researcher's beliefs, activities, and questions when using the quantitative and qualitative approaches.

QUANTITATIVE AND QUALITATIVE RESEARCH APPROACHES

Beliefs

Chapter 2 introduces the reader to the quantitative approach in nursing research. Quantitative approaches are grounded by beliefs that humans are a composite of many body systems that can be objectively measured, one at a time or in combination. As one reads and critiques quantitative studies, it is often apparent that the researcher has focused on measuring one or more human characteristics (e.g., psychological, physiological, social), striving to isolate the characteristics of interest and gain a clear, context-free picture. A context-free picture is achieved by eliminating or controlling variables that may interfere with the variables being studied.

In contrast, qualitative approaches embrace the wholeness of humans, focusing on human experience in naturalistic settings. The researcher using this approach believes that unique humans attribute meaning to their experiences and experiences evolve from life context. **Life context** is the matrix of human-human-environment relationships emerging over the course of day-to-day living. From this perspective, one person's experience of pain is distinct from another's and can be known by the individual's subjective description of it.

The researcher interested in studying the lived experience of pain for the adolescent with rheumatoid arthritis will spend time in the adolescent's natural settings, such as home and school, to uncover the meaning of pain as it extends beyond the facts of the number of medications taken or a rating on a Likert scale. This approach is grounded in the belief that fac-

If your beliefs are:

| Researcher beliefs | Humans are biopsychosocial beings, known by their biological, psychological, and social characteristics.

Truth is objective reality that can be experienced with the senses and measured by the researcher. | or | Humans are complex beings who attribute unique meaning to their life situations. They are known by their personal expressions.

Truth is the subjective expression of reality as perceived by the participant and shared with the researcher. Truth is context laden. |

then you'll ask questions, such as:

| Example questions | What is the difference in blood pressure and heart rate for adolescents who are angry compared to those who are not angry? | or | What is the structure of the lived experience of anger for adolescents? |

and select approaches:

| Approaches | **Quantitative/deductive** | or | **Qualitative/inductive** |

leading to research activities:

| Research activities | Researcher selects a representative (of population) sample and determines size before collecting data.

Researcher uses an extensive approach to collect data.

Questionnaires and measurement devices are preferably administered in one setting by an unbiased individual to control for extraneous variables.

Primarily deductive analysis is used, generating a numerical summary that allows the researcher to reject or accept the null hypothesis. | or | Researcher selects participants who are experiencing the phenomenon of interest and collects data until saturation is reached.

Researcher uses an intensive approach to collect data.

Researcher conducts interviews and participant or nonparticipant observation in environments where participants usually spend their time. Researcher bias is acknowledged and set aside.

Primarily inductive analysis is used, leading to a narrative summary, which synthesizes participant information, creating a description of human experience. |

Critical Thinking Decision Path   Selecting a research process.

tual objective data do not capture the human experience. Rather, the meaning of the adolescent's pain emerges within the context of personal history, current relationships, and future plans as the individual lives daily life in dynamic interaction with environment. That is, the experience of pain is believed to be a unique personal experience that is context laden.

Research Activities

The activities of the researcher using the quantitative approach are discussed throughout Part Two of this text. The Critical Thinking Decision Path contrasts some of these familiar activities with those used in the qualitative approach. Rather than determining sample size before initiation of the study, data collection is terminated when saturation is reached. **Data saturation** occurs when the information being shared with the researcher becomes repetitive. That is, the ideas conveyed by the participant have been shared before by other participants, and inclusion of additional participants does not result in new ideas. Generally, the number of participants, when using the qualitative approach, is smaller than the number of subjects needed when using the quantitative approach. Fewer subjects are intensively studied (qualitative) as compared with a larger number extensively studied (quantitative).

The research activities of each approach reflect the previously discussed beliefs about the importance of context. Whereas qualitative approaches strive to eliminate extraneous variables, qualitative approaches explore all dimensions of human uniqueness that may aid the researcher in understanding the meaning of the experience for the participant. The researcher is the major instrument, conducting interviews, observing, and gathering data. The researcher's unique interaction in the participants' setting contributes to the meaning uncovered. It is the researcher's responsibility to recognize personal biases and set them aside. Researcher bias will color what is learned by covertly directing observation and interview, as well as shading interpretation of the data. The researcher goes where the data lead.

In spite of this rigorous attention to the researcher as an instrument, what a participant shares with one researcher may not be exactly what would be shared with another. This subjective expression cocreated by researcher and participant is in contrast to the objective measurement valued by quantitative approaches.

The researcher using the qualitative approach begins collecting bits of information and piecing them together, building a mosaic or a picture of the human experience being studied. As with a mosaic, when one steps away from the work, the whole picture emerges. This whole picture transcends the bits and pieces and cannot be known from any one bit or piece. In presenting the narrative summary, the researcher strives to capture the human experience and present it so that others can understand it. This inductive analysis contrasts with the primarily deductive analysis used in quantitative approaches. Deductive analysis begins with a picture and seeks to explore pieces of the picture by testing the relationship of one piece with another.

Research Questions

The choice to use either quantitative or qualitative methods is guided by the research question. Generally, questions that suggest a test of relationship or difference are addressed through a quantitative approach. Questions that suggest an exploration of a human experience are addressed through a qualitative approach. The questions noted in Table 9-1 were posed by the

Table 9-1		

Comparison of Two Studies Examining Postpartum Depression: The Quantitative and Qualitative Approaches

	MATERNITY BLUES AND POSTPARTUM DEPRESSION	THE LIVED EXPERIENCE OF POSTPARTUM DEPRESSION: A PHENOMENOLOGICAL STUDY
Subjects	n = 49 Primiparous American-born women who had uncomplicated pregnancies and vaginal deliveries	n = 7 Mothers who attended a local postpartum depression support group; 4 were primiparous, and 3 were multiparous; 4 had vaginal and 3 had cesarean deliveries
Data collectors	Four trained research assistants who had no health-related education to "ensure that they would not become confounding variables"	The researcher was the data collector (see Instruments)
Instruments	Stein's Maternity Blues Scale, a 13-symptom self-rated scale with acceptable reliability and validity; Beck Depression Inventory, measuring 21 categories of symptoms and attitudes and reporting well-established reliability and validity	Researcher interviewed the subjects and scheduled follow-up interviews to be sure that participants agreed with her interpretation of their experiences; before each interview the researcher recalled and transcénded her biases to capture the participant's reality
Analysis/summary	Deductive analysis was accomplished through inferential statistics: "No significant differences were found at 1, 6, and 12 weeks postpartum in the mean depression scores for mothers who were discharged after the customary length of hospital stay"	Inductive analysis was conducted by using the phenomenological method; the meaning of participants' descriptions was distilled and synthesized into 11 themes, including loneliness, obsessive thoughts of being a bad mom, fear and guilt over pondering harming infant, inability to concentrate, and insecurity leading to a need to be mothered herself

same researcher, Beck, about postpartum depression. When using a quantitative approach, Beck, Reynolds, and Rutowski (1992) raised a question of relationship between variables (maternity blues and postpartum depression) and a question of difference between groups (early discharge versus customary discharge). In contrast, when using a qualitative approach, Beck (1992) was interested in the lived experience of postpartum depression. Table 9-1 compares the two studies, highlighting the previously discussed differences in quantitative and qualitative approaches.

In each of these studies, Beck used a different research approach to study the same topic, postpartum depression. She was guided by her research questions. In each instance, she embraced a different set of values and activities to add to the body of nursing knowledge of postpartum depression. Clearly, no nurse is either a quantitative or a qualitative researcher. Although most nurse researchers tend to use one or the other research approach repeatedly, their choice of approach is guided by their questions. For instance, although Beck continues to report qualitative research (1993; 1996a) her recent questions have led her to yet another research method. She has recently reported two metaanalyses, one that addresses the effects of postpartum depression on maternal-infant interaction (1995) and one that addresses the predictors of postpartum depression (1996b).

QUALITATIVE APPROACH AND NURSING SCIENCE

Qualitative research is particularly well suited to study the human experience of health, a central concern of nursing science. Because qualitative methods focus on the whole of human experience and the meaning ascribed by individuals living the experience, these methods permit broader understanding and deeper insight into complex human behaviors than what might be obtained from surveys or other linear measures of perceptions (Lincoln, 1992). Two examples are cited to emphasize the capacity of qualitative methods to guide nursing practice and to contribute to instrument and theory development.

Resnick (1996) explored the factors that helped motivate clients in a geriatric rehabilitation unit and factors that decreased motivation. This study was done through a series of interviews at 3- to 5-day intervals to allow informants time to experience rehabilitation. Emergent themes that described factors that increased motivation included having goals; using humor, caring, and kindness; believing in the competence of staff and in rehabilitation; getting encouragement; basic personality; and "power-with" relationships. Factors that seemed to decrease motivation included dominating, responses to domination, and believing that rehabilitation was not necessary. In-depth exploration of the themes revealed that the domination experienced by informants led to feelings of valuelessness and hopelessness, a sense of "power over" rather than the more desirable "power with" or empowerment. Domination by caregivers in the geriatric rehabilitation setting may indeed lead to compliance, but when the domination stops and patients go home, they are no longer motivated. Resistance to domination expressed by study informants caused staff to reevaluate their methods and consider changes to improve the nature of the program.

The results of Resnick's work (1996), or of any study of individuals living with health changes, may effectively communicate insights that contribute to high-quality nursing care. Thus qualitative nursing studies generate rich, descriptive data and promote increased sensitivity to the health experiences of others. Information obtained from in-depth qualitative studies may also provide the researcher with descriptive categories that can be used to construct a quantitative instrument—one that is based on subjects' actual experiences rather than the judgment of outsiders.

Qualitative studies also may serve the purpose of conceptualization or theory development. Wing (1995) explored the phenomenon of denial, a characteristic of alcoholism and other drug abuse that must be understood to facilitate the recovery process. Data collection involved participant-observation and a series of semistructured interviews with 42 individuals in a treatment center. Wing generated a theory that explains that process by which recovering alcoholics transcend denial. The process occurs in the following five progressive stages:

1. Reacting to the critical event
2. Role disaffiliation
3. Ambiguous anticipation
4. Peer affiliation
5. Acceptance

Qualitative methods have direct relevance to nursing practice in that they move beneath the surface of outcomes to uncover life processes that contributed to the outcome. A knowledge of these life processes increases understanding and provides a basis for intervention that may enhance quality of life (Munhall, 1992). For instance, description of the life processes that influence motivation for rehabilitation in elders or support recovery from substance abuse could provide valuable information to guide nursing intervention.

FOUR QUALITATIVE RESEARCH METHODS

Thus far an overview distinguishing the quantitative from the qualitative research approach has been presented. The contribution of qualitative study to nursing science has been introduced. These topics provide a foundation for examining the four qualitative methods discussed in this chapter. The phenomenological, grounded theory, ethnographic, and historical methods are briefly contrasted in Table 9-2. More detailed comparison of these methods is provided for the consumer of nursing research throughout this chapter. Parse, Coyne, and Smith (1985) suggested that research methods, whether quantitative or qualitative, include the following five basic elements:

1. Identifying the phenomenon
2. Structuring the study
3. Gathering the data
4. Analyzing the data
5. Describing the findings

Each qualitative method is defined, followed by a discussion of these five basic elements. The factors that distinguish the methods are highlighted, and research examples are presented, providing critiquing direction for the beginning research consumer.

Phenomenological Method

The **phenomenological method** is a process of learning and constructing the meaning of human experience through intensive dialogue with persons who are living the experience. The researcher's goal is to understand the meaning of the experience as it is lived by the partici-

Table 9-2

Comparison of Qualitative Methods: Essence, Foundation, and Questions

METHOD	ESSENCE OF METHOD	FOUNDATION	EXAMPLE QUESTIONS FROM PUBLISHED STUDIES
Phenomenological	Description of the individual's "lived experience"	Philosophy	What is the meaning of comfort as an everyday experience for individuals who have traumatic injuries or life-threatening illness? (Morse, Bottorff, and Hutchinson, 1995)
			What is the meaning of aging for elders living in a community in Valencia, Spain? (Rendon et al, 1995)
Grounded theory	Systematic set of procedures used to arrive at theory about basic social processes in groups	Symbolic interaction and the social sciences	How do family caregivers experience their role in home settings? (Boland and Sims, 1996)
			What is the experience of family members living with a member with depression? (Badger, 1996)
Ethnographic	Descriptions of cultural groups or subgroups	Cultural anthropology	How do adolescents in juvenile detention make decisions about substance abuse? (Anderson, 1996)
			What are the issues of legitimacy that emerge in the experience of work-related back injury? (Tarasuk and Eakin, 1995)

			EXAMPLE QUESTIONS
Table 9-2—cont'd			
Comparison of Qualitative Methods: Essence, Foundation, and Questions			
METHOD	ESSENCE OF METHOD	FOUNDATION	EXAMPLE QUESTIONS FROM PUBLISHED STUDIES
Historical	Systematic compilation of data to describe some past event	Philosophy, art, and science	How do turn-of-the-century nursing perspectives on venereal disease provide a context for current nursing issues? (Temkin, 1994)
			How did nurses actively influence the development of ICUs through observation and triage, as well as seeking out necessary knowledge? (Fairman, 1992)

pant. The critiquer will notice that recent literature often links hermeneutic with phenomenological methods, so that there are fewer studies that are identified as using only phenomenological methods. The common core uniting the methods is their focus on pursuing meaning through a dialogical process. The phenomenological method will be discussed for the critiquer. Husserl developed the phenomenological method of inquiry, in part as a response to the popular philosophers of the time who believed that experimental methods could be used to study all human phenomena (Jennings, 1986). These philosophers focused on objectivity and what could be observed as a basis for establishing truth. Husserl was driven to establish a rigorous science that found truth in the lived experience.

Identifying the Phenomenon

Because the focus of the phenomenological method is the lived experience, the researcher is likely to choose this method when studying some dimension of day-to-day existence for a particular group of individuals. For instance, the nurse may be interested in the experience of hope for the patient who has cancer or the experience of anger for persons who have heart disease. Smith (1995) studied the lived experience of staying healthy in rural African American families. Her research report is used to guide the critiquer's understanding of the phenomenological method.

Structuring the Study

For the purpose of describing structuring, the following topics are addressed: the research question, the researcher's perspective, and sample selection. The issue of human subjects' protection has been suggested as a dimension of structuring (Parse, Coyne, and Smith, 1985); this issue is discussed generally with ethics in a subsequent section of the chapter.

Research question. Research questions that warrant the use of the phenomenological method are those that query the lived experience, such as, "What is the experience of hope for persons who have cancer?" or "How do persons who have heart disease experience anger?" Smith's (1995) research question was, "What is the meaning of staying healthy in the low income rural African American family?" Participants were volunteers who (1) had children in a Head Start Program, (2) identified themselves as African American, (3) had an annual income below $15,000, (4) resided in the same rural community, and (5) defined their family as one that was staying healthy. The question the researcher posed to the participants was, "When you identified your family as one that is staying healthy, what thoughts or feelings did you have that made you decide that this is true?"

HELPFUL HINT

Although the research question may not always be explicitly reported, it may be identified by evaluating the study purpose or the question/statement posed to the participants.

Researcher's perspective. When using the phenomenological method, the researcher's perspective is **bracketed**. That is, the researcher identifies personal biases about the phenomenon of interest to clarify how personal experience and beliefs may color what is heard and reported. The researcher is expected to set aside personal biases—to bracket them—when engaged with the participants. By becoming aware of personal biases, the researcher is more likely to be able to pursue issues of importance introduced by the participant, rather than leading the participant to issues deemed important by the researcher.

Smith (1995) sets her personal biases aside by reviewing the theoretical perspectives that guide her work. She believes that health is a process and she uses Newman's theory of nursing, which accepts health and illness as dimensions of complex human phenomena. By making her theoretical perspective explicit, she allows the reader to identify how her perspective may influence her findings.

Sample selection. The reader of a phenomenological study report will find that the selected sample will be living the experience the researcher is querying, or the sample may have lived the experience in their past. Because phenomenologists believe that each individual's history is a dimension of the present, a past experience will exist in the present moment. Even when a participant is describing an experience occurring in the present the critiquer will notice that remembered information is being gathered by the researcher using the phenomenological method.

Data Gathering

Written or oral data may be collected when using the phenomenological method. The researcher may pose the query in writing and ask for a written response or may schedule a time to interview the participant and tape-record the interaction. In either case the researcher may return to ask for clarification of written or tape-recorded transcripts. To some extent, the particular data collection strategy is guided by the choice of specific analysis technique. Different analyses techniques require a differing number of interviews. For most analyses techniques, data saturation guides decisions regarding how many interviews are enough. However, van

Kaam's (1969) analyses technique proposes a strategy for using the phenomenological method when the researcher has a large number of written transcripts.

Smith (1995) used the Giorgi modification of the phenomenological method of analysis. She audio-taped interviews, which were then transcribed for analysis. She interviewed 10 family participant groups, involving 21 family members.

Data Analysis

There are several techniques for data analysis when using the phenomenological method. For detailed information about specific techniques, the critiquer is referred to original sources (Colaizzi, 1978; Giorgi, Fischer, and Murray, 1975; Spiegelberg, 1976; van Kaam, 1969). Although the techniques are slightly different from each other, there is a general pattern of moving from the participant's description to the researcher's synthesis of all participants' descriptions. The steps generally include the following:

1. Thorough reading and sensitive presence with the entire transcription of the participant's description
2. Identification of shifts in participant thought resulting in division of the transcription into thought segments
3. Specification of the significant phrases in each thought segment, using the words of the participant
4. Distillation of each significant phrase to express the central meaning of the segment in the words of the researcher
5. Preliminary synthesis of central meanings of all thought segments for each participant with a focus on the essence of the phenomenon being studied
6. Final synthesis of the essences that have surfaced in all participant's descriptions, resulting in an exhaustive description of the **lived experience**

Smith (1995) provided examples of the words of the participants leading the reader through the steps of the analyses to arrive at the final synthesis of the meaning of staying healthy for these participants. An example of a participants' words was: "I believe that if you take care of yourself, God will take care of you and bless you, but if you don't do things that you know you should, He will take that blessing. But, if you don't know, you can't help it." The meaning derived by the researcher was: "Knowing what is right involves being responsible and accountable. Following the rules about healthcare is integral to following his religious beliefs and staying healthy." The researcher's final synthesis included an understanding that staying healthy centered on finding an inner feeling of knowing what to do; . . . "families became more conscious of their own abilities and what was important in their lives." She then linked her findings to Newman's theory, noting how the findings support the theory.

Describing the Findings

When using the phenomenological method, the researcher provides the reader with a path of information leading from the research question, through samples of participant's words, researcher's interpretation, and leading to the final synthesis that narratively elaborates the lived experience. When reading the report of a phenomenological study, the critiquer will find that detailed descriptive language is used to convey the complex meaning of the lived experience.

Grounded Theory Method

The critiquer who is assessing a study that uses the **grounded theory method** finds an inductive approach that implements a systematic set of procedures to arrive at theory about basic social processes. The emergent theory is based on observations and perceptions of the social scene and evolves during data collection and analysis in the actual research process (Strauss and Corbin, 1994). The aim of the grounded theory approach is to discover underlying social forces that shape human behavior. This method is used to construct theory where no theory exists or in situations when existing theory fails to explain a set of circumstances.

Symbolic interaction is the theoretical base for grounded theory. Symbolic interactionist tradition holds that the relationship between self and society is an ongoing process of symbolic communication, whereby individuals create a social reality. George Herbert Mead, social psychologist, is credited with originating this tradition in the early twentieth century.

Glaser and Strauss (1967) developed the systematic approach to the study of interactions, known as the *grounded theory method,* to bridge a perceived gap between theory and research and the consequent undervaluing of qualitative studies. In this method, theory remains closely connected to data through descriptive examples that provide direct empirical evidence that the theory fits the phenomenon under investigation. Theory generated in this manner may then serve as a conceptual framework on which to base a testable hypothesis and subsequent quantitative studies. Grounded theory may also be used to extend or elaborate on a previously developed theory.

Developed originally as a sociologist's tool to investigate interactions in social settings, the grounded theory method, or procedure, is not bound to that discipline. Investigators from different disciplines may study the same phenomenon from varying perspectives (Strauss and Corbin, 1994). As an example, in an area of study such as chronic illness, a nurse might be interested in coping patterns within families, a psychologist in personal adjustment, and a sociologist in group behavior in health care settings. Theory generated by each discipline will reflect the discipline and will serve the discipline in explaining the phenomenon.

Identifying the Phenomenon

Researchers typically use the grounded theory method when they are interested in social processes from the perspective of human interactions. The basic social process, or core category that is the foundation of a theory, is often expressed as a gerund, indicating change across time as social reality is negotiated. For example, Pursley-Crotteau and Stern (1996) studied *creating a new life,* or the developmental process that occurs when perinatal women experience treatment for cocaine crack use. Price (1993) studied *self-managing* with a group of diabetic patients. Price's study (1993) will be elaborated as a way of introducing the research consumer to the grounded theory method.

Structuring the Study

Research question. Research questions appropriate for the grounded theory method are those that address basic social process. They tend to be action oriented or change oriented, such as, "How do parents of children with development delay/mental retardation experience the parenting process?" (Seideman and Kleine, 1995) or "How do family members experience living with a member with depression?" (Badger, 1996). "Transformed parenting" and "family transformation," processes revealed in these studies, are evidence of change-orientation. In a grounded theory study, the research question can be a statement or a broad question that permits in-depth explanation of the phenomenon. For instance, the reader will recognize Price's question implied in the statement that her study addressed: "How patients learn self-management through applying diabetes information and how they adapt it to their lives" (Price, 1993).

Researcher's perspective. The grounded theorist is interested in providing a study of the processes that occur as individuals interact with others in the social setting in response to life circumstances. The researcher will bring some knowledge of the literature to the study, but the critiquer will notice that an exhaustive literature review is not done. This allows theory to emerge directly from data. For example, Price (1993) notes that other studies of self-management of diabetes use *a priori* models related to compliance, behavior modification, or cognitive style to explain and predict patient behaviors. However, the current study (Price, 1993) provides a description of factors and processes that emerge as diabetes self-management is learned. Price (1993) indicates that self-management was examined from the patients' perspective, but such factors as social circumstances and doctors' orders are investigated to provide sufficient depth for theory generation. Thus grounded theory is more likely to be sensitive to contextual values and not merely to the researcher's values (Strauss and Corbin, 1994).

Another important aspect of the researcher's perspective is concern that theory remain connected to or "grounded in" the data. Price (1993) initially intended to study the concept of uncertainty within chronic illness as experienced by adults in an outpatient setting. However, as the data emerged, the concept of uncertainty was found to be subsumed by the broader central theme, learning self-management.

Sample selection. Sample selection involves choosing participants who are experiencing the circumstance and selecting events and incidents related to the social process under investigation. Price recruited adult diabetics through a diabetes newsletter distributed in the area. Enrollment criteria required that the participants be diagnosed with diabetes mellitus for at least 1 year but no longer than 10 years. All of the 18 subjects required two or more injections of insulin daily, and all were monitoring their own blood glucose level. Thus the participants had a period for learning and they had specific activities or tasks that were required for self-management. Price also describes other factors or variables, such as age, education, marital status, and whether the participants were involved in support groups or had attended formal diabetes education classes.

Data Gathering

In the grounded theory method, the critiquer will find that data are collected through interviews and through skilled observations of individuals interacting in a social setting. Interviews are audio-taped and then transcribed, and observations are recorded as field notes. Open-ended questions are used initially to identify concepts.

Price (1993) interviewed each participant twice for approximately 2 hours each time. Most of the interviews were in the participants' homes. The interview questions were based on the researcher's clinical experience and focused on aspects of uncertainty. Questions were developed "to probe the areas of diagnosis, treatment, prognosis, and perceived disruptions of body changes and social interactions due to chronic disease." Examples of questions include the following:

- "What about diabetes worries you the most?"
- "What about diabetes is/remains puzzling or confusing? Are those things always confusing or puzzling?"
- "Are there other areas of uncertainties or unknowns that you often have to deal with that we have not talked about?"

Data Analysis

A major feature of the grounded theory method is that data collection and analysis occur simultaneously. The process requires systematic, detailed record keeping using field notes and transcribed interview tapes. Hunches about emerging patterns in the data are noted in memos, and the researcher directs activities in the field by pursuing these hunches. This technique, called **theoretical sampling**, is used to select experiences that will help the researcher test ideas and gather complete information about developing concepts. The researcher begins by noting indicators or actual events, actions, or words in the data. Concepts, or abstractions, are developed from the indicators (Strauss, 1987).

The initial analytical process is called *open coding* (Strauss, 1987). Data are examined carefully line by line, broken down into discrete parts, and compared for similarities and differences (Strauss and Corbin, 1990). Data are compared with other data continuously as they are acquired during research. This is a process called the **constant comparative method.** Codes in the data are clustered to form categories. The categories are expanded and developed or collapsed into one another. Theory is constructed through this systematic process. As a result, data collection, analysis, and theory generation have a direct reciprocal relationship (Strauss and Corbin, 1990).

Related literature, both technical and nontechnical, is reviewed continuously throughout data collection and analysis. All literature is treated as data and is compared with the researcher's developing theory as it progresses. When critiquing a study using grounded theory, expect to find, at the end of the report, the researcher's grounded theory formally related to and incorporated with existing knowledge.

In describing data analysis, Price (1993) listed the following phrases or indicators:

- "I *trust my body* about 90% of the time."
- "I feel like I am fairly *well tuned in to my body.*"
- "I am always *listening,* running checks on how I feel; there is *never a time when I am not thinking about it.*"

These phrases were coded as "body trust" and "body listening." Through an intense coding process around a single theme called *axial coding,* "body listening" was developed in depth. The researcher noted when "body listening" occurred and what physical cues were monitored. The theme "body listening" was central to the process under investigation and was elevated to the status of a category, "experiencing body changes through 'body listening.'" Through the next process, selective coding, 11 categories were collapsed into 4 major categories—personal considerations, monitoring, cognitive skills, and control. Through this rigorous process and further consultation with the subjects, the core category was identified as "learning self-management of diabetes." A model depicting the sequential steps in the process was described, and the four factors were found to be operative at each stage of the model and to be important to the direction of movement between the stages.

 HELPFUL HINT
The critiquer must not find dimensions of the method, such as axial coding, explicitly identified in the manuscript.

Describing the Findings

Grounded theory studies are reported in sufficient detail to provide the reader with the steps in the process and the logic of the method. Price (1993) takes the reader through the steps of data collection, theoretical sampling, constant comparisons, and three levels of coding to a schematic model that depicts the process. Reports of grounded theory studies use descriptive language to ensure that the theory reported in the findings remains connected to the data.

Ethnographic Method

The **ethnographic method** focuses on scientific descriptions of cultural groups. The critiquer should know that the goal of the ethnographer is to understand the natives' view of their world or the emic view. The **emic** (insiders') **view** is contrasted to the **etic** (outsiders') **view** obtained when the researcher uses quantitative analyses of behavior (Parse, Coyne, and Smith, 1985). The ethnographic approach requires that the researcher enter the world of the study participants to watch what happens, listen to what is said, ask questions, and collect whatever data are available. The term *ethnography* is used to mean both the research technique and the product of that technique, the study itself (Atkinson and Hammersley, 1994).

Sanday (1989) notes that ethnography is at least as old as the work of Herodotus, the ancient Greek ethnographer, who recorded the infinite variety and strangeness he saw in other cultures. Modern ethnographic tradition is based in cultural anthropology and the works of Malinowski (1922), Mead (1928), and Boas (1948). Nurses use the method to study cultural variations in health and to study patient groups as subcultures within larger social contexts.

Identifying the Phenomenon

The critiquer may expect that the phenomenon in an ethnographic study will vary in scope from a long-term study of a very complex culture, such as that of the Aborigines, to a shorter-term study of a phenomenon within subunits of cultures, such as comparison of health and healing philosophies of nurses and alternative healers (Engebretson, 1996), ways adolescents in juvenile detention make decisions about substance abuse (Anderson, 1996), and use of an urban senior center as a haven for the social health of elders (Kaufman, 1995). Kleinman (1992) notes the clinical utility of ethnography in describing the "local world" of groups of patients who are experiencing a particular phenomenon, such as suffering. The local worlds of patients have cultural, political, economic, institutional, and social-relational dimensions in much the same way that larger complex societies have these units of analysis. Mayo's (1992) study of the phenomenon of lifelong patterns of physical activity among African-American women is used as an example throughout the presentation of ethnography.

Structuring the Study

Research question. When reviewing the report of ethnographic research, notice that questions are asked about lifeways or particular patterns of behavior within the social context of a culture or subculture. Culture is viewed as the system of knowledge and linguistic expressions used by social groups that allows the researcher to interpret or make sense of the world (Aamodt, 1991). Ethnographic nursing studies address questions that concern how cultural knowledge, norms, values, and other contextual variables influence one's health experience. Uphall (1992) asked, "How do nurses from various health care settings (government, private, missions, industrial and nongovernmental organizations) perceive collaboration between indigenous and cosmopolitan health care systems?" Other possible ethnographic questions include "What does comforting mean in Hispanic families?" "What are patient and nurse roles like in intensive care units?" and "What are the meanings of health and illness care to migrant workers?" Often the research question is implied in the purpose statement. As an example, Mayo (1992) constructed her study to ask, "What are the lifelong patterns of physical activity among black working women?"

Researcher's perspective. When using the ethnographic method, the researcher's perspective is that of an interpreter entering an alien world and attempting to make sense of that world from the insider's point of view (Agar, 1986). Like phenomenologists and grounded theorists, ethnographers make their own beliefs explicit and bracket, or set aside, their personal biases as they seek to understand the world view of others. Mayo (1992) identifies the cultural-ecological orientation as a frame of reference for her study of the physical activity practices of African-American working women. This perspective holds that definitions of health are derived by cultural groups using scientific information, common sense, and personal experience (Kleinman, 1980). Mayo (1992) further notes, "Despite the widespread availability of information about the health promoting benefits of physical activity more than one half of all American women and two thirds of African-American women are sedentary."

Sample selection. The ethnographer selects a cultural group who are living the phenomenon under investigation. The researcher gathers information from general informants and from key informants. **Key informants** are individuals who have special knowledge, status, or communication skills and who are willing to teach the ethnographer about the phenomenon (Crabtree and Miller, 1992). Mayo (1992) initiated contact with potential informants through personal directors, occupational health nurses, and professional acquaintances. She conducted 51 unstructured interviews and identified a study group of 24 African-American working women.

HELPFUL HINT
Managing personal bias is an expectation of researchers using all the methods discussed in this chapter.

Data Gathering
Ethnographic data gathering involves participant observation or immersion in the setting, informant interviews, and interpretation by the researcher of cultural patterns (Crabtree and Miller, 1992). According to Boyle (1991), ethnographic research in nursing as in other disciplines always involves "face-to-face interviewing, with data collection and analysis taking place

in the natural setting." Thus fieldwork is a major focus on the method. Other techniques may include obtaining life histories and collecting material items reflective of the culture. Photographs and films of the informants in their world can be used as data sources. Spradley (1979) identified three categories of questions for ethnographic inquiry: descriptive, or broad, open-ended questions; structural, or in-depth questions that expand and verify the unit of analysis; and contrast questions, or ones that further clarify and provide criteria for exclusion.

Through participant observation, Mayo (1992) gathered information about the physical activity practices of a subsample of 13 women during such activities as aerobic dance, walking, jogging, weight lifting, and floor exercises. Interview questions ranged from the open-ended: "Tell me about your physical activity, starting at whatever age you want; describe your experiences, and what you have done in the past or do now in terms of activity" to the specific: "What things, such as people, your own feelings, the time of year, facility availability, or finances, help or block your participation in physical activity?"

Data Analysis

As with the grounded theory method, data are collected and analyzed simultaneously. Data analysis proceeds through several levels as the researcher looks for the meaning of cultural symbols on the informants' language. Analysis begins with a search for **domains** or symbolic categories that include smaller categories. Language is analyzed for semantic relationships, and structural questions are formulated to expand and verify data. Mayo (1992) used the biomedical labels *cardiorespiratory, muscular,* and *metabolic* to group the emic criteria for physical fitness supplied by the informants. For example, such terms as *conditioned, better balance, better shape all over, in good shape,* and *flexible* constituted the category of muscular. Analysis proceeds through increasing levels of complexity and includes taxonomic analysis or in-depth verification of domains, componential analysis or analysis for contrasts among categories, and theme analysis or uncovering of cultural themes. The data, grounded in the informants' reality and synthesized by the researcher, lead eventually to hypothetical propositions about the cultural phenomenon under investigation. Mayo (1992) proceeded through the levels of analysis to conceptualize the idea that physical activity behaviors among African-American women reflect a process of nongenetic adaptation to social and physical environmental conditions. The management of physical activity was further described by Lazarus and Folkman's (1984) concept of coping. The reader is encouraged to consult Spradley (1979); Leininger (1985); or Parse, Coyne, and Smith (1985) for detailed descriptions of the ethnographic analysis process.

Describing the Findings

Ethnographic studies yield large quantities of data amassed as field notes of observations, interview transcriptions, and other artifacts, such as photographs. When critiquing, be aware that the report of findings usually provides examples from data, thorough description of the analytical process, and statements of the hypothetical propositions and their relationship to the ethnographer's frame of reference. Complete ethnographies may be published as monographs.

Historical Method

The **historical research method** is a systematic approach for understanding the past through collection, organization, and critical appraisal of facts. One of the goals of the researcher using historical methodology is to shed light on the past so that it can guide the present and the future.

The historical method is embedded in philosophy, art, and science (Cramer, 1992). Nursing's focus on historical methodology was led by Teresa E. Christy, who established it as a legitimate method of inquiry more than a decade ago (Schweer, 1982). Christy elaborated the method (1975) and the need (1981) for historical research long before most nurse scholars accepted it as a legitimate research method. Historical methodology can emerge from within the quantitative or qualitative approach. However, the nature of history is fundamentally narrative (qualitative) rather than numerical (quantitative).

Identifying the Phenomenon

The historical method requires that the phenomenon of interest is a past event that can be circumscribed to permit distinction from other events. Roberts' (1996) study of the use ancillary personnel to augment existing nursing practice in Britain between 1914 and 1918 is cited for the critiquer to highlight the process of using historical methods. Roberts (1996) presents data linking the phenomenon of dilution (a process of adding nonskilled volunteers to do skilled work) with the emergence of registration to ensure appropriate credentialing of skilled nurses.

Structuring the Study

Research question. When critiquing, expect to find the research question embedded in the phenomenon to be studied. The question is implicitly rather than explicitly stated. Roberts' (1996) study question is embedded in what she labels hers hypothesis: ". . . registration is seen as a vehicle for protecting the emerging privileges and expanding employment markets of qualified nursing personnel."

Researcher's perspective. Christy (1975) notes that the researcher's first responsibility is to understand the information being acquired without imposing his or her own interpretation. The researcher does this by being aware of personal biases that may color the interpretation. The report of historical research provides no documentation of this step of the research process.

Sample selection. In historical research, sample selection is accomplished by identifying data sources (Sarnecky, 1990). The more clearly a researcher delineates the phenomenon, the more specifically data sources can be identified. All possible sources of data will be listed by the researcher. Data may include written or video documents, interviews with persons who witnessed the phenomenon, photographs, and any other artifacts that shed light on the phenomenon. Once again, the research report does not reveal all the data sources that were explored.

Data Gathering

Once a list of possible data sources has been composed, the researcher will begin the process of learning what is available. Sometimes pivotal information cannot be retrieved and must be eliminated from the list of possible sources. To determine which data sources were used when reviewing a published study, the reader will look at the reference list. Roberts (1996) used British government reports, nursing journals published during the period, and the Nurses Registration Act of 1919, to name only a few of her sources. She may have wanted to talk with some individuals who had lived through the volunteer experience, but sources who can recall the significant events and engage in dialogue are not always available.

Sources of data may be primary or secondary. **Primary sources** are eyewitness accounts provided by varying sorts of communication appropriate to the time. These may include but are not limited to original documents, films, letters, diaries, records, artifacts, periodicals, or tapes. In contrast, **secondary sources** provide a view of the phenomenon from another's perspective rather than a first-hand account.

Data Analysis

Data will be analyzed first for importance and then for validity and reliability. To judge importance, the researcher separates what is (1) of clear value from (2) the "mildly interesting" and (3) the unimportant (Sarnecky, 1990). The unimportant will be discarded as data sources and data of clear value are included. Mildly interesting data require further review before they are included or discarded.

Validity of documents is established by external criticism; reliability is established by internal criticism. **External criticism** judges the authenticity of the data source. The researcher seeks to ensure that the data source is what it seems to be. For instance, if the researcher is reviewing a handwritten letter of Florence Nightingale, some of the validity issues are the following:

- Are the ink, paper, and wax seal on the envelope representative of Nightingale's time?
- Is the wax seal one that Nightingale used in other authentic data sources?
- Is the writing truly Nightingale's?

Only if the data source passes the test of external criticism does the researcher begin internal criticism. **Internal criticism** concerns the reliability of information within the document (Christy, 1975). To judge reliability, the researcher must familiarize himself or herself with the time in which the data emerged. A sense of the context and language of the time is essential to understanding a document. The meaning of a word in one era may not be equivalent to the meaning in another era. Knowing the language, customs, and habits of the historical period is critical for judging reliability.

The researcher assumes that a primary source provides a more reliable account than a secondary source (Christy, 1975). The further a source moves from providing an eyewitness account, the more questionable is its reliability. The researcher using historical methods attempts to establish fact, probability, or possibility (Box 9-1).

 HELPFUL HINT
When critiquing the historical method, do not expect to find a report of data analysis but simply a description of findings synthesized into a continuous narrative.

Describing the Findings

The findings of an historical study are presented as a well-synthesized chronicle. The entire manuscript is the description of findings. "If the synthesis is successful, the reader thinks the research and the writing have been effortless. The reader is never aware of the painstaking work, the careful attention to detail, nor the arduous pursuit of clues endured by the writer of history" (Christy, 1975). Roberts' (1996) report chronicles the context for the emergence of registration for nurses in Britain. She synthesizes the social, political, and professional environments that influenced the decision to initiate credentialing through registration. It is as

Box 9-1	Establishing Fact, Probability, and Possibility With the Historical Method

Fact

Two independent primary sources that agree with each other

or

One independent primary source that receives critical evaluation and one independent secondary source that is in agreement and receives critical evaluation and no substantive conflicting data

Probability

One primary source that receives critical evaluation and no substantive conflicting data

or

Two primary sources that disagree about particular points

Possibility

One primary source that provides information but is not adequate to receive critical evaluation

or

Only secondary or tertiary sources

Modified from Christy TE: The methodology of historical research: a brief introduction, *Image J Nurs Sch* 24(3):189-192, 1975.

though she has woven many historical perspectives into a whole, which enhances understanding.

QUALITATIVE APPROACH: NURSING METHODOLOGY

The qualitative methodologies that are elaborated throughout this chapter are derived from other disciplines, such as sociology, anthropology, and philosophy. The discipline of nursing borrowed these methodologies to conduct research. However, as the discipline matured, methodology based on nursing ontology (belief system) emerged. Madeleine Leininger (1985, 1988, 1996), Rosemarie Rizzo Parse (1992; 1996) and Margaret Newman (1994) are examples of nurse theorists who have created research methods specific to their theories. Table 9-3 compares the methodology of these theorists. Each method was developed over years and tested by other researchers. Each attempts to advance nursing knowledge through inquiry that is congruent with her theory.

ISSUES IN QUALITATIVE RESEARCH

Case Study Methodology: Under Used but Promising

The **case study method** focuses on a selected contemporary phenomenon over time to provide an in-depth description of its essential dimensions and processes. Many of the phenomenon of interest to nursing lend themselves to case study methodology. The experience of be-

Table 9-3			
Nursing Research Methodology			
	LEININGER	PARSE	NEWMAN
Theory	Culture Care	Human Becoming	Health As Expanding Consciousness
Research methodology	Ethnonursing is centered on learning from people about their beliefs, experiences, and culture care information (Leininger, 1996)	Parse's research methodology is the study of universal health experiences through true presence both with participants sharing life stories and with transcribed data to uncover meaning (Parse, 1992, 1996)	Newman's method focuses on pattern recognition and utilizes multiple interviews, involving interviewer-interviewee collaboration to arrive at recognized life patterns (Newman, 1994)
Example of research question(s)	What are the meanings and expressions of health to older Greek-Canadian widows? What Greek folk health and illness care beliefs and practices are prevalent with Greek-Canadian widows? (Rosenbaum, 1991)	What is the structure of the lived experience of suffering? (Daly, 1995)	What is the evolving pattern of selected persons diagnosed as HIV positive? (Lamendola and Newman, 1994)

coming a parent, living through a natural disaster such as a hurricane, or living with a chronic illness are some examples. Although these phenomenon are often studied using the qualitative research approach, case study research methodology is seldom used. Lewis (1995) is a recent exception. Not only did she use case study research methodology, but she also combined qualitative and quantitative approaches. She studied the premenstrual syndrome in one individual over the course of 13 menstrual cycles, collecting quantitative information with a menstrual symptom checklist and qualitative information with a journal narrative. Using this methodology, she was able to uncover symptom patterns and enhance understanding of patterns through the individual's interpretation of self and environment recorded in the journal. Case study methodology promises to offer another qualitative avenue for nursing investigation in the future. It may offer an ideal methological vehicle for joining quantitative and qualitative approaches.

Ethics

Inherent in all research is the demand for the protection of human subjects. This demand exists for both quantitative and qualitative research approaches. Human subjects' protection as applicable to the quantitative approach is discussed in Chapter 11. These basic tenets hold true for the qualitative approach. However, several characteristics of qualitative methodologies outlined in Table 9-4 generate unique concerns and necessitate an expanded view of protecting human subjects.

Naturalistic Setting

The concerns that arise when research is conducted in naturalistic settings focus on the issue of the need to gain consent. Some fieldwork models allow that the researcher collect data without informing participants. Johnson (1992) notes, "Many research ethical committees would automatically fail to grant access to studies where the proposed sample will not be able to choose between being included or excluded from the investigation." For nurses, this circumstance is most likely to occur when collecting data in public settings, where the researcher can easily gain entry as an accepted member of the community without explanation.

Emergent Nature of Design

The emergent nature of the research design emphasizes the need for ongoing negotiation of consent with the participant. In the course of a study, situations change and what was aggreable at the beginning may become intrusive. Sometimes, as data collection proceeds and new

Table 9-4

Characteristics of Qualitative Research Generating Ethical Concerns

CHARACTERISTICS	ETHICAL CONCERNS
Naturalistic setting	Some researchers using methods that rely on participant observation may believe that consent is not always possible or necessary.
Emergent nature of design	Planning for questioning and observation emerges over the time of the study. Thus it is difficult to inform the participant precisely of all potential threats before he or she agrees to participate.
Researcher-participant interaction	Relationships developed between the researcher and participant may blur the focus of the interaction.
Researcher as instrument	The researcher is the study instrument, collecting data and interpreting the participant's reality.

information emerges, the study shifts direction in a way that is not acceptable to the participant. For instance, if the researcher were present in a family's home during a time that marital discord arose, the family may choose to renegotiate the consent. Lipson (1994) highlights the need for reciprocity, questioning the responsibility of researchers to their participants. Consent is an ongoing reciprocal process. The opportunity to renegotiate consent establishes a relationship of trust and respect characteristic of the ethical conduct of research.

Researcher-Participant Interaction

The nature of the researcher-participant interaction over time introduces the possibility that the research experience becomes a therapeutic one. Although the idea of research-as-practice is endorsed by some (Newman, 1994; Wilde, 1992), it is generally not accepted. It is useful for the researcher to be mindful of the role and gently guide participants to focus on the purpose of the researcher-participant experience. In spite of this focus, it is possible that therapeutic value will be derived by the participant, but the researcher will not have made therapeutic intervention the priority.

Researcher as Instrument

The responsibility to remain true to the data requires that the researcher acknowledge any personal bias, interpreting findings in a way that accurately reflects the participant's reality. This is a serious ethical obligation. To accomplish this, the researcher may return to the subjects at critical interpretive points and ask for clarification or validation.

Credibility, Auditability, and Fittingness

Quantitative studies are reliability and validity of instruments, as well as internal and external validity criteria, as measures of scientific rigor (see Critical Thinking Decision Path, p. 217), but these are not appropriate for qualitative work. The rigor of qualitative methodology is judged by unique criteria appropriate to the research approach. Credibility, auditability, fittingness, and confirmability are scientific rigor criteria proposed by Guba and Lincoln (1981). Although lists of specific criteria vary slightly (Leininger, 1994; Lincoln and Guba, 1985; Morse and Field, 1995), the general themes of credibility, auditability, and fittingness persist as criteria for judging the scientific rigor of qualitative research. The meaning of credibility, auditability, fittingness, and confirmability is briefly explained in Table 9-5. As can be seen, confirmability is ensured when the other criteria have been met.

Triangulation

Triangulation is the expansion of research methods in a single study or multiple studies to enhance diversity, enrich understanding, and accomplish specific goals. There are several perspectives about triangulation. Morse (1991) provides one perspective, a combination of methods labeled *simultaneous* or *sequential triangulation*. Simultaneous triangulation is the combination of qualitative and quantitative methods in one study at the same time. In sequential triangulation, only one approach is used in a study, but the researcher conducts multiple studies using different approaches in each. Beck used sequential triangulation, beginning

Table 9-5

Criteria for Judging Scientific Rigor: Credibility, Auditability, Fittingness, and Confirmability

CRITERIA	CRITERIA CHARACTERISTICS
Credibility	Truth of findings as judged by participants and others within the discipline
Auditability	Accountability as judged by the adequacy of information leading the reader from the research question and raw data through various steps of analysis to the interpretation of findings
Fittingness	Faithfulness to everyday reality of the participants, described in enough detail so that others in the discipline can evaluate importance for their own practice, research, and theory development
Confirmability	Findings that reflect implementation of creditability, auditability, and fittingness standards

with a quantitative approach followed by qualitative work (see Table 9-1). In simultaneous and sequential triangulation each combination is made for distinct reasons (Table 9-6).

Denzin (1978) provides another perspective, identifying four basic types of triangulation: data, investigator, theory, and methodological. Janesick (1994) has expanded Denzin's view to include interdisciplinary triangulation (Table 9-7). This perspective is very different than that suggested by Morse (1991). It proposes diversity beyond methodological diversity. Both of these perspectives of triangulation offer to enrich understanding of human phenomena. However, the simultaneous use of multiple methods in a single study generates questions.

The fundamental differences cited in the Critical Thinking Decision Path on p. 217 suggest the confusion a researcher may experience with one foot in qualitative and one in quantitative methods for a single study. Still, there is an intrinsic drive for nurses to substantiate the description of lived experience with hard data—or perhaps, it is a mandate to substantiate hard data with descriptions of lived experience. In our current health care climate, with its focus on patient outcomes, the individual meaning ascribed to health has increasing value. Who is best prepared to identify desirable outcomes? What research models can most effectively be used to accomplish this task? Nursing is challenged to create unique research models capable of addressing the complexity of humans, while maintaining the integrity of its belief systems.

Computer Management of Qualitative Data

At the completion of data collection, the qualitative researcher is faced with volumes of data requiring sorting, coding, and synthesizing. The researcher reports may use one of the computer programs that are available to assist with the task of data management. Unlike computer programs used with quantitative data, these programs do not analyze data. Data analysis and interpretation is the task of the researcher. However, data can be managed by computers (Taft,

Table 9-6

Simultaneous and Sequential Combinations of Quantitative and Qualitative Research Methods: Rationale and Examples

COMBINATION	RATIONALE	EXAMPLE
Simultaneous		
Qualitative + quantitative	There is a qualitative foundation, and quantitative methods are used to provide complementary information.	The researcher is interested in the experience of feeling depressed after the loss of a spouse. Phenomenological methods could be used to address the research question: administration of a depression scale would provide complementary information.
Quantitative + qualitative	There is a quantitative foundation, and qualitative methods are used to provide complementary information.	The researcher is testing hypotheses about depression after the death of a spouse. The phenomenological method is used to uncover the experience for a select group who acknowledge feelings of depression.
Sequential		
Qualitative → quantitative	Findings from qualitative investigation lead to use of the quantitative approach.	The researcher has described the experience of feeling depressed after the death of a spouse. The themes emerging from the data are used to create a depression scale. The scale is tested for reliability and validity.
Quantitative → qualitative	Findings from quantitative investigation lead to use of the qualitative approach.	The researcher has tested hypotheses linking the death of a spouse with depression and found no significant relationships. A qualitative study is undertaken to uncover the experience of living through the death of one's spouse in an effort to let the data lead to common thoughts and feelings.

Modified from Morse JM: Approaches to qualitative-quantitative methodological triangulation, *Nurs Res* 40(1):120-123, 1991.

Table 9-7	
Types of Triangulation	
TYPE	EXPLANATION
Data triangulation	The use of a variety of data sources in a study
Investigator triangulation	The use of several different researchers or evaluators
Theory triangulation	The use of multiple perspectives to interpret a single set of data
Methodological triangulation	The use of multiple methods to study a single problem
Multidisciplinary triangulation	The use of multiple disciplines to inform the research process

Data from Denzin NK: *The research act: a theoretical introduction to sociological methods,* ed 2, New York, 1978, Mc-Graw-Hill; Janesick VJ: The dance of qualitative research design: metaphor, methodolatry, and meaning. In Denzin NK, Lincoln YS, eds: *Handbook of qualitative research,* Thousand Oaks, Calif, 1994, Sage.

1993; Tesch, 1991). Reid (1992) distinguishes the following three data management functions:

1. Data preparation: entry of data from field notes, interviews, and various other sources; cleaning of data to ensure that spelling is correct and data are easy to evaluate
2. Data identification: dividing data into meaningful segments for analysis/synthesis
3. Data manipulation: searching for particular words or phrases and sorting them from the text

Sandelowski (1995) emphasizes the concurrence of data collection, analysis, preparation, and interpretation. Although data collection, analysis, and preparation may be computer assisted, interpretation requires the thoughtful presence of the researcher and cannot be accomplished with a computer. The critiquer will want to carefully evaluate the synthesized product, noting faithfulness to the participant's descriptions and integration into a meaningful whole.

CRITIQUING QUALITATIVE RESEARCH

Although general criteria for critiquing qualitative research are proposed in the Critiquing Criteria box, each qualitative method has unique characteristics that influence what the research consumer may expect in the published research report. The proposed general criteria are most useful for critiquing studies using the phenomenological, grounded theory, and ethnographic methods. They are less relevant for critiquing research using the historical method.

The criteria for critiquing are formatted to evaluate the selection of the phenomenon, the structure of the study, data gathering, data analysis, and description of the findings. Each question of the criteria focuses on factors that are discussed throughout the chapter. The credibility (criteria 13 and 14), auditability (criteria 15), and fittingness (criteria 12) of the study are addressed by specific criteria (see Chapter 18 for additional discussion of critiquing qualitative research).

CRITIQUING CRITERIA

IDENTIFYING THE PHENOMENON

1. Is the phenomenon focused on human experience within a natural setting?
2. Is the phenomenon relevant to nursing and/or health?

STRUCTURING THE STUDY

Research Question

3. Does the question specify a distinct process to be studied?
4. Does the question identify the context (participant group/place) of the process that will be studied?
5. Does the choice of a specific qualitative method fit with the research question?

Researcher's Perspective

6. Are the biases of the researcher reported?
7. Do the researchers provide a structure of ideas that reflect their beliefs?

Sample Selection

8. Is it clear that the selected sample is living the phenomenon of interest?

DATA GATHERING

9. Are data sources and methods for gathering data specified?
10. Is there evidence that participant consent is an integral part of the data gathering process?

DATA ANALYSIS

11. Can the dimensions of data analysis be identified and logically followed?
12. Does the researcher paint a clear picture of the participant's reality?
13. Is there evidence that the researcher's interpretation captured the participant's meaning?
14. Have other professionals confirmed the researcher's interpretation?

DESCRIBING THE FINDINGS

15. Are examples provided to guide the reader from the raw data to the researcher's synthesis?
16. Does the researcher link the findings to existing theory or literature, or is a new theory generated?

KEY POINTS

- Qualitative research is the investigation of human experiences in naturalistic settings, pursuing meanings that inform theory, practice, and further research.
- Qualitative research studies are guided by research questions.
- Data saturation occurs when the information being shared with the researcher becomes repetitive.

- Qualitative research methods include five basic elements: identifying the phenomenon, structuring the study, gathering the data, analyzing the data, and describing the findings.
- The phenomenological method is a process of learning and constructing the meaning of human experience through intensive dialogue with persons who are living the experience.
- The grounded theory method is an inductive approach that implements a systematic set of procedures to arrive at theory about basic social processes.
- The ethnographic method focuses on scientific descriptions of cultural groups.
- The historical method is the systematic compilation of data and the critical presentation, evaluation, and interpretation of facts regarding people, events, and occurrences of the past.
- The case study method focuses on a selected contemporary phenomenon over time to provide an in-depth description of its essential dimensions and processes.
- Ethical issues in qualitative research involve issues related to the naturalistic setting, emergent nature of the design, researcher-participant interaction, and researcher as instrument.
- Credibility, auditability, fittingness, and confirmability are criteria for judging the scientific rigor of a qualitative research study.
- Triangulation refers to strategies for combining research methods and/or approaches.
- Qualitative research data can be managed through the use of computers, but data interpretation must be done by the researcher.

CRITICAL THINKING CHALLENGES

Barbara Krainovich-Miller

? Discuss how the qualitative researcher knows when "data saturation" has occurred. Offer explanations from your life experience that are similar to the experience of data saturation.

? How would you answer your classmate in research class who insists that it is impossible for researchers to "bracket" their personal biases about the phenomenon they are going to study. Use examples from your own clinical experience in your response.

? You are asked to defend why qualitative studies do not include hypotheses. Include in your argument whether or not you think qualitative studies warrant the same recognition as true experimental studies.

? How would the researcher use information gathered via computer-based searches and the Internet in various qualitative designs?

REFERENCES

Aamodt AA: Ethnography and epistemology: generating nursing knowledge. In Morse JM, ed: *Qualitative nursing research: a contemporary dialogue,* Newbury Park, Calif, 1991, Sage.

Agar MH: *Speaking of ethnography,* Beverly Hills, Calif, 1986, Sage.

Anderson NLR: Decisions about substance abuse among adolescents in juvenile detention, *Image J Nurs Sch* 28(1):65-70, 1996.

Atkinson P, Hammersley M: Ethnography and participant observation. In Denzin NK, Lincoln YS, eds: *Handbook of qualitative research,* Thousand Oaks, Calif, 1994, Sage.

Badger TA: Family members' experience living with members with depression, *West J Nurs Res* 18(2):149-171, 1996.

Beck CT: The lived experience of postpartum depression: a phenomenological study, *Nurs Res* 41(3):166-170, 1992.

Beck CT: Teetering on the edge: a substantive theory of postpartum depression, *Nurs Res* 42(1):42-48, 1993.

Beck CT: The effects of postpartum depression on maternal-infant interaction: a metaanalysis, *Nurs Res* 44(5):298-304, 1995.

Beck CT: Post partum depressed mothers' experiences interacting with their children, *Nurs Res* 45(2):98-104, 1996a.

Beck CT: A meta-analysis of predictors of postpartum depression, *Nurs Res* 45(1):297-303, 1996b.

Beck CT, Reynolds MA, Rutowski P: Maternity blues and postpartum depression, *J Obstet Gynecol Neonatal Nurs* 21(4):287-293, 1992.

Boas F: *Race, language, and culture,* New York, 1948, MacMillan.

Boland DL, Sims SL: Family care giving at home as a solitary journey, *Image J Nurs Sch* 28(1):55-58, 1996.

Boyle JS: Field research: a collaborative model for practice and research. In Morse JM, ed: *Qualitative nursing research: a contemporary dialogue,* Newbury Park, Calif, 1991, Sage.

Christy TE: The methodology of historical research: a brief introduction, *Image J Nurs Sch* 24(3):189-192, 1975.

Christy TE: The need for historical research in nursing, *Image J Nurs Sch* 4:227-228, 1981.

Colaizzi P: Psychological research as a phenomenologist views it. In Valle RS, King M, eds: *Existential phenomenological alternatives for psychology,* New York, 1978, Oxford University Press.

Crabtree BF, Miller WL, eds: *Doing qualitative research,* Newbury Park, Calif, 1992, Sage.

Cramer S: The nature of history: meditations on Clio's craft, *Nurs Res* 41(1):4-7, 1992.

Daly J: The lived experience of suffering. In Parse RR, ed: *Illuminations: the human becoming theory in practice and research,* New York, 1995, NLN.

Denzin NK: *The research act: a theoretical introduction to sociological methods,* ed 2, New York, 1978, McGraw-Hill.

Denzin NK, Lincoln YS: Introduction: entering the field of qualitative research. In Denzin NK, Lincoln YS, eds: *Handbook of qualitative research,* Thousand Oaks, Calif, 1994, Sage.

Engebretson J: Comparison of nurses and alternative healers, *Image J Nurs Sch* 28(2):95-99, 1996.

Fairman J: Watchful vigilance: nursing care, technology, and the development of intensive care units, *Nurs Res* 41(1):56-58, 1992.

Giorgi A, Fischer CL, Murray EL, eds: *Duquesne studies in phenomenological psychology,* Pittsburgh, 1975, Duquesne University Press.

Glaser BG, Strauss AL: *The discovery of grounded theory: strategies for qualitative research,* Chicago, 1967, Aldine.

Guba E, Lincoln Y: *Effective evaluation,* San Francisco, 1981, Jossey-Bass.

Janesick VJ: The dance of qualitative research design: metaphor, methodolatry, and meaning. In Denzin NK, Lincoln YS, eds: *Handbook of qualitative research,* Thousand Oaks, Calif, 1994, Sage.

Jennings JL: Husserl revisited: the forgotten distinction between psychology and phenomenology, *Am Psychol* 41(11):1231-1240, 1986.

Johnson M: A silent conspiracy: some ethical issues of participant observation in nursing research, *Int J Nurs Stud* 29(2):213-233, 1992.

Kaufman KS: Center as haven: findings of an urban ethnography, *Nurs Res* 44(4):231-236, 1995.

Kleinman A: *Patients and healers in the context of culture,* Berkeley, 1980, University of California Press.

Kleinman A: Local worlds of suffering: an interpersonal focus for ethnographies of illness experience, *Qual Health Res* 2(2):127-134, 1992.

Lamendola FP, Newman ME: The paradox of HIV/AIDS as expanding consciousness, *Adv Nurs Sci* 16(3):13-21, 1994.

Lazarus R, Folkman S: *Stress appraisal, and coping,* New York, 1984, Springer.

Leininger MM: Ethnography and ethnonursing: models and modes of qualitative data analysis. In Leininger MM, ed: *Qualitative research methods in nursing,* Orlando, 1985, Grune & Stratton.

Leininger MM: *Qualitative research methods in nursing,* New York, 1985, Grune & Stratton.

Leininger MM: Leininger's theory of nursing: cultural care diversity and universality, *Nurs Sci Q* 1(4):152-160, 1988.

Leininger MM: Evaluation criteria and critique of qualitative research studies. In Morse JM, ed: *Critical issues in qualitative research methods,* Thousand Oaks, Calif, 1994, Sage.

Leininger MM: Culture care theory, *Nurs Sci Q* 9(2):71-78, 1996.

Lewis L: One year in the life of a woman with premenstrual syndrome: a case study, *Nurs Res* 44(2):111-116, 1995.

Lincoln YS: Sympathetic connections between qualitative methods and health research, *Qual Health Res* 2(4):375-391, 1992.

Lincoln YS, Guba EG: *Naturalistic inquiry,* Newbury Park, Calif, 1985, Sage.

Lipson JG: Ethical issues in ethnography. In Morse JM, ed: *Critical issues in qualitative research methods,* Thousand Oaks, Calif, 1994, Sage.

Malinowski B: *1961. Argonauts of the Western Pacific,* New York, 1922, EP Dutton.

Mayo K: Physical activity practices among American black working women, *Qual Health Res* 2(3):318-333, 1992.

Mead M: *1949. Coming of age in Samoa,* New York, 1928, New American Library, Mentor Books.

Morse JM: Approaches to qualitative-quantitative methodological triangulation, *Nurs Res* 40(1):120-123, 1991.

Morse JM, Bottorff JL, Hutchinson S: The paradox of comfort, *Nurs Res* 44(1):14-19, 1995.

Morse JM, Field PA: *Qualitative research methods for health professionals,* ed 2, Thousand Oaks, Calif, 1995, Sage.

Munhall PL: Holding the Mississippi River in place and other implications for qualitative research, *Nurs Outlook* 40(6):257-262, 1992.

Newman M: *Health as expanding consciousness,* ed 2, New York, 1994, NLN.

Parse RR: Human becoming: Parse's theory of nursing, *Nurs Sci Q* 5(1):35-42, 1992.

Parse RR: The human becoming theory: challenges in practice and research, *Nurs Sci Q* 9(2):55-60, 1996.

Parse RR, Coyne AB, Smith MJ: *Nursing research: qualitative methods,* Bowie, Md, 1985, Brady.

Price MJ: An experiential model of learning diabetes self-management, *Qual Health Res* 3(1):29-54, 1993.

Pursley-Crotteau S, Stern PN: Creating a new life: dimensions of temperance in perinatal co-caine crack users, *Qual Health Res* 6(3):350-367, 1996.

Reid AO: Computer management strategies for text data. In Crabtree BF, Miller WL, eds: *Doing qualitative research,* Newbury Park, Calif, 1992, Sage.

Rendon DC: The lived experience of aging in community-dwelling elders in Valencia, Spain: a phenomenological study, *Nurs Sci Q* 8(4):152-157, 1995.

Resnick B: Motivation in geriatric rehabilitation, *Image J Nurs Sch* 28(1):41-45, 1996.

Roberts J: British nurses at war 1914-1918: ancillary personnel and the battle for registration, *Nurs Res* 45(3):167-172, 1996.

Rosenbaum JN: The health meanings and practices of older Greek-Canadian widows, *J Adv Nurs* 16:1320-1327, 1991.

Sanday RR: The ethnographic paradigm(s). In Van Maanen J, ed: *Qualitative methodology,* Newbury Park, Calif, 1989, Sage.

Sandelowski M: Qualitative analysis: what it is and how to begin, *Res Nurs Health* 18:371-375, 1995.

Sarnecky MT: Historiography: a legitimate research methodology for nursing, *Adv Nurs Sci* 12(4):1-10, 1990.

Schweer KD: Lessons from nursing's historian: a tribute to Teresa E Christy, EdD, FAAN (1927-1982), *Image J Nurs Sch* 14(3):66, 1982.

Seideman RY, Kleine PF: A theory of transformed parenting: parenting a child with developmental delay/mental retardation, *Image J Nurs Sch* 44(1):38-44, 1995.

Smith CA: The lived experience of staying healthy in rural African-American families, *Nurs Sci Q* 8(1):17-21, 1995.

Spiegelberg H: *The phenomenological movement,* vols I and II, The Hague, 1976, Martinus Nijhoff.

Spradley JP: *The ethnographic interview,* New York, 1979, Holt, Rinehart, & Winston.

Strauss AL: *Qualitative analysis for social scientists,* New York, 1987, Cambridge University Press.

Strauss A, Corbin J: *Basics of qualitative research: grounded theory procedures and techniques,* Newbury Park, Calif, 1990, Sage.

Strauss A, Corbin J: Grounded theory methodology. In Denzin NK, Lincoln YS, eds: *Handbook of qualitative research,* Thousand Oaks, Calif, 1994, Sage.

Taft LB: Computer-assisted qualitative research, *Res Nurs Health* 16:379-383, 1993.

Tarasuk V, Eakin JM: The problem of legitimacy in the experience of work-related back injury, *Qual Health Res* 5(2):204-221, 1995.

Temkin E: Turn-of-the-century nursing perspectives on venereal disease, *Image J Nurs Sch* 26(3):207-211, 1994.

Tesch R: Computer programs that assist in the analysis of qualitative data: an overview, *Qual Health Res* 1(3):309-325, 1991.

Uphall MJ: Nursing perceptions of collaboration with indigenous healers in Swaziland, *Int J Nurs Stud* 29(1):27-36, 1992.

van Kaam A: *Existential foundations in psychology,* New York, 1969, Doubleday.

Wilde V: Controversial hypotheses on the relationship between researcher and informant in qualitative research, *J Adv Nurs* 17:234-242, 1992.

Wing DM: Transcending alcoholic denial, *Image J Nurs Sch* 27(2):121-126, 1995.

Sampling

Judith Haber

Key Terms

accessible
  population
convenience
  sampling
data saturation
delimitations
element
eligibility criteria
matching
multistage (cluster)
  sampling

network sampling
  (snowballing)
nonprobability
  sampling
population
probability
  sampling
purposive sampling
quota sampling
random selection
representative
  sample

sample
sampling
sampling frame
sampling interval
sampling unit
simple random
  sampling
stratified random
  sampling
systematic
  sampling
target population

Learning Outcomes

After reading this chapter the student should be able to do the following:

- Identify the purpose of sampling.
- Define population, sample, and sampling.
- Compare and contrast a population and a sample.
- Discuss the eligibility criteria for sample selection.
- Define nonprobability and probability sampling.
- Identify the types of nonprobability and probability sampling strategies.
- Compare the advantages and disadvantages of specific nonprobability and probability sampling strategies.
- Discuss the factors that influence determination of sample size.
- Discuss the procedure for drawing a sample.
- Identify the criteria for critiquing a sampling plan.
- Use the critiquing criteria to evaluate the sampling section of a research report.

Sampling is the process of selecting representative units of a population for study in a research investigation. Although sampling is a complex process, it is a familiar one. In our daily lives we gather knowledge, make decisions, and formulate predictions based on sampling procedures. For example, nursing students may make generalizations about the overall quality of nursing professors as a result of their exposure to a sample of nursing professors during their undergraduate programs. Patients may make generalizations about a hospital's food during a 1-week hospital stay. It is apparent that limited exposure to a limited portion of these phenomena forms the basis of our conclusions and so much of our knowledge and decisions are based on our experience with samples.

Scientists also derive knowledge from samples. Many problems in scientific research cannot be solved without employing sampling procedures. For example, when testing the effectiveness of a medication for patients with cancer, the drug is administered to a sample of the population for whom the drug is potentially appropriate. The scientist must come to some conclusions without administering the drug to every known patient with cancer or every laboratory animal in the world. But because human lives are at stake, the scientist cannot afford to arrive casually at conclusions that are based on the first dozen patients available for study. The consequences of arriving at erroneous conclusions or making inaccurate generalizations from a small, nonrepresentative sample are much more severe in scientific investigations than in everyday life. Consequently, research methodologists have expended considerable effort to develop sampling theories and procedures that produce accurate and meaningful information. Essentially, researchers sample representative segments of the population, because it is rarely feasible or necessary to sample the entire population of interest to obtain relevant information.

This chapter will familiarize the research consumer with the basic concepts of sampling as they primarily pertain to the principles of quantitative research design, nonprobability and probability sampling, sample size, and the related critiquing process. Sampling issues that relate to qualitative research designs are discussed mainly in Chapter 9.

SAMPLING CONCEPTS

Population

A **population** is a well-defined set that has certain specified properties. A population can be composed of people, animals, objects, or events. For example, if a researcher is studying undergraduate nursing students, the type of educational preparation of the population must be specified. In this instance the population consists of undergraduate students enrolled in a generic baccalaureate nursing program. Examples of other possible populations might be all male patients admitted to hospital X for prostatectomies for treatment of prostate cancer during the year 1997, all children with asthma in the state of New York, or all men and women with a diagnosis of bipolar disorder in the United States. These examples illustrate that a population may be broadly defined and potentially involve millions of people or narrowly specified to include only several hundred people.

The reader of a research report should consider whether the researcher has identified the population descriptors that form the basis for the **eligibility criteria** that are used to select the sample from the array of all possible units, whether people, objects, or events. Let us consider the population previously defined as undergraduate nursing students enrolled in a generic baccalaureate program. Would this population include both part-time and full-time students?

Would it include students who had previously attended another nursing program? What about foreign students? Would freshmen through seniors qualify? Insofar as it is possible, the researcher must demonstrate that the exact criteria used to decide whether an individual would be classified as a member of a given population have been specifically delineated. The population descriptors that provide the basis for eligibility criteria should be evident in the sample; that is, the characteristics of the population and the sample should be congruent. The degree of congruence is evaluated to assess the representativeness of the sample. For example, if a population were defined as full-time, American-born, senior nursing students enrolled in a generic baccalaureate nursing program, the sample would be expected to reflect these characteristics.

Think about the concept of eligibility criteria applied to a research study where the subjects are patients. For example, participants in a study investigating inpatient self-management of bipolar disorder (Pollack, 1996) had to meet the following eligibility criteria:

1. Age—between 18 and 65 years of age
2. Medication—receiving lithium carbonate, carbamazapine, and/or valproic acid for treatment of their bipolar disorder
3. Status—sufficiently stable to be interviewed
4. Treatments—not receiving electroconvulsive treatment
5. Activity level—ambulatory
6. Language competence—English speaking
7. Physician endorsement—MD prescription permitting participation in study protocol
8. Awareness of diagnosis—have been told their diagnosis
9. Comorbid conditions—no evidence of organic brain disorder or known terminal illness

Eligibility criteria may also be viewed as **delimitations,** or those characteristics that restrict the population to a homogeneous group of subjects. Examples of delimitations include the following: gender, age, marital status, socioeconomic status, religion, ethnicity, level of education, age of children, health status, and diagnosis. In a study evaluating the efficacy of absorbent products for women with mild to moderate urinary incontinence (Baker and Norton, 1996), the researchers established the following delimitations:

- Women who were currently using three or more extraabsorbency incontinent pads a day to control their incontinence, indicating incontinence of a moderate to severe degree
- Symptoms such as dysuria or vaginitis
- Inability to comply with record keeping
- Subjects would be dropped from the study if more than 75% of the study pads were soaked, indicating incontinence of a moderate to severe degree

These delimitations were selected because of their potential effect on the accurate evaluation of eight different absorbent pads for use by community-dwelling women with mild to moderate urinary incontinence. Let us consider the criterion of degree of incontinence. If women with mild to moderate and moderate to severe urinary incontinence were both included and grouped together in the sample, the researchers would have two groups for whom the efficacy of the absorbent pads may be very different (especially in a community-dwelling context) because of the incontinence variable, and hence the accuracy of the findings may be distorted. Heterogeneity of this sample group would inhibit the researchers' ability to interpret the findings meaningfully and make generalizations. It is much wiser to study only one homogeneous group or include specific groups as distinct subsets of the sample and study the groups comparatively. For example, in a study investigating the effectiveness of retention control training in increasing bladder capacity and eliminating enuresis (Ronen and Abraham, 1996), two age groups of children were used. The final sample consisted of 30 enuretic children divided into two age groups, 15 younger children ages 4.7 to 6.1 years and 15 older children ages 6.2 to 9 years, that were studied comparatively. You should remember that delimitations are not established in a casual or meaningless way, but they are established to control for extraneous variability or bias. Each delimitation should have a rationale, presumably related to a potential contaminating effect on the dependent variable. The careful establishment of sample delimitations will increase the precision of the study and contribute to the accuracy and generalizability of the findings (see Chapter 6).

The population criteria establish the **target population;** that is, the entire set of cases about which the researcher would like to make generalizations. A target population might include all undergraduate nursing students enrolled in generic baccalaureate programs in the United States. It often is not feasible, because of time, money, and personnel, to pursue using a target population. An **accessible population,** one that meets the population criteria and that is *available,* is used instead. For example, an accessible population might include all full-time generic baccalaureate students attending school in Pennsylvania. Pragmatic factors must also be considered when identifying a potential population of interest.

It is important to know that a population is not restricted to human subjects. It may consist of hospital records; blood, urine, or other specimens taken from patients at a clinic; historical documents; or laboratory animals. For example, a population might consist of all the urine specimens collected from patients in the Crestview Hospital antepartum clinic or all of the patient charts on file at the Day Surgery Center. It is apparent that a population can be defined in a variety of ways. The important point to remember is that the basic unit of the population must be clearly defined, because the generalizability of the findings will be a function of the population criteria.

HELPFUL HINT
Often researchers do not clearly identify the population under study, or the population is not clarified until the discussion section when the effort is made to discuss the group (population) to which the study findings can be generalized.

Samples and Sampling

Sampling is a process of selecting a portion of the designated population to represent the entire population. A **sample** is a set of elements that make up the population; an **element** is the most basic unit about which information is collected. The most common element in nursing research is individuals, but other elements, such as places or objects, can form the basis of a sample or population. A **sampling unit** is the element or set of elements used for selecting the sample. Sometimes the sampling unit and the element represent the same thing, and other times it is more efficient to use a unit larger than the element for sampling purposes. For example, a researcher was planning a study that compared the effectiveness of different nursing interventions on the healing rate of decubitus ulcers. Four hospitals, each using a different treatment protocol, were identified as the sampling units rather than the nurses themselves or the treatment alone.

The purpose of sampling is to increase the efficiency of a research study. The novice reviewer of research reports must realize that it would not be feasible to examine every element or unit in the population. When sampling is properly done it allows the researcher to draw inferences and make generalizations about the population without examining each unit in the population. Sampling procedures that entail the formulation of specific criteria for selection ensure that the characteristics of the phenomena of interest will be, or are likely to be, present in all of the units being studied. The researcher's efforts to ensure that the sample is representative of the target population puts the researcher in a stronger position to draw conclusions from the sample findings that are generalizable to the population.

After having reviewed a number of research studies, you will recognize that samples and sampling procedures vary in terms of merit. The foremost criterion in evaluating a sample is its representativeness. A **representative sample** is one whose key characteristics closely approximate those of the population. If 70% of the population in a study of child-rearing practices consisted of women and 40% were full-time employees, a representative sample should reflect these characteristics in the same proportions.

It must be understood that there is no way to guarantee that a sample is representative without obtaining a database about the entire population. Because it is difficult and inefficient to assess a population, the researcher must employ sampling strategies that minimize or control for sample bias. If an appropriate sampling strategy is used, it almost always is possible to obtain a reasonably accurate understanding of the phenomena under investigation by obtaining data from a sample.

TYPES OF SAMPLES

Sampling strategies are generally grouped into two categories: nonprobability sampling and probability sampling. In **nonprobability sampling,** elements are chosen by nonrandom methods. The drawback of this strategy is that there is no way of estimating the probability that each element has of being included in the samples. Essentially there is no way of ensuring that every element has a chance for inclusion in the nonprobability sample. Probability sampling uses some form of random selection when choosing the sample units. This type of sample enables the researcher to estimate the probability that each element of the population will be included in the sample. **Probability sampling** is the more rigorous type of sampling strategy, and it is more likely to result in a representative sample. The remainder of this section is devoted to a discussion of different types of nonprobability and probability sampling strategies. A summary of sampling strategies appears in Table 10-1. You may wish to refer to this table as the various nonprobability and probability strategies are discussed in the following sections.

HELPFUL HINT

Research articles are not always explicit about the type of sampling strategy that was used. If the sampling strategy is not specified, assume that a convenience sample was used for a quantitative study and a purposive sample was used for a qualitative study.

Table 10-1

Summary of Sampling Strategies

SAMPLING STRATEGY	EASE OF DRAWING SAMPLE	RISK OF BIAS	REPRESENTATIVENESS OF SAMPLE
Nonprobability			
Convenience	Very easy	Greater than any other sampling strategy	Because samples tend to be self-selecting, representativeness is questionable
Quota	Relatively easy	Contains unknown source of bias that affects external validity	Builds in some representativeness by using knowledge about the population of interest
Purposive	Relatively easy	Bias increases with greater heterogeneity of the population; conscious bias is also a danger	Very limited ability to generalize because sample is handpicked
Probability			
Simple random	Laborious	Low	Maximized; probability of nonrepresentativeness decreases with increased sample size
Stratified random	Time consuming	Low	Enhanced
Cluster	Less time consuming than simple or stratified	Subject to more sampling errors than simple or stratified	Less representative than simple or stratified
Systematic	More convenient and efficient than simple, stratified, or cluster sampling	Bias in the form of nonrandomness can be inadvertently introduced	Less representative if bias occurs as a result of coincidental nonrandomness

Nonprobability Sampling

The nonprobability sampling strategy is less rigorous than the probability sampling strategy, and it tends to produce less accurate and less representative samples. However, most samples, not only in nursing research but also in other disciplines, are nonprobability samples. Although such samples are more feasible for the researcher to obtain, the use of nonprobability samples does limit the ability of the researcher to make generalizations about the findings. The three major types of nonprobability sampling are the following: convenience, quota, and purposive sampling strategies.

Convenience Sampling

Convenience sampling is the use of the most readily accessible persons or objects as subjects in a study. The subjects may include volunteers, the first 25 patients admitted to hospital X with a particular diagnosis, all people who enrolled in program Y during the month of September, or all students enrolled in course Z at a particular university during 1997. The subjects are convenient and accessible to the researcher and are thus called a *convenience sample.* For example, a researcher studying adjustment of women with systemic lupus erythematosus (SLE) used a convenience sample of women ranging in age from 23 to 65 years of age who met the criteria for SLE as defined by the American Rheumatism Association and who volunteered to participate in the study (Failla et al, 1996). Another researcher studying the effect of group patient education on cardiac rehabilitation used all patients transferred from the coronary care unit to the intermediate coronary care unit in hospital X between September and December 1996.

The advantage of a convenience sample is that it is easier for the researcher to obtain subjects. The researcher may have to be concerned only with obtaining a sufficient number of subjects who meet the same criteria.

The major disadvantage of a convenience sample is that the risk of bias is greater than in any other type of sample (see Table 10-1). The problem of bias is related to the fact that convenience samples tend to be self-selecting; that is, the researcher ends up obtaining information only from the people who volunteer to participate. In this case the following questions must be raised: What motivated some of the people to participate and others to not participate? What kind of data would have been obtained if nonparticipants had also responded? How representative are the people who did participate in relation to the population? For example, a researcher may stop people on a street corner to ask their opinion on some issue; place advertisements in the newspaper; or place signs in local churches, community centers, or supermarkets indicating that volunteers are needed for a particular study. For example, in a study examining social support networks, level of social support, and perceived physical health of older rural adults, subjects were recruited from senior centers, church groups, advertisements in newspapers and on the radio, and posters placed in local stores (Johnson, 1996). Because acquiring research subjects is a problem that confronts many nurse researchers, innovative recruitment strategies may be used. For example, a researcher may even offer to pay the participants for their time. A unique method of accessing and recruiting subjects is the use of on-line computer networks available on personal computers (Wilmoth, 1995).

The evaluator of a research report should recognize that the convenience sample, although the most common, is the weakest form of sampling strategy with regard to generalizability. Its use should be avoided whenever possible. When a convenience sample is used, caution should be exercised in analyzing and interpreting the data. When critiquing a research study that has employed this sampling strategy, the reviewer will be justifiably skeptical about the external validity of the findings (see Chapter 6).

Quota Sampling

Quota sampling refers to a form of nonprobability sampling in which knowledge about the population of interest is used to build some representativeness into the sample (see Table 10-1). A quota sample identifies the strata of the population and proportionally represents the strata in the sample. For example, the data in Table 10-2 reveal that 20% of the 5000 nurses in city X are diploma graduates, 40% are associate degree students, and 40% are baccalaureate graduates. Each stratum of the population should be proportionately represented in the sample. In this case the researcher used a proportional quota sampling strategy and decided to sample 10% of a population of 5000, or 500 nurses. Based on the proportion of each stratum in the population, 100 diploma graduates, 200 associate degree graduates, and 200 baccalaureate graduates were the quotas established for the three strata. The researcher recruited subjects who met the eligibility criteria of the study until the quota for each stratum was filled. In other words, once the researcher obtained the necessary 100 diploma, 200 associate degree, and 200 baccalaureate graduates, the sample was complete.

The researcher systematically ensures that proportional segments of the population are included in the sample. The quota sample is not randomly selected—that is, once the proportional strata have been identified, the researcher obtains subjects until the quota for each stratum has been filled—but it does increase the representativeness of the sample. This sampling strategy addresses the problem of overrepresentation or underrepresentation of certain segments of a population in a sample.

The characteristics chosen to form the strata are selected according to a researcher's judgment based on knowledge of the population and the literature review. The criterion for selection should be a variable that would reflect important differences in the dependent variables under investigation. Age, gender, religion, ethnicity, medical diagnosis, socioeconomic status, level of completed education, and occupational rank are among those variables that are likely to be important stratifying variables in nursing research investigations.

The critiquer of a research study seeks to determine whether the sample strata appropriately reflect the population under consideration and whether the stratifying variables are ho-

Table 10-2			

Numbers and Percentages of Students in Strata of a Quota Sample of 5000 Graduates of Nursing Programs in City X

	DIPLOMA GRADUATES	ASSOCIATE DEGREE GRADUATES	BACCALAUREATE GRADUATES
Population	1000 (20%)	2000 (40%)	2000 (40%)
Strata	100	200	200

mogeneous enough to ensure a meaningful comparison of differences among strata. Even when the preceding factors have been addressed by the researcher, the evaluator must remember that as a nonprobability sample, the quota strategy contains an unknown source of bias that affects external validity.

The problem is that those who choose to participate may not be typical of the population with regard to the variables being measured. There is no way to assess the biases that may be operating. In cases where the phenomena under investigation are relatively homogeneous within the population, the risk of bias may be minimal. However, in heterogeneous populations the risk of bias is great.

Purposive Sampling

Purposive sampling is an increasingly common strategy in which the researcher's knowledge of the population and its elements is used to handpick the cases to be included in the sample. The researcher usually selects subjects who are considered to be typical of the population. For example, in a qualitative research study by Beck (1996) examining the meaning of postpartum depressed mothers' interactions with their infants and older children, a purposive sample of mothers who had been diagnosed as having postpartum depression and were or had been under the care of a therapist or psychiatrist was used, because they were typical of the population under consideration and could illuminate the phenomenon being studied (see Chapters 9 and 18).

A purposive sample is used also when a highly unusual group is being studied, such as a population with a rare genetic disease such as Tay-Sachs disease. In this case the researcher would describe the sample characteristics precisely to ensure that the reader will have an accurate picture of the subjects in the sample.

In another situation the researcher may wish to interview individuals who reflect different ends of the range of a particular characteristic. For example, a researcher investigates the psychosocial needs in individuals who test positive for the human immunodeficiency virus (HIV) but have no symptoms, in comparison with individuals who have active acquired immunodeficiency syndrome (AIDS).

Today, computer networks such as on-line services can be of great value in helping researchers access and recruit subjects for purposive samples. One researcher used the Prodigy Cancer Support Group Bulletin Board and personal mailbox to aid in subject access and accrual when testing the psychometric properties of the Sexual Behaviors Questionnaire (Wilmoth, 1995). A posting was placed on the Cancer Support Group Bulletin Board, and within 24 hours, 11 replies had been received. Several respondents were participants in breast cancer support groups and offered to distribute copies of the questionnaires to support group members. This method contributed 4% of the sample in an inexpensive and timely way.

The researcher who uses a purposive sample assumes that errors of judgment in overrepresenting or underrepresenting elements of the population in the sample will tend to balance out. However, there is no objective method for determining the validity of this assumption. The evaluator must be aware of the fact that the more heterogeneous the population, the greater the chance of bias being introduced in the selection of a purposive sample. As indicated in Table 10-1, conscious bias in the selection of subjects remains a constant danger. As such, the findings from a study using a purposive sample should be regarded with caution. As with any nonprobability sample, the ability to generalize is very limited. The following are several instances when a purposive sample may be appropriate:

- The effective pretesting of newly developed instruments with a purposive sample of divergent types of people
- The validation of a scale or test with a known-groups technique
- The collection of exploratory data in relation to an unusual or highly specific population, particularly when the total target population remains an unknown to the researcher
- The collection of descriptive data as in qualitative studies that seek to describe the lived experience of a particular phenomenon, such as postpartum depression, caring, hope, or surviving childhood sexual abuse

Even when the use of a purposive sample is appropriate, the researcher, as well as the critiquer, should be cognizant of the limitations of this sampling strategy.

Probability Sampling

The primary characteristic of probability sampling is the random selection of elements from the population. **Random selection** occurs when each element of the population has an equal and independent chance of being included in the sample. Four commonly used probability sampling strategies are simple random sampling, stratified random sampling, cluster sampling, and systematic sampling.

Random selection of sample subjects should not be confused with *random assignment* of subjects. The latter, as discussed in Chapter 7, refers to the assignment of subjects to either an experimental or a control group on a purely random basis.

Simple Random Sampling

Simple random sampling is a laborious and carefully controlled process. Because the more complex probability designs incorporate the principles of simple random sampling in their procedures, the principles of this strategy are presented.

The researcher defines the population (a set), lists all of the units of the population (a **sampling frame**), and selects a sample of units (a subset) from which the sample will be chosen. For example, if American hospitals specializing in respiratory problems were the sampling unit, a list of all such hospitals would be the sampling frame. If certified clinical specialists constituted the accessible population, a list of those nurses would be the sampling frame.

Once a list of the population elements has been developed, the best method of selecting a sample is to employ a table of random numbers containing columns of digits, such as the one appearing in Figure 10-1. Such tables can be generated by computer programs. After assigning consecutive numbers to units of the population, the researcher starts at any point on the table of random numbers and reads consecutive numbers in any direction (horizontally, vertically, or diagonally). When a number is read that corresponds with the written unit on a card, that unit is chosen for the sample. The investigator continues to read until a sample of the desired size is drawn. The advantages of simple random sampling are the following:

- The sample selection is not subject to the conscious biases of the researcher.

1000 random integers between 0 and 99																			
40	23	0	29	10	94	17	58	12	85	13	25	80	84	72	74	54	63	55	31
32	98	49	23	74	97	51	42	21	87	48	64	54	38	84	68	14	17	35	48
84	34	84	14	53	65	67	37	2	45	84	21	71	34	10	80	72	27	11	13
86	37	24	89	23	4	44	40	72	81	44	69	25	44	34	34	34	75	50	50
50	58	85	8	22	24	73	20	63	35	60	87	91	92	96	80	19	22	87	24
1	87	43	82	9	31	40	88	33	28	82	73	18	6	48	64	59	45	34	3
21	19	42	76	84	67	29	68	8	66	93	89	96	28	12	14	38	47	52	65
32	66	33	21	81	97	39	76	67	27	97	22	76	89	41	11	91	29	6	66
16	82	42	75	35	42	92	90	77	24	21	8	36	16	5	54	89	51	57	85
74	32	63	65	93	96	18	36	82	72	39	69	37	97	51	17	36	71	38	30
50	94	4	66	17	37	10	53	8	29	67	74	88	38	11	59	60	91	56	17
71	47	81	18	53	98	7	87	29	37	22	93	13	6	95	7	95	71	14	6
71	93	48	16	33	19	46	21	60	44	52	91	52	58	10	9	41	31	35	18
20	94	13	99	45	6	53	54	1	25	79	28	1	48	36	26	68	37	59	7
75	22	69	56	62	40	64	45	40	99	94	14	98	84	22	38	24	87	43	71
16	87	41	0	88	83	11	37	71	78	22	39	43	37	75	84	84	11	55	58
92	90	80	2	30	37	85	55	56	50	3	71	24	13	62	74	82	44	90	32
96	89	31	32	37	45	70	67	80	55	58	9	55	60	61	55	86	44	27	77
38	29	36	94	65	39	56	29	29	65	88	13	71	38	71	8	81	66	31	44
20	6	61	66	90	13	70	60	92	53	87	49	34	42	14	47	75	33	26	9
63	44	94	21	14	13	41	80	39	72	29	3	25	89	44	88	13	49	18	58
13	32	93	90	31	75	86	95	18	51	61	59	84	95	67	54	40	30	29	63
26	35	48	81	19	24	36	36	76	16	46	5	93	41	97	46	79	54	95	49
89	74	96	95	94	69	31	60	16	69	76	42	28	71	69	34	46	55	20	42
50	39	28	64	20	68	60	33	92	82	61	70	5	68	95	88	12	85	18	94
55	86	5	96	87	69	75	93	54	79	0	57	45	8	86	59	25	21	9	29
75	35	1	2	86	62	70	83	85	13	97	37	13	73	16	38	36	23	54	11
74	50	1	77	87	92	68	87	57	36	17	47	0	97	78	72	72	45	54	51
34	24	35	13	26	42	22	75	47	2	34	87	15	50	65	27	5	72	28	68
73	33	42	65	91	24	44	84	71	55	70	1	27	30	8	61	65	61	18	92
7	55	12	6	61	17	23	95	91	58	60	30	35	61	34	27	75	44	35	64
10	94	18	4	3	19	21	37	28	55	76	25	10	29	80	64	8	81	20	32
20	48	92	87	95	58	57	73	42	1	12	81	94	85	63	97	24	19	93	51
81	10	92	49	70	15	76	4	36	92	62	99	78	32	86	74	43	22	98	46
66	67	82	94	67	75	16	88	84	98	0	52	37	0	43	9	0	51	2	62
64	92	36	11	3	52	44	65	45	67	97	86	92	2	50	5	93	66	73	40
36	29	98	46	88	23	28	44	8	71	69	43	53	16	87	21	56	23	37	24
15	11	82	30	59	94	23	30	40	25	87	26	24	30	44	53	33	65	72	55
89	57	49	79	83	88	42	45	41	93	38	24	15	80	97	18	61	12	13	42
23	36	65	9	64	26	93	37	26	44	42	17	45	68	27	77	74	56	49	34
9	93	90	61	45	40	75	85	64	66	36	89	72	43	99	90	92	10	10	85
53	94	30	31	62	92	82	30	94	56	40	4	50	53	9	74	87	2	36	36
18	69	77	38	89	78	30	68	71	92	22	93	91	74	52	1	97	69	71	42
50	20	76	36	6	20	75	56	36	5	14	70	9	78	23	33	91	33	25	72
30	46	1	10	16	72	69	26	94	39	80	36	36	68	92	74	22	74	41	42
59	47	7	92	77	55	2	12	5	24	0	30	25	62	83	36	92	96	36	75
93	22	3	20	82	44	16	69	98	72	30	57	77	15	90	29	32	38	3	48
9	55	27	41	40	94	77	14	54	10	25	75	1	74	72	15	69	80	33	58
70	8	3	5	46	89	28	86	40	6	25	40	81	26	63	97	87	48	26	41
19	6	89	31	80	60	13	89	17	69	38	93	58	55	54	69	74	33	8	55

Figure 10-1   A table of random numbers.

- The representativeness of the sample in relation to the population characteristics is maximized.
- The differences in the characteristics of the sample and the population are purely a function of chance.
- The probability of choosing a nonrepresentative sample decreases as the size of the sample increases.

Simple random sampling was used in a study examining the relationship between nursing care requirements and nursing resource consumption in home health care using both an intensity index and nursing diagnoses. Using a table of random numbers, a random sample of 306 patient records was drawn from patients dismissed during a 6-month period who received at least three nursing visits at home from a specific home health care agency.

Consumers must remember that despite the utilization of a carefully controlled sampling procedure that minimizes error, there is no guarantee that the sample will be representative. Factors such as sample heterogeneity and subject dropout may jeopardize the representativeness of the sample despite the most stringent random sampling procedure.

The major disadvantage of simple random sampling is that it is a time-consuming and inefficient method for obtaining a random sample. Consider the task of listing all of the baccalaureate nursing students in the United States. In addition, it may be impossible to obtain an accurate or complete listing of every element in the population. Imagine trying to obtain a list of all completed suicides in New York City for the year 1997. It often is the case that although suicide may have been the cause of death, another cause, such as cardiac failure, appears on the death certificate. It would be difficult to estimate how many elements of the target population would be eliminated from consideration. The issue of bias would definitely enter the picture despite the researcher's best efforts. Thus the evaluator of a research paper must exercise caution in generalizing from reported findings, even when random sampling is the stated strategy, if the target population has been difficult or impossible to list completely.

Stratified Random Sampling

Stratified random sampling requires that the population be divided into strata or subgroups. The subgroups or subsets that the population is divided into are homogeneous. An appropriate number of elements from each subset are randomly selected, on the basis of their proportion in the population. This strategy's goal is to achieve a greater degree of representativeness. Stratified random sampling is similar to the proportional stratified quota sampling strategy discussed earlier in the chapter. The major difference is that stratified random sampling uses a random selection procedure for obtaining sample subjects. Figure 10-2 provides an example that illustrates the use of stratified random sampling.

The population is stratified according to any number of attributes, such as age, gender, ethnicity, religion, socioeconomic status, or level of completed education. The variables selected to make up the strata should be adaptable to homogeneous subsets with regard to the attributes being studied. The following criteria can be used for decision making in the selection of a stratified sample:

- Is there a critical variable or attribute that provides a logical basis for stratifying the sample?
- Does the population list contain sufficient information about the attributes that will be used to divide the sample into subsets?

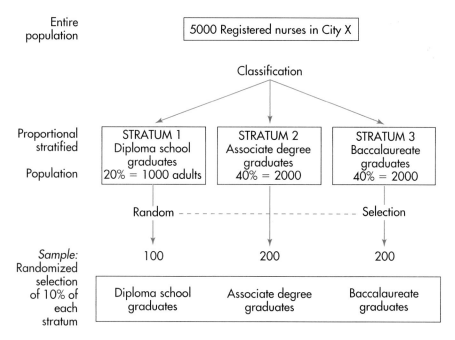

Figure 10-2   Subject selection using a proportional stratified random sampling strategy.

- Is it appropriate for each subset to be equal in size, or is it more appropriate for each subset to be proportionally stratified based on the proportion of each subset in the population?
- If proportional sampling is being used, is there a sufficient number of subjects in each subset for basing meaningful comparisons?
- Once the subset comparison has been determined, are random procedures used for selection of the sample?

As illustrated in Table 10-1, there are several advantages to a stratified sampling strategy: (1) the representativeness of the sample is enhanced; (2) the researcher has a valid basis for making comparisons among subsets if information on the critical variables has been available; and (3) the researcher is able to oversample a disproportionately small stratum to adjust for their underrepresentation, statistically weigh the data accordingly, and continue to be able to make legitimate comparisons.

The obstacles encountered by a researcher using this strategy include the following: (1) the difficulty of obtaining a population list containing complete critical variable information; (2) the time-consuming effort of obtaining multiple enumerated lists; and (3) the time and money involved in carrying out a large-scale study using a stratified sampling strategy. The critiquer needs to question the appropriateness of this sampling strategy to the problem under investigation. For example, in a posthospitalization telephone survey evaluating patient-centered care outcomes, 17 midwestern hospitals were selected from a pool of 69 acute care institutions in a single metropolitan area using a stratified random sampling strategy. The stratification was based on location (inner-city, urban, and suburban) and the annual number of adult nonpsychiatric, nonobstetrical admissions (Minnick et al, 1995). It is appropriate for the researcher to strive to represent all strata proportionately in the study sample. When 3 of the original 17 hospitals in the example on p. 259 refused to participate in the study, they were replaced within the original sampling framework to retain the representativeness of each stratum.

Multistage Sampling (Cluster Sampling)

Multistage (cluster) sampling involves a successive random sampling of units (clusters) that progress from large to small and meet sample eligibility criteria. The first stage sampling unit consists of large units or clusters. The second stage sampling unit consists of smaller units or clusters. Third stage sampling units are even smaller. For example, if a sample of clinical nurse specialists (CNSs) is desired, the first sampling unit would be a random sample of hospitals, obtained from an American Hospital Association list, who meet the eligibility criteria (e.g., size, type). The second stage sampling unit would consist of a list of CNSs practicing at each hospital selected in the first stage—the list obtained from the vice president for nursing at each hospital. The criteria for inclusion in the list of CNSs were (1) certified CNS with at least 2 years experience as a CNS; (2) at least 50% of the CNS's time must be spent in providing direct patient care; and (3) full-time employment at the hospital. The second stage sampling strategy called for random selection of two CNSs from each hospital who met the previously mentioned eligibility criteria.

When multistage sampling is used in relation to large national surveys, states are used as the first stage sampling unit, proceeding at successively smaller units like counties, cities, districts, and blocks as the second stage sampling unit, and then households as the third stage sampling unit.

Sampling units or clusters can be selected by simple random or stratified random sampling methods. Suppose that the hospitals, described in the example above, were grouped into four strata according to size (number of beds): (1) 200 to 299; (2) 300 to 399; (3) 400 to 499; and (4) 500 or more. Stratum 1 comprised 25% of the population; stratum 2 comprised 30% of the population; stratum 3 comprised 20% of the population; and stratum 4 comprised 25% of the population. This means that either a simple random or a proportional, stratified sampling strategy is used to randomly select hospitals that would proportionately represent the population of hospitals in the American Hospital Association list.

The main advantage of cluster sampling, as illustrated in Table 10-1, is that it is considerably more economical in terms of time and money than other types of probability sampling, particularly when the population is large and geographically dispersed or when a sampling frame of the elements is not available. There are two major disadvantages: (1) more sampling errors tend to occur than with simple random or stratified random sampling; and (2) the appropriate handling of the statistical data from cluster samples is very complex.

The reader who is evaluating a research report will need to consider whether the use of cluster sampling is justified in light of the research design, as well as other pragmatic matters, such as economy.

Systematic Sampling

Systematic sampling refers to a sampling strategy that involves the selection of every "kth" case drawn from a population list at fixed intervals, such as every tenth member listed in the directory of the American Association of Critical Care Nurses. Systematic sampling might be used to sample every "kth" person to enter a hospital lobby or to be hospitalized with a diagnosis of AIDS in 1997. When systematic sampling is used, the population must be narrowly defined as consisting, for example, of all those people entering or leaving for the sample to be considered as a probability sample. If senior citizens were sampled systematically on entering a hospital lobby, the resulting sample would not be called a probability sample, because not every senior citizen would have a chance of being selected. As such, systemic sampling can sometimes represent a nonprobability sampling strategy.

However, systematic sampling strategies can be designed to fulfill the requirements of a probability sample. First, the listing of the population (sampling frame) must be random in relation to the variable of interest. For example, subjects were being selected from every tenth hospital room for a study on patient satisfaction with nursing care. Every tenth room happens to be a private room in the hospital where the study is being conducted. It is possible that the responses of patients in private rooms with regard to patient satisfaction might be different from those of patients in semiprivate rooms. Because of the nonrandom arrangement of the rooms, bias may have been introduced.

Second, the first element or member of the sample must be selected randomly. In this case the researcher, who has a population list or sampling frame, first divides the population *(N)* by the size of the desired sample *(n)* to obtain the sampling interval width *(k)*. The **sampling interval** is the standard distance between the elements chosen for the sample. For example, to select a sample of 50 family nurse practitioners from a population of 500 family nurse practitioners, the sampling interval would be as follows:

$$k = \frac{500}{50} = 100$$

Essentially, every tenth case on the family nurse practitioner list would be sampled. Once the sampling interval has been determined, the researcher uses a table of random numbers (see Figure 10-1) to obtain a starting point for the selection of the 50 subjects. If the population size is 500 and a sample size of 50 is desired, a number between 1 and 500 is randomly selected as the starting point. In this instance, if the first number is 51, the family nurse practitioners corresponding to numbers 51, 61, 71, and so forth, would be included in the sample of 50. Another procedure recommended in many texts is to randomly select the first element from within the first sampling interval. If the sampling interval is 5, a number between 1 and 5 would be selected as the random starting point. For example, the number 3 is randomly chosen. Keeping in mind the sampling interval of 5, the next elements selected would correspond to the numbers 8, 13, 18, and so on, until the sample was obtained. Although this latter procedure is technically correct, choosing a random starting point from across the total population of elements is more attractive because every element has a chance to be chosen for the sample during the first selection step.

Systematic and simple random sampling are essentially the same type of procedure. The advantage of systematic sampling is that the results are obtained in a more convenient and efficient manner (see Table 10-1). The disadvantage of systematic sampling is that bias in the form of nonrandomness can inadvertently be introduced to the procedure. This problem may occur if the population list is arranged so that a certain type of element is listed at intervals that coincide with the sampling interval. Let us say that if every tenth nursing student on a population list of all types of nursing students in Texas were a baccalaureate student and the sampling interval was 10, baccalaureate students would be overrepresented in the sample. Cyclical fluctuations are also a factor. For example, if a list is kept of nursing students using the college library each day, a biased sample will probably be obtained if every seventh day is chosen as the sampling interval, because fewer and perhaps different nursing students probably study in the library on Sundays than on weekdays. Therefore caution must be exercised about departures from randomness as they affect the representativeness of the sample and, as a result, affect the external validity of the study.

The critiquer will want to note whether a satisfactory random selection procedure was carried out. If randomization was not used, the systematic sampling may have become a nonprobability quota sample. It is important to be cognizant of this issue, because the implications related to interpretation and generalizability are drastically altered if the evaluator is dealing with a nonprobability sample.

Special Sampling Strategies

Several special sampling strategies are used in nonprobability sampling. **Matching** is a special strategy used to construct an equivalent comparison sample group by filling it with subjects who are similar to each subject in another sample group in relation to such preestablished variables as age, gender, level of education, medical diagnosis, or socioeconomic status. Theoretically, any variable other than the independent variable that could affect the dependent variable should be matched. In reality, the more variables matched, the more difficult it is to obtain an adequate sample size. For example, matching was used in a study that sought to determine if a group of women who developed severe preeclampsia had a higher midtrimester mean arterial pressure (MAP-2) than a matched group of women who remained normotensive throughout pregnancy and the puerperium. Each group was matched in relation to parity, race, maternal age, and date of delivery to obtain two equivalent groups with respect to those variables (Atterbury, Groome, and Baker, 1996).

Networking sampling, sometimes referred to as *snowballing*, is a strategy used for locating samples difficult or impossible to locate in other ways. This sampling strategy takes advantage of social networks and the fact that friends tend to have characteristics in common. When a researcher has found a few subjects with the needed eligibility criteria, they are asked for their assistance in getting in touch with others with similar criteria. For example, Stevens (1994) used networking and snowballing to obtain participants for a study investigating the health care experiences of a racially and economically diverse sample of lesbians. A core of 8 informants who were knowledgeable and influential members of African-American, Latina, Asian/Pacific Islander, and Euro-American subgroups of the San Francisco lesbian community collaborated with the Euro-American, lesbian-identified researcher to, among other things, devise sampling strategies. Their endorsement of the project, contacts with community members, referral efforts, and word-of-mouth referrals by interview participants capture the essence of the networking (snowball effect) sampling strategy that resulted in a racially and economically diverse sample of 45 lesbians. Today, on-line computer networks, as described in the section on purposive sampling, can be used to assist researchers in acquiring otherwise difficult to locate subjects, thereby taking advantage of the networking or snowball effect. The Critical Thinking Decision Path illustrates the relationship between the type of sampling strategy and the appropriate generalizability.

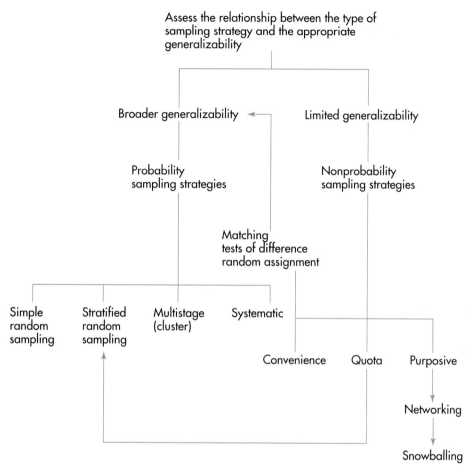

Critical Thinking Decision Path   Assessing the relationship between the type of sampling strategy and the appropriate generalizability.

> **HELPFUL HINT**
> Look for a brief discussion of the sampling strategy in the *Methods* section of a research article. Sometimes there is a separate subsection with the heading *Sample, Subjects,* or *Study Participants.* A description of the characteristics of the actual sample often does not appear until the results section of a research article.

SAMPLE SIZE

There is no single rule that can be applied to the determination of a sample's size. When arriving at an estimate of sample size, many factors, such as the following, must be considered:

- The type of design used
- The type of sampling procedure used
- The type of formula used for estimating optimum sample size

- The degree of precision required
- The heterogeneity of the attributes under investigation
- The relative frequency of occurrence of the phenomenon of interest in the population; that is, a common versus a rare health problem
- The projected cost of using a particular sampling strategy

The sample size should be determined before the study is conducted. A general rule of thumb is always to use the largest sample possible. The larger the sample, the more representative of the population it is likely to be; smaller samples produce less accurate results.

The exception to this principle occurs when using certain qualitative designs. In this case, sample size is not predetermined. Sample sizes in qualitative research tend to be small because of the large volume of verbal data that must be analyzed and because this type of design tends to emphasize intensive and prolonged contact with subjects (Streubert and Carpenter, 1995). Subjects are added to the sample until **data saturation** is reached; that is, new data no longer emerge during the data collection process. Fittingness of the data is a more important concern than representativeness of subjects (see Chapter 9).

The principle of "larger is better" holds true for both probability and nonprobability samples. Results based on small samples (under 10) tend to be unstable—the values fluctuate from one sample to the next. Small samples tend to increase the probability of obtaining a markedly nonrepresentative sample. As the sample size increases, the mean more closely approximates the population values and thus introduces less sampling error.

An example of this concept is illustrated by a study in which the average monthly sleeping pill consumption is being investigated for patients on a rehabilitation unit after a cerebrovascular accident. The data in Table 10-3 indicate that the population consists of 20 patients whose average consumption of sleeping pills is 15.15 per month. Two simple random samples with sample sizes of 2, 4, 6, and 10 have been drawn from the population of 20 patients. Each sample average in the right-hand column represents an estimate of the population average, which is known to be 15.15. In most cases the population value is unknown to the researchers, but because the population is so small, we could calculate it. As we examine the data in Table 10-3, we note that with a sample size of 2, the estimate might have been wrong by as much as 8 sleeping pills in sample 1B. As the sample size increases, the averages get closer to the population value, and the differences in the estimates between samples A and B also get smaller. Large samples permit the principles of randomization to work effectively; that is, to counterbalance atypical values in the long run.

It is possible to estimate the sample size with the use of a statistical procedure known as *power analysis* (Cohen, 1977). It is beyond the scope of this chapter to describe this complex procedure in great detail, but a simple example will illustrate its use. A researcher wants to determine the effect of nurse preoperative teaching on patient postoperative anxiety. Patients are randomly assigned to an experimental group or a control group. How many patients should be used in the study? When using power analysis the researcher must estimate how large a difference will be observed between the groups; that is, the difference in the mean amount of postoperative anxiety after the experimental preoperative teaching program. If a small difference is expected, the sample would need to be large (in this case 196 patients in each group) to ensure that the differences will actually be revealed in a statistical analysis. If a medium-size difference is expected, the total sample size would be 128—64 in each group. When expected differences are large, it does not take a very large sample to ensure that differences will be re-

Table 10-3

Comparison of Population and Sample Values and Averages in Study of Sleeping Pill Consumption

NUMBER IN GROUP	GROUP	NUMBER OF SLEEPING PILLS CONSUMED (VALUES EXPRESSED MONTHLY)	AVERAGE
20	Population	1, 3, 4, 5, 6, 7, 9, 11, 13, 15, 16, 17, 19, 21, 22, 23, 25, 27, 29, 30	15.15
2	Sample 1A	6, 9	7.5
2	Sample 1B	21, 25	23.0
4	Sample 2A	1, 7, 15, 25	12.0
4	Sample 2B	5, 13, 23, 29	17.5
6	Sample 3A	3, 4, 11, 15, 21, 25	13.3
6	Sample 3B	5, 7, 11, 19, 27, 30	16.5
10	Sample 4A	3, 4, 7, 9, 11, 13, 17, 21, 23, 30	13.8
10	Sample 4B	1, 4, 6, 11, 15, 17, 19, 23, 25, 27	14.8

vealed through statistical analysis. Power analysis is an advanced statistical technique that is used increasingly by researchers and is a requirement for external funding (Polit and Sherman, 1990). When it is not used, research studies may be based on samples that are too small. When samples are too small, the researcher may have unsupported hypotheses and may commit a type I error of rejecting a null hypothesis when it should have been accepted (see Chapter 15). A researcher may also commit a type II error of accepting a null hypothesis when it should have been rejected if the sample is too small (see Chapter 15).

Despite the principles related to determining sample size that have been identified, the consumer should be aware that large samples do not ensure representativeness or accuracy. A large sample cannot compensate for a faulty research design. The proportion of the population that is sampled does not provide a guarantee of accurate results. It is often possible to obtain accurate results from only a small fraction of a large population. For example, a 10% probability sample of a population containing 1500 elements will yield more precise results than a nonprobability 0.01% sample of a population with 100,000 elements.

The critiquer should evaluate the sample size in terms of whether it adequately represents the elements and subsets of the population. Unless representativeness is ensured, all the data in the world become inconsequential.

HELPFUL HINT

Remember to look for some rationale about the sample size and those strategies the researcher has used (e.g., matching, test of differences on demographic variables) to ascertain or build in sample representativeness.

SAMPLING PROCEDURES

Criteria for drawing a sample vary according to the sampling strategy. Regardless of which strategy is used, it is important that the procedure be systematically organized. This will eliminate the bias that occurs when sample selection is carried out inconsistently. Bias in sample representativeness and generalizability of findings are important sampling issues that have generated national concern. Many of the landmark adult health studies, such as the Framingham heart study and the Baltimore longitudinal study on aging historically excluded women as subjects. Despite the all-male samples, the findings of these studies were generalized from males to *all* adults despite the lack of female representation in the samples. Similarly, the use of largely Euro-American subjects in medication clinical trials limits the identification of variant responses to drugs in ethnic or racially distinct groups (Kudzma, 1992). Findings based on Euro-American data cannot be generalized to African Americans, Asians, Hispanics, or any other cultural group (Campinha-Bacote, 1997). Consequently, careful identification of the target population is a crucial step in the process. If a researcher wants to be able to draw conclusions about psychosocial stressors related to *all* patients with a first-time myocardial infarction, then both males *and* females must be included in the target population. When a researcher wants to be able to draw conclusions about the incidence of extrapyramidal side effects of haloperidol (Haldol) in African-American psychiatric patients compared to Euro-American, the target population must be diverse. Sometimes the target population has to be gender-specific, as when studying breast or prostate cancer or aspects of pregnancy or menopause.

Several general steps, as illustrated in Figure 10-3, can be identified that will ensure a consistent approach by the researcher. Initially the target population must be identified; that is, the entire group of people or objects about whom the researcher wants to draw conclusions or make generalizations. The target population may consist of all male patients with a first-time

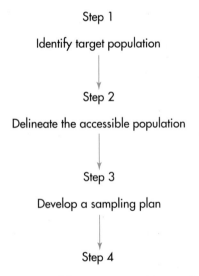

Step 1

Identify target population

Step 2

Delineate the accessible population

Step 3

Develop a sampling plan

Step 4

Obtain approval from Institutional Review Board

Figure 10-3   Summary of general sampling procedure.

myocardial infarction, all children with acute leukemia, all pregnant teenagers, or all doctoral students in the United States. Next, the accessible portion of the target population must be delineated. An accessible population might consist of all CNSs in the state of California, all male patients with AIDS admitted to hospital X during 1996, all pregnant teenagers in a specific prenatal clinic, or all children with acute leukemia under care at a specific hospital specializing in oncology. Then a sampling plan or a protocol for actually selecting the sample from the accessible population is formulated. The researcher makes decisions about how subjects will be approached, how the study will be explained, and who will select the sample—the researcher or a research assistant. Regardless of who implements the sampling plan, consistency in how it is done is of paramount importance. The reader of a research study will want to find a description of the sample, as well as the sampling procedure, in the report. On the basis of the appropriateness of what has been reported, the critiquer is able to make judgments about the soundness of the sampling protocol, which of course will affect the interpretations made about the findings. Finally, once the accessible population and sampling plan have been established, permission is obtained from the institution's research board. This permission provides free access to the desired population.

When an appropriate sample size and sampling strategy have been used, the researcher can feel more confident that the sample is representative of the accessible population; however, it is more difficult to feel confident that the accessible population is representative of the target population. Are CNSs in California representative of all CNSs in the United States? It is impossible to be sure about this. Researchers must exercise judgment when assessing typicality. Unfortunately there are no guidelines for making such judgments, and there is even less basis for the critiquer to make such decisions. The best rule of thumb to use when evaluating the representativeness of a sample and its generalizability to the target population is to be realistic and conservative about making sweeping claims relative to the findings.

HELPFUL HINT

Remember to evaluate the appropriateness of the generalizations made about the study findings in light of the target population, the accessible population, the type of sampling strategy, and the sample size.

CRITIQUING THE SAMPLE

The criteria for critiquing the sampling technique of a study are presented in the Critiquing Criteria box. The research consumer approaches the sample section of a research report with a different perspective than does the researcher. The consumer must raise two questions. The first question asks, "If this study were to be replicated, would there be enough information presented about the nature of the population, the sample, the sampling strategy, and sample size of another investigator to carry out the study?" The second question asks, "Are the previously mentioned factors appropriate in light of the particular research design, and if not, which factors require modification, especially if the study is to be replicated?"

Sampling is considered to be one important aspect of the methodology of a research study. As such, data pertaining to the sample usually appear in the *Methodology* section of the research report. The sampling content presented should reflect the outcome of a series of decisions based on sampling criteria appropriate to the design of the study, as well as the options

CRITIQUING CRITERIA

1. Have the sample characteristics been completely described?
2. Can the parameters of the study population be inferred from the description of the sample?
3. To what extent is the sample representative of the population as defined?
4. Are criteria for eligibility in the sample specifically identified?
5. Have sample delimitations been established?
6. Would it be possible to replicate the study population?
7. How was the sample selected? Is the method of sample selection appropriate?
8. What kind of bias, if any, is introduced by this method?
9. Is the sample size appropriate? How is it substantiated?
10. Are there indications that rights of subjects have been ensured?
11. Does the researcher identify the limitations in generalizability of the findings from the sample to the population? Are they appropriate?
12. Does the researcher indicate how replication of the study with other samples would provide increased support for the findings?

and limitations inherent in the context of the investigation. The following discussion will highlight several sampling criteria that the research consumer will want to consider when evaluating the merit of a sampling strategy as it relates to a specific research study.

Initially the parameters or attributes of the study population should clearly specify to what population the findings may be generalized. Generally the target population of the study is not specifically identified by the researcher, but the nature of it is implied in the description of the accessible population and/or the sample. For example, if a researcher states that 100 subjects were randomly drawn from a population of married primiparas who vaginally delivered full-term infants at hospital X during 1997, the critiquer is able to specifically evaluate the parameters of the population. Demographic characteristics of the sample, such as age, gender, diagnosis, ethnicity, religion, and marital status, should also be presented in either a tabled or a narrative summary, because they provide further explication about the nature of the sample and enable the critiquer to evaluate the sampling procedure more accurately. For example, in a study by Miller and Champion (1996) titled *Mammography in Older Women: One-Time Adherence and Three-Year Adherence to Guidelines,* the authors present detailed data summarizing demographic variables of importance. These data are reproduced as follows:

The age range of the women as 50 to 89 years (M = 65.7 years). Years of education varied from 5 to 26 years (M = 13.6 years). The sample was 75% White, 22% Black, and 3% missing or other. Median income fell in the $30,000 to $40,000 range, with 18% having incomes of $15,000 or less. A majority of women were married (55%), 24% were widowed, 12% divorced or separated, and 7% never married. Nearly half of the sample were retired, 24% were employed full-time, and 10% had always been full-time homemakers.

This example illustrates how a detailed description of the sample provides the critiquer with a frame of reference about the study population and sample and generates questions to be raised. For instance, the reader will note the variability in the range of subject age (50 to 89). The evaluator who has this demographic sample information available is able to question a sampling strategy that does not also consider the differential effect of age on one-time mammography use and 3-year adherence to professional mammography screening guidelines. It would seem logical that there might be a difference in health practices such as mammography for women in a 50- to 60-year-old cohort versus a 70- to 80-year-old cohort.

It is also helpful if the researcher has presented a rationale for having elected to study one type of population versus another. For example, why did the previously cited study focus only on married primiparas who vaginally delivered full-term infants, as opposed to unmarried women or women who had had cesarean births? In a research study that uses a nonprobability sampling strategy, it is particularly important to fully describe the population and the sample in terms of who the study subjects are, the way they were chosen, and the reason they were chosen. If these criteria are adhered to, the degree of heterogeneity or homogeneity of the sample can be determined. The use of a homogeneous sample minimizes the amount of sampling error introduced, a problem particularly common in nonprobability sampling.

Next, the defined representativeness of the population should be examined. Probability sampling is clearly the ideal sampling procedure for ensuring the representativeness of a study population. Use of random selection procedures, such as simple random, stratified, cluster, or systematic sampling strategies, minimizes the occurrence of conscious and unconscious biases, which, of course, would affect the researcher's ability to generalize about the findings from the sample to the population. The evaluator should be able to identify the type of probability strategy used and to determine whether the researcher adhered to the criteria for a particular sampling plan. In experimental and quasiexperimental studies the evaluator must know also whether or how the subjects were assigned to groups. If the criteria have not been followed, the reader would have a valid basis for being cautious about the proposed conclusions of the study.

Although random selection is the ideal in establishing the representativeness of a study population, more often realistic barriers, such as institutional policy, inaccessibility of subjects, lack of time or money, and current state of knowledge in the field, necessitate the use of nonprobability sampling strategies. Many important research problems that are of interest to nursing do not lend themselves to experimental design and probability sampling. This is particularly true with qualitative research designs. A well-designed, carefully controlled study using a nonprobability sampling strategy can yield accurate and meaningful findings that make a significant contribution to nursing's scientific body of knowledge. As the critiquer, you need to ask a philosophical question: "If it is not possible or appropriate to conduct an experimental or quasiexperimental investigation that uses probability sampling, should the study be abandoned?" The answer usually suggests that it is better to carry out the investigation and be fully aware of the limitations of the methodology than to lose the knowledge that can be gained. The researcher is always able to move on to subsequent studies that either replicate the study or use more stringent design and sampling strategies to refine the knowledge derived from a nonexperimental study.

The greatest difficulty in nonprobability sampling stems from the fact that not every element in the population has an equal chance of being represented in the sample. Therefore it is likely that some segment of the population will be systematically underrepresented. If the population is homogeneous on critical characteristics, systematic bias will not be very important. However, few of the attributes that researchers are interested in are sufficiently homogeneous to render sampling bias an irrelevant consideration.

Next, the sampling plan's suitability to the research design should be evaluated. Experimental and quasiexperimental design use some form of random selection or random assignment of subjects to groups (see Chapter 7). The critiquer evaluates whether the researcher adhered to the principles of random selection and assignment. Lack of adherence to such principles compromises the representativeness of the sample and the external validity of the study. The following are questions the evaluator might pose relative to this issue:

- Has a random selection procedure been identified, such as a table of random numbers?
- Has the appropriate random sampling plan been selected; that is, has a proportional stratified sampling plan been selected instead of a simple random sampling plan in a study where there are three distinct occupational levels that appear to be critical variables for stratification?
- Has the particular random sampling plan been carried out appropriately; that is, if a cluster sampling strategy was used, did the sampling units logically progress from the largest to the smallest?

Random sampling should not be looked on as a cure-all. Sometimes bias is inadvertently introduced even when the principle of random selection is used.

Nonexperimental designs often use nonprobability sampling strategies. In this instance the question that can be raised by the critiquer is whether a nonexperimental design and a related nonprobability sampling plan were most appropriate for this study. It is sometimes true that if the researcher had used another type of design or sampling plan, he or she could have constructed a stronger study that would have allowed greater confidence to be placed in the findings and greater generalizability. However, the critiquer is rarely in a position to know what factors entered into the decision to plan one type of study versus another.

When critiquing qualitative research designs, the evaluator would apply criteria related to sampling strategies that are relevant for a particular type of qualitative study. In general, sampling strategies are purposive, because the study of specific phenomenon in their natural setting is emphasized; any subject belonging to a specified group is considered to represent that group. For example, when a qualitative study such as *Male Survivors of Childhood Sexual Abuse* (Draucker and Petrovic, 1996) is conducted, the specified group is male survivors who had experienced healing from the trauma of childhood sexual abuse. The goal of the researcher is to establish the meaning of their slices of life; that is, the typicality or atypicality of the observed events, behaviors, or responses in the lives of the male survivors (see Chapter 9).

Then the evaluator should determine whether the sample size is appropriate and whether its size is justifiable. It no longer is unusual for the researcher to indicate in a research article how the sample size was determined; this is also seen commonly in doctoral dissertations. The method of arriving at the sample size and the rationale should be briefly mentioned. For example, a researcher may state in a very detailed way:

Power analysis, using the expected proportion of quitters, based on previous smoking cessation research, was used to estimate the minimum sample size (Cohen, 1977). Given a moderate effect size (0.5, which was likely at the postprogram measure), a power of 0.80, and an alpha of 0.05, a sample of 100 subjects would suffice. Thus drawing a sample of 100 subjects, 50 per group from a pool of 600 eligible women was deemed possible and adequate (Pletsch, Howe, and Tenney, 1995).

The importance of this example lies not in understanding every technical word cited, but rather in understanding that this type of statement or some abbreviated form of it meets the criteria stated at the beginning of the paragraph and should be evident on the research report.

Other considerations with respect to sample size, especially where the sample size appears to be small or inadequate and there is no stated rationale for the size, are the following:

- How will the sample size affect the accuracy of the results?
- Are any subsets or cells of the sample overrepresented or underrepresented?
- Are any of the subsets so small as to limit meaningful comparisons?
- Has the researcher examined the effect of attrition or dropouts on the results?
- Has the researcher recognized and identified any limitations posed by the size of the sample?

Essentially, these criteria demand that the critiquer carefully scrutinize several important elements pertaining to sample size that have implications for the generalizability of the findings. Keep in mind that qualitative studies will not discuss predetermining sample size or method for arriving at sample size. Rather, sample size will tend to be small and a function of data saturation (see Chapter 11).

Finally, evidence that the rights of human subjects have been protected should appear in the sample section of the research report. The critiquer will evaluate whether permission was obtained from an institutional review board that reviewed the study relative to the maintenance of ethical research standards (see Chapter 11). For example, the review board examines the research proposal to determine whether the introduction of an experimental procedure may be potentially harmful and therefore undesirable. The critiquer also examines the report for evidence of informed consent of subjects, as well as protection of confidentiality or anonymity. It is highly unusual for research studies not to demonstrate evidence of having met these criteria. Nevertheless, the careful evaluator will want to be certain that ethical standards that protect sample subjects have been maintained.

It is evident that there are many factors to consider when critiquing the sample section of a research report. The type and appropriateness of the sampling strategy become crucial elements in the analysis and intepretation of data, in the conclusions derived from the findings, and in the generalizability of the findings from the sample to the population. As stated earlier in this chapter, the major purpose of sampling is to increase the efficiency of a research study by using a sample that is representative of the particular population so that every element need not be studied, and yet generalizing the findings from the sample to the population. The critiquer needs to justify that the sampling strategy used provided a valid basis for feeling confident of the findings and their generalizability.

KEY POINTS

- Sampling is a process that selects representative units of a population for study. Researchers sample representative segments of the population, because it is rarely feasible or necessary to sample entire populations of interest to obtain accurate and meaningful information.
- A population is a well-defined set that has certain specified properties. A population may consist of people, objects, or events.

- Researchers establish eligibility criteria; these are descriptors of the population and provide the basis for selection into a sample. Eligibility criteria, also referred to as *delimitations,* include the following: age, gender, socioeconomic status, level of education, religion, and ethnicity.
- The researcher must identify the target population; that is, the entire set of cases about which the researcher would like to make generalizations. However, because of the pragmatic constraints, the researcher usually utilizes an accessible population, one that meets the population criteria and is available.
- A sample is a set of elements that makes up the population.
- A sampling unit is the element or set of elements used for selecting the sample. The foremost criterion in evaluating a sample is the representativeness or congruence of characteristics with the population.
- Sampling strategies consist of nonprobability and probability sampling.
- In nonprobability sampling the elements are chosen by nonrandom methods. Types of nonprobability sampling include convenience, quota, and purposive sampling.
- Probability sampling is characterized by the random selection of elements from the population. In random selection each element in the population has an equal and independent chance of being included in the sample. Types of probability sampling include simple random, stratified random, cluster, and systematic sampling.
- Sample size is a function of the type of sampling procedure being used, the degree of precision required, the type of sample estimation formula being used, the heterogeneity of study attributes, the relative frequency of occurrence of the phenomena under consideration, and cost.
- Criteria for drawing a sample vary according to the sampling strategy. Systematic organization of the sampling procedure minimizes bias. The target population is identified, the accessible portion of the target population is delineated, permission to conduct the research study is obtained, and a sampling plan is formulated.
- The critiquer of a research report evaluates the sampling plan for its appropriateness in relation to the particular research design. Completeness of the sampling plan is examined in light of potential replicability of the study. The critiquer evaluates whether the sampling strategy is the strongest plan for the particular study under consideration.
- An appropriate systematic sampling plan will maximize the efficiency of a research study. It will increase the accuracy and meaningfulness of the findings and enhance the generalizability of the findings from the sample to the population.

CRITICAL THINKING CHALLENGES
Barbara Krainovich-Miller

? A research classmate asks the instructor the following question: "Why isn't it better to study an entire population of patients with lung cancer instead of using the research technique of sampling?" How would you answer this question? Include examples that will help the student see it from your point of view.

? A quasiexperimental study indicates that it used a convenience sample with random assignment. How is this possible? Would this be a nonprobability or probability sample? If you agree that this is a legitimate sampling technique, present both the advantages and the disadvantages; if you disagree, indicate your rationale.

❓ Your research class is having a debate on probability versus nonprobability sampling regarding desirability and feasibility. You are assigned to present the pros of nonprobability sampling in nursing research. What arguments would you use?

❓ Discuss the principle of "larger is better" and its relationship to "networking" sampling and the sample size of qualitative studies. Include in your discussion the concept of "data saturation," as well as the use of computer technology.

REFERENCES

Atterbury JL, Groome LJ, Baker SL: Elevated midtrimester mean arterial blood pressure in women with severe preeclampsia, *Appl Nurs Res* 9(4):161-166, 1996.

Baker J, Norton P: Evaluation of absorbent products for women with mild to moderate urinary incontinence, *Appl Nurs Res* 9(1):29-36, 1996.

Beck CT: Postpartum depressed mothers' experiences interacting with their children, *Nurs Res* 45(2):98-104, 1996.

Campinha-Bacote J: Understanding the influence of culture. In Haber J et al: *Comprehensive psychiatric nursing,* ed 5, St Louis, 1997, Mosby.

Cohen J: *Statistical power analysis for the behavioral sciences,* rev ed, New York, 1977, Academic Press.

Draucker CB, Petrocvic K: Male survivors of childhood sexual abuse, *Image* 28(4):325-330, 1996.

Failla S et al: Adjustment of women with systemic lupus erythematosus, *Appl Nurs Res* 9(2):87-96, 1996.

Johnson JE: Social support and physical health in the rural elderly, *Appl Nurs Res* 9(2):61-66, 1996.

Kudzma E: Drug response: all bodies are not created equal, *Am J Nurs* 92:1248-1251, 1992.

Miller AM, Champion VL: Mammography in older women: one-time adherence and three-year adherence to guidelines, *Nurs Res* 45(4):239-245, 1996.

Minnick A et al: An analysis of posthospitalization telephone survey data, *Nurs Res* 44(6):371-375, 1995.

Pletsch PK, Howe C, Tenney M: Recruitment of minority subjects for intervention research, *Image* 27(3):211-215, 1995.

Polit DF, Sherman RE: Statistical power in nursing research, *Nurs Res* 39(6):365-368, 1990.

Pollack LE: Inpatient self-management of bipolar disorder, *Appl Nurs Res* 9(2):71-79, 1996.

Ronen T, Abraham Y: Retention control training in the treatment of younger versus older enuretic children, *Nurs Res* 45(2):78-82, 1996.

Stevens PE: Lesbians' health-related experiences of care and noncare, *West J Nurs Res* 16(6):639-659, 1994.

Streubert HJ, Carpenter DR: *Qualitative research in nursing,* Philadelphia, 1995, JB Lippincott.

Wilmoth MC: Computer networks as a source of research subjects, *West J Nurs Res* 17(3):335-338, 1995.

ADDITIONAL READINGS

Demi AS, Warren NA: Issues in conducting research with vulnerable families, *West J Nurs Res* 17(2):188-202, 1995.

Floyd JA: Systematic sampling: theory and clinical methods, *Nurs Res* 42(5):290-293, 1993.

Kerlinger FN: *Foundations of behavioral research,* New York, 1986, Holt, Rinehart & Winston.

Knapp TR: The overemphasis on power analysis, *Nurs Res* 45(6):379-381, 1996.

Timmerman GM: The art of advertising for research subjects, *Nurs Res* 45(6):339-340, 1996.

Yam M: Teaching nursing students to critique research for gender bias, *West J Nurs Res* 16(6):724-727, 1994.

Yarandi HN: Planning sample sizes: comparison of factor level means, *Nurs Res* 40(1):57-58, 1991.

Legal and Ethical Issues

Judith Haber

Key Terms

animal rights
anonymity
assent
beneficence
benefits
confidentiality
consent
ethics

informed consent
institutional review boards
   (IRBs)
justice
product testing
respect for persons
risk-benefit ratio
risks

Learning Outcomes

After reading this chapter the student should be able to do the following:

- Describe the historical background that led to the development of ethical guidelines for the use of human subjects in research.
- Identify the essential elements of an informed consent form.
- Evaluate the adequacy of an informed consent form.
- Describe the institutional review board's role in the research review process.
- Identify populations of subjects who require special legal and ethical research considerations.
- Appreciate the nurse researcher's obligations to conduct and report research in an ethical manner.
- Describe the nurse's role as patient advocate in research situations.
- Discuss the nurse's role in ensuring that FDA guidelines for testing of medical devices are followed.
- Discuss animal rights in research situations.
- Critique the ethical aspects of a research study.

Listen, Martin. I am aware that the technique of experimenting on humans without their consent is against any traditional concept of medical ethics. But I believe the results justify the methods. Seventeen young women have unknowingly sacrificed their lives. That is true. But it has been for the betterment of society and the future guarantee of the defense superiority of the United States. From the point of view of two hundred million Americans, it is a very small one. Think of how many young women will-fully take their lives each year, or how many people kill themselves on the highways, and to what end? Here these seventeen women have added something to society, and they have been treated with compassion (Cook, 1981).

"When people rely on rules to protect them from harm, they are not interested in pieces of paper, but in the conduct of the people who are supposed to be governed by the rules" (Hanks, 1984a). It is not just rules and regulations dealing with the involvement of human subjects in research that ensure that research will be conducted legally and ethically. Researchers themselves and caregivers providing care to patients, who also happen to be research subjects, must be fully committed to the tenets of informed consent and patients' rights. The principle "the ends justify the means" must never be tolerated. Researchers and caregivers of research subjects must take every precaution to protect people being studied from physical or mental harm or discomfort. It is not always clear what constitutes harm or discomfort.

The focus of this chapter is the legal and ethical considerations that must be addressed before, during, and after the conduct of research. Informed consent, institutional review boards, and research involving vulnerable populations—the elderly, pregnant women, children, prisoners, persons with AIDS, and animals—are discussed. The nurse's role as patient advocate, whether functioning as researcher, caregiver, or research consumer, is addressed.

ETHICAL AND LEGAL CONSIDERATIONS IN RESEARCH: AN HISTORICAL PERSPECTIVE

Past Ethical Dilemmas in Research

Ethical and legal considerations with regard to research first received attention after World War II. When the then U.S. Secretary of State and Secretary of War learned that the trials for war criminals would focus on justifying the atrocities committed by Nazi physicians as "medical research," the American Medical Association was asked to appoint a group to develop a code of ethics for research that would be asked as a standard for judging the medical atrocities committed by physicians on concentration camp prisoners.

The 10 rules included in what was called the Nuremberg Code appear in Box 11-1. Its definitions of the terms *voluntary, legal capacity, sufficient understanding,* and *enlightened decision* have been the subject of numerous court cases and presidential commissions involved in setting ethical standards in research (Creighton, 1977). The code that was developed requires informed consent in all cases but makes no provisions for any special treatment of children, the elderly, or the mentally incompetent. Several other international standards have followed, the most notable of which was the Declaration of Helsinki, which was adopted in 1964 by the World Medical Assembly and then later revised in 1975 (Levine, 1979).

In the United States, federal guidelines for the ethical conduct of research involving human subjects were not developed until the 1970s. Some of the most atrocious, and hence memorable, examples of unethical research studies took place in the United States as recently as the 1970s. These examples are highlighted in Table 11-1. They are sad reminders of our own tar-

---

Box 11-1   Articles of the Nuremberg Code

1. The voluntary consent of the human subject is absolutely essential.
2. The study should be such as to yield fruitful results for the good of society, unprocurable by other means of study, and not random and unnecessary in nature.
3. The experiment should be so designed and based on the results of animal experimentation and knowledge of the natural history of the disease or other problems under study that the anticipated results will justify the performance of the experiment.
4. The experiment should be conducted to avoid all unnecessary physical and mental suffering and injury.
5. No experiment should be conducted where there is a prior reason to believe that death or disabling injury will occur.
6. The degree of risk to be taken should never exceed that determined by the humanitarian importance of the problem to be solved by the experiment.
7. Proper preparations should be made and adequate facilities provided to protect the subject against . . . injury, disability, or death.
8. The experiment should be conducted only by scientifically qualified persons.
9. The human subject should be at liberty to bring the experiment to an end.
10. During the experiment, the scientist . . . if he has probable cause to believe that a continuation of the experiment is likely to result in injury, disability, or death to the experimental subject . . . will bring it to a close.

Modified from Katz J: *Experimentation with human beings,* New York, 1972, Russell Sage Foundation.

---

nished research heritage and illustrate the human consequences of not adhering to ethical research standards.

The conduct of harmful, illegal research made additional controls necessary. In 1973 the Department of Health, Education, and Welfare published the first set of proposed regulations on the protection of human subjects. The most important provision was a regulation mandating that an institutional review board (IRB) functioning in accordance with specifications of the department must review and approve all studies. The National Research Act, passed in 1974 (Public Law 93-348), created the National Commission for the Protection of Human Subjects of Biomedical and Behavioral Research. A major charge of the Commission was to identify the basic principles that should underlie the conduct of biomedical and behavioral research involving human subjects and develop guidelines to ensure that research is conducted in accordance with those principles (Levine, 1986). Three ethical principles were identified as relevant to the conduct of research involving human subjects: the principles of **respect for persons, beneficence,** and **justice.** They are defined in Box 11-2. Included in a report issued in 1979, called the *Belmont Report,* these principles provided the basis for regulations affecting research sponsored by the federal government. The *Belmont Report* also served as a model for many of the ethical codes developed by scientific disciplines (National Commission, 1978).

In 1980 the Department of Health and Human Services developed a set of regulations in response to the Commission's recommendations. These regulations were published in 1981

Table 11-1

Highlights of Unethical Research Studies Conducted in the United States

RESEARCH STUDY	YEAR(S)	FOCUS OF STUDY	ETHICAL PRINCIPLE VIOLATED
Hyman vs. Jewish Chronic Disease Hospital case	1965	Doctors injected aged and senile patients with their cancer cells to study their rejection response.	Informed consent was not obtained, and there was no indication that the study had been reviewed and approved by an ethics committee. The two physicians claimed that they did not wish to evoke emotional reactions or refusals to participate by informing the subjects of the nature of the study (Hershey and Miller, 1976).
Milledgeville, Georgia, case	1969	Investigational drugs were used on mentally disabled children without first obtaining the opinion of a psychiatrist.	There was no review of the study protocol or institutional approval of the program before implementation (Levine, 1986).
Tuskegee, Alabama, syphilis study	1932-1973	For 40 years the United States Public Health Service conducted a study using two groups of poor black male sharecroppers. One group consisted of those who had untreated syphilis; the other group was judged to be free of the disease. Treatment was withheld from the group having syphilis even after penicillin became generally available and accepted as effective treatment in the 1950s. Steps were taken to prevent the subjects from obtaining it. The researcher wanted to study the untreated disease.	Many of the subjects who consented to participate in the study were not informed about the purpose and procedures of the research. Others were unaware that they were subjects. The degree of risk outweighed the potential benefit. Withholding of known effective treatment violates the subjects' right to fair treatment and protection from harm (Levine, 1986).

Table 11-1—cont'd

Highlights of Unethical Research Studies Conducted in the United States

RESEARCH STUDY	YEAR(S)	FOCUS OF STUDY	ETHICAL PRINCIPLE VIOLATED
San Antonio contraceptive study	1969	In a study examining the side effects of oral contraceptives, 76 impoverished Mexican-American women were randomly assigned to an experimental group receiving birth control pills or a control group receiving placebos. Subjects were not informed about the placebo and attendant risk of pregnancy. Eleven subjects became pregnant, 10 of whom were in the placebo control group.	Principles of informed consent were violated; full disclosure of potential risk, harm, results, or side effects was not evident in the informed consent document. The potential risk outweighed the benefits of the study. The subjects' right to fair treatment and protection from harm was violated (Levine, 1986).
Willowbrook Hospital	1972	Mentally incompetent children ($n = 350$) were not admitted to Willowbrook Hospital, a residential treatment facility, unless parents consented to their children being subjects in a study examining the natural history of infectious hepatitis and the effect of gamma globulin. The children were deliberately infected with the hepatitis virus under various conditions; some received gamma globulin; others did not.	Principle of voluntary consent was violated. Parents were coerced to consent to their children's participation as research subjects. Subjects or their guardians have a right to self-determination; that is, they should be free of constraint, coercion, or undue influence of any kind. Many subjects feel pressured to participate in studies if they are in powerless, dependent positions (Rothman, 1982).

Continued

Table 11-1—cont'd

Highlights of Unethical Research Studies Conducted in the United States

RESEARCH STUDY	YEAR(S)	FOCUS OF STUDY	ETHICAL PRINCIPLE VIOLATED
UCLA Schizophrenia Medication Study	1983 to present	In a study examining the effects of withdrawing psychotropic medications of 50 patients under treatment for schizophrenia, 23 subjects suffered severe relapses after their medication was stopped. The goal of the study was to determine if some schizophrenics might do better without medications that, themselves, had deleterious side effects.	Although all subjects signed informed consent documents, they were not informed about how severe their relapses might be, or that they could suffer worsening symptoms with each recurrence. Principles of informed consent were violated; full disclosure of potential risk, harm, results, or side effects was not evident in the informed consent document. The potential risk outweighed the benefits of the study. The subjects' right to fair treatment and protection from harm was violated (Hilts, 1995).

Box 11-2   Basic Ethical Principles Relevant to the Conduct of Research

Respect for persons: People have the right to self-determination and to treatment as autonomous agents. Thus they have the freedom to participate or not participate in research. Persons with diminished autonomy are entitled to protection.

Beneficence: An obligation to do no harm and maximize possible benefits. Persons are treated in an ethical manner when their decisions are respected, they are protected from harm, and efforts are made to secure their well-being.

Justice: Human subjects should be treated fairly. An injustice occurs when benefit to which a person is entitled is denied without good reason or when a burden is imposed unduly.

and revised in 1983 (Department of Health and Human Services, 1983). These regulations include the following:

- General requirements for informed consent
- Documentation of informed consent
- IRB review of research proposals
- Exempt and expedited review procedures for certain kinds of research
- Criteria for IRB approval of research

These regulations are discussed in the sections on informed consent and institutional review later in this chapter.

In 1992 the National Institutes of Health (NIH) Office of Research Integrity was established to set standards for dealing with allegations of scientific misconduct. In 1993, Congress passed the NIH Revitalization Act which, among other provisions, created a 12-member Commission on Research Integrity to propose new procedures for addressing scientific misconduct. A report, "Integrity and Misconduct in Research," issued by the Commission in 1995, proposed a new definition of scientific misconduct, additional protection for "whistle blowers," and a set of guidelines for handling allegations of scientific misconduct (Commission on Research Integrity, 1995; Ryan, 1996). In 1996, President Clinton appointed members of the National Bioethics Advisory Commission, which provides guidance to federal agencies on the ethical conduct of current and future human biological and behavioral research.

Current and Future Ethical Dilemmas in Research

On a national level, the ethical dilemmas in research for the present and twenty-first centuries will be in the area of biotechnology, of animals for research, and the creation of an organizational culture that values and nurtures research ethics and the rights of people who engage in research either as investigators or subjects (Pranulis, 1996). For example, the Human Genome Project is an international research project initiated by Congress in 1988 (National Center for Human Genome Research, 1990). The goal of this subject is to map the estimated 50,000 to 100,000 genes in the human genome by the year 2005 and thereby identify the complete genetic makeup of humans (Green and Waterson, 1991). In 1993 the U.S. Government ended a 5-year moratorium and began approving animal patents. Patents have been issued to organizations for the development of "transgenic" or genetically engineered animals suited to research in humans (Andrews, 1993). Another use of animals for research is in the area of xenograft transplantation. In 1992 three liver transplants were done using two baboons and one pig. In 1993 a man dying of acquired immunodeficiency syndrome (AIDS) received a bone marrow transplant from a baboon (Altman, 1994). Several centers have obtained approval from their IRBs to perform xenograft transplants. The **ethics,** as well as the risks and benefits of this type of human/animal research, are still in question; the issue is very controversial.

Other areas of research that engender much discussion and controversy are fetal tissue research and use of women who are of childbearing potential as subjects in drug/therapeutic studies. In 1993 an executive order lifted the government's ban on fetal tissue research. This allows the resumption of research into the testing of fetal tissue for use in the treatment of such diseases as Parkinson's.

In the past, women of childbearing potential were denied access to participation as subjects in drug or potentially therapeutic studies because of the unknown potentially harmful effects of drugs and other therapies that were in various stages of testing on fetuses. Guidelines related to the inclusion of pregnant women as research subjects have been even more stringent. This policy has led to the exclusion of women from many important drug and research studies over the years. Currently researchers seeking funds from the NIH have to justify excluding women from such studies (Burd, 1993).

In 1993, the NIH issued guidelines requiring grantees to include enough women in clinical trials to determine whether and how experimental drugs affect them differently from men (Larson, 1994). And, in 1994, the Food and Drug Administration (FDA) allowed researchers to include AIDS-infected pregnant women, without the father's consent, in studies to determine whether the drug AZT would prevent transmission of the virus from mother to fetus (Walker, 1996).

Over the next decade many questions and controversies will arise in relation to the risks and benefits of the just-mentioned areas of research and as a result of ever-increasing technology in health care in areas that have not been defined as yet. Although these areas of research may seem far removed from nursing research and patient care, they will affect the type of patients nurses will care for and the type of clinical research nurses will conduct.

EVOLUTION OF ETHICS IN NURSING RESEARCH

The evolution of ethics in nursing research can be traced back to 1897 and the constitution of the Nurses' Associated Alumnae Organization. One of the first purposes of this organization was to establish a code of ethics for the nursing profession. In 1900, Isabel Hampton Robb wrote *Nursing Ethics: For Hospital and Private Use.* In describing moral laws by which people must abide, she states:

Etiquette, speaking broadly, means a form of behavior or manners expressly or tacitly required on particular occasions. It makes up the code of polite life and includes forms of ceremony to be observed, so that we invariably find in societies that a certain etiquette is required and observed either tacitly or by expressed agreement.

Clearly, Hampton Robb's comments reflect the norms of Victorian society. However, they highlight an historical concern for ethical actions by nurses as health care providers (Robb, 1900).

In 1967 the American Nurses Association (ANA) charged its Committee on Research Studies with the task of developing guidelines for the nurse researcher in clinical research. In 1968 the ANA Board of Directors approved the statement titled "The Nurse in Research: ANA Guidelines on Ethical Values." Not only were basic principles regarding the use of human subjects endorsed, but the role of the nurse as investigator, as well as practitioner, was also described.

The ANA established the Commission on Nursing Research in 1970. By doing so, it publicly affirmed nursing's obligation to support the advancement of scientific knowledge and reflected a commitment to support two sets of human rights: (1) the rights of qualified nurses to engage in research and have access to resources necessary for implementing scientific investigation and (2) the rights of all persons who are participants in research performed by investigators whose studies impinge on the patient care provided by nurses. The ANA emphasized human rights in terms of three domains: (1) right to freedom from intrinsic risk or injury, (2) right to privacy and dignity, and (3) right to anonymity.

The ANA's *Human Rights Guidelines for Nursing in Clinical and Other Research,* published in 1975, reflects the nursing profession's code of ethics for research. Box 11-3 provides a summary of this document, one that helps ensure that research maintains ethical, as well as scientific, rigor. This document is relevant for all nurses; the nurse as a researcher or caregiver must assure patients that their human rights will be safeguarded. In fact, nurses, when interviewing

---

Box 11-3   American Nurses Association Human Rights Guidelines for Nurses in Clinical and Other Research

Guideline I: Right to Self-Determination
Implementation: Where research participation is a condition of employment, nurses must be informed in writing of the nature of the activity involved in advance of employment. If nurses are not so informed, they must be given the opportunity of not participating in the research.
Potential of risk to others must be clarified in relation to the types of risk involved, the ways of recognizing when risk is present, and the ways in which to counteract potential and unnecessary danger.
Guideline 2: Right to Freedom from Risk or Harm
Implementation: Investigators must ensure freedom of risk from harm by estimating the potential physical or emotional risk and benefit involved. Vulnerable and captive subjects, such as students, patients, prisoners, mentally incompetent, children, the elderly, and the poor, must be carefully monitored for sources of potential risk of injury so they can be protected.
Guideline 3: Scope of Application
Implementation: Guidelines for protection of human rights apply to all individuals, that is, subjects involved in research activities. The use of subjects with limited civil freedom can usually be justified only when there is benefit to them or others in similar circumstances.
Guideline 4: Responsibilities to Support Knowledge Development
Implementation: Nurses have an obligation to support the development of knowledge that expands the depth and breadth of the scientific knowledge or base of nursing practice.
Guideline 5: Informed Consent
Implementation: The right to self-determination is protected when informed consent is obtained from the prospective subject or legal guardian.
Guideline 6: Participation on Institutional Review Boards
Implementation: As professionals accountable to the public who are the consumers of health care, nurses have an obligation to support the inclusion of nurses on institutional review boards (IRBs). Nurses also have an obligation to serve on IRBs to review ethical implications of proposed and ongoing research. All studies involving data collection from humans, animals, or records should be reviewed by a review board of health professionals and community representatives who ensure the protection of subject rights.

From American Nurses Association: *Guidelines for nurses in clinical and other research,* Kansas City, Mo, 1975, ANA.

for potential employment, should ask what is expected of them in terms of research responsibilities. For example, nurses might ask:

- Are nurses required to collect data or administer medications or treatments in double-blind clinical trials?
- Are written research protocols available as references?
- Has the IRB ruled on each protocol?
- Are nurses free to decline to participate without jeopardizing their position?
- What channels exist for addressing ethical concerns with regard to research being conducted?

Clearly, ignorance and naivete vis a vis ethical and legal guidelines for the conduct of research must never be an excuse for a nurse's failure to be familiar with and act on behalf of the patients whose human rights must, at all times, be safeguarded. Nurse researchers are often among the most responsible and conscientious investigators when it comes to respecting the rights of human subjects. All nurses should be aware that the tenets of the ANA's *Code for Nurses* (1985), currently undergoing revision, are integral with the *ANA Human Rights Guidelines for Nursing in Clinical and Other Research* mentioned earlier.

Fowler (1988), a nurse ethicist, calls for an international code of ethics for nursing research. She raises many ethical questions that nurses around the world need to address now and in the future. Davis (1990) supports the concept of shared values among all nurses, stating that many of nursing's shared values are found in their professional codes. Some countries have their own code; others use the International Council of Nurses (ICN) Code for Nurses.

PROTECTION OF HUMAN RIGHTS

Human rights are the claims and demands that have been justified in the eyes of an individual or by a group of individuals. The term refers to the following five rights outlined in the ANA (1985) guidelines:

1. Right to self-determination
2. Right to privacy and dignity
3. Right to anonymity and confidentiality
4. Right to fair treatment
5. Right to protection from discomfort and harm

These rights apply to everyone involved in a research project, including research team members who may be involved in data collection, practicing nurses involved in the research setting, and subjects participating in the study. As consumers of research read a research article, they must realize any issues highlighted in Table 11-2 should have been addressed and resolved before a research study is approved for implementation.

HELPFUL HINT
Recognize that the right to personal privacy may be more difficult to protect when carrying out qualitative studies because of the small sample size and because the subjects' verbatim quotes are often used in the results/findings section of the research report to highlight the findings.

Procedures for Protecting Basic Human Rights

Informed Consent

Informed consent illustrated by the ethical principles of respect and its related right to self-determination are outlined in Box 11-4 and Table 11-2. Nurses need to understand elements of informed consent so that they are knowledgeable participants in obtaining informed consents from patients and/or in critiquing this process as it is presented in research articles.

Informed consent is the legal principle that, at least in theory, governs the patient's ability to accept or reject individual medical interventions designed to diagnose or treat an illness. It is also a doctrine that determines and regulates participation in research (Pranulis, 1996; Silva, 1995). The Code of Federal Regulations (1983) defines the meaning of informed consent:

The knowing consent of an individual or his/her legally authorized representative, under circumstances that provide the prospective subject or representative sufficient opportunity to consider whether or not to participate without undue inducement or any element of force, fraud, deceit, duress, or other forms of constraint or coercion.

No investigator may involve a human being as a research subject before obtaining the legally effective informed consent of a subject or legally authorized representative. Prospective subjects must have time to decide whether to participate in a study. The researcher must not coerce the subject into participating. Nor may researchers collect data on subjects who have explicitly refused to participate in a study. An ethical violation of this principle is illustrated by a large-scale study about women with breast cancer in which the outcomes for mastectomy versus lumpectomy were compared. A 1994 audit in study records indicated that medical data on at least three dozen women were collected and analyzed without authorization, against their expressed wishes (Snowden, 1994).

The language of the consent form must be understandable. For example, the reading level should be no greater than eighth grade for adults and the use of technical research language should be avoided (Rempusheski, 1991). According to the Code of Federal Regulations, subjects should in no way be asked to waive their rights or release the investigator from liability for negligence.

The elements that need to be contained in an informed consent are listed in Box 11-4. It is important to note that many institutions require additional elements. A sample of an informed consent form is presented in Figure 11-1.

HELPFUL HINT

Remember that research reports rarely provide readers with detailed information regarding the degree to which the researcher adhered to the ethical principles, such as informed consent, because of space limitations in journals that make it impossible to describe all aspects of a study. Failure to mention procedures to safeguard subjects' rights does not necessarily mean that such precautions were not taken.

Most investigators obtain consent through personal discussion with potential subjects. This process allows the person to obtain immediate answers to questions. However, consent forms, written in narrative or outline form, highlight elements that both inform and remind subjects of the nature of the study and their participation (Pranulis, 1996).

Table 11-2

Protection of Human Rights

BASIC HUMAN RIGHT	DEFINITION
Right to self-determination	Based on the ethical principle of respect for persons; people should be treated as autonomous agents who have the freedom to choose without external controls. An autonomous agent is one who is informed about a proposed study and is allowed to choose to participate or not to participate (Brink, 1992); subjects have the right to withdraw from a study without penalty.
	Subjects with diminished autonomy are entitled to protection. They are more vulnerable because of age, legal or mental incompetence, terminal illness, or confinement to an institution.
	Jusification for use of vulnerable subjects must be provided.
Right to privacy and dignity	Based on the principle of respect, privacy is the freedom of a person to determine the time, extent, and circumstances under which private information is shared or withheld from others.
Right to anonymity and confidentiality	Based on the principle of respect, anonymity exists when the subject's identity cannot be linked, even by the researcher, with his or her individual responses (ANA, 1985).
	Confidentiality means that individual identities of subjects will not be linked to the information they provide and will not be publicly divulged.

VIOLATION OF BASIC HUMAN RIGHT	EXAMPLE
A subject's right to self-determination is violated through the use of coercion, covert data collection, and deception. ■ Coercion occurs when an overt threat of harm or excessive reward is presented to ensure compliance. ■ Covert data collection occurs when people become research subjects and are exposed to research treatments without knowing it. ■ Deception occurs when subjects are actually misinformed about the purpose of the research. ■ Potential for violation of the right to self-determination is greater for subjects with diminished autonomy; they have decreased ability to give informed consent and are vulnerable.	Subjects may feel that their care will be adversely affected if they refuse to participate in research. The Jewish Chronic Disease Hospital Study (see Table 11-1) is an example of a study in which patients and their doctors did not know that cancer cells were being injected. In the Milgrim (1963) Study, subjects were deceived when asked to administer electric shocks to another person; the person was really an actor who pretended to feel the shocks. Subjects administering the shocks were very stressed by participating in this study though they were not administering shocks at all. The Willowbrook Study (see Table 11-1) is an example of how coercion was used to obtain parental consent of vulnerable mentally retarded children who would not be admitted to the institution unless the children participated in a study in which they were deliberately injected with the hepatitis virus.
The Privacy Act of 1974 was instituted to protect subjects from such violations. These occur most frequently during data collection when invasive questions are asked that might result in loss of job, friendships, or dignity or might create embarrassment and mental distress. It also may occur when subjects are unaware that information is being shared with others.	Subjects may be asked personal questions such as "Were you sexually abused as a child?" "Do you use drugs?" "What are your sexual preferences?" When questions are asked using hidden microphones or hidden tape recorders, the subjects' privacy is invaded because they have no knowledge that the data are being shared with others. Subjects also have a right to control access of others to their records.
Anonymity is violated when the subjects' responses can be linked with their identity.	Subjects are given a code number instead of using names for identification purposes. Subjects' names are never used when reporting findings.
Confidentiality is breached when a researcher, by accident or by direct action, allows an unauthorized person to gain access to study data that contain information about subject identity or responses that create a potentially harmful situation for subjects.	Breaches of confidentiality with regard to sexual preference, income, drug use, prejudice, or personality variables can be harmful to subjects. Data are analyzed as group data so that individuals cannot be identified by their responses.

Continued

Table 11-2—cont'd

Protection of Human Rights

BASIC HUMAN RIGHT	DEFINITION
Right to fair treatment	Based on the ethical principle of justice, people should be treated fairly and should receive what they are due or owed.
	Fair treatment is equitable selection of subjects and their treatment during the research study. This includes selection of subjects for reasons directly related to the problem studied versus convenience, compromised position, or vulnerability. It also includes fair treatment of subjects during the study, including fair distribution of risks and benefits regardless of age, race, or socioeconomic status.
Right to protection from discomfort and harm	Based on the ethical principle of beneficence, people must take an active role in promoting good and preventing harm in the world around them, as well as in research studies.
	Discomfort and harm can be physical, psychological, social, or economic in nature.
	There are five categories of studies based on levels of harm and discomfort:
	1. No anticipated effects
	2. Temporary discomfort
	3. Unusual level of temporary discomfort
	4. Risk of permanent damage
	5. Certainty of permanent damage

VIOLATION OF BASIC HUMAN RIGHT	EXAMPLE
Injustices with regard to subject selection have occurred as a result of social, cultural, racial, and gender biases in society. Historically, research subjects often have been obtained from groups of people who were regarded as having less "social value," the poor, prisoners, slaves, the mentally incompetent, and the dying. Often subjects were treated carelessly, without consideration of physical or psychological harm.	The Tuskegee Syphilis Study (1973), the Jewish Chronic Disease Study (1965), the San Antonio Contraceptive Study (1969), and the Willowbrook Study (1972) (see Table 11-1) all provide examples related to unfair subject selection. Investigators should not be late for data collection appointments, should terminate data collection on time, should not change agreed upon procedures or activities without consent, and should provide agreed upon benefits such as a copy of the study findings or a participation fee.
Subjects' right to be protected is violated when researchers know in advance that harm, death, or disabling injury will occur and thus the benefits do not outweigh the risk.	Temporary physical discomfort involving minimal risk include fatigue or headache; emotional discomfort includes the expense involved in traveling to and from the data collection site. Studies examining sensitive issues, such as rape, incest, or spouse abuse, might cause unusual levels of temporary discomfort by opening up current and/or past traumatic experiences. In these situations, researchers assess distress levels and provide debriefing sessions during which the subject may express feelings and ask questions. The researcher has the opportunity to make referrals for professional intervention. Studies having the potential to cause permanent damage are more likely to be medical rather than nursing in nature. A recent clinical trial of a new drug, a monoclonal antibody endotoxin (Centocor), was suspended when preliminary findings revealed a higher mortality rate for the treatment group versus the placebo group. Evaluation of the data led to termination of the trial. In some research, such as the Tuskegee Syphilis Study or the Nazi medical experiments, subjects experienced permanent damage or death.

Box 11-4   Elements of Informed Consent

1. A statement that the study involves research.
2. An explanation of the purposes of the research, delineating the expected duration of the subject's participation.
3. A description of the procedures to be followed, and identification of any procedures which are experimental.
4. A description of any reasonably foreseeable risks or discomforts to the subject.
5. A description of any benefits to the subject or to others that may reasonably be expected from the research.
6. A disclosure of appropriate alternative procedures or course of treatment, if any, that might be advantageous to the subject.
7. A statement describing the extent to which anonymity and confidentiality of the records identifying the subject will be maintained.
8. For research involving more than minimal risk, an explanation as to whether any medical treatments are available if injury occurs and, if so, what they consist of, or where further information may be obtained.
9. An explanation about who to contact for answers to questions about the research and researcher subjects' rights, and who to contact in the event of a research-related injury to the subject.
10. A statement that participation is voluntary, that refusal to participate will not involve any penalty or less benefit to which the subject is otherwise entitled, and the subject may discontinue participation at any time without penalty or loss of otherwise entitled benefits.

From Code of Federal Regulations: Protection of human subjects, 45 CFR 46, *OPRR Reports,* Revised March 8, 1983.

Assurance of **anonymity** and **confidentiality** (defined in Table 11-2) is usually conveyed in writing. This is sometimes difficult in unique research situations that capture the public's attention, for example, that involving Dr. Barney Clark, the first recipient of an artificial heart. More recently, when physicians at Loma Linda University Hospital in California transplanted a baboon's heart into a 2-week old infant, the identity of the infant was protected; she was known only as Baby Fae.

The consent form must be signed and dated by the subject. The presence of witnesses is not always necessary but does constitute evidence that the subject concerned actually signed the form. In cases where the subject is a minor or is physically or mentally incapable of signing the consent, the legal guardian or representative must sign. The investigator also signs the form to indicate commitment to the agreement.

Generally the signed informed consent form is given to the subject. The researcher should keep a copy also. Some research, such as a retrospective chart audit, may not require informed consent—only institutional approval. Or in some cases, where minimal risk is involved, the investigator may have to provide the subject only with an information sheet and verbal explanation. In other cases, such as a volunteer convenience sample, completion and return of re-

---

Informed Consent

The Caldwell Medical Center
Code No. _____

I understand that I am being treated with the drug *cis*-platin, which may cause the unpleasant side effects of nausea and vomiting. Treatment to control these side effects includes using various medications, reducing the intake of food and fluids before chemotherapy, maintaining a quiet environment, and accepting support from others. In addition, I understand that using various coping strategies is helpful to persons in similar situations.

I understand that the purpose of this study is to help clients learn some coping techniques and evaluate how their use affects the occurrence of nausea and vomiting after *cis*-platin is administered. If I agree to participate in this research study, I understand that I will be randomly assigned to one of the following three nursing treatment programs:

1. I will meet with one of the investigators before I receive my chemotherapy. We will discuss my experience and the methods that other clients and I have found helpful.

or

2. I will meet with one of the investigators before I receive my chemotherapy. I will follow directions for practicing a technique that produces, under my own control, a state of altered consciousness called *self-hypnosis.* I will be asked to practice this technique during and after receiving my chemotherapy. I will be expected to practice this technique daily so that I may learn to use it without being directed by another person.

or

3. I will be given the customary nursing care that is rendered to every client taking the drugs that I am receiving.

In addition, if necessary, I will receive only the medication Reglan to control nausea and vomiting.

I understand that in no case will I receive less than the usual standard and expected level of nursing care that I am already receiving.

I understand that if I am selected to be in Group 2, a simple test to determine my susceptibility to this technique will be performed. Most people are susceptible, but if I am not and I wish to continue in the study, I will be randomly assigned to one of the two remaining groups.

I understand that this research study has been discussed with my physician and that he or she is aware of my participation. The treatments prescribed to control the side effects of nausea and vomiting will not be altered if I participate in this study.

Continued

Figure 11-1 Example of an informed consent form.

Informed Consent—cont'd

I understand that a nurse investigator will be in my room while my chemotherapy is ending and for 4 hours after the treatment. I understand that nursing care will be provided by the nurses on the unit and not by the nurse-investigator. The research nurse will be taking notes on my reactions to the chemotherapy. Once an hour she will ask me to rate my nausea. I can expect that this will take only a few minutes of my time and that, if I am sleeping, I will not be awakened.

I have been told that this routine will be followed for three courses of chemotherapy, during three separate hospitalizations.

I understand that the benefits from this treatment are that I may experience less nausea and vomiting or fewer of the feelings of being sick to my stomach that often occur with *cis*-platin. There are no side effects or risks from my participation.

My participation is voluntary and I may choose to not participate or to withdraw at any time without jeopardizing my future treatment.

My identity will not be revealed in any way. My name will be encoded so that I will remain anonymous.

I also understand that if I believe I have sustained an injury as a result of participating in this research study, I may contact the investigators, Ms. B. J. Simon at 608-0011 or B. A. Smith at 124-6142, or the Office of the Institutional Review Board at 124-2500 so that I can review the matter and identify the medical resources that may be available to me.

I understand the following statements:
1. The Caldwell Medical Center will furnish whatever emergency medical care that the medical staff of this hospital determine to be necessary.
2. I will be responsible for the cost of such emergency care personally, through my medical insurance, or by another form of coverage.
3. No monetary compensation for wages lost as a result of an injury will be paid to me by The Caldwell Medical Center.
4. I will receive a copy of this consent form.

_____   _____
Date   Patient

_____   _____
Witness   Investigator

The Institutional Review Board of the Caldwell Medical Center has approved the solicitation of subjects for participation in this research proposal.

Figure 11-1—cont'd   Example of an informed consent form.

search instruments provide evidence of consent. The IRB will help to advise on exceptions to these guidelines, cases in which the IRB might grant waivers or amend its guidelines in other ways. The IRB makes the final determination as to the most appropriate documentation format. Research consumers should note whether and what kind of evidence of informed consent has been provided in a research article.

HELPFUL HINT

Note that researchers often do not obtain written, informed consent when the major means of data collection is through self-administered questionnaires. The researcher usually assumes applied consent in such cases; that is, the return of the completed questionnaire reflects the respondent's voluntary consent to participate.

Institutional Review Board

Institutional review boards (IRBs) are boards that review research projects to assess that ethical standards are met in relation to the protection of the rights of human subjects. The National Research Act (1974) requires that such agencies as universities, hospitals, and other health agencies applying for a grant or contract for any project or program that involves the conduct of biomedical or behavioral research involving human subjects must submit with their application assurances that they have established an IRB, sometimes called a human subjects committee, which reviews the research projects and protects the rights of the human subjects (Code of Federal Regulations, 1983). At agencies where no federal grants or contracts are awarded, there is usually a review mechanism similar to an IRB process, such as a research advisory committee.

The National Research Act requires that the IRB have at least five members of various backgrounds to promote complete and adequate project review. The members must be qualified by virtue of their expertise and experience and reflect professional, gender, racial, and cultural diversity. Membership must include one member whose concerns are primarily nonscientific (lawyer, clergy, ethicist) and at least one member from outside the agency.

The IRB is responsible for protecting subjects from undue risk and loss of personal rights and dignity. For a research proposal to be eligible for consideration by an IRB, it must already have been approved by a departmental review group such as a nursing research committee that attests to the proposal's scientific merit and congruence with institutional policies, procedures, and mission. The IRB reviews the study's protocol to ensure that it meets the requirements of ethical research that appear in Box 11-5. Most boards provide guidelines or instructions for researchers that include steps to be taken to receive IRB approval. For example, guidelines for writing a standard consent form or criteria for qualifying for an expedited rather than a full IRB review may be made available. The IRB has the authority to approve research, require modifications, or disapprove a research study. A researcher must receive some form of IRB approval before beginning to conduct research. Institutional review boards have the authority to suspend or terminate approval of research that is not conducted in accordance with IRB requirements or that has been associated with unexpected serious harm to subjects.

IRBs also have mechanisms for reviewing research in an expedited manner where there is minimal risk to research subjects (Code of Federal Regulations, 1983). An expedited review usually shortens the length of the review process. Keep in mind that although a researcher may determine that a project involves minimal risk, the IRB makes the final determination and the

---

Box 11-5 Code of Federal Regulations for IRB Approval of Research Studies

To approve research, the IRB must determine that the following Code of Federal Regulations has been satisfied:
1. The risks to subjects are minimized.
2. The risks to subjects are reasonable in relation to anticipated benefits.
3. The selection of the subjects is equitable.
4. Informed consent, in one of several possible forms, must be and will be sought from each prospective subject or the subject's legally authorized representative.
5. The informed consent form must be properly documented.
6. Where appropriate, the research plan makes adequate provision for monitoring the data collected to ensure subject safety.
7. Where appropriate, there are adequate provisions to protect the privacy of subjects and the confidentiality of data.
8. Where some or all of the subjects are likely to be vulnerable to coercion or undue influence, such as persons with acute or severe physical or mental illness or persons who are economically or educationally disadvantaged, appropriate additional safeguards are included.

---

research may not be undertaken until then. A full list of research categories eligible for expedited review is available from any IRB office. It includes the following:

- Collection of hair and nail clippings in a nondisfiguring manner
- Collection of excreta and external secretions including sweat
- Recording of data on subjects 18 years or older, using noninvasive procedures routinely employed in clinical practice
- Voice recordings
- Study of existing data, documents, records, pathological specimens, or diagnostic data

An expedited review does not automatically exempt the researcher from obtaining informed consent.

The *Federal Register* is a publication that contains updated information about federal guidelines for research involving human subjects. Every researcher should consult an agency's research office to ensure that the application being prepared for IRB approval adheres to the most current requirements. Nurses who are critiquing published research should be conversant with current regulations to determine whether ethical standards have been met. The Critical Thinking Decision Path illustrates the ethical decision-making process an IRB might use in evaluating the risk/benefit ratio of a research study.

Protecting Basic Human Rights of Vulnerable Groups

Researchers are advised to consult their agency's IRB for the most recent federal and state rules and guidelines when considering research involving vulnerable groups such as the elderly, children, pregnant women, the unborn, those who are emotionally or physically disabled, prison-

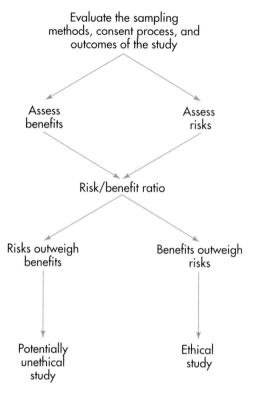

Evaluate the sampling
methods, consent process, and
outcomes of the study

Assess
benefits

Assess
risks

Risk/benefit ratio

Risks outweigh
benefits

Benefits outweigh
risks

Potentially
unethical
study

Ethical
study

Critical Thinking Decision Path   Evaluating the risk/benefit ratio of a research study.

ers, the deceased, students, and persons with AIDS (Demi and Warren, 1995). In addition, researchers should consult the IRB before planning research that potentially involves an over-subscribed research population, such as organ transplantation patients, AIDS patients, or "captive" and convenient populations, such as prisoners. It should be emphasized that use of special populations does not preclude undertaking research; extra precautions must be taken, however, to protect their rights (Levine, 1995). Davis (1981) reminds us that a society can be judged by the way it treats its most vulnerable people—a point worth remembering in research that involves children, the elderly, and other vulnerable groups.

Mitchell discussed the National Commission's concept of **assent** versus **consent** in regard to pediatric research. Assent contains the following three fundamental elements:

1. A basic understanding of what the child will be expected to do and what will be done to the child
2. A comprehension of the basic purpose of the research
3. An ability to express a preference regarding participation

In contrast to assent, consent requires a relatively advanced level of cognitive ability. Informed consent reflects competency standards requiring abstract appreciation and reasoning regarding the information provided. The issue of assent versus consent is an interesting one when one determines at what age children can make meaningful decisions about participating in research. In terms of the work by Piaget regarding cognitive ability, children at age 6 and older can participate in giving assent. Children at age 14 and older, although not legally authorized to give sole consent unless they are emancipated minors, can make such decisions as capably as adults (Mitchell, 1984).

Federal regulations require parental permission whenever a child is involved in research unless otherwise specified, for example, in cases of child abuse or mature minors at minimal risk (Broome and Stieglitz, 1992; Levine, 1995). If the research involves more than minimal risk and does not offer direct benefit to the individual child, both parents must give permission. When individuals reach maturity, usually at 18 years of age in cases of research, they may render their own consent. They may do so at a younger age if they have been legally declared emancipated minors. Questions regarding this should be addressed by the IRB and/or research administration office and not left to the discretion of the researcher to answer.

Dubler (1987), as an advocate for the vulnerable elderly who are of increasing dependence and declining cognitive ability, states that elders are precisely the class of persons who were historically and are potentially vulnerable to abuse and for whom the law must struggle to fashion specific protections. The issue of the legal competence of elders is often raised (Alt-White, 1995). There is no issue if the potential subject can supply legally effective informed consent. Competence is not a clear "black or white" situation. The complexity of the study may affect one's ability to consent to participate. For example, an elderly person may be able to consent to participate in a simple observation study but not in a clinical drug trial.

The issue of the necessity of requiring the elderly to provide consent often arises. Dubler (1993) refers to the research regulations that provide that requirements for some or all of the elements of informed consent may be waived for the following:

1. The research involves no more than minimal risk to the subjects
2. The waiver or alteration will not adversely affect the rights and welfare of the subjects
3. The research could not feasibly be carried out without the waiver or alteration
4. Whenever appropriate, the subjects will be provided with additional pertinent information after participation.

No vulnerable population may be singled out for study because it is simply convenient. For example, prisoners may not be studied simply because they are an available and convenient group. Prisoners may be studied if the study pertains to them, that is, studies concerning the effects and processes of incarceration. Students are often a convenient group. They must not be singled out as research subjects because of convenience; the research questions must have some bearing on their status as students.

Researchers and patient caregivers involved in research with vulnerable people are well advised to seek advice from appropriate IRBs, clinicians, lawyers, ethicists, and others. In all cases, the burden should be on the investigator to show the IRB that it is appropriate to involve vulnerable subjects in research.

HELPFUL HINT

Keep in mind that researchers rarely mention explicitly that the study participants were vulnerable subjects or that special precautions were taken to appropriately safeguard the human rights of this vulnerable group. Research consumers need to be attentive to the special needs of groups who may be unable to act as their own advocates or are unable to adequately assess the risk/benefit ratio of a research study.

SCIENTIFIC FRAUD AND MISCONDUCT

Fraud

Periodically articles reporting unethical actions of researchers appear in the professional and lay literature. Data may have been falsified or fabricated or subjects may have been coerced to participate in a research study (Abdellah, 1990; Hawley and Jeffers, 1992; Kevles, 1996). In a climate of "publish or perish" in academic and scientific settings and declining research dollars, there is increasing pressure on academics and scientists to produce significant research findings. Job security and professional recognition are coveted, essential, and often predicated on being a productive scientist and prolific writer. These pressures have been known to overpower some people, who then take shortcuts, fabricate data, and falsify findings to advance their positions.

The risks are many, including harming research subjects or basing clinical practice on false data. Nurses, as advocates of patient welfare and professional practice, should be aware that, albeit ideally rare, there are occasions when misconduct of the researcher is observed or suspected. In such cases, nurses must be advised to contact the appropriate group, such as the IRB, to ensure that this matter receives appropriate attention and review.

Misconduct

Of equal importance is the issue of basing practice on reports that appear in journals, where subsequent research and reports on those subjects change the scientific basis for practice. Journals may print corrections or further research in follow-up reports that are buried, obscure, or underreported. A physician, Lawrence K. Altman (1988), stated, "Such shortcomings are critically important because the thousands of journals that cover a range of specialties are the central reservoir of scientific knowledge. They are the standard references for crediting discoveries and determining treatments." It is incumbent on nurses as patient advocates and research consumers to keep up to date on scientific reports related to nursing practice and adjust practice as directed by ever-evolving research findings.

Unauthorized Research

At times, ad hoc or informal and unauthorized research does go on, including product testing. Although the testing may seem to be harmless, again it is not the purview of the investigator to make that determination. Nurses must carefully avoid being involved in unauthorized research for a number of reasons, including the following (Hanks, 1984b):

- These treatments or methods of care are usually not monitored as closely for untoward effects, hence exposing the client to unwarranted risk
- Clients' rights to informed consent in clinical trials are not protected
- The success or failure of these unrecorded trials contributes nothing to the organized scientific knowledge of the efficacy or complications of the treatment
- The lack of independent quality supervision allows deviations from the adopted experimental program that may eliminate the program's effectiveness.

Sometimes the nurse plays the dual role of researcher and caregiver. In that situation, the nurse must question whether there may be risks inherent in the research that do not exist in the care. Even when these risks are clearly identified—and they must be—the caregiver must be comfortable that the level of risk is acceptable and that the **benefits** outweigh the **risks.** Patients must feel comfortable in refusing to participate in the caregiver's research while continuing to require the nurse's care. It must be made clear to patients that they may refuse to participate or withdraw from the study at any time without consequence or compromise to their care or relationship to the institution. The nurse in this dual role must consider whether the research will incur additional expense for the patient, whether that is warranted, and whether the subject has been apprised of such expenses.

PRODUCT TESTING

Nurses are often approached by manufacturers to test products on patients. Moore (1984) points out that all nurses should be aware of the FDA guidelines and regulations for testing of medical devices before they initiate any form of clinical testing. Medical devices are classified under Section 513 in the Federal Food, Drug and Cosmetic Act according to the extent of control necessary to ensure safety and effectiveness of each device. Classes related to product testing are defined in Table 11-3.

It is important that nurses be aware of their own institution's policies for **product testing.** The class of the product will obviously make a difference to the institution's position. If a nurse suspects that, for example, a Class II device is being tested in an ad hoc or unauthorized manner and without patient consent, this should be discussed with a supervisor or other appropriate authorities.

LEGAL AND ETHICAL ASPECTS OF ANIMAL EXPERIMENTATION

The federal laws that have been written to protect **animal rights** in research emanate from an interesting history of attitudes toward animals and the value people place on them. Animal activists (e.g., the Animal Liberation Front) and antivivisectionist societies began to gain considerable public attention in the 1970s. Of interest, however, is the fact that the oldest piece of legislation controlling animal experimentation goes back to 1876 in the United Kingdom. With the increase in the use of animals in research after World War II, a number of states passed legislation called "pound seizure laws" that allowed and even mandated the release of unclaimed animals from pounds to laboratories. The first pound seizure law was enacted in 1949; not until 1972 was the first law of that type repealed. In 1966 in the United States, the first Laboratory Animal Welfare Act was passed. The act did not deal with what we consider today to be some of the most salient issues related to animal experimentation (e.g., pain management), and amendments continued to be passed to address these concerns. The 1970 Act provided for the establishment of an institutional Animal Care and Use Committee (ACUC), one member of which must be a veterinarian. The United States Department of Agriculture (USDA) oversees compliance with animal welfare acts and holds institutions' administration accountable for such compliance.

In 1985 President Reagan signed PL 99-108, which contains the "Improved Standards for the Laboratory Animals' Act." Provisions in the series of acts and amendments to acts pertaining to animal experimentation include, but are by no means limited to, the list that appears in Box 11-6 (PHS Policy on Humane Care, 1985).

Table 11-3

Classes Related to Product Testing

CLASSES	EXAMPLES
Class I: general controls Included in Class I are devices whose safety and effectiveness can be reasonably guaranteed by the general controls of the Good Manufacturing Practices Regulations. The Regulations part of the act ensures that manufacturers will follow specific guidelines for packaging, storing, and providing specific product instructions.	Ostomy supplies
Class II: performance standards General controls are insufficient in this case to ensure safety and efficacy of the product, and the manufacturer must provide this assurance in the form of information.	Cardiac pacemakers, sutures, surgical metallic mesh, and biopsy needles
Class III: premarket approval This class includes devices whose safety and effectiveness are insufficiently ensured by general controls and for which performance standards are insufficient to ensure safety and effectiveness. These products are represented to be life sustaining or life supporting, are implanted into the body, or present a potential, unreasonable risk of illness or injury to the patient. Devices in this class are required to have approved applications for premarket approval. Extensive laboratory, animal, and human studies, which often require 2 to 3 years to complete, are required for Class III devices.	Heart valves, bone cements, contact lenses, and implantable devices left in the body for 30 days or longer

This section serves only as an introduction to the concept of legal/ethical issues related to animal experimentation. Principles of protection of animal rights in research have evolved over time. Animals, unlike humans, cannot give informed consent, but other conditions related to their welfare must not be ignored. Nurses who encounter the use of animals in research should be alert to their rights.

CRITIQUING THE LEGAL AND ETHICAL ASPECTS OF A RESEARCH STUDY

Research articles and reports often do not contain detailed information regarding the degree to which or all of the ways in which the investigator adhered to the legal/ethical principles presented in this chapter. Space considerations in articles preclude extensive documentation of all legal and ethical aspects of a research study. Lack of written evidence

---

Box 11-6 Basic Provisions of Acts Pertaining to Animal Experimentation

1. The transportation, care, and use of animals should be in accordance with the Animal Welfare Act and other applicable federal laws, guidelines, and policies.
2. Procedures involving animals should be designed and performed with consideration of their relevance to human or animal health, the advancement of knowledge, or the good of society.
3. The animals selected for a procedure should be of an appropriate species and quality and the minimum number required to obtain valid results. Methods such as mathematical models, computer simulation, and in vitro biological systems should be considered.
4. Proper use of animals, including the avoidance or minimization of discomfort, distress, and pain when consistent with sound scientific practices, is imperative. Unless the contrary is established, investigators should consider the procedures that cause pain or distress in human beings may cause pain or distress in other animals.
5. Procedures with animals that may cause more than temporary or slight pain or distress should be performed with appropriate sedation, analgesia, or anesthesia. Surgical or other painful procedures should not be performed on unanesthetized animals paralyzed by chemical agents.
6. Animals that would otherwise suffer severe or chronic pain or distress that cannot be relieved should be painlessly killed at the end of the procedure or, if appropriate, during the procedure.
7. The living conditions of animals should be appropriate for their species and contribute to their health and comfort. Normally the housing, feeding, and care of all animals used for biomedical purposes must be directed by a veterinarian or other scientist trained and experienced in the proper care, handling, and use of the species being maintained or studied. In any case, veterinary care shall be provided as indicated.
8. Investigators and other personnel shall be appropriately qualified and experienced for conducting procedures on living animals. Adequate arrangements shall be made for their in-service training, including the proper and humane care and use of laboratory animals.
9. Where exceptions are required in relation to the provision of these principles, the decisions should not rest with the investigators directly concerned but should be made, with regard to principle 2, by an appropriate review group, such as an institutional animal research committee. Such exceptions should not be made solely for the purposes of teaching or demonstration.

---

regarding the protection of human rights does not imply that appropriate steps were not taken.

The Critiquing Criteria box provides guidelines for evaluating the legal-ethical aspects of a research report. Although research consumers reading a research report will not see all areas explicitly addressed in the research article, they should be aware of them and should determine that the researcher has addressed them before gaining IRB approval to conduct the study. A

CRITIQUING CRITERIA

1. Was the study approved by IRB or other agency committee members?
2. Is there evidence that informed consent was obtained from all subjects or their representatives? How was it obtained?
3. Were the subjects protected from physical or emotional harm?
4. Were the subjects or their representatives informed about the purpose and nature of the study?
5. Were the subjects or their representatives informed about any potential risks that might result from participation in the study?
6. Did the benefits of the study outweigh the risks?
7. Were subjects coerced or unduly influenced to participate in this study? Did they have the right to refuse to participate or withdraw without penalty? Were vulnerable subjects used?
8. Were appropriate steps taken to safeguard the privacy of subjects? How have data been kept anonymous and/or confidential?

nurse who is asked to serve as a member of an IRB will find the critiquing criteria useful in evaluating the legal-ethical aspects of the research proposal.

Information about the legal-ethical considerations of a study is usually presented in the *Methods* section of a research report. The subsection on the sample or data collection methods is the most likely place for this information. The author most often indicates in a few sentences that informed consent was obtained and that approval from an IRB or similar committee was granted. It is likely that a paper will not be accepted for publication without such a discussion. This also makes it almost impossible for unauthorized research to be published. Therefore when a research article provides evidence of having been approved by an external review committee, the reader can feel confident that the ethical issues raised by the study have been thoroughly reviewed and resolved.

To protect subject and institutional privacy, the locale of the study frequently is described in general terms in the sample subsection section of the report. For example, the article might state that data were collected at a 350-bed community hospital in the Northeast, without mentioning its name. Protection of subject privacy may be explicitly addressed by statements indicating that anonymity or confidentiality of data was maintained or that grouped data were used in the data analysis.

Determining whether participants were subjected to physical or emotional risk is often accomplished indirectly by evaluating the study's methods section. The reader evaluates the **risk-benefit ratio,** that is, the extent to which the benefits of the study are maximized and the risks are minimized such that subjects are protected from harm during the study.

For example, the study by Rudy et al (1995) compared the effect of a low-technology/case management special care unit with a traditional high-technology/primary nursing intensive care unit on long-term critically ill patient outcomes such as length of stay, mortality, readmission, complications, satisfaction, and cost. Results from this 4-year clinical trial demonstrate that nurse case managers in a special care unit setting can produce patient outcomes equal to or better than those in the traditional intensive care unit environment for long-term critically ill clients while showing significant cost savings, thereby demonstrating low or no risk and benefit to both patients and health care institution.

In another example, the study by Ward, Berry, and Misiewicz (1996), investigating concerns about analgesics among patients and family caregivers in a hospice setting, compared the concerns of subjects and their family caregivers associated with underutilization of analgesics. The benefits to the participants were increased knowledge about barriers (e.g., exaggerated fears of addiction) to effective palliative pain management that occur because of concerns that are unique to each member of the patient and caregiver dyad about reporting pain and hesitancy using analgesics. Risk is minimized because patient subjects were all taking palliative analgesics, their usual regimen was not being altered, and many were already not experiencing effective pain control from their current pain management protocol. The evaluator could infer from a description of the method that the benefits were greater than the risks and subjects were protected from harm. The findings of the study, which highlighted the need for individualized patient and family caregiver pain management education and accurate and systematic pain assessment, have the potential to benefit the effectiveness of pain management for other terminally ill people. The obligation to balance the risks and benefits of a study is the responsibility of the researcher. However, the research consumer reading a research report also should be confident that subjects have been protected from harm.

When considering the special needs of vulnerable subjects, research consumers should be sensitive to whether the special needs of groups, unable to act on their own behalf, have been addressed. For instance, has the right of self-determination been addressed by the informed consent protocol identified in the research report? For example, in a study by Armer (1996) exploring factors influencing adjustment among relocating rural elders, the study was approved by the institutional committee for review of research involving human subjects, as well as the management and owners of the elderly congregate residence. The purpose of the study was explained to the residents at a pot luck dinner at the residence. Residents were individually recruited, and 34 of 38 completed informed consent forms. When qualitative studies are reported, verbatim quotes from informants often are incorporated into the findings section of the article. In such cases the reader will evaluate how effectively the author protected the informant's identity, either by using a fictitious name or withholding information such as age, gender, occupation, or other potentially identifying data.

It should be apparent from the preceding sections that although the need for guidelines for the use of human and animal subjects in research is evident and the principles themselves are clear, there are many instances when the nurse must use best judgment both as a patient advocate and as a researcher when evaluating the ethical nature of a research project. In any research situation, the basic guiding principle of protecting the patient's human rights must always apply. When conflicts arise, the nurse must feel free to raise suitable questions with appropriate resources and personnel. In an institution these may include contacting the researcher first and then, if there is no resolution, the director of nursing research and the chairperson of the IRB. In cases where ethical considerations in a research article are in question, clarification from a colleague, agency, or IRB is indicated. The nurse should pursue his or her concerns until satisfied that the patient's rights and his or her rights as a professional nurse are protected.

KEY POINTS

- Ethical and legal considerations in research first received attention after World War II during the Nuremberg Trials, from which developed the Nuremberg Code. This became the standard for research guidelines protecting the human rights of research subjects.
- The National Research Act, passed in 1974, created the National Commission for the Protection of Human Subjects of Biomedical and Behavioral Research. The findings, contained in the *Belmont Report,* discuss three basic ethical principles (respect for persons, beneficence, and justice), which underlie the conduct of research involving human subjects. Federal regulations developed in response to the Commission's report provide guidelines for informed consent and IRB protocols.
- The American Nurses Association's Commission on Nursing Research published *Human Rights Guidelines for Nursing in Clinical and Other Research* in 1975, for protection of human rights of research subjects. It is relevant to nurses as researchers, as well as caregivers. The ANA *Code for Nurses* is integral with the Research Guidelines.
- Protection of human rights includes (1) right to self-determination, (2) right to privacy and dignity, (3) right to anonymity and confidentiality, (4) right to fair treatment, and (5) right to protection from discomfort and harm.
- Procedures for protecting basic human rights include gaining informed consent, which illustrates the ethical principle of respect, and obtaining IRB approval, which illustrates the ethical principles of respect, beneficence, and justice.
- Special consideration should be given to studies involving vulnerable populations, such as children, the elderly, prisoners, and those who are mentally or physically disabled.
- Scientific fraud or misconduct represents unethical conduct and must be monitored as part of professional responsibility. Informal, ad hoc, or unauthorized research may expose patients to unwarranted risk and may not protect subject rights adequately.
- Nurses who are asked to be involved in product testing should be aware of FDA guidelines and regulations for testing medical devices before becoming involved in product testing and, perhaps, violating guidelines for ethical research.
- Animal rights need to be protected, and regulations for animal research have evolved over time. Nurses who encounter the use of animals in research should be alert to their rights.
- Nurses as consumers of research must be knowledgeable about the legal-ethical components of a research study so they can evaluate whether appropriate protection of human or animal rights has been ensured by a researcher.

CRITICAL THINKING CHALLENGES
Barbara Krainovich-Miller

? Your state government is interested in determining the number of babies infected with the human immunodeficiency virus (HIV) as needs assessment for future health care delivery planning. A state-wide study is funded that will include the testing of all newborns for HIV, but the mothers will not be told that the test is being done, nor will they be told the results. Using the basic ethical principles found in Box 11-2, defend or refute this practice.

❧ The IRB of your health care agency does not include a nurse and you think it should. You discuss this with your supervisor and she states that it really isn't necessary because the IRB uses strict guidelines. What essential arguments and explanations should you include in your proposal for including a nurse on your institution's IRB?

❧ A qualitative researcher intends to conduct a phenomenological study on caring and use informants who are severely and persistently mentally ill who attend an outpatient clinic. The IRB denies the study indicating that informed consent cannot be obtained and that these patients will not be able to tolerate an interview. What assumptions have the members of this IRB made? If you were the researcher and you were given the opportunity to address their concerns, what would you say? Include information from Table 11-2.

❧ How do you see computer database searchers and the WWW assisting researchers in conducting ethical studies? Do you think IRBs can use this technology to assist them in their goals?

REFERENCES

Abdellah F: Scientific misconduct: myth or reality? *J Prof Nurs* 6(1):61-63, 1990.

Altman LK: A flaw in the research process: uncorrected errors in journals. Medical science, *The New York Times,* May 31, 1988.

Altman LK: Baboon cells might repair AIDS-ravaged immune systems, *The New York Times,* B6, July 19, 1994.

Alt-White AC: Obtaining informed consent from the elderly, *West J Nurs Res* 17(6):700-705, 1995.

American Nurses Association: *Guidelines for nurses in clinical and other research,* Kansas City, Mo, 1975, ANA.

American Nurses Association: *Code for nurses with interpretive statements,* Kansas City, Mo, 1985, ANA.

Andrews EL: U.S. resumes granting patents on genetically altered animals, *The New York Times,* C1, February 3, 1993.

Armer JM: An exploration of factors influencing adjustment among relocating rural elders, *Image* 28(1):35-39, 1996.

Brink PJ: Autonomy versus do no harm, *West J Nurs Res* 14(3):264-266, 1992.

Broome ME, Stieglitz KA: The consent process and children, *Res Nurs Health* 15:147-152, 1992.

Burd S: Scientists oppose diversity rule for clinical trials in NIH bill, *Chronicle of Higher Education,* A26, April 7, 1993.

Code of Federal Regulations: Protection of human subjects, 45 CFR 46, *OPRR Reports,* Revised March 8, 1983.

Commission on Research Integrity: *Integrity and misconduct in research,* Washington, DC, 1995, USDHHS.

Cook R: *Brain,* New York, 1981, Signet.

Creighton H: Legal concerns of nursing research, *Nurs Res* 26(4):337-340, 1977.

Davis A: Ethical issues in gerontological nursing research, *Geriatr Nurs* 2:267-272, 1981a.

Davis A: Ethical similarities internationally, *West J Nurs Res* 12(5):685-688, 1990.

Demi AS, Warren NA: Issues in conducting research with vulnerable families, *West J Nurs Res* 12(2):188-202, 1995.

Department of Health and Human Services: *Department of Health and Human Services rules and regulations*, 45CF46, Title 45, Pt 46, *Fed Regul* March 8, 1983.

Dubler NN: Legal judgments and informed consent in geriatric research, *J Am Geriatr Soc* 35:545-549, 1987.

Dubler NN: Personal communication, 1993.

Fowler MDM: Ethical issues in nursing research: a call for an international code of ethics for nursing research, *West J Nurs Res* 3(10):352-355, 1988.

Green E, Waterson R: The human genome project: prospects and implications for clinical medicine, *JAMA* 266:1966-1975, 1991.

Hanks GE: *Implementing human research regulations: second biennial report on the adequacy and uniformity of federal rules and policies and of their implementation, for the study of ethical problems in medicine and biomedical and behavioral research, March 1983*, 1984a.

Hanks GE: The dangers of ad hoc protocols, *J Clin Oncol* 2:1177-1178, 1984b.

Hawley DJ, Jeffers JM: Scientific misconduct as a dilemma for nursing, *Image* 24(1):51-55, 1992.

Hershey N, Miller RD: *Human experimentation and the law,* Germantown, Md, 1976, Aspen.

Hilts PJ: Agency faults a UCLA study for suffering of mental patients, *The New York Times,* A1, 11, March 9, 1995.

Katz J: *Experimentation with human beings,* New York, 1972, Russell Sage Foundation.

Kevles DJ: An injustice to a scientist is reversed, and we learn some lessons, *Chronicle of Higher Education,* B1-2, July 5, 1996.

Larson E: Exclusion of certain groups from clinical research, *Image* 26(3):185-190, 1994.

Levine RJ: Clarifying the concepts of research ethics, *Hastings Cent Rep* 93(3):21-26, 1979.

Levine RJ: *Ethics and regulation of clinical research,* ed 2, Baltimore-Munich, 1986, Urban and Schwartzenberg.

Levine FJ: Consent for research on children, *Chronicle of Higher Education,* B1-2, November 10, 1995.

Mitchell K: Protecting children's rights during research, *Pediatr Nurs* 10:9-10, 1984.

Moore L: Conducting clinical trials, *J Enterostom Ther* 11:229-232, 1984.

National Center for Human Genome Research: *National Center for Human Genome Research: Annual Report I-FY 1990,* Bethesda, Md, 1990, Department of Health and Human Services, Public Health Service, National Institutes of Health.

National Commission for the Protection of Human Subjects of Biomedical and Behavioral Research: *Belmont report: ethical principles and guidelines for research involving human subjects,* DHEW Pub No 05, Washington, DC, 1978, US Government Printing Office, 78-0012.

Pranulis MF: Protecting rights of human subjects, *West J Nurs Res* 18(4):474-478, 1996.

Public Health Service Policy on Humane Care in Use of Lab Animals by Awardee Institution: *NIH guidelines for grants and contracts,* 14(8), June 25, 1985.

Rempusheski VF: Elements, perceptions, and issues of informed consent, *Appl Nurs Res* 4(4):201-204, 1991.

Robb IH: *Nursing ethics: for hospital and private use,* Milwaukee, Wi, 1900, GN Gaspar.

Rothman DJ: Were Tuskegee and Willowbrook studies in nature? *Hastings Cent Rep* 12(2):5-7, 1982.

Rudy EB et al: Patient outcomes for the chronically critically ill: special care unit versus intensive care unit, *Nurs Res* 44(6):324-331, 1995.

Ryan K: Scientific misconduct in perspective: the need to improve accountability, *Chronicle of Higher Education,* B1-2, July 19, 1996.

Silva MC: *Ethical guidelines in the conduct, dissemination, and implementation of nursing research,* Washington, DC, 1995, American Nurses Publishing.

Snowden J: Breast cancer study monitored patients against their wishes, *Houston Chronicle,* A22, December 17, 1994.

Walker PV: Government may ease limits on research on pregnant women, *Chron Higher Educ* June 21, 1996.

Ward SE, Berry PE, Misiewicz H: Concerns about analgesics among patients and family caregivers in a hospice setting, *Res Nurs Health* 19:205-211, 1996.

ADDITIONAL READINGS

Beecher HK: Ethics and clinical research, *N Engl J Med* 274:1354-1360, 1966a.

Beecher HK: Consent in clinical experimentation: myth and reality, *J Am Med Assoc* 195:34-35, 1966b.

Blancett SS, Flanagan A, Young RK: Duplicate publication in the nursing literature, *Image* 27(1):51-56, 1995.

Cooper C: Principle-oriented ethics and the ethic of care: a creative tension, *Adv Nurs Sci* 14(2):22-31, 1991.

Davis AJ: The clinical nurses' role in informed consent, *J Prof Nurs* 4:88-91, 1988.

Davis AJ: Clinical nurses' ethical decision making in situations of informed consent, *Adv Nurs Sci* 11:63-69, 1989.

Department of Health and Human Services: *Policy on informing those tested about HIV sero status,* May, 1988.

Levine RJ: Research involving children: an interpretation of the new regulations, *IRB Rev Human Subj Res* 5:1-5, 1983.

Melnick VL et al: Clinical research in senile dementia of the Alzheimer type: suggested guidelines addressing the ethical and legal issues, *J Am Geriatr Soc* 32:531-536, 1984.

Orlans FB, Simmonds RC, Dodds WJ: Effective animal care use committees, *Lab Animal Sci* 1987 (special issue).

Rothman D: Ethics and human experimentation: Henry Beecher revisited, *N Engl J Med* 317:1195-1199, 1987.

Rothman D: *Strangers at the bedside,* New York, 1991, Basic Books.

Rowen AH: *Of mice, models and men: a critical evaluation of animal research,* Albany, NY, 1984, State University of New York Press.

Twomey JG: Investigating pediatric HIV research ethics in the field, *West J Nurs Res* 16(4):404-413, 1994.

Wheeler DL: Making amends to radiation victims, *Chronicle of Higher Education,* A10-11, October 13, 1995.

Data Collection Methods

Margaret Grey

Key Terms

close-ended items
concealment
consistency
content analysis
external criticism
internal criticism
interrater reliability
intervention

interviews
Likert scales
objective
open-ended item
operational
   definition
operationalization
physiological
   measurement

questionnaires
reactivity
records or available
   data
scale
scientific
   observation
social desirability
systematic

Learning Outcomes

After reading this chapter the student should be able to do the following:

- Define the types of data collection methods used in nursing research.
- List the advantages and disadvantages of each of these methods.
- Critically evaluate the data collection methods used in published nursing research studies.

Nurses use all of their senses when collecting data from the patients for whom they provide care. Nurse researchers also have available many ways to collect information about their research subjects. The major difference between the data collected when performing patient care and the data collected for the purpose of research is that the data collection methods employed by researchers need to be **objective** and **systematic.** By *objective,* we mean that the data must not be influenced by another who collects the information; by *systematic,* we mean that the data must be collected in the same way by everyone who is involved in the collection procedure.

The methods that researchers use to collect information about subjects are the identifiable and repeatable operations that define the major variables being studied. **Operationalization** is the process of translating the concepts that are of interest to a researcher into observable and measurable phenomena. There may be a number of ways to collect the same information. For example, a researcher interested in measuring anxiety physiologically could do so by measuring sweat gland activity or by administering an anxiety scale, such as the State-Trait Anxiety Scale for Children (Speilberger, 1973). The researcher could also observe children to see whether they displayed anxious behavior. The method chosen by the researcher would depend on a number of decisions regarding the problem being studied, the nature of the subjects, and the relative costs and benefits of each method.

This chapter's purpose is to familiarize the student with the various ways the researchers collect information from and about subjects. The chapter provides nursing research consumers with the tools for evaluating the selection, utilization, and practicality of the various ways of collecting data.

MEASURING VARIABLES OF INTEREST

To a large extent the success of a study depends on the quality of the data collection methods chosen and employed. Researchers have many types of methods available for collecting information from subjects in research studies. Determining what measurement to use in a particular investigation may be the most difficult and time-consuming period in study design. In addition, because nursing research is still developing, researchers are beginning to have an array of quality instruments with adequate reliability and validity (see Chapter 13) from which to choose. This aspect of the research process demands painstaking efforts of the researcher. Thus the process of evaluating and selecting the available tools to measure variables of interest is of critical importance to the potential success of the study. In this section the selection of measures and the implementation of the data collection process are discussed. An algorithm that influences a researcher's choice of data collection methods is diagrammed in the Critical Thinking Decision Path.

You will find that researchers can use many different ways to collect information about phenomena of interest to nurses. We are interested in biological and physical indicators of health, such as blood pressure and heart rates, but nurses are also interested in complex psychosocial questions presented by patients. Psychosocial variables, such as anxiety, hope, social support, and self-concept, may be measured by several different techniques, such as observation of behavior or self-reports of feelings or attitudes by means of interviews or questionnaires. Researchers may also use data that have already been collected for another purpose, such as records, diaries, or other media, to study phenomena of interest.

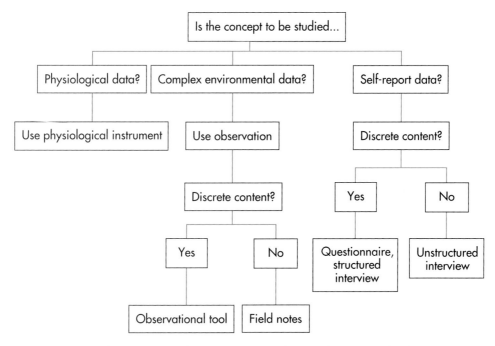

Critical Thinking Decision Path   Data collection methods.

As you can surmise, choosing the most appropriate method and instrument is difficult. The method must be appropriate to the problem, the hypothesis, the setting, and the population. For example, if a researcher is interested in studying the behavior of 3-year-old children in day care, it probably would not be sensible to provide the children with some kind of paper-and-pencil test. Although the children might be able to draw on the paper, they would not be likely to answer written questions appropriately.

Selection of the data collection method begins during the literature review. In Chapter 4 one purpose of the review noted is to provide clues to instrumentation. As the literature review is conducted, the researcher begins to explore how previous investigators defined and operationalized variables similar to those of interest in the current study. The researcher uses this information to define conceptually the variables to be studied. Once a variable has been defined conceptually, the researcher returns to the literature to define the variable operationally. This **operational definition** translates the conceptual definition into behaviors or verbalizations that can be measured for the study. In this second literature review the researcher searches for measuring instruments that might be used as is or adapted for use in the study. If instruments are available, the researcher needs to obtain permission for their use from the author.

An example may illustrate the relationship of the conceptual and operational definitions. Stress research is popular with researchers from many disciplines, including nursing. Definitions of stressors may be psychological, social, or physiological. If a researcher is interested in studying stressors, the researcher needs first to define what he or she means by the concept of stressor. For example, Holmes and Rahe (1967) defined the stressful life event as any occurrence that required change or adaptation. This definition implies that it is the event that is stressful, not how the individual appraises the event. According to this conceptual definition, the researcher could use a life-event checklist (operational definition) to determine the degree of stress encountered by subjects in the study. If the researcher disagreed with this definition and supported the definition that events are stressful only when individuals appraise them as such (Lazarus and Folkman, 1984), another approach to measurement would be consistent with that view. McCain et al (1996) used a cognitive appraisal framework in developing their stress management program for men with the human immunodeficiency virus (HIV), so they measured stress levels and coping in a method consistent with that view.

It is sometimes the case that no suitable measuring device exists, so the researcher needs to decide whether the variable is important to the study and whether a new device should be constructed. This is often a problem in nursing research, because many variables of interest have not been studied. The construction of new instruments for data collection that have reasonable reliability and validity (see Chapter 13) is a most difficult task. Sometimes researchers decide not to study a variable if no suitable measuring device exists; at other times the researcher may decide to invest time and energy in tool development. Either decision is acceptable depending on the goals of the study and the goals of the researcher.

Whether the researcher uses available methods or creates new ones, once the variables have been operationally defined in a manner consistent with the aims of the study, the population to be studied, and the setting, the researcher will determine how the data collection phase of the study will be implemented. This decision deals with how the instruments for data collection will be given to the subjects. Consistency is the most important issue in this phase.

Consistency means that the data are collected from each subject in the study in exactly the same way or as close to the same way as possible. Consistency can minimize the bias introduced when more than one person collects the data. Thus the researcher must consider ways to minimize subjects' anxiety and to maintain their motivation to complete the data collection process (Weinert and Burman, 1996), and data collectors must be carefully trained and supervised (Collins et al, 1988). To ensure consistency in data collection, researchers must rehearse data collectors in the methods to be used in the study so that each person collects the information in the same way. Information about how to observe and collect data often is included in a kind of "cookbook" protocol for the research project. A researcher may spend several months developing the protocol and training research assistants to collect data systematically and reliably. If data collectors are used, the reader should expect to see some comment about their training and the consistency with which they collected the data for the study. For example, in the study by Rudy et al (1995; see Appendix C), the procedure by which the consistency of measurement was ensured is clearly presented. Nurses were trained in the scoring of some instruments, such as the Acute Physiological and Chronic Health Evaluation II instrument so that they could accurately extract data from patients' charts. Another example of the importance of training data collectors is provided by Wikblad and Anderson (1995) in their study comparing three wound dressings in patients undergoing heart surgery. These researchers needed to be accurate in their assessment of surgical wound healing and used a photograph of the wound as the data. Wounds were rated by observers in several categories, such as redness, healing, and blisters. Agreement between raters was calculated using the kappa statistic. The index of agreement in this study was 0.81, and the percent agreement between rates was 91%. These demonstrate a high level of agreement between the two observers. **Interrater**

reliability (see Chapter 13) is the consistency of observations between two or more observers; it often is expressed as a percentage of agreement among raters or observers or a coefficient of agreement that considers the element of chance (coefficient kappa).

HELPFUL HINT

Remember that the researcher may not always present complete information about the way the data were collected, especially when established tools were used. To learn about the tool that was used, the reader may need to consult the original article describing the tool.

DATA COLLECTION METHODS

In general, data collection methods can be divided into the following five types: physiological, observational, interviews, questionnaires, and records or available data. Each of these methods has a specific purpose, as well as certain pros and cons inherent in its use. Each type of data collection method is discussed, and then its respective uses and problems are discussed.

Physiological or Biological Measurements

In everyday practice, nurses collect physiological data about patients, such as their temperature, pulse rate, and blood pressure. Such data frequently are useful to nurse researchers as well, as in the study by Caudell and Gallucci (1995). The purpose of the study was to measure neuroendocrine, immunological, and psychosocial variables before and after the application of a particular stressor. To study this problem, it was important for the researchers to provide the stressful stimulus in the same manner to all subjects, and then measure the physiological and psychosocial variables at similar intervals for all subjects. The study used both psychosocial instruments (mood, stress appraisal, stress symptoms) and physiological measurements (urine catecholamines, plasma catecholamines, cortisol, autonomic nervous system activity, natural killer cell activity).

The study by Caudell and Gallucci (1995) is an excellent example of the use of a particular type of data collection method—physiological. **Physiological measurement** and biological measurement involve the use of specialized equipment to determine physical and biological status of subjects. Frequently such measures also require specialized training. Such measures can be physical, such as weight or temperature; chemical, such as blood glucose level; microbiological, as with cultures; or anatomical, as in radiological examinations. What separates these measurements from others used in research is that they require the use of special equipment to make the observation. We can say, "This subject feels warm," but to determine how warm the subject is requires the use of a sensitive instrument, a thermometer.

Erickson, Meyer, and Woo (1996) did a study to determine the clinical accuracy of clinical dot thermometers. They compared temperature measurements with chemical dot thermometers and electronic thermometers at the oral site in 27 adults and the axillary site in 44 adults and 34 young children in critical care units. They found that the chemical dot thermometers provided good temperature estimates, although there were variations by site and by age of the subjects. The study required careful standardization of the procedures so that the instruments were all used in the same way, which are reported in the article.

Physiological or biological measurement is particularly suited to the study of several types of nursing problems. The aforementioned example is typical of studies dealing with ways to improve the performance of certain nursing actions, such as measuring and recording of patients' physiological data. Physiological measures may be important criteria for determining the effectiveness of certain nursing actions. An experimental study by Gift, Moore, and Soeken (1992) tested the effectiveness of a taped relaxation message in reducing dyspnea and anxiety in patients with chronic obstructive pulmonary disease. The authors used a combination of measures, including a portable skin temperature monitor and a peak flow meter to determine airway obstruction. They found that the taped relaxation message was effective in reducing airway obstruction, as well as feelings of anxiety and dyspnea. This study (Gift, Moore and Soeken, 1992) illustrates a type of research that is a priority for the National Institute for Nursing Research: studies of the interface between biology and behavior (termed *biobehavioral interface*). The study of neuroendocrine response to stress would also be a study of this type (Caudell and Gallucci, 1995).

The advantages of using physiological data collection methods include their objectivity, precision, and sensitivity. Such methods are generally quite objective because unless there is a technical malfunction, two readings of the same instrument taken at the same time by two different nurses are likely to yield the same result. Because such instruments are intended to measure the variable being studied, they offer the advantage of being precise and sensitive enough to pick up subtle variations in the phenomenon of interest. It is also unlikely that a subject in a study can deliberately distort physiological information.

Physiological measurements are not without inherent disadvantages, however. Some instruments, if they are not available through a hospital, may be quite expensive to obtain. In addition, such instruments often require specialized knowledge and training to be used accurately. Another problem with such measurements is that just by using them, the variable of interest may be changed. Although some researchers think of these instruments as being nonintrusive, the presence of some types of devices might change the measurement. For example, the presence of a heart rate monitoring device might make some patients anxious and increase their heart rate. In addition, nearly all types of measuring devices are affected in some way by the environment. Even a simple thermometer can be affected by the subject drinking something hot immediately before the temperature is taken. Thus it is important to consider whether the researcher controlled such environmental variables in the study. Finally, there may not be a physiological way to measure the variable of interest. Occasionally researchers try to force a physiological parameter into a study in an effort to increase the precision of measurement. However, if the device does not really measure the phenomenon of interest, the validity of its use is suspect.

Observational Methods

Sometimes nurse researchers are interested in determining how subjects behave under certain conditions. For example, the researcher might be interested in how children respond to painful situations. We might ask children how painful an experience was, but they may not be able to answer the question, may not be able to quantify the amount of pain, or may distort their responses to please the researcher. Therefore sometimes observing the subject may give a more accurate picture of the behavior in question than asking the patient.

Although observing the environment is a normal part of living, **scientific observation** places a great deal of emphasis on the objective and systematic nature of the operation. The researcher is not merely looking at what is happening but rather is watching with a trained eye for certain specific events. To be scientific, observations must fulfill the following four conditions:

1. The observations undertaken are consistent with the study's specific objectives.
2. There is a standardized and systematic plan for the observation and the recording of data.
3. All of the observations are checked and controlled.
4. The observations are related to scientific concepts and theories.

Observation is particularly suitable as a data collection method in complex research situations that are best viewed as total entities and that are difficult to measure in parts, such as studies dealing with the nursing process, parent-child interactions, or group processes. In addition, observational methods can be the best way to operationalize some variables of interest in nursing research studies, particularly individual characteristics and conditions, such as traits and symptoms, verbal and nonverbal communication behaviors, activities and skill attainment, and environmental characteristics.

A study of health beliefs and social influences on the home safety practices of mothers of preschool children was conducted by Russell and Champion (1996). Because asking mothers to describe the safety precautions they had taken at home would likely miss some important information and thus that data would not be reliable or valid, the researchers used two observational tools to measure the presence of home-safety hazards. The observational tools were adapted from an observation instrument and measured the presence or absence of several observable categories of potential injurious situations. The researchers note that there was consistency of recording of these observations between observers, because the interrater reliability ranged from 90% to 96.7% In the study the researchers demonstrated that health beliefs, social influence, and demographic and experiential variables accounted for 51% of the variance in observed hazard accessibility.

Observational methods can be distinguished also by the role of the observer. This role is determined by the amount of interaction between the observer and those being observed. Each of the following four basic types of observational roles is distinguishable by the amount of concealment or intervention implemented by the observer:

1. Concealment without intervention
2. Concealment with intervention
3. No concealment without intervention
4. No concealment with intervention

These methods are illustrated in Figure 12-1, and examples are given later. **Concealment** refers to whether the subjects know that they are being observed, and **intervention** deals with whether the observer provokes actions from those who are being observed. The study of the effect of a strategy to promote night sleep in hospitalized 3- to 8-year-old children, conducted by White et al (1990), is an excellent example of no concealment with intervention. The researchers were not concealed in their observations of sleep behavior, but they did intervene with the children by varying the bedtime ritual. Suppose the researcher believed that by being open to the subjects, the subjects' behavior would change. For example, if these researchers wanted to replicate their studies with older children who might be more suggestive in response to the presence of a known investigator, the researchers might employ concealment with intervention. When a researcher is concerned that the subjects' behavior will change as a result of being observed, the

Concealment

	Yes	No
Yes	Researcher hidden Some intervention	Researcher open Some intervention
No	Researcher hidden No intervention	Researcher open No intervention

Intervention

Figure 12-1   Types of observational roles in research.

type of observation most commonly employed is that of concealment without intervention. In this case the researcher watches the subjects without their knowledge of the observation, but he or she does not provoke them into action. Often such concealed observations use hidden television cameras, audiotapes, or one-way mirrors. Concealment without intervention often is used in observational studies of children. You may be familiar with rooms with one-way mirrors, where a researcher can observe the behavior of the occupants of the room without being observed by them. Such studies allow for the observation of children's natural behavior and often are used in developmental research. No concealment without intervention also is commonly used for observational studies. In this case the researcher obtains informed consent from the subject to be observed and then simply observes his or her behavior. This is the type of observation done in the Russell and Champion (1996) study.

Observing subjects without their knowledge may violate assumptions of informed consent, and therefore researchers face ethical problems with this type of approach. However, sometimes there is no other way to collect such data and the data collected are unlikely to have negative consequences for the subject; therefore the disadvantages of the study are outweighed by the advantages. Further, the problem often is handled by informing subjects after the observation and allowing them the opportunity to refuse to have their data included in the study and to discuss any question they might have. This process is called *debriefing*.

When the observer is neither concealed nor intervening, the ethical question is not a problem. Here the observer makes no attempt to change the subjects' behavior and informs them that they are to be observed. Because the observer is present, this type of observation allows a greater depth of material to be studied than if the observer is separated from the subjects by an artificial barrier, such as a one-way mirror. Participant observation is a commonly used observational technique where the researcher functions as a part of a social group to study the group in question. The problem with this type of observation is **reactivity**, the Hawthorne effect, or the distortion created when the subjects change behavior because they are being observed.

In the study by White et al (1990), the researchers used unconcealed observation, because the children and parents had given full consent for participation in the study. They also performed an intervention—the use of recorded stories by parents or a stranger or the presence of a parent—so the method was no concealment with intervention. No concealment with intervention is employed when the researcher is observing the effects of some intervention introduced for scientific purposes. Because the subjects know that they are participating in a research study, there are few problems with ethical concerns, but reactivity is a problem with this type of study.

Concealed observation with intervention involves staging a situation and observing the behaviors that are evoked in the subjects as a result of the intervention. Because the subjects are unaware of their participation in a research study, this type of observation has fallen into disfavor and rarely is used in nursing research.

Observations may be structured or unstructured. Unstructured observational methods, such as those suggested by West, Bondy, and Hutchinson (1991) for working with the elderly, are not characterized by a total absence of structure but usually involve collecting descriptive information about the topic of interest. In participant observation the observer keeps field notes that record the activities, as well as the observer's interpretations of these activities. Field notes usually are not restricted to any particular type of action or behavior; rather, they intend to paint a picture of a social situation in a more general sense. Another type of unstructured observation is the use of anecdotes. Anecdotes are not necessarily funny but usually focus on the behaviors of interest and frequently add to the richness of research reports by illustrating a particular point. On the other hand, structured observations, such as the tools used to observe home hazards in the Russell and Champion (1996) study, involve specifying in advance what behaviors or events are to be observed and preparing forms for record keeping, such as categorization systems, checklists, and rating scales. Whichever system is employed, the observer watches the subject and then marks on the recording form what was seen. In any case, the observations must be similar among the observers (see earlier discussion and Chapter 13 for an explanation of interrater reliability). Thus it is important that observers be trained to be consistent in their observations and ratings of behavior.

Scientific observation has several advantages as a data collection method, the main one being that observation may be the only way for the researcher to study the variable of interest. For example, what people say they do often is not what they really do. Therefore if the study is designed to obtain substantive findings about human behavior, observation may be the only way to ensure the validity of the findings. In addition, no other data collection method can match the depth and variety of information that can be collected when using these techniques. Such techniques also are quite flexible in that they may be used in both experimental and nonexperimental designs and in laboratory and field studies.

HELPFUL HINT

Sometimes a researcher may carefully train observers or data collectors, but the research report does not address this. Often the length of research reports dictates that certain information cannot be included. Readers can often assume that if reliability data are provided, then appropriate training occurred.

As with all data collection methods, observation also has its disadvantages. We mentioned the problems of reactivity and ethical concerns when we discuss the concealment and intervention dimensions. In addition, data obtained by observational techniques are vulnerable to the bias of the observer. Emotions, prejudices, and values all can influence the way that behaviors and events are observed. In general, the more the observer needs to make inferences and judgments about what is being observed, the more likely it is that distortions will occur. Thus in judging the adequacy of observational methods, it is important to consider how observational tools were constructed and how observers were trained and evaluated.

Interviews and Questionnaires

Subjects in a research study often have information that is important to the study and that can be obtained only by asking the subject. Such questions may be asked orally by a researcher in person or over the telephone in an interview, or they may be asked in the form of a paper-and-pencil test. Both interviews and questionnaires have the purpose of asking subjects to report data for themselves, but each has unique advantages and disadvantages as well. **Interviews** are a method of data collection where a data collector questions a subject verbally. Interviews may be face-to-face or performed over the telephone, and they may consist of open-ended or close-ended questions. On the other hand, **questionnaires** are paper-and-pencil instruments designed to gather data from individuals about knowledge, attitudes, beliefs, and feelings. Survey research relies almost entirely on questioning subjects with either interviews or questionnaires, but these methods of data collection also can be used in other types of research. No matter what type of study is conducted, the purpose of questioning subjects is to seek information. This information may be of either direct interest, such as the subject's age, or indirect interest, such as when the researcher uses a combination of items to estimate to what degree the respondent has some trait or characteristic. An intelligence test is an example of how an individual item is combined with several others to develop an overall scale intelligence. When items of indirect interest are combined to obtain an overall score, the measurement tool is called a *scale*. The investigator determines the content of an interview or questionnaire from the literature review (see Chapter 4). When evaluating these methods, the reader should consider the content of the schedule, the individual items, and the order of the items. The basic standard for evaluating the individual items in an interview or questionnaire is that the item must be clearly written so that the intent of the question and the nature of the information sought are clear to the respondent. The only way to know whether the questions are understandable to the target respondents is to pilot test them in a similar population. Items also must ask only one question, be free of suggestions, and use correct grammar. Items also may be open-ended items or close-ended items. **Open-ended items** are used when the researcher wants the subjects to respond in their own words or when the researcher does not know all of the possible alternative responses. **Close-ended items** are used when there is a fixed number of alternative responses. Many scales use a fixed response format called a *Likert scale.*

Likert scales are lists of statements on which respondents indicate, for example, whether they "strongly agree," "agree," "disagree," or "strongly disagree." Sometimes more fine distinctions are given or there may be a neutral category. The use of the neutral category, however, sometimes creates problems because it often is the most frequent response and this response is difficult to interpret. Fixed-response items also can be used for questions requiring a "yes" or "no" response or when there are categories, such as with income. Structured, fixed-response items are best used when the question has a fixed number of responses and the respondent is to choose the one closest to the right one. Fixed-response items have the advantage of simplifying the respondent's task and the researcher's analysis, but they may miss some important information about the subject. Unstructured response formats allow such information to be included but require a special technique to analyze the responses. This technique is called **content analysis** and is a method for the objective, systematic, and quantitative description of communications and documentary evidence.

Box 12-1 shows a few items from a survey of pediatric nurse practitioners (Grey and Flint, 1989). The first items are taken from a list of similar items, and they are both closed and of a Likert-type format. Note that respondents are asked to choose how strongly they agree with

Box 12-1	Examples of Close-Ended and Open-Ended Questions

Close-Ended (Likert-Type Scale)

A. How satisfied are you with your current position?
    1. Very satisfied
    2. Moderately satisfied
    3. Undecided
    4. Moderately dissatisfied
    5. Very dissatisfied

B. To what extent do the following factors contribute to your current level of positive satisfaction?

	Not at all	Very little	Somewhat	Moderate amount	A great deal
1. % of time in patient care	1	2	3	4	5
2. Types of patients	1	2	3	4	5
3. % of time in educational activity	1	2	3	4	5
4. % of time in administration	1	2	3	4	5

Close-Ended

A. On an average, how many clients do you see in one day?
    1. 1 to 3
    2. 4 to 6
    3. 7 to 9
    4. 10 to 12
    5. 13 to 15
    6. 16 to 18
    7. 19 to 20
    8. More than 20

B. How would you characterize your practice?
    1. Too slow
    2. Slow
    3. About right
    4. Busy
    5. Too busy

Open-Ended

A. Are there incentives that the National Association of Pediatric Nurse Associates and Practitioners ought to provide for members that are currently not being done?

_____

_____

_____

_____

each item. In using these questions in the survey, we are forcing the respondent to choose from only these answers because we think that these will be the only responses. The only possible alternative response is to skip the item and leave it blank. On the other hand, sometimes we have no idea or we have only a limited idea of what the respondent will say, or we want the answer in the respondent's own words, as with the second set of items. Here, the respondent may also leave the item blank but we are not forcing the subject to make a particular response.

Interviews and questionnaires commonly are used in nursing research. Both are strong approaches to gathering information for research, because they approach the task directly. In addition, both have the ability to obtain certain kinds of information, such as the subjects' attitudes and beliefs, that would be difficult to obtain without asking the subject directly. All methods that involve verbal reports, however, share a problem with accuracy. There is often no way to know whether what we are told is indeed true. For example, people are known to respond to questions in a way that makes a favorable impression. This response style is known as **social desirability.** Because there is no way to tell whether the respondent is telling the truth or responding in a socially desirable way, the researcher usually is forced to assume that the respondent is telling the truth.

Questionnaires and interviews also have some specific purposes, advantages, and disadvantages. Questionnaires and paper-and-pencil tests are most useful when there is a finite set of questions to be asked and the researcher can be assured of the clarity and specificity of the items. Questionnaires are desirable tools when the purpose is to collect information. If questionnaires are too long, they are not likely to be completed. Face-to-face techniques or interviews are best used when the researcher may need to clarify the task for the respondent or is interested in obtaining more personal information from the respondent. Telephone interviews allow the researcher to reach more respondents than face-to-face interviews, and they allow for more clarity than questionnaires.

HELPFUL HINT

Remember, sometimes researchers make trade-offs when determining the measures to be used. For example, a researcher may want to learn about an individual's attitudes regarding practice; practicalities may preclude using an interview, so a questionnaire may be used instead.

Grey et al (1995) used a combination of interview and questionnaires to study the psychological, social, and physiological adaptation in children and adolescents with diabetes over the first 2 years after diagnosis. One of the measures of social adaptation is the Child and Adolescent Adjustment Profile, which is a parent interview measuring the social role performance of children and adolescents in the areas of productivity, peer relations, dependency, hostility, and withdrawal. Obtaining a more complete evaluation of the adaptation of the children, however, required that the children also report on their own feelings. This was accomplished by using the Self-Perception Profile for Children, which is a questionnaire dealing with children's feelings of competence in several areas. Thus the researchers were able to report both the children's and their parents' accounts of the child's overall adaptation. This use of multiple measures gives a more complete picture than the use of just one measure.

Researchers face difficult choices when determining whether to use interviews or questionnaires. The final decision is often based on what instruments are available and their relative costs and benefits.

Both face-to-face and telephone interviews offer some advantages over questionnaires. All things being equal, interviews are better than questionnaires because the response rate is almost always higher and this helps to eliminate bias in the sample (see Chapter 10). Respondents seem to be less likely to hang up the telephone or to close the door in an interviewer's face than to throw away a questionnaire. Another advantage of the interview is that some people, such as children, the blind, and the illiterate, could not fill out a questionnaire but they could participate in an interview. With an interview, the data collector knows who is giving the answers. When questionnaires are mailed, for example, anyone in the household could be the person who supplies the answers.

Interviews also allow for some safeguards to be built into the interview situation. Interviewers can clarify misunderstood questions and observe the level of the respondent's understanding and cooperativeness. In addition, the researcher has strict control over the order of the questions. With questionnaires, the respondent can answer questions in any order. Sometimes changing the order of the questions can change the response.

Finally, interviews allow for richer and more complex data to be collected. This is particularly so when open-ended responses are sought. Even when close-ended response items are used, interviews can probe to understand why a respondent answered in a particular way. Questionnaires also have certain advantages. They are much less expensive to administer than interviews, because interviews may require the hiring and training of interviewers. Thus if a researcher has a fixed amount of time and money, a larger and more diverse sample can be obtained with questionnaires. Questionnaires also allow for complete anonymity, which may be important if the study deals with sensitive issues. Finally, the fact that no interviewer is present assures the researcher and the reader that there will be no interviewer bias. Interviewer bias occurs when the interviewer unwittingly leads the respondent to answer in a certain way. This problem is especially pronounced in studies that use unstructured interview formats. A subtle nod of the head, for example, could lead a respondent to change an answer to correspond with what the researcher wants to hear.

Badger (1996) used relatively unstructured interview methods to study family members' experiences in living with a member with depression. These unstructured interviews allowed the researchers to obtain a more complete picture of the experiences of the subjects than would be provided by either a more structured interview or a questionnaire.

Records or Available Data

All of the data collection methods discussed thus far concern the ways that nurse researchers gather new data to study phenomena of interest. Not all studies, though, require a researcher to acquire new information. Sometimes existing information can be examined in a new way to study a problem. The use of records and available data sometimes is considered to be primarily the province of historical research, but hospital records, care plans, and existing data sources, such as the census, are frequently used for collecting information. What sets these studies apart from a literature review is that these available data are examined in a new way, are not merely summarized, and answer specific research questions. **Records or available data,** then, are forms of information that are collected from existing materials, such as hospital records, historical documents, or videotapes, and are used to answer research questions in a new manner. Much of the data analyzed in the Rudy et al study (1995; see Appendix C) consisted of available data, such as mortality and length of stay statistics and hospital charges and costs.

The use of available data has certain advantages. Because the data collection step of the research process often is the most difficult and time consuming, the use of available records often allows for a significant savings of time. If the records have been kept in a similar manner over time, as with the National Health and Examination Surveys, analysis of these records allows for the examination of trends over time. In addition, the use of available data decreases problems of reactivity and response set bias. The researcher also does not have to ask individuals to participate in the study.

On the other hand, institutions are sometimes reluctant to allow researchers to have access to their records. If the records are kept so that an individual cannot be identified, this is usually not a problem. However, the Privacy Act, a federal law, protects the rights of individuals who may be identified in records. Another problem that affects the quality of available data is that the researcher has access only to those records that have survived. If the records available are not representative of all of the possible records, the researcher may have a problem with bias. Often there is no way to tell whether the records have been saved in a biased manner, and the researcher has to make an intelligent guess as to their accuracy. For example, a researcher might be interested in studying socioeconomic factors associated with the suicide rate. These data are frequently underreported because of the stigma attached to suicide, and so the records would be biased.

Another problem is related to the authenticity of the records. The distinction of primary and secondary sources is as relevant here as it was in discussing the literature review (see Chapter 4). A book, for example, may have been ghostwritten but credit accorded to the known author. It may be difficult for the researcher to ferret out these types of subtle biases.

Nonetheless, records and available data constitute a rich source of data for study. Aber and Hawkins (1992) provide an interesting example of the use of available data in studying the image of nurses in advertisements. In this study the researchers were interested in determining whether nurses were portrayed in advertising as professionals or as physician helpers. They examined 313 different advertisements in medical and nursing journals by using a standardized content analysis. They found that nurses were portrayed as sex objects, ornaments, and physicians' handmaidens.

CONSTRUCTION OF NEW INSTRUMENTS

As already mentioned in this chapter, researchers sometimes cannot locate an instrument or method with acceptable reliability and validity to measure the variable of interest. This often is the case when testing a part of a nursing theory or when evaluating the effect of a clinical intervention. A recent example is provided by the work of Gilmer et al (1993), who were interested in assessing functional status of the elderly for a series of studies of nursing interventions. They developed and tested the Iowa Self-Assessment Inventory to measure seven functional characteristics of the elderly: economic resources, cognitive status, mobility, physical health, emotional balance, social support, and trusting others. Then the items were tested for readability and the items were combined into a test that could be tested and piloted.

Tool development is complex and time consuming. It consists of the following steps:

- Define the construct to be measured
- Formulate the items
- Assess the items for content validity

- Develop instructions for respondents and users
- Pretest and pilot test the items
- Estimate reliability and validity

To define the construct to be measured requires that the researcher develop an expertise in the construct. This requires an extensive review of the literature and of all tests and measurements that deal with related constructs. The researcher will use all of this information to synthesize the available knowledge so that the construct can be defined.

Once defined, the individual items measuring the construct can be developed. The researcher will develop many more items than are needed to address each aspect of the construct or subconstruct. The items are evaluated by a panel of experts in the field so that the researcher is assured that the items measure what they are intended to measure (content validity; see Chapter 13). Eventually the number of items will be decreased, because some items will not work as they were intended and they will be dropped. In this phase the researcher needs to ensure consistency among the items, as well as consistency in testing and scoring procedures.

Finally, the researcher administers or pilot tests the new instrument by giving it to a group of people who are similar to those who will be studied in the larger investigation. The purpose of this analysis to determine the quality of the instrument as a whole (reliability and validity), as well as the ability of each item to discriminate individual respondents (variance in item response). The researcher also may administer a related instrument to see if the new instrument is sufficiently different from the older one.

It is important that researchers who invest significant amounts of time in tool development publish those results. This type of research serves not only to introduce other researchers to the tool but also to ultimately enhance the field, because our ability to conduct meaningful research is limited only by our ability to measure important phenomena.

HELPFUL HINT

Note whether a newly developed paper-and-pencil test was pilot tested to determine preliminary evidence of reliability and validity.

Savedra et al (1995) developed the Adolescent Pediatric Pain Tool (APPT; Savedra et al, 1993) to measure pain in children and adolescents but found that they needed to add a temporal dimension to the measurement. To do so, they conducted a study in two phases. First, they tested the usefulness of a dot matrix format to assist children and adolescents to communicate the change in their pain over time. They also generated a list of words related to onset, duration, and changing pattern of pain. Then they examined the validity of the list of words and the representation by the dot matrix format by asking children to rate pain experiences associated with short- and long-term painful events.

CRITIQUING DATA COLLECTION METHODS

Evaluating the adequacy of data collection methods from written research reports is often problematic for new nursing research consumers. This is because the tool itself is not available for inspection and the reader may not feel comfortable about judging the adequacy of the method without seeing it. However, a number of questions can be asked as you read to judge the method chosen by the researcher. These questions are listed in the Critiquing Criteria box.

CRITIQUING CRITERIA

1. Are all of the data collection instruments clearly identified and described?
2. Is the rationale for their selection given?
3. Is the method used appropriate to the problem being studied?
4. Is the method used appropriate to the clinical situation?
5. Are the data collection procedures similar for all subjects?

PHYSIOLOGICAL MEASUREMENT

1. Is the instrument used appropriate to the research problem and not forced to fit it?
2. Is a rationale given for why a particular instrument was selected?
3. Is there a provision for evaluating the accuracy of the instrument and those who use it?

OBSERVATIONAL METHODS

1. Who did the observing?
2. Were the observers trained to minimize any bias?
3. Was there an observational guide?
4. Were the observers required to make inferences about what they saw?
5. Is there any reason to believe that the presence of the observers affected the behavior of the subjects?
6. Were the observations performed using the principles of informed consent?

INTERVIEWS

1. Is the interview schedule described adequately enough to know whether it covers the subject?
2. Is there clear indication that the subjects understood the task and the questions?
3. Who were the interviewers, and how were they trained?
4. Is there evidence of any interviewer bias?

QUESTIONNAIRES

1. Is the questionnaire described well enough to know whether it covers the subject?
2. Is there evidence that subjects were able to perform the task?
3. Is there clear indication that the subjects understood the questionnaire?
4. Are the majority of the items appropriately close- or open-ended?

AVAILABLE DATA AND RECORDS

1. Are the records that were used appropriate to the problem being studied?
2. Are the data examined in such a way as to provide new information and not summarize the records?
3. Has the author addressed questions of internal and external criticism?
4. Is there any indication of selection bias in the available records?

All studies should have clearly identified data collection methods. The conceptual and operational definitions of each important variable should be present in the report. Sometimes it is useful for the researcher to explain why a particular method was chosen. For example, if the study dealt with young children, the researcher may explain that a questionnaire was deemed to be an unreasonable task, so an interview was chosen.

Once you have identified the method chosen to measure each variable of interest, you should decide if the method used was the best way to measure the variable. If a questionnaire was used, for example, you might wonder why the decision was made not to use an interview. In addition, consider whether the method was appropriate to the clinical situation. Does it make sense to interview patients in the recovery room, for example?

Once you have decided whether all relevant variables are operationalized appropriately, you can begin to determine how well the method was carried out. For studies using physiological measurement, it is important to determine whether the instrument was appropriate to the problem and not forced to fit it. The rationale for selecting a particular instrument should be given. For example, it may be important to know that the study was conducted under the auspices of a manufacturing firm that provided the measuring instrument. In addition, provision should be made to evaluate the accuracy of the instrument and those who use it.

Several considerations are important when reading studies that use observational methods. Who were the observers, and how were they trained? Is there any reason to believe that different observers saw events or behaviors differently? Remember that the more inferences the observers are required to make, the more likely there will be problems with biased observations. Also consider the problem of reactivity; in any observational situation, the possibility exists that the mere presence of the observer could change the behavior in question. What is important here is not that reactivity could occur, but rather how much reactivity could affect the data. Finally, consider whether the observational procedure was ethical. The reader needs to consider whether subjects were informed that they were being observed, whether any intervention was performed, and whether subjects had agreed to be observed.

Interviews and questionnaires should be clearly described to allow the reader to decide whether the variables were adequately operationalized. Sometimes the researcher will reference the original report about the tool, and the reader may wish to read this study before deciding if the method was appropriate for the present study. The respondents' task should be clear. Thus provision should be made for the subjects to understand both their overall responsibilities and the individual items. Who were the interviewers in the interview situation? Does the researcher explain how they were trained to decrease any interviewer bias?

Available data are subject to internal and external criticism. **Internal criticism** deals with the evaluation of the worth of the records. Internal criticism primarily refers to the accuracy of the data. The researcher should present evidence that the records are genuine. **External criticism** is concerned with the authenticity of the records. Are the records really written by the first author? Finally, the reader should be aware of the problems with selective survival. The researcher may not have an unbiased sample of all of the possible records in the problem area, and this may have a profound effect on the validity of the results.

Finally, the reader should consider the data collection procedure. Is any assurance provided that all of the subjects received the same information? In addition, it is important to try to determine whether all of the information was collected in the same way for all of the subjects in the study.

Once you have decided that the data collection method used was appropriate to the problem and the procedures were appropriate to the population studied, the reliability and validity of the instruments themselves need to be considered. These characteristics are discussed in the next chapter.

KEY POINTS

- Data collection methods are described as being both objective and systematic. The data collection methods of a study provide the operational definitions of the relevant variables.
- Types of data collection methods include physiological, observational, interviews, questionnaires, and available data or records. Each method has advantages and disadvantages.
- Physiological measurements are those methods that use technical instruments to collect data about patients' physical, chemical, microbiological, or anatomical status. Such instruments are particularly suited to the study of the effectiveness of nursing care and the ways to improve the provision of nursing care. Physiological measurements are objective, precise, and sensitive. However, they may be very expensive and they may distort the variable of interest.
- Observational methods frequently are used in nursing research when the variables of interest deal with events or behaviors. Scientific observation requires preplanning, systematic recording, controlling the observations, and relationship to scientific theory. This method is best suited to research problems that are difficult to view as a part of a whole. Observers may be passive or active and concealed or obvious. Observational methods have several advantages, the most important one being the flexibility of the method to measure many types of situations. In addition, observation allows for a great depth and breadth of information to be collected, depending on the problem being studied. Observation has several disadvantages, too. Reactivity, or the distortion of data as a result of the observer's presence, is a common problem in nonconcealed observations. If the observer is concealed, however, there are ethical considerations. Finally, observations may be biased by the person who is doing the observing.
- Interviews and questionnaires are the most commonly used data collection methods in nursing research. Both have the purpose of asking subjects to report data for themselves. Items on questionnaire and interview schedules may be of direct or indirect interest and can be combined into scales. Scales provide an estimate of the degree to which the respondent possesses some trait or characteristic. Either open-ended or close-ended questions may be used when asking subjects questions. The form of the question should be clear to the respondent, free of suggestion, and grammatically correct.
- Questionnaires, or paper-and-pencil tests, are particularly useful when there are a finite number of questions to be asked and the researcher is sure that the questions are clear and specific. Questionnaires also are much less costly in time and money to administer to a large number of subjects, particularly if the subjects are geographically widespread. Another advantage of questionnaires over interviews is that questionnaires have the potential to be completely anonymous. In addition, there is no possibility of interviewer bias.
- Interviews are best used when a large response rate and an unbiased sample are important, because the refusal rate for interviews is much less than that for questionnaires. In-

terviews also allow for some portions of the population who would be precluded by the use of a questionnaire, such as children and the illiterate, to participate in the study. An interviewer can clarify the questions and maintain the order of the questions for all participants.

■ Records and available data also are an important source for research data. The use of available data may save the researcher considerable time and money when conducting a study. This data collection method reduces problems with both reactivity and ethical concerns. However, records and available data are subject to problems of availability, authenticity, and accuracy.

■ A critical evaluation of data collection methods should emphasize the appropriateness, objectivity, and consistency of the method employed.

CRITICAL THINKING CHALLENGES

Barbara Krainovich-Miller

❓ Physiological measurements are objective, precise, and sensitive. Discuss factors that might impact on their validity and feasibility.

❓ A student in research class asks why nurses who participate in a clinical research study in the role of a data collector or perform a "treatment intervention" need to be trained. What important factors or rationale would you offer to support the establishment of interrater reliability?

❓ Observational methods are a frequent data collection method in nursing research. Discuss what makes nurses perfect potential candidates for this role and what are the disadvantages of using this method.

❓ Discuss how the Internet can play a role in critiquing and refining data collection methods. Include any ethical implications you might anticipate.

REFERENCES

Aber CSM, Hawkins JW: Portrayal of nurses in advertisements in medical and nursing journals, *Image J Nurs Sch* 24:289-293, 1992.

Badger TA: Family members' experiences living with members with depression, *West J Nurs Res* 18:149-171, 1996.

Caudell KA, Gallucci BB: Neuroendocrine and immunological responses of women to stress, *West J Nurs Res* 17:672-692, 1995.

Collins C et al: Interviewer training and supervision, *Nurs Res* 37:122-124, 1988.

Erickson RS, Meyer LT, Woo TM: Accuracy of chemical dot thermometers in critically ill adults and young children, *Image J Nurs Sch* 28:23-28, 1996.

Gift AG, Moore T, Soeken K: Relaxation to reduce dyspnea and anxiety in COPD patients, *Nurs Res* 41:242-245, 1992.

Gilmer JS et al: Instrument format issues in assessing the elderly: the Iowa Self-Assessment Inventory, *Nurs Res* 42:297-299, 1993.

Grey M, Flint S: 1988 NAPNAP membership survey: characteristics of member's practice, *J Pediatr Health Care* 3:336-341, 1989.

Grey M et al: Psychosocial status of children with diabetes over the first two years, *Diabetes Care* 18:1330-1336, 1995.

Holmes TH, Rahe RH: The social readjustment rating scale, *J Psychosom Res* 11:213-218, 1967.

Lazarus RS, Folkman S: Coping and adaptation. In Gentry WD, ed: *The handbook of behavioral medicine,* New York, 1984, Guildford.

McCain NL et al: The influence of stress management training in HIV disease, *Nurs Res* 45:246-253, 1996.

Rudy EB et al: Patient outcomes for the chronically critically ill: special care unit versus intensive care unit, *Nurs Res* 44:324-331, 1995.

Russell KM, Champion VL: Health beliefs and social influence in home safety practices of mothers with preschool children, *Image J Nurs Sch* 28:59-64, 1996.

Savedra MC et al: Assessment of postoperative pain in children and adolescents using the Adolescent Pediatric Pain Tool, *Nurs Res* 42:5-9, 1993.

Savedra MC et al: A strategy to assess the temporal dimension of pain in children and adolescents, *Nurs Res* 44:272-276, 1995.

Speilberger CD: *Manual for the state-trait anxiety inventory for children,* Palo Alto, Calif, 1973, Consulting Psychologists.

Weinert C, Burman M: Nurturing longitudinal samples, *West J Nurs Res* 18:360-364, 1996.

West M, Bondy E, Hutchinson S: Interviewing institutionalized elders: Threats to validity, *Image J Nurs Sch* 23:171-176, 1991.

White MA et al: Sleep onset latency and distress in hospitalized children, *Nurs Res* 39(3):134-139, 1990.

Wikblad K, Anderson B: A comparison of three wound dressings in patients undergoing heart surgery, *Nurs Res* 44(5):312-316, 1995.

ADDITIONAL READINGS

Butz AM, Alexander C: Use of health diaries with children, *Nurs Res* 40:59-61, 1991.

Cowan MJ: Measurement of heart rate variability, *West J Nurs Res* 17:32-48, 1995.

DeKeyser FG, Puch LC: Assessment of the reliability and validity of biochemical measures, *Nurs Res* 39:314-317, 1990.

Hutchinson S, Wilson HS: Validity threats in scheduled semistructured research interviews, *Nurs Res* 41:117-119, 1992.

Jones EJ, Kay M: Instrumentation in cross-cultural research, *Nurs Res* 41:186-188, 1992.

Knapp TR, Brown JK: Ten measurement commandments that often should be broken, *Res Nurs Health* 18:465-469, 1995.

Morse JM: Approaches to qualitative-quantitative methodological triangulation, *Nurs Res* 40:120-123, 1991.

Nield M, Kim MJ: The reliability of magnitude estimation for dyspnea measurement, *Nurs Res* 40:17-19, 1991.

Strickland OL, Waltz CF: *Measurement of nursing outcomes: measuring client outcomes,* vol 1, New York, 1988, Springer.

Waltz CF, Strickland OL: *Measurement of nursing outcomes: measuring client outcomes,* vol 2, New York, 1988, Springer.

Reliability and Validity

Geri LoBiondo-Wood ■ Judith Haber

Key Terms

chance errors
  (random errors)
concurrent validity
construct validity
content validity
contrasted-groups
  approach
  (known-groups
  approach)
convergent validity
criterion-related
  validity
Cronbach's alpha
divergent validity

equivalence
error variance
face validity
factor analysis
homogeneity
  (internal
  consistency)
hypothesis-testing
  validity
interrater reliability
item to total
  correlation
Kuder-Richardson
  (KR-20)
  coefficient

multitrait-
  multimethod
  approach
parallel or
  alternate form
  reliability
predictive validity
reliability
split-half reliability
stability
systematic error
  (constant error)
test-retest
  reliability
validity

Learning Outcomes

After reading this chapter the student should be able to do
the following:

- Discuss how measurement error can affect the outcomes
  of a research study.
- Discuss the purposes of reliability and validity.
- Define reliability.
- Discuss the concepts of stability, equivalence, and
  homogeneity as they relate to reliability.
- Compare and contrast the estimates of reliability.
- Define validity.
- Compare and contrast content, criterion-related, and
  construct validity.
- Identify the criteria for critiquing the reliability and
  validity of measurement tools.
- Use the critiquing criteria to evaluate the reliability and
  validity of measurement tools.

easurement of nursing phenomena is a major concern of nursing researchers. Unless measurement tools validly and reliably reflect the concepts of the theory being tested, conclusions drawn from the empirical phase of the study will be invalid and will not advance the development of nursing theory and practice. Issues of reliability and validity are of central concern to the researcher, as well as the critiquer of research. From either perspective the measurement tools that are used in a research study must be evaluated in terms of the extent to which reliability and validity have been established. Many new constructs are relevant to nursing theory, and a growing number of established measurement instruments are available to researchers. However, investigators frequently face the challenge of developing new instruments and, as part of that process, establishing the reliability and validity of those tools. The growing importance of measurement issues, tool development, and related issues such as reliability and validity is evident in the recent publication of the *Journal of Nursing Measurement,* which commenced publication in 1993.

In other contexts investigators use tools that have been developed by researchers in nursing or other disciplines. They must evaluate the tools they select to be certain that they are valid and reliable measures—that they accurately operationalize the constructs being tested.

The critiquer of research, when reading research studies and reports, must assess the reliability and validity of the instruments used in the study to determine the soundness of these selections in relation to the constructs under investigation. The appropriateness of the tools and the extent to which reliability and validity are demonstrated have a profound influence on the findings and the internal and external validity of the study. Invalid measures produce invalid estimates of the relationships between variables, thus affecting internal validity. The use of invalid measures produces inaccurate generalizations to the populations being studied, thus affecting external validity and the ability to apply or not apply research findings in clinical practice. As such, the assessment of reliability and validity is an extremely important skill for you, as a critiquer of nursing research, to develop.

Regardless of whether a new or already developed measurement tool is used in a research study, evidence of reliability and validity is of crucial importance to the research investigator and evaluator. Box 13-1 identifies several computer resources that research consumers can use to access and evaluate the reliability and validity of measurement instruments used in research studies.

The purpose of this chapter is to examine the major types of reliability and validity and demonstrate the applicability of these concepts to the development, selection, and evaluation of measurement tools in nursing research.

RELIABILITY, VALIDITY, AND MEASUREMENT ERROR

Researchers may be concerned about whether the scores that were obtained for a sample of subjects were consistent, true measures of the behaviors and thus an accurate reflection of the differences between individuals. The extent of variability in test scores that is attributable to error rather than a true measure of the behaviors would be the **error variance.**

An observed test score that is derived from a set of items actually consists of the true score plus error (Figure 13-1). The error may be either chance error or random error, or it may be what is known as systematic error. Validity is concerned with systematic error, whereas reliability is concerned with random error (Waltz, Strickland, and Lenz, 1991). **Chance** or **ran-**

Box 13-1	Computer Resources for Accessing and Evaluating the Validity and Reliability of Measurement Instruments*

- *Health and Psychosocial Instruments (HaPI)*
Behavioral Measurement Database Services
Pittsburgh, PA
412-687-6850
A CD-ROM database of measurement instruments in the areas of health and behavioral sciences
- *1997 Guide to Behavioral Resources on the Internet*
Faulkner & Gray, Inc.
11 Penn Plaza
New York, NY 10001
1-800-535-8403
http://www.faulknergray.com
A print guide to more than 500 Internet resources devoted to mental health and behavioral research, including research tools
- *Online Journal of Knowledge Synthesis for Nursing*
  - Full-text articles
  - Full-text searches
  - Hypertext navigation
  - Links to CINAHL and MEDLINE
  - Tables and figures
- *Virginia Henderson International Nursing Library*
  Includes the following databases:
  - Registry of nurse researchers
  - Registry of research projects
  - Registry of research results
Sigma Theta Tau International Nursing Honor Society
550 West North Street
Indianapolis, IN 46202
317-634-8171
http://stti-web.iupui.edu/
- *CINAHL CD-ROM or Online Services*
Access to searches in nursing and 17 allied health disciplines
CINAHL Information Systems
1509 Wilson Terrace
Glendale, CA 91206
1-800-959-7167
http://www.cinahl.com/

*See Chapter 4 for detailed information about computer resources.

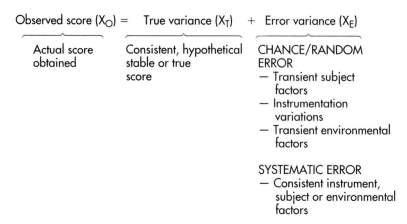

Figure 13-1   Components of observed scores.

dom errors are errors that are difficult to control, such as a respondent's anxiety level at the time of testing. Random errors are unsystematic in nature. Random errors are a result of a transient state in the subject, in the context of the study, or in the administration of the instrument (Jennings and Rogers, 1989). For example, perceptions or behaviors that occur at a specific point in time, such as anxiety, are known as a state or transient characteristic and are often beyond the awareness and control of the examiner. Another example of random error is in a study that measures blood pressure. Random error could occur by misplacement of the cuff, not waiting for a specific time period before taking the blood pressure, or random placement of the arm in relationship to the heart while measuring blood pressure.

Systematic or **constant error** is measurement error that is attributable to relatively stable characteristics of the study population that may bias their behavior and/or cause incorrect instrument calibration. Such error has a systematic biasing influence on the subjects' responses and thereby influences the validity of the instruments. For instance, level of education, socioeconomic status, social desirability, response set, or other characteristics may influence the validity of the instrument by altering measurement of the "true" responses in a systematic way.

For example, a subject who wants to please the investigator may constantly answer items in a socially desirable way, thus making the estimate of validity inaccurate. Systematic error occurs also when an instrument is improperly calibrated. Consider a scale that consistently weighs a person 2 pounds less than the actual body weight. The scale could be quite reliable (i.e., capable of reproducing the precise measurement), but the result is consistently invalid.

HELPFUL HINT
Research articles vary considerably in the amount of detail included about reliability and validity. When the focus of a study is tool development, psychometric evaluation, including extensive reliability and validity data, is carefully documented and appears throughout the article rather than briefly in the *Instruments* section of other research studies.

VALIDITY

Validity refers to whether a measurement instrument accurately measures what it is supposed to measure. When an instrument is valid, it truly reflects the concept it is supposed to measure.

A valid instrument that is supposed to measure anxiety does so; it does not measure some other construct, such as stress. A reliable measure can consistently rank participants on a given construct, such as anxiety, but a valid measure correctly measures the construct of interest. A measure can be reliable but not valid. Let us say that a researcher wanted to measure anxiety in patients by measuring their body temperatures. The researcher could obtain highly accurate, consistent, and precise temperature recordings, but such a measure could not be a valid indicator of anxiety. Thus the high reliability of an instrument is not necessarily congruent with evidence of validity. However, a valid instrument is reliable. An instrument cannot validly measure the attribute of interest if it is erratic, inconsistent, and inaccurate.

There are three major kinds of validity that vary according to the kind of information provided and the purpose of the investigator—content, criterion-related, and construct validity. A critiquer of research articles will want to evaluate whether sufficient evidence of validity is present and whether the type of validity is appropriate to the design of the study and instruments used in the study.

Content Validity

Content validity represents the universe of content, or the domain of a given construct. The universe of content provides the framework and basis for formulating the items that will adequately represent the content. When an investigator is developing a tool and issues of content validity arise, the concern is whether the measurement tool and the items it contains are representative of the content domain the researcher intends to measure. The researcher begins by defining the concept and identifying the dimensions that are the components of the concept. Those items that reflect the concept and its dimensions are formulated.

When the researcher has completed this task, the items are submitted to a panel of judges who are considered to be experts about this concept. Researchers typically request that the judges indicate their agreement with the scope of the items and the extent to which the items reflect the concept under consideration (Berk, 1990).

Carruth (1996) developed a caregiver reciprocity scale (CRS), a tool for measuring reciprocal intergenerational exchanges of assistance and support. On the basis of a review of the literature and interviews with 12 adults, the children or in-laws of elderly parents, 109 items were developed to reflect exchanges within the caregiving context and/or among family members directly or indirectly involved with caregiving. Items were deleted if they were not congruent with the theoretical rationale or if they were redundant, poorly worded, neutral in tone, or lacking probable response variation. Initial content validity was undertaken with 50 items that were submitted to a panel of 10 experts in instrument development and/or gerontological nursing. Panel members were asked to rate each item for clarity and fit with the subscale label and definition, determine whether the item fit conceptually with the caregiver reciprocity, and determine whether the conceptual domain of each subscale had been adequately represented by the set of items. Each expert was asked to rate the relevance of all items on the instrument independently, using a 4-point rating scale ranging from not relevant to very relevant. Content validity indexes (CVIs), indicating percent of agreement between experts for each item, subscale, and total instrument, were calculated. Although consensus existed for the concept of reciprocity, there was no agreement about the extent to which each item reflected the two subscales. Therefore, items were rewritten and a second panel of 8 experts was asked to examine the revised 35-item instrument for content validity. Using the same procedure, all items were judged to reflect the overall concept of caregiver reciprocity. Thirty-two items with a preestablished CVI level of 0.80 or greater were retained on the CRS.

A subtype of content validity is face validity. **Face validity** is a rudimentary type of validity that verifies basically that the instrument gives the appearance of measuring the concept. It is an intuitive type of validity in which colleagues or subjects are asked to read the instrument and evaluate the content in terms of whether it appears to reflect the concept the researcher intends to measure. This procedure may be useful in the tool development process in relation to determining readability and clarity of content. However, it should in no way be considered a satisfactory alternative to other types of validity. Dimmitt (1995) conducted an instrumentation study to, in part, develop and perform initial psychometric evaluation of a Spanish-language version of the Adult Self-Perception Scale (ASPP) as a tool to enable investigation of self-concept and abuse for rural Mexican-American women. Face validity in relation to the Spanish version's readability and language meaning of content was appropriately determined before any other psychometric testing.

Criterion-Related Validity

Criterion-related validity indicates to what degree the subject's performance on the measurement tool and the subject's actual behavior are related. The criterion is usually the second measure, which assesses the same concept under study.

Two forms of criterion-related validity are concurrent and predictive. **Concurrent validity** refers to the degree of correlation of two measures of the same concept administered at the same time. A high correlation coefficient indicates agreement between the two measures. **Predictive validity** refers to the degree of correlation between the measure of the concept and some future measure of the same concept. Because of the passage of time, the correlation coefficients are likely to be lower for predictive validity studies.

Neelon et al (1996) assessed concurrent validity of the NEECHAM Confusion Scale by correlating NEECHAM scores with those from the Mini–Mental Status Exam (MMSE). Acute confusion and/or delirium were assessed according to the DSM-III-R criteria. These are two well-established tools for the assessment of confusion and/or delerium in adults. Significant positive correlations between the NEECHAM and the MMSE ($r = 0.87$) and significant negative correlations between the NEECHAM and the DSM-III-R ($r = -0.91$) provided support for the concurrent validity of the NEECHAM. Macnee and Talsma (1995) assessed predictive validity of the Barriers to Cessation Scale (BCS), a tool to measure barriers to smoking cessation. The relevant criterion to be predicted by the BCS was success versus relapse in efforts at smoking cessation. Statistically significant scores for subjects who subsequently abstained versus those who relapsed in efforts at smoking cessation provide support for the predictive validity of the BCS. Significant differences were noted in initial (T1) BCS scores, $F(2, 139) = 3.4$, $P < 0.05$, between subjects ($n = 103$) who reported smoking at T2 (8 weeks later), reported that they were in the process of quitting at T2 ($n = 30$), or reported that they were nonsmokers at T2 ($n = 9$). Tukey's post-hoc comparisons indicated that individuals who were quitters at T2 had significantly lower initial BCS scores ($m = 19$) compared to individuals who were smokers at T2 ($m = 24.6$).

Construct Validity

Construct validity is based on the extent to which a test measures a theoretical construct or trait. It attempts to validate a body of theory underlying the measurement and testing of the hypothesized relationships. Empirical testing confirms or fails to confirm the relationships that would be predicted among concepts and, as such, provides greater or lesser support for the construct validity of the instruments measuring those concepts. The establishment of construct validity is a complex process, often involving several studies and several approaches. The hypothesis testing, factor analytical, convergent and divergent, and contrasted-groups approaches are discussed.

Hypothesis-Testing Approach

When **hypothesis-testing validity** is used, the investigator uses the theory or concept underlying the measurement instrument's design to develop hypotheses regarding the behavior of individuals with varying scores on the measure, to gather data to test the hypotheses, and to make inferences, on the basis of the findings, concerning whether the rationale underlying the instrument's construction is adequate to explain the findings.

For example, Leidy and Darling-Fisher (1995) used a hypothesis-testing approach to establish the construct validity of the Modified Erikson Psychosocial Stage Inventory (MEPSI) across four diverse samples, healthy young adults, hemophilic men, healthy older adults, and older adults with chronic obstructive pulmonary disease (COPD). The MEPSI is a survey measure designed to assess the strength of psychosocial attributes that arise from progression through Erikson's eight stages of development. As illustrated in Table 13-1, Leidy and Darling-Fisher derived four hypotheses that represented propositions related to measurement of psychosocial attribute strength and a theoretically related concept that could be used to assess the construct validity of the MEPSI. As predicted, the MEPSI total correlated significantly with indicators of adaptation to parenthood, social adjustment, self-transcendence, and need for satisfaction thereby lending support for the hypotheses and, as such, preliminary support for the theoretical basis and conceptual accuracy of the MEPSI. The results of some of the other analyses related to demographic variables (age, gender, and health) are in contrast to study predictions, which suggests the need for additional construct validity studies.

Convergent and Divergent Approaches

Two strategies for assessing construct validity include convergent and divergent approaches.

Convergent validity refers to a search for other measures of the construct. Sometimes two or more tools that theoretically measure the same construct are identified, and both are administered to the same subjects. A correlational analysis is performed. If the measures are positively correlated, convergent validity is said to be supported. In the development of the Cardiac Event Threat Questionnaire (CTQ), Bennett et al (1996) established convergent validity by correlating the CTQ with the Profile of Mood States (POMS), given that a key attribute of threat is the association with negatively toned emotions. The statistically significant but moderate correlation of 0.28 between the CTQ and the POMS supported the idea that the

Table 13-1

Pearson Correlation Coefficients Between Relevant Variables and MEPSI* Subscales and Total Scale by Study and Gender

	STUDY, RELATED CONSTRUCT, AND GENDER						
	1 (ADAPTATION TO PARENTHOOD)		2 (SOCIAL ADJUST-MENT)	3 (SELF-TRANSCENDENCE)		4 (NEED SATISFACTION)	
SCALE	WOMEN (n = 205)	MEN (n = 196)	MEN (n = 134)	WOMEN (n = 59)	MEN (n = 41)	WOMEN (n = 49)	MEN (n = 57)
Trust	0.49†	0.43†	0.58†	0.32‡	0.14	0.50†	0.34†
Autonomy	0.47†	0.40†	0.57†	0.45†	0.46‡	0.44†	0.37†
Initiative	0.36†	0.45†	0.46†	0.33‡	0.45‡	0.29‡	0.23
Industry	0.37†	0.40†	0.49†	0.29	0.54†	0.50†	0.42†
Identity	0.53†	0.43†	0.62†	0.40†	0.64†	0.50†	0.48†
Intimacy	0.47†	0.34†	0.61†	0.49†	0.27	0.41†	0.17
Generativity	0.42†	0.49†	0.52†	0.47†	0.48†	0.48†	0.54†
Integrity	0.52†	0.41†	0.54†	0.29	0.40	0.53†	0.55†
MEPSI* total	0.56†	0.52†	0.65†	0.48†	0.54†	0.60†	0.46†

From Leidy NK, Darling-Fisher CS: Reliability and validity of the modified Erikson psychosocial stage inventory in diverse samples, *West J Nurs Res* 17(2):168-187, 1995.

**MEPSI,* Modified Erikson Psychosocial Stage Inventory.

†$P < 0.01$.

‡$P < 0.05$.

CTQ was measuring threat related to cardiac events. More recently, causal modeling has been used to establish convergent validity. In the development of the CRS (discussed earlier), Carruth (1996) established convergent validity using the causal modeling approach. As illustrated in Table 13-2, several indicators have been recommended to assess convergent validity: item loadings, composite reliability, average variance extracted by each construct, examining standard error, and *t* values. Table 13-2 presents data indicating significant findings between the CRS factor structure and the relevant causal modeling indicators, thereby offering support for the convergent validity of the items in each factor of the CRS.

Divergent validity uses measurement approaches that differentiate one construct from others that may be similar. Sometimes researchers search for instruments that measure the opposite of the construct. If the divergent measure is negatively related to other measures, validity for the measure is strengthened. More recently, the data from a factor analysis being conducted for other validity purposes can be used to determine divergent (sometimes called *discriminant*) validity. Carruth (1996) assessed the discriminant validity of the four factors (subscales) of the CRS by examining the correlations between each factor or subscale that appears in Table 13-2.

A specific method of assessing convergent and divergent validity is the **multitrait-multimethod approach.** Similar to the approach described, this method, proposed by Campbell and Fiske (1959), also involves examining the relationship between indicators that should

Table 13-2

Estimated LISREL Parameters of Construct Validity

	STANDARDIZED LOADINGS	ITEM/COMPOSITE RELIABILITY	$2 \times SE$	VARIANCE EXTRACTED ESTIMATE
Warmth and regard				
		0.89*		0.48
#2	0.52	0.27	†	
#10	0.70	0.48	0.40	
#12	0.76	0.58	0.42	
#21	0.60	0.35	0.37	
#22	0.71	0.51	0.40	
#25	0.67	0.45	0.39	
#28	0.70	0.49	0.40	
#30	0.82	0.66	0.43	
#33	0.74	0.54	0.41	
Intrinsic rewards of giving				
		0.83*		0.49
#1	0.62	0.38	†	
#13	0.64	0.40	0.29	
#17	0.74	0.55	0.30	
#29	0.76	0.60	0.30	
#32	0.74	0.55	0.30	
Love and affection				
		0.88*		0.64
#4	0.77	0.60	†	
#5	0.73	0.53	0.18	
#8	0.90	0.80	0.18	
#15	0.81	0.65	0.18	
Balance within family caregiving				
		0.77*		0.47
#6	0.72	0.51	†	
#19	0.69	0.48	0.24	
#20	0.75	0.56	0.24	
#34	0.56	0.31	0.23	

From Carruth AK: Development and testing of the caregiver reciprocity scale, *Nurs Res* 45(2):92-97, 1996.
*Denotes composite reliabilities.
†Denotes value not estimated (parameter constrained at 1.0 in LISREL).

measure the same construct and between those that should measure different constructs. However, a variety of measurement strategies are used. For example, anxiety could be measured by the following:

- Administering the State-Trait Anxiety Inventory
- Recording blood pressure readings
- Asking the subject about anxious feelings
- Observing the subject's behavior

The results of one of these measures should then be correlated with results of each of the others in a multitrait-multimethod matrix (Waltz, Strickland, and Lenz, 1991). A study designed to develop, validate, and norm a measure of dimensions of interpersonal relationships including social support, reciprocity, and conflict by Tilden, Nelson, and May (1990) used the multitrait-multimethod approach to validity assessment. The two traits of social support and conflict of the Interpersonal Relationship Inventory (IPRI) were each measured with two different methods—a subject self-report tool and an investigator observation visual analog rating. Reciprocity was not included because of its high correlation with social support.

The use of multiple measures of a concept decreases systematic error. A variety of data collection methods, such as self-report, observation, interview, and collection of physiological data, will also diminish the effect of systematic error.

Contrasted-Groups Approach

When the **contrasted-groups approach** (sometimes called the **known-groups approach**) to the development of construct validity is used, the researcher identifies two groups of individuals who are suspected to score extremely high or low in the characteristic being measured by the instrument. The instrument is administered to both the high- and low-scoring group, and the differences in scores obtained are examined. If the instrument is sensitive to individual differences in the trait being measured, the mean performance of these two groups should differ significantly and evidence of construct validity would be supported. A t test or analysis of variance is used to statistically test the difference between the two groups. In the study by Dimmitt (1995) that sought to develop and assess the psychometric properties of the ASPS, the contrasted-groups approach was used to identify differences between known abused ($n = 58$) and nonabused ($n = 126$) groups on self-concept. Participants indicating abuse scored significantly lower ($P < 0.05$) on dimensions of morality, sociability, and global self-worth than did those who were not abused. Dimmitt (1995) states that this finding is consistent with previous studies that have described low self-concept for individuals experiencing abuse.

Factor Analytical Approach

A final approach to assessing construct validity is factor analysis. This is a procedure that gives the researcher information about the extent to which a set of items measures the same underlying construct or dimension of a construct. **Factor analysis** assesses the degree to which the individual items on a scale truly cluster together around one or more dimensions. Items designed to measure the same dimension should load on the same factor; those designed to measure differing dimensions should load on different factors (Anastasi, 1988; Nunnally, 1978). This analysis will indicate also whether the items in the instrument reflect a single construct or several constructs.

A factor analysis was carried out by Bennett et al (1996) during the establishment of construct validity of the CTQ, an instrument developed to measure threat related to cardiac events. The final CTQ consisted of 37 items. A confirmatory factor analysis of the CTQ was conducted to assess the factor structure of the CTQ and, hence, the construct validity. A five-factor solution was sought, based on previous research identifying five factors related to cardiac threat. Findings from the factor analysis indicate that the five-factor structure of the CTQ, presented in Table 13-3, is similar to the five categories suggested in earlier work by Bennett (1993) and that are consistent with types of threat identified in Lazarus and Folkman's (1984) theory of stress and coping, a theoretical foundation of this study.

HELPFUL HINT

When validity data about the measurement instruments used in a study are not included in a research article, you have no way of determining whether the intended concept is actually being captured by the measurement tool. In such a case before you use the results, it is important to go back to the original source to check the instrument's validity.

The Critical Thinking Decision Path will help you assess the appropriateness of the type of validity and reliability selected for use in a particular research study.

RELIABILITY

Reliable people are people whose behavior can be relied on to be consistent and predictable. **Reliability** of a research instrument likewise is defined as the extent to which the instrument yields the same results on repeated measures. Reliability is then concerned with consistency, accuracy, precision, stability, equivalence, and homogeneity. Concurrent with the questions of validity or after they are answered, the researcher and the critiquer of research ask the question of how reliable is the instrument? A reliable measure is one that can produce the same results if the behavior is measured again by the same scale. Reliability then refers to the proportion of accuracy to inaccuracy in measurement. In other words, if we use the same or comparable instruments on more than one occasion to measure a set of behaviors that ordinarily remain relatively constant, we would expect similar results if the tools are reliable. The three main attributes of a reliable scale are stability, homogeneity, and equivalence. The stability of an instrument refers to the instrument's ability to produce the same results with repeated testing. The homogeneity of an instrument means that all the items in a tool measure the same concept or characteristic. An instrument is said to exhibit equivalence if the tool produces the same results when equivalent or parallel instruments or procedures are used. Each of these attributes and the means to estimate them will be discussed. Before these are discussed an understanding of how to interpret reliability is essential.

Reliability Coefficient Interpretation

Because all the attributes of reliability are concerned with the degree of consistency between scores that are obtained at two or more independent times of testing, they often are expressed in terms of a correlation coefficient. The reliability coefficient ranges from 0 to 1. The reliability coefficient expresses the relationship between the error variance, true variance, and the observed

Table 13-3

Factor Loadings of Cardiac Event Threat Questionnaire (CTQ) Items (n = 270)

	FACTOR 1: FATIGUE	FACTOR 2: GENERAL HEALTH	FACTOR 3: DISEASE-SPECIFIC SYMPTOMS	FACTOR 4: WORK	FACTOR 5: FAMILY
Not being able to do things I used to do	0.74				
My loss of strength	0.72				
Needing more rest than usual	0.74				
Being more tired than usual	0.71				
Feeling dependent	0.61				
Feeling weak	0.61				
My inability to sleep	0.58				
The special diet I am supposed to follow	0.49				
Doing jobs around the house	0.45				
Side effects of medications I am taking	0.44				
My condition in general		0.75			
The entire situation		0.68			
My arteries being blocked		0.60			
My future		0.54			
Needing more procedures or surgery		0.52			
Developing other medical problems		0.52			
Getting back to a normal life		0.52			
Cost of my health care		0.50			
Paying my bills		0.45			
Tingling in my chest			0.76		
Pain in my chest			0.68		
Pain in my arms			0.66		
Irregular heartbeats			0.53		
Medical care I receive			0.51		
My cholesterol level			0.48		
Returning to a stressful job				0.83	
Returning to work				0.75	
Being asked to do heavy physical work at my job				0.73	
My cigarette smoking				0.42	
The effects of my condition on my children					0.79
Caring for my children					0.68
Not being with my family					0.50
Eigenvalue	10.43	1.98	1.75	1.62	1.38
Variance explained	32.6	6.2	5.5	5.1	4.3

From Bennett SJ et al: Development of an instrument to measure threat related to cardiac events, *Nurs Res* 45(5)266-270, 1996.

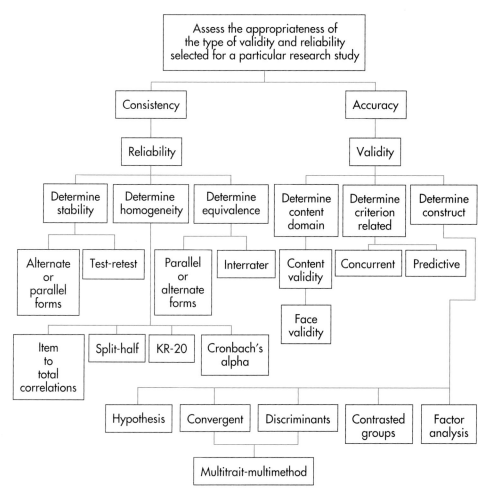

Critical Thinking Decision Path   Determining the appropriate type of validity and reliability selected for a study.

score. A zero correlation indicates that there is no relationship. When the error variance in a measurement instrument is low, the reliability coefficient will be closer to 1. The closer to 1 the coefficient is, the more reliable the tool. For example, a reliability coefficient of a tool is reported to be 0.89. This tells you that the error variance is small and the tool has little measurement error. On the other hand, if the reliability coefficient of a measure is reported to be 0.49, the error variance is high and the tool has a problem with measurement error. For a tool to be considered reliable, a level of 0.70 or higher is considered to be an acceptable level of reliability. The interpretation of the reliability coefficient depends on the proposed purpose of the measure. There are five major tests of reliability that can be used to calculate a reliability coefficient. The test(s) used depends on the nature of the tool. They are known as test-retest, parallel or alternate form, item-total correlation, split-half, Kuder-Richardson (KR-20), Cronbach's alpha, and interrater reliability. These tests are discussed as they relate to the attributes of stability, equivalence, and homogeneity (Box 13-2). There is no best means to assess reliability in relationship to stability, homogeneity, and equivalence. The critiquer of research should be aware that the method of reliability that the researcher uses should be consistent with the investigator's aim.

Stability

An instrument is thought to be stable or to exhibit **stability** when the same results are obtained on repeated administration of the instrument. Researchers are concerned with the stability of an instrument when they want the instrument to be able to measure the concept consistently over a period of time. Measurement over time is important when an instrument is used in a longitudinal study and therefore will be used on several occasions. Stability is also a consideration when the researcher is conducting an intervention study that is designed to affect an alteration in a specific variable. In this case the instrument is administered once and again later after the alteration or change intervention has been completed. The tests that are used to estimate stability are test-retest and parallel or alternate form.

Test-Retest Reliability

Test-retest reliability is the administration of the same instrument to the same subjects under similar conditions on two or more occasions. Scores on the repeated testing are compared. This comparison is expressed by a correlation coefficient, usually a Pearson r (see Chapter 15). The interval between repeated administrations varies and depends on the phenomenon being measured. For example, if the variable that the test measures is related to the developmental stages in children, the interval between tests should be short. The amount of time over which the variable was measured should also be recorded in the report. An example of an instrument that was tested for test-retest reliability is the Barriers Questionnaire (BQ) used in the study by Ward, Berry, and Misiewicz (1996) that investigated concerns about analgesics among patients and family caregivers in a hospice setting. Test-retest reliability for the BQ, which measures eight concerns about reporting pain and using analgesics, was obtained in a previous

---

Box 13-2   Measures Used to Test Reliability

Stability
Test-retest reliability
Parallel or alternate form

Homogeneity
Item-total correlation
Split-half reliability
Kuder-Richardson coefficient
Cronbach's alpha

Equivalence
Parallel or alternate form
Interrater reliability

study (Ward and Gatwood, 1994) over a 1-week period for 56 subjects. Test-retest correlations were 0.90 for the total scale and ranged from 0.61 to 0.81 for the subscales. The magnitude of the correlation for the total scale supports the idea that the BQ has the attribute of stability. Because the lowest mentioned correlation for the subscales is 0.61, the critiquer would want to examine the test-retest data from the previous study before drawing definitive conclusions about the overall stability of items in the BQ.

Parallel or Alternate Form

Parallel or alternate form reliability is applicable and can be tested only if two comparable forms of the same instrument exist. It is like test-retest reliability in that the same individuals are tested within a specific interval, but it differs because a different form of the same test is given to the subjects on the second testing. Parallel forms or tests contain the same types of items that are based on the same domain or concept, but the wording of the items is different. The development of parallel forms is desired if the instrument is intended to measure a variable for which a researcher believes that "test-wiseness" will be a problem. For example, there are two alternate forms of the Partner Relationship Inventory (Hoskins, 1988) that may be used in a repeated-measures design. An item on one scale ("I am able to tell my partner how I feel") is consistent with the paired item on the second form ("My partner tries to understand my feelings"). Practically speaking, it is difficult to develop alternate forms of an instrument when one considers the many issues of reliability and validity of an instrument. If alternate forms of a test exist, they should be highly correlated if the measures are to be considered reliable.

HELPFUL HINT
When a longitudinal design with multiple data collection points is being conducted, look for evidence of test-retest or parallel form reliability.

Homogeneity

Another attribute of an instrument related to reliability is the **internal consistency** or **homogeneity** with which the items within the scale reflect or measure the same concept. This means that the items within the scale correlate or are complementary to each other. This also means that a scale is unidimensional. A unidimensional scale is one that measures one concept. The Life Support Preferences Questionnaire (LSPQ) (Beland and Froman, 1995), a tool that measures attitudes about life support decisions, is an example of a unidimensional scale. The results of the factor analysis, set for a two-factor solution, indicate that all items loaded on a single factor with an internal consistency estimated at 0.94. The internal consistency of items allows the investigator to tally the items and obtain a total score for the concept. The total score is then used in the analysis of data. Homogeneity can be assessed by using one of four methods: item-total correlations, split-half reliability, Kuder-Richardson (KR-20) coefficient, or Cronbach's alpha.

HELPFUL HINT
When the characteristics of a study sample differ significantly from the sample in the original study, check to see if the researcher has reestablished the reliability of the instrument with the current sample.

Item to Total Correlations

Item to total correlations measure the relationship between each of the items and the total scale. When item to total correlations are calculated, a correlation for each item on the scale is generated (Table 13-4). Items that do not achieve a high correlation may be deleted from the instrument. Usually in a research study, not all the item to total correlations are reported unless the study is a report of a methodological study. Typically the lowest and highest correlations are reported. An example of an item to total correlation report is illustrated in the study by Macnee and Talsma (1995) in which item to total correlations were computed for the 19 item BCS in two studies, Study 1 and Study 3. In Study 1, the item to total score correlations ranged between 0.30 and 0.57. In Study 3, they ranged from 0.27 to 0.60, with the exception of the first item on the scale, "weight gain," which correlated 0.14 with the total score. Given that uncorrected item to total correlations above 0.25 are considered indicative of acceptable internal consistency (Nunnally, 1978), these results, with the exception of "weight gain," support the reliability of the BCS.

The investigators eliminate items that have too low a correlation, whereas they examine others to ensure that they are high enough to be measuring the same concept without being redundant. If item to total correlations are found to be too high, they are considered to be redundant and therefore not complementary to each other (Anastasi, 1988). This is unlike the other errors of reliability in which a higher correlation is generally a better correlation.

Split-Half Reliability

Split-half reliability involves dividing a scale into two halves and making a comparison. The halves may be odd-numbered and even-numbered items or a simple division of the first from the second half, or items may be randomly selected as to the halves that will be analyzed opposite one another. The split-half provides a measure of consistency in terms of sampling the content. The two halves of the test or the contents in both halves are assumed to be comparable, and a reliability coefficient is calculated. If the scores for the two halves are approximately equal, the test may be considered reliable. A formula called the *Spearman-Brown formula* is one method used to calculate the reliability coefficient. In a study investigating the appraisal of pain and coping in cancer patients, Arathuzik (1991) obtained a split-half reliability rating of 0.85 from a pilot test of the Pain Experience Inventory with 30 patients with metastatic breast cancer who were experiencing pain.

Table 13-4

Examples of Item to Total Correlations from Computer-Generated Data

ITEM	ITEM TO TOTAL CORRELATION
1	0.5096
2	0.4455
3	0.4479
4	0.4369
5	0.4139
6	0.4016

Kuder-Richardson (KR-20) Coefficient

The **Kuder-Richardson (KR-20) coefficient** is the estimate of homogeneity used for instruments that have a dichotomous response format. A dichotomous response format is one in which the question asks for a "yes/no" or a "true/false" response. The technique yields a correlation that is based on the consistency of responses to all the items of a single form of a test that is administered one time. In a study investigating relationships among spirituality, perceived social support, death anxiety, and nurses' willingness to care for acquired immunodeficiency syndrome (AIDS) patients, Sherman (1996) uses the Templer Death Anxiety Scale (TDAS) (Templer, 1970), one of the most widely used measures of conscious death anxiety. Because the response format for the TDAS is binary ("true/false"), the KR-20 was used to determine the original internal consistency of the 15 items. A KR-20 reliability coefficient of 0.76 indicated a moderate level of internal consistency reliability. Because the original data was based on a sample of 31 college students and Sherman's study sample consisted of registered nurses, a pilot study was conducted and a reliability coefficient of 0.78 was calculated. However, when a KR-20 was calculated in the actual study, the reliability coefficient was computed at 0.63, certainly lower than was anticipated based on the results of the pilot study. In the discussion section of this article, Sherman (1996) does comment on the low internal consistency reliability of the TDAS, suggesting that the "true/false" format that limits response possibilities may contribute to this phenomenon. She proposes that reformulation of the tool using a Likert scale format (see Chapter 8) may allow a researcher to better detect the real feelings of an individual and thereby increase the reliability of the TDAS.

Cronbach's Alpha

The fourth and most commonly used test of internal consistency is **Cronbach's alpha**. Many tools used to measure psychosocial variables and attitudes have a Likert scale response format. A Likert scale format asks the subject to respond to a question on a scale of varying degrees of intensity between two extremes. The two extremes are anchored by responses such as "strongly agree" to "strongly disagree" or "most like me" to "least like me." The points between the two extremes may range from 1 to 5 or 1 to 7. Subjects are asked to circle the response closest to how they feel. Figure 13-2 provides examples of items from

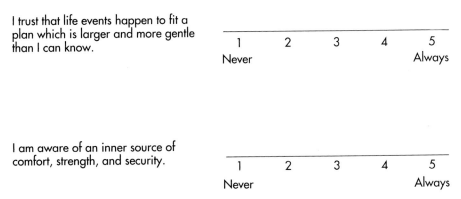

Figure 13-2   Examples of a Likert Scale. (Redrawn from Roberts KT, Aspy CB: Development of the serenity scale, *J Nurs Measure* 1(2):145-164, 1993.)

a tool that uses a Likert scale format. Cronbach's alpha compares each item in the scale simultaneously with each other. Examples of reported Cronbach's alpha are in Box 13-3.

> **HELPFUL HINT**
>
> If a research article provides information about the reliability of a measurement instrument but does not specify the type of reliability, it is probably safe to assume that internal consistency reliability was assessed using Cronbach's alpha.

Equivalence

Equivalence is either the consistency or agreement among observers using the same measurement tool or the consistency or agreement among alternate forms of a tool. An instrument is thought to demonstrate equivalence when two or more observers have a high percentage of agreement of an observed behavior or when alternate forms of a test yield a high correlation. There are two methods to test equivalence: interrater reliability and alternate or parallel form.

Interrater Reliability

Some measurement instruments are not self-administered questionnaires but are direct measurements of observed behavior. Instruments that depend on direct observation of a behavior that is to be systematically recorded need to be tested for interrater reliability. To accomplish **interrater reliability,** two or more individuals should make an observation or one observer observe the behavior on several occasions. The observers should be trained or oriented to the definition of the behavior to be observed. In the method of direct observation of behavior, the consistency or reliability of the observations between observers is extremely important. In the instance of interrater reliability, the reliability or consistency of the observer is tested rather than the reliability of the instrument. Interrater reliability is expressed as a percentage of agreement between scorers or as a correlation coefficient between the scores assigned to the observed behaviors.

Box 13-3   Examples of Reported Cronbach's Alpha

Perlow M (p 206, 1992): "The Perlow Self Esteem Survey (PSES) had a Cronbach's alpha of .86. The alpha value is quite high, indicating that . . . the PSES has demonstrated internal consistency."

Affonso DD et al (p 341, 1994): "Cronbach's alpha coefficients for the Cognitive Adaptation to Stressful Events scale (CASE) were high. Scores ranged from .94 to .96 across 6 assessment points."

Allred CA et al (p 176, 1994): "The item internal consistency as measured by Cronbach's alpha and based on all seven items of the Perceived Environmental Uncertainty Questionnaire (PEUQ) was .81. An alpha coefficient of at least .70 is adequate for an instrument in the early stages of development."

In the study *Patient Outcomes for the Chronically Critically Ill: Special Care Unit Versus Intensive Care Unit* (Rudy et al, 1995) the researchers carefully monitored interrater reliability, because four out of six instruments used in the study depended on accurate abstraction of data from the patient record. Each member of the research team who participated in data collection was trained by the project director and had to achieve a 90% agreement on each measurement tool before independent data were collected. In addition a detailed rule book was kept so that reliability could be maintained. Interrater reliability was checked on a random selection of 10% of records and maintained at 90% agreement between coders. Whenever agreement dropped below 90%, differences in scoring were analyzed and resolved, usually through the construction of additional coding rules.

Another example of interrater reliability is given in the study conducted by Wikblad and Anderson (1995), who studied the differential effect on healing of three wound dressings in patients undergoing heart surgery. The first use of interrater reliability in this study consisted of five nurses from each of the units used in the study who were trained to examine the dressings. They rated the following parameters: (1) how well the incision could be seen through the dressing, (2) how much the dressing had loosened, (3) number of bandage changes and the reasons for those changes, (4) pain at removal of dressing on fifth day, and (5) difficulty in removing the dressing. They compared their results and discussed ratings that differed from each other. This procedure was repeated on five new patients until there was 100% agreement in their ratings. The second use of interrater reliability consisted of evaluation of color photographs of the wound taken on day 5 after surgery. The actual evaluation was done by two independent raters, neither of whom was aware of the experimental conditions. The interrater reliability was calculated by use of the kappa coefficient. The kappa coefficient for ratings of wound healing was 0.81, and the agreement between the two raters was 91%. For ratings of redness, the agreement was 85% (kappa coefficient = 0.73).

Parallel or Alternate Form
Parallel or alternate form was described under the heading "Stability." Use of parallel forms is then a measure of stability and equivalence. The procedures for assessing equivalence using parallel forms are the same.

CRITIQUING RELIABILITY AND VALIDITY

Reliability and validity are two crucial aspects in the critical appraisal of a measurement instrument. Criteria for critiquing reliability and validity are presented in the Critiquing Criteria box. The reviewer evaluates an instrument's level of reliability and validity and the manner in which they were established. In a research report the reliability and validity for each measure should be presented. If these data have not been presented at all, the reviewer must seriously question the merit and use of the tool and the study's results.

In an article about the proliferation of unreliable and invalid questionnaires, Rempusheski (1990) stresses that when psychometric principles in general, but including those related to reliability and validity, are violated, the product (i.e., the instrument used) impacts on the profession, the organization, and the individuals within the organization. It is the ethical responsibility of the critiquer to question the reliability and validity of instruments used in research studies and to examine the findings in light of the quality of the instruments used and the data

CRITIQUING CRITERIA

1. Was an appropriate method used to test the reliability of the tool?
2. Is the reliability of the tool adequate?
3. Was an appropriate method(s) used to test the validity of the instrument?
4. Is the validity of the measurement tool adequate?
5. If the sample from the developmental stage of the tool was different from the current sample, were the reliability and validity recalculated to determine if the tool is still adequate?
6. Have the strengths and weaknesses of the reliability and validity of each instrument been presented?
7. Are strengths and weaknesses of instrument reliability and validity appropriately addressed in the *Discussion, Limitations,* or *Recommendations* sections of the report?

presented. The following discussion highlights key areas related to reliability and validity that should be evident to the critiquer in a research article.

Appropriate reliability tests should have been performed by the developer of the measurement tool and should then have been included by the current user in the research report. If the initial standardization sample and the current sample have different characteristics, the reader would expect (1) that a pilot study for the present sample would have been conducted to determine if the reliability was maintained or (2) that a reliability estimate was calculated on the current sample. For example, if the standardization sample for a tool that measures "satisfaction in an intimate heterosexual relationship" comprises undergraduate college students and if an investigator plans to use the tool with married couples, it would be advisable to establish the reliability of the tool with the latter group.

The investigator determines which type of reliability procedures are used in the study, depending on the nature of the measurement tool and how it will be used. For example, if the instrument is to be administered twice, the critiquer might determine that test-retest reliability should have been used to establish the stability of the tool. If an alternate form has been developed for use in a repeated-measures design, evidence of alternate form reliability should be presented to determine the equivalence of the parallel forms. If the degree of internal consistency among the items is relevant, an appropriate test of internal consistency should be presented. In some instances more than one type of reliability will be presented, but the evaluator should determine whether all are appropriate. For example, the Kuder-Richardson formula implies that there is a single right or wrong answer, making it inappropriate to use with scales that provide a format of three or more possible responses. In such cases another formula is applied, such as Cronbach's coefficient alpha formula. Another important consideration is the acceptable level of reliability, which varies according to the type of test. Coefficients of reliability of 0.70 or higher are desirable. The validity of an instrument is limited by its reliability; that is, less confidence can be placed in scores from tests with low reliability coefficients.

Satisfactory evidence of validity is probably the most difficult item for the reviewer to ascertain. It is this aspect of measurement that is most likely to fall short of meeting the required criteria. Validity studies are time consuming, as well as complex, and sometimes researchers will settle for presenting minimal validity data. Therefore the critiquer should closely examine the item content of a tool when evaluating its strengths and weaknesses and try to find conclusive evidence of content validity. However, in the body of a research article it is most unusual to have more than a few sample items available for review. Because that is the case, the critiquer should determine whether the appropriate assessment of content validity was used to meet the researcher's goal. Such procedures provide the reviewer with assurance that the tool is psychometrically sound and that the content of the items is consistent with the conceptual framework and construct definitions. Construct and criterion-related validity are some of the more precise statistical tests of whether the tool measures what it is supposed to measure. Ideally an instrument should provide evidence of content validity, as well as criterion-related or construct validity, before a reviewer invests a high level of confidence in the tool.

The reader would also expect to see the strengths and weaknesses of instrument reliability and validity presented in the *Discussion, Limitations,* and/or *Recommendations* section of a research article. In this context the reliability and validity might be discussed in relation to other tools devised to measure the same variable. The relationship of the findings to strengths and weaknesses in instrument reliability and validity would be another important discussion point. Finally, recommendations for improving future studies in relation to instrument reliability and validity should be proposed (Rempusheski, 1990). For example, in the *Instruments* and *Discussion* sections of a study investigating examining relationships among spirituality, perceived social support, death anxiety, and nurses' willingness to care for AIDS patients, Sherman (1996) appropriately reports the weaknesses in reliability of the TDAS. She states that although the TDAS is often cited in the literature, the low internal consistency reliability of the scale (0.76) supports the recommendation that the instrument be pilot tested on the specific sample to which it will be administered. Because of the marginally acceptable reliability of the TDAS and because the study sample (registered nurses) was different from the original sample (college students) used for establishing reliability, a pilot study, yielding a marginally acceptable reliability coefficient of 0.78, was conducted using a sample of 30 nurses enrolled in a doctoral course. Sherman goes on, however, to comment that in the actual study, the TDAS's reliability coefficient of 0.63 was lower than anticipated, based on the results of the pilot study. Although Sherman appropriately addresses the low reliability of TDAS in relation to the psychometric properties of the tool and makes recommendations about revising the response format, she does not address this weaknesses in relation to the hypotheses and the findings of the study.

As you can see, the area of reliability and validity is complex. These aspects of research reports can be evaluated to varying degrees. The research consumer should not feel inhibited by the complexity of this topic but may use the guidelines presented in this chapter to systematically assess the reliability and validity aspects of a research study. Collegial dialogue also is an approach to evaluating the merits and shortcomings of an existing, as well as a newly developed, instrument that is reported in the nursing literature. Such an exchange promotes the understanding of methodologies and techniques of reliability and validity, stimulates the acquisition of a basic knowledge of psychometrics, and encourages the exploration of alternative methods of observation and the use of reliable and valid tools in clinical practice.

KEY POINTS

- Reliability and validity are crucial aspects of conducting and critiquing research.
- Validity refers to whether an instrument measures what it is purported to measure, and it is a crucial aspect of evaluating a tool.
- Three types of validity are content validity, criterion-related validity, and construct validity.
- The choice of a validation method is important and is made by the researcher on the basis of the characteristics of the measurement device in question and its utilization.
- Reliability refers to the accuracy/inaccuracy ratio in a measurement device.
- The major tests of reliability are the following: test-retest, parallel or alternate form, split-half, item to total correlation, Kuder-Richardson, Cronbach's alpha, and interrater reliability.
- The selection of a method for establishing reliability will depend on the characteristics of the tool, the testing method that is used for collecting data from the standardization sample, and the kinds of data that are obtained.

CRITICAL THINKING CHALLENGES

Barbara Krainovich-Miller

- Do you agree or disagree with the following statement: "Much of nursing's research 'sits on shelves in libraries.'" Support your position with examples.
- There are several classic research utilization (RU) demonstration projects. Discuss the similarities and differences among these classic RU projects. Include in your discussion the Agency for Health Care Policy Research (AHCPR) Guidelines for various clinical problems. Include what technology you might use to assist you in your answer.
- Discuss the differences between an individual clinical model of research utilization and an organizational model of RU. Given the various settings you have used during your clinical educational experience, support which model you think would work best in these settings.
- Discuss the role of technology in implementing the steps of RU. Do you think the review of the literature is the same for developing a research proposal as it is for implementing the steps of RU? Support your position.

REFERENCES

Affonso DD et al: Cognitive adaptation to stressful events during pregnancy and postpartum: development and testing of the CASE instrument, *Nurs Res* 43(6):338-343, 1994.

Allred CA et al: A measure of perceived environmental uncertainty in hospitals, *West J Nurs Res* 16(2):169-182, 1994.

Anastasi A: *Psychological testing*, ed 6, New York, 1988, Macmillan.

Arathuzik MD: The appraisal of pain and coping in cancer patients, *West J Nurs Res* 13(6):714-731, 1991.

Beland DK, Froman RD: Preliminary validation of a measure of life support preferences, *Image* 24(4):307-310, 1995.

Bennett SJ: Relationships among selected antecedent variables and coping effectiveness in post-myocardial infarction patients, *Res Nurs Health* 16:131-139, 1993.

Bennett SJ et al: Development of an instrument to measure threat related to cardiac events, *Nurs Res* 45(5):266-270, 1996.

Berk RA: Importance of expert judgment in content-related validity evidence, *West J Nurs* 12(5):659-671, 1990.

Campbell D, Fiske D: Convergent and discriminant validation by the matrix, *Psychol Bull* 53:273-302, 1959.

Carruth AK: Development and testing of the caregiver reciprocity scale, *Nurs Res* 45(2):92-97, 1996.

Dimmitt J: Adult self-perception profile (ASPP) Spanish translation and reassessment for a rural minority population, *West J Nurs Res* 17(2):203-217, 1995.

Hoskins CN: *The partner relationship inventory,* Palo Alto, Calif, 1988, Consulting Psychologists Press.

Jennings BM, Rogers S: Managing measurement error, *Nurs Res* 38:186-187, 1989.

Lazarus RS, Folkman S: *Stress, appraisal, and coping,* New York, 1984, Springer.

Leidy NK, Darling-Fisher CS: Reliability and validity of the modified Erikson psychosocial stage inventory in diverse samples, *West J Nurs Res* 17(2):168-187, 1995.

Macnee CL, Talsma A: Development and testing of the barriers to cessation scale, *Nurs Res* 44(4):214-219, 1995.

Neelon VJ et al: The NEECHAM confusion scales: construction, validation, and clinical testing, *Nurs Res* 45(6):324-329, 1996.

Nunnally JC: *Psychometric theory,* New York, 1978, McGraw-Hill.

Perlow M: Validity and reliability of the PSES, *West J Nurs Res* 14(2):201-210, 1992.

Rempusheski VF: The proliferation of unreliable and invalid questionnaires, *Appl Nurs Res* 3(4):174-176, 1990.

Roberts KT, Aspy CB: Development of the serenity scale, *J Nurs Measure* 1(2):145-164, 1993.

Rudy EB et al: Patient outcomes for the chronically critically ill: special care unit versus intensive care unit, *Nurs Res* 44(6):324-331, 1995.

Sherman DW: Nurses' willingness to care for AIDS patients and spirituality, social support, and death anxiety, *Image* 28(3):205-213, 1996.

Templer DI: The construction and validation of a death anxiety scale, *J Gen Psychol* 82:165-177, 1970.

Tilden VP, Nelson CA, May BA: The IPR inventory: development and psychometric characteristics, *Nurs Res* 39(6):337-343, 1990.

Waltz C, Strickland O, Lenz E: *Measurement in nursing research,* ed 3, Philadelphia, 1991, FA Davis.

Ward SE, Berry PE, Misiewicz H: Concerns about analgesics among patients and family caregivers in a hospice setting, *Res Nurs Health* 19:205-211, 1996.

Ward S, Gatwood J: Concerns about reporting pain and using analgesics: a comparison of persons with and without cancer, *Cancer Nurs* 17:200-206, 1994.

Wikblad K, Anderson B: A comparison of three wound dressings in patients undergoing heart surgery, *Nurs Res* 44(5):312-316, 1995.

ADDITIONAL READINGS

Berk RA: Importance of expert judgment in content-related validity evidence, *West J Nurs Res* 12(5):659-671, 1990.

Grubba CJ, Popovich B, Jirovec MM: Reliability and validity of the Popovich scale in home health care assessments, *Appl Nurs Res* 3(4):161-163, 1990.

Laschinger HKS: Intraclass correlations as estimates of interrater reliability in nursing research, *West J Nurs Res* 14(2):246-251, 1992.

Reineck C: Nursing research instruments: pathway to resources, *Appl Nurs Res* 4(1):34-45, 1991.

Thomas SD, Hathaway DK, Arheart KL: Face validity, *West J Nurs Res* 14(1):109-112, 1992.

Weinert C, Tilden VP: Measures of social support: assessment of validity, *Nurs Res* 39(4):212-216, 1990.

Descriptive Data Analysis

Ann Bello

Key Terms

descriptive
statistics
frequency
distribution
interval
measurement
kurtosis
levels
of measurement
mean
measurement

measures of
central tendency
measures of
variability
median
modal percentage
modality
mode
nominal
measurement
normal curve

ordinal
measurement
percentile
range
ratio measurement
semiquartile range
(semiinterquartile
range)
standard deviation
(SD)
Z score

Learning Outcomes

After reading this chapter the student should be able to do the following:

- Define descriptive statistics.
- State the purposes of descriptive statistics.
- Identify the levels of measurement in a research study.
- Describe a frequency distribution.
- List measures of central tendency and their use.
- List measures of variability and their use.
- Critically analyze the descriptive statistics used in published research studies.

After carefully collecting data, the researcher is faced with the task of organizing the individual pieces of information so that the meaning is clear. It would be neither practical nor helpful to the reader to list individually each piece of data collected. The researcher must choose methods of organizing the raw data based both on the kind of data collected and on the hypothesis that was tested.

Statistical procedures are used to give organization and meaning to data. Procedures that allow researchers to describe and summarize data are known as **descriptive statistics.** Procedures that allow researchers to estimate how reliably they can make predictions and generalize findings based on the data are known as inferential statistics (see Chapter 15). Descriptive statistical techniques reduce data to manageable proportions by summarizing them, and they also describe various characteristics of the data under study. Descriptive techniques include measures of central tendency, such as mode, median, and mean; measures of variability, such as modal percentage, range, and standard deviation (SD); and some correlation techniques, such as scatter plots. The research consumer does not need detailed knowledge of how to calculate these statistics but does need an understanding of their meaning, use, and limitations.

Measures of central tendency describe the average member of the sample, whereas **measures of variability** describe how much dispersion is in the sample. If a researcher reported that the average age of one nursing class was 22 years, with the youngest member 18 and the oldest 25, and that in another nursing class students had an average age of 22 years, but the youngest member was 17 and the oldest 45, the reader would form a very different picture of the two classes. In both cases the average member of the sample was the same, but in the second class there was much greater variation or dispersion in the age of the members of the class.

Descriptive statistics may be presented in several ways in a research report. The data may be reported in words in the text of the report or summarized in tables or graphs. Whatever the method of presentation, the report should give the reader a clear and orderly picture of the research results.

This chapter and the next are designed to provide an understanding of statistical procedures. This chapter focuses on the understanding and evaluation of descriptive statistical procedures, and the next chapter discusses inferential statistical procedures. To evaluate the appropriateness of the statistical procedures used in a study, the research consumer should have an understanding of the **levels of measurement** that are appropriate to each statistical technique.

LEVELS OF MEASUREMENT

Measurement is the assignment of numbers to objects or events according to rules (Pedhazur and Schmelkin, 1991). Every event that is assigned a specific number must be similar to every other event assigned that number. For example, male subjects may be assigned the number 1 and female subjects the number 2. The measurement level is determined by the nature of the object or event being measured. Levels of measurement in ascending order are nominal, ordinal, interval, and ratio. The levels of measurement are the determining factors of the type of statistics to be used in analyzing data.

The higher the level of measurement, the greater the flexibility the researcher has in choosing statistical procedures. Every attempt should be made to use the highest level of measurement possible so that the maximum amount of information will be obtained from the data as highlighted in Table 14-1. The Critical Thinking Decision Path illustrates the relationship between levels of measurement and appropriate choice of specific descriptive statistics.

Table 14-1

Summary Table

MEASUREMENT	DESCRIPTION	MEASURES OF CENTRAL TENDENCY	MEASURES OF VARIABILITY
Nominal	Classification	Mode	Modal percentage, range, frequency distribution
Ordinal	Relative rankings	Mode, median	Range, percentile, semi-quartile range, frequency distribution
Interval	Rank ordering with equal intervals	Mode, median, mean	Range, percentile, semiquartile range, standard deviation
Ratio	Rank ordering with equal intervals and absolute zero.	Mode, median, mean	All

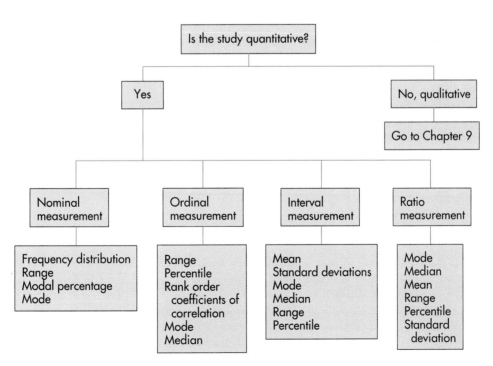

Critical Thinking Decision Path   Descriptive statistics.

Nominal Measurement

Nominal measurement is used to classify objects or events into categories. The categories are mutually exclusive; the object or event either has the characteristic or does not have it. The numbers assigned to each category are nothing more than labels; such numbers do not indicate more or less of a characteristic. Nominal level measurement can be used to categorize a sample on such information as gender, hair color, marital state, or religious affiliation. In Ward, Berry, and Misiewicz's (1996) study of concerns about the use of analgesics among hospice patients and their caregivers, there are several examples of nominal level measurement, including marital status, cancer site, caregiver relationship to patient, and sex (see Appendix D). The nominal level of measurement allows the least amount of mathematical manipulation. Most commonly the frequency of each event is counted, as well as the percent of the total each category represents. In Table 1 of their study, Ward, Berry, and Misiewicz (1996) summarize the marital status of participants by their status as patient or caregiver (see Appendix D).

Ordinal Measurement

Ordinal measurement is used to show relative rankings of objects or events. The numbers assigned to each category can be compared, and a member of a higher category can be said to have more of an attribute that one in a lower category. The intervals between numbers on the scale are not necessarily equal, nor is zero an absolute zero. For example, ordinal measurement is used to formulate class rankings where one student can be ranked higher or lower than another. However, the difference in actual grade point average between students may differ widely. In the study by Rudy et al (1995; see Appendix C) patient outcomes for the chronically critically ill measured severity of illness using an ordinal level measure, the APACHE II. Based on the assumption that the severity of illness can be quantified, this instrument predicts the risk of death. The range of possible scores is 0 to 71. A low number reflects less risk of death and a high number more risk of death. However, it is not possible to say a score of 71 represents 71 times more risk than a score of 0.

Ordinal level data are limited in the amount of mathematical manipulation possible. In addition to what is possible with nominal data, medians, percentiles, and rank order coefficients of correlation can be calculated.

Interval Measurement

Interval measurement shows rankings of events or objects on a scale with equal intervals between the numbers. The zero point remains arbitrary. For example, interval measurements are used in measuring temperatures on the Fahrenheit scale. The distances between degrees are equal, but the zero point is arbitrary.

In many areas in the social sciences, including nursing, there is much controversy over the classification of the level of measurement of intelligence, aptitude, and personality tests, with some regarding these measurements as ordinal and others as interval. The research consumer needs to be aware of this controversy and to look at each study individually in terms of how the data are analyzed (Knapp, 1990, 1993). Interval level data allow more manipulation of data, including the addition and subtraction of numbers and the calculation of means. This additional manipulation is why many want to argue for the higher classification level. The Barriers Questionnaire (BQ) is used as an interval measure by Ward, Berry, and Misiewicz (1996) in their study of concern about the use of analgesics in hospice patients and their caregivers.

Ratio Measurement

Ratio measurement shows rankings of events or objects on scales with equal intervals and absolute zeros. The number represents the actual amount of the property the object possesses. This is the highest level of measurement, but it is usually achieved only in the physical sciences. Examples of ratio level data are height, weight, pulse, and blood pressure. Rudy et al's (1995) study used ratio measurement in reporting length of stay in the hospital (see Appendix C).

All mathematical procedures can be performed on data from ratio scales. Therefore the use of any statistical procedure is possible as long as it is appropriate to the design of the study (see Chapter 15).

HELPFUL HINT
The descriptive statistics calculated must be appropriate to both the purpose of the study and the level of measurement.

FREQUENCY DISTRIBUTION

One of the most basic ways of organizing data is in a **frequency distribution.** In a frequency distribution the number of times each event occurs is counted or the data are grouped and the frequency of each group is reported. An instructor reporting the results of an examination could report the number of students receiving each grade or could group the grades and report the number in each group. Table 14-2 shows the results of an examination given to a class of 51 students. The results of the examination are reported in several ways. The columns on the left give the raw data tally and the frequency for each grade, whereas the columns on the right give the grouped-data tally and grouped frequencies. Rudy et al's (1995) study of outcomes of chronically critically ill patients, rather than reporting the results for each patient, groups the patients by care site and reports the results for each care site (see Appendix C).

When data are grouped, it is necessary to define the size of the group or the interval width so that no score will fall into two groups. The grouping of the data in Table 14-2 prevents overlap; each score falls into only one group. If the grouping had been 70 to 80 and 80 to 90, scores of 80 would have fallen into two categories. The grouping should allow for a precise presentation of the data without serious loss of information. Very large interval widths lead to loss of data information and may obscure patterns in the data. If the test scores in Table 14-2 had been grouped as 40 to 69 and 70 to 99, the pattern of the scores would have been obscured.

Information about frequency distributions may be presented in the form of a table, such as Table 14-2, or in graphic form. Figure 14-1 illustrates the most common graphic forms: the histogram and the frequency polygon. The two graphic methods are similar in that both plot scores or percentages of occurrence against frequency. The greater the number of points plotted, the smoother the resulting graph. The shape of the resulting graph allows for observations that will further describe the data.

Table 14-2

Frequency Distribution

INDIVIDUAL			GROUP		
SCORE	TALLY	FREQUENCY	SCORE	TALLY	FREQUENCY
90	|	1	>89	|	1
88	|	1			
86	|	1	80-89	⅃⅂ℸ ⅃⅂ℸ ⅃⅂ℸ	15
84	⅃⅂ℸ |	6			
82	||	2	70-79	⅃⅂ℸ ⅃⅂ℸ ⅃⅂ℸ ⅃⅂ℸ |||	23
80	⅃⅂ℸ	5			
78	⅃⅂ℸ	5			
76	|	1	60-69	⅃⅂ℸ ⅃⅂ℸ	10
74	⅃⅂ℸ ||	7			
72	⅃⅂ℸ ||||	9	<59	||	2
70	|	1			
68	|||	3			
66	||	2			
64	||||	4			
62	|	1			
60		0			
58	|	1			
56		0			
54	|	1			
52		0			
50		0			
TOTAL		51			51

Mean, 73.1; standard deviation, +12.1; median, 74; mode, 72; range, 36 (54-90).

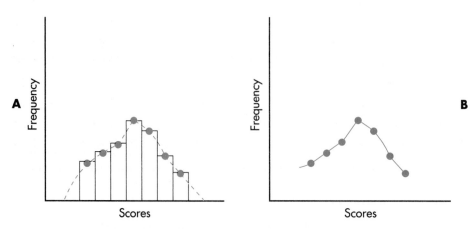

Figure 14-1   Frequency distributions. **A,** Histogram; **B,** frequency polygon.

MEASURES OF CENTRAL TENDENCY

Measures of central tendency answer questions such as "What does the average nurse think?" and "What is the average temperature of patients on a unit?" They yield a single number that describes the middle of the group. They summarize the members of a sample. Therefore they are known as summary statistics and are sample specific. Because they are sample specific, they change with each sample. Table 14-3 shows how Ward, Berry, and Misiewicz (1996), in their study of hospice patients and their caregivers concerns about analgesics, list means and SDs for each subscale and the total score on the BQ by patient and caregiver. These scores represent the average of each subscore and the total score and the amount of variation in each group on each of the reported scores. For example, the patient group had an average fear of addiction of 2.34 with an SD (variation) of 1.39. This means that 68% of the patient group scored between 0.95 and 3.73 on the measure of fear of addiction to analgesics.

Summary statistics also may be reported in narrative form as illustrated by the following excerpt from Badger's (1996) study of family members' experiences of living with members with depression.

Purposeful sampling was used to recruit 11 English-speaking family members who were living or who had recently lived with someone with depression. A combination of advertising at a local mental health clinic and network/snowball sampling in which initial informants referred others to the study was used. Of the family members, 9 were women, and 10 were White. A total of 7 family members were wives of men with depression, 2 were husbands of women with depression, and 2 were parents of children (1 son, 1 daughter) with depression. The mean age of the family members was 46 years (ranging from 32 to 61). Of the family members, 8 were married, and the mean number of years married was 18.8. A total of 8 had at least a baccalaureate education, and annual incomes ranged from below the poverty level to above $50,000.

Table 14-3

Illustration of Data Reporting: Mean (SD) BQ Subscale and Total Scores for Patients and Caregivers

SCALE	PATIENT	CAREGIVER	t
Fear of addiction	2.34 (1.39)	2.26 (1.18)	−0.35
Fatalism about pain relief	1.29 (1.05)	0.96 (1.01)	−1.80
Concern about drug tolerance	1.39 (1.35)	1.27 (1.25)	−1.41
Desires to be a good patient	1.73 (1.59)	0.83 (1.00)	−3.20*
Concern about side effects	2.50 (1.00)	2.57 (0.83)	0.35
Fear of injections	1.52 (1.27)	1.97 (1.64)	1.50
Concern about distracting MD	1.67 (1.28)	1.06 (1.09)	−2.15
Concern pain signifies disease progress	2.59 (1.39)	2.68 (1.53)	0.32
BQ total score	1.94 (0.85)	1.80 (0.61)	−0.92

From Ward SE, Berry PE, Misiewicz H: Concerns about analgesics among patients and family caregivers in a hospice setting, *Res Nurs Health* 19:209, 1996.

*$P < 0.01$.

The characteristics of a sample in a study are described in terms of summary statistics. The mean test score ($\overline{X} = 73.1$) reported in Table 14-2 is an example of such a statistic. If a different group of students was given the same test, it is likely that the mean would be different. The term *average* is a nonspecific, general term. In statistics there are three measures of central tendency: the mode, the median, and the mean. Depending on the distribution, these measures may not all give the same answer to the question, "What is the average?" Each measure of central tendency has a specific use and is most appropriate to specific kinds of measurement and types of distributions.

> **HELPFUL HINT**
> Careful review of the description of the sample will aid in deciding whether the study results are relevant to the population with whom the reader is working.

Mode

The **mode** is the most frequent score or result, and it can be obtained by inspection of the frequency distribution table or graph. A distribution can have more than one mode. The number of modes contained in a distribution is called the *modality* of the distribution. Figures 14-2, *A* and 14-3 show unimodal or one-peak distributions. Figure 14-2, *B,* shows a bimodal or two-peaked distribution. Multimodal distributions having two or more peaks are shown in Figure 14-2, *B* and *D.* Table 14-4 illustrates how the change in a few scores can change the modality of a distribution from unimodal to bimodal. The mode is most appropriately used with nominal data but can be used with all levels of measurement (see Table 14-1). It cannot be used for any subsequent calculations, and it is unstable; that is, the mode can fluctuate widely from sample to sample from the same population. A change in just one score in Table 14-2 would change the mode from 72.

Median

The **median** is the middle score or the score where 50% of the scores are above it and 50% of the scores are below it. The median is not sensitive to extremes in high and low scores. In the series of scores in Table 14-2 the twenty-sixth score will always be the median regardless of how high the highest or low the lowest score. It is best used when the data are skewed (see "Normal Distribution" in this chapter) and the researcher is interested in the "typical" score. For example, if age is a variable and there is a wide range with extreme scores that may affect the mean, it would be appropriate to also report the median. The median is easy to find by either inspection or calculation and can be used with ordinal or higher data as shown in Table 14-1.

Mean

The **mean** is the arithmetical average of all the scores and is used with interval or ratio data (see Table 14-1). It is what is usually thought of when the term *average* is used in general conversation and is the most widely used measure of central tendency. Most tests of significance use the mean (see Chapter 15). The mean is affected by every score but is more stable than the median

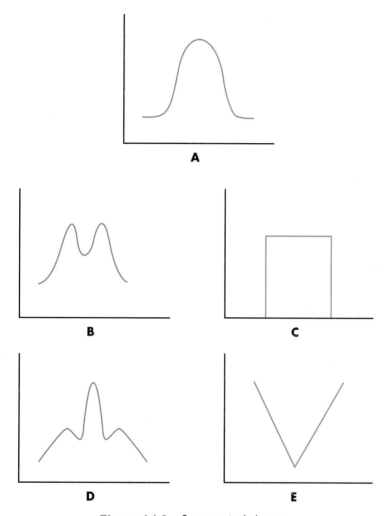

Figure 14-2 Symmetrical shapes.

or mode, and of the three measures of central tendency, it is the most constant or least affected by chance. The larger the sample size, the less affected the mean will be by a single extreme score. The mean is generally considered the single best point for summarizing data. In Table 14-4 the mean is the least affected by the change in the distribution from unimodal to bi-modal.

When one compares the measures of central tendency, the mean is the most stable and the median the most typical of these statistics. If the distribution is symmetrical and unimodal, the mean, median, and mode will coincide. If the distribution is skewed, the mean will be pulled in the direction of the long tail of the distribution. With a skewed distribution, all three statistics should be reported. For example, national income in the United States is skewed. The mean wage differs from the median wage, because the large salaries are so much greater than the low salaries.

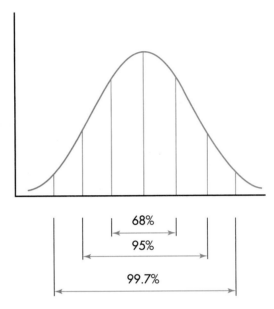

Figure 14-3 The normal distribution (mesokurtosis) and associated standard deviations.

Table 14-4			

Measures of Central Tendency

SCORE	FREQUENCY	MEASURE
35	JHT	
36	JHT III	Mode
37	IIII	Median, mean
38	JHT	
39	JHT	
40	JHT I	
35	JHT	
36	JHT III	Mode
37	III	Mean
38	IIII	Median
39	JHT III	Mode
40	JHT	

> **HELPFUL HINT**
> Of the three measures of central tendency, the mean is the most stable, least affected
> by extremes, and most useful for other calculations. The mean can only be calculated
> with interval and ratio data.

NORMAL DISTRIBUTION

The concept of the normal distribution is a theoretical one, based on the observation that data
from repeated measures of interval or ratio level data group themselves about a midpoint in a distribution in a manner that closely approximates the **normal curve** illustrated in Figure 14-3. In
addition, if the means of a large number of samples of the same interval or ratio data are calculated and plotted on a graph, that curve also approximates the normal curve. This tendency of
the means to approximate the normal curve is termed the *sampling distribution of the means.* The
mean of the sampling distribution of the means is the mean of the population (see Chapter 15).

The normal curve is one that is symmetrical about the mean and is unimodal. The mean,
median, and mode are equal. An additional characteristic of the normal curve is that a fixed
percentage of the scores falls within a given distance of the mean. As shown in Figure 14-3,
about 68% of the scores or means will fall within 1 SD of the mean; 95% within 2 SD of the
mean; and 99.7% within 3 SD of the mean.

Skewness

Not all samples of data approximate the normal curve. Some samples are nonsymmetrical and
have the peak off center. If one tail is longer than the other, the distribution is described in terms
of skew. In a positive skew the bulk of the data are at the low end of the range and there is a longer
tail pointing to the right or the positive end of the graph. World-wide individual income has a
positive skew, with most individuals in the low-to-moderate range and very few in the upper
range. The mean in a positive skew is to the right of the median. In a negative skew the bulk of the
data are in the high range and there is a longer tail pointing to the left or the negative end of the
graph. Age at death in the United States has a negative skew, because most deaths occur at older
ages. In a negative skew the mean is to the left of the median. Figure 14-4 illustrates positive and
negative skew. In each diagram the peak is off center and one tail is longer.

Symmetry

When the two halves of a distribution are folded over and they can be superimposed on each other,
the distribution is said to be *symmetrical.* In other words, the two halves of the distribution are mirror
images of each other. The overall shape of the distribution does not affect symmetry. Although the
shapes in Figure 14-2 are different, they are all symmetrical; however, only Figure 14-2, *A,* approximates the normal curve. Symmetry and modality are independent. Look at Figures 14-2, *A,* and 14-
3. These are all unimodal, but Figure 14-4 is skewed, whereas Figure 14-2, *A,* is symmetrical.

Kurtosis

Kurtosis is related to the peakness or flatness of a distribution. The peakness or flatness of a
distribution is related to the spread of the data. The farther the data are spread out on a scale,

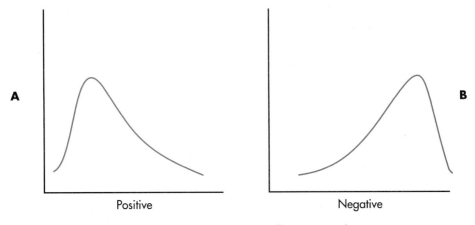

Figure 14-4   **A,** Positive skew; **B,** negative skew.

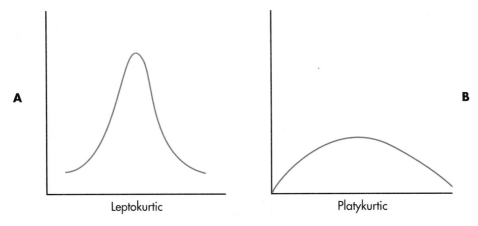

Figure 14-5   Kurtosis. **A,** Leptokurtosis; **B,** platykurtosis.

the flatter the peak. The distribution that peaks sharply is called *leptokurtic,* whereas a broad, flat distribution is called *platykurtic.* Figure 14-5 illustrates kurtosis. Neither the leptokurtic nor the platykurtic distributions approximate the normal curve or mesokurtic distribution.

INTERPRETING MEASURES OF VARIABILITY

Variability or dispersion is concerned with the spread of data. Samples with the same mean could differ in both distribution (kurtosis) and skew. Variability measures answer the questions "Is the sample homogeneous or heterogeneous?" and "Is the sample similar or different?" If a researcher measures oral temperatures in two samples, one sample drawn from a healthy population and one sample from a hospitalized population, it is possible that the two samples will have the same mean. However, it is likely that there will be a wider range of temperatures in the hospitalized sample than in the healthy sample. Measures of variability are used to describe these differences in the dispersion of data.

As with measures of central tendency, the various measures of variability are appropriate to specific kinds of measurement and types of distributions.

Modal percentage is used with nominal data and is the percentage of cases in the mode. A high modal percentage is indicative of decreased variability.

HELPFUL HINT
Remember that descriptive statistics related to variability will enable you to evaluate the homogeneity or heterogeneity of a sample.

Range

The **range** is the simplest but most unstable measure of variability. Range is the difference between the highest and lowest scores. A change in either of these two scores would change the range. The range should always be reported with other measures of variability. The range in Table 14-2 is 36, but this could easily change with an increase or decrease in the high score of 90 or the low score of 54.

Semiquartile Range

The **semiquartile range (semiinterquartile range)** indicates the range of the middle 50% of the scores. It is more stable than the range, because it is less likely to be changed by a single extreme score. It lies between the upper and lower quartiles, the upper quartile being the point below which 75% of the scores fall and the lower quartile being the point below which 25% of the scores fall. The middle 50% of the scores in Table 14-2 lies between 68 and 78, and the semiquartile range is 10.

Percentile

A **percentile** represents the percentage of cases a given score exceeds. The median is the 50% percentile, and in Table 14-2 it is a score of 74. A score in the 90th percentile is exceeded by only 10% of the scores. The zero percentile and the 100th percentile are usually dropped.

Standard Deviation

The **standard deviation (SD)** is the most frequently used measure of variability, and it is based on the concept of the normal curve (see Figure 14-3). It is a measure of average deviation of the scores from the mean and as such should always be reported with the mean. It takes all scores into account and can be used to interpret individual scores. Because the mean ($\overline{X}$) and standard deviation (SD) for the examination in Table 14-2 was 73.1 ± 12.1, a student should know that 68% of the grades were between 85.1 and 61. If the student received a grade of 88, he would know he did better than most of the class, whereas a grade of 58 would indicate he did not do as well as most of the class. Table 14-3, from the study by Ward, Berry, and Misiewicz (1996) reports the means and SDs of each subscale and the total score on the BQ by patient and caregiver. As illustrated in this table, the mean total score for the patient group was 1.94 and the SD was 0.85. This means that 68% of the patient group total scores would be expected to fall between 1.09 and 2.79. This table allows the reader to inspect the data and get a feel for the variation the data contain.

The SD is used in the calculation of many inferential statistics (see Chapter 15). One limitation of the SD is that it is expressed in terms of the units used in the measurement and cannot be used to compare means that have different units. If researchers were interested in the relationship between height measured in inches and weight measured in pounds, it would be necessary for them to convert the height and weight measurements to standard units or Z scores.

Z Scores

The **Z score** is used to compare measurements in standard units. Each of the scores is converted to a Z score, and then the Z scores are used to examine the relative distance of the scores from the mean. A Z score of 1.5 means that the observation is 1.5 SD above the mean, whereas a score of −2 means that the observation is 2 SD below the mean. By using Z scores, a researcher can compare results from scales that use different units, such as height and weight.

Many measures of variability exist. The modal frequency is the easiest to calculate, but the SD is the most useful. The SD and the semiquartile range always exist and are unique for each sample. The SD is the most stable statistic. Transformation of scores to Z scores allows comparison between scores that have different measurement units.

CORRELATION

Correlations are used to answer the question "To what extent are the variables related?" Correlations are used most commonly with ordinal or higher level data. Most correlations are discussed in Chapter 15, but here we will briefly mention scatter plots, which are visual representations of the strength and magnitude of the relationship between two variables. Figure 14-6 illustrates a perfect positive correlation, a perfect negative correlation, and no correlation. In most research, correlation results lie between these extremes. The strength of the correlation is demonstrated by

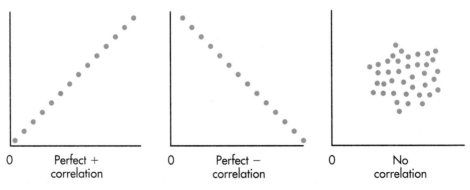

Figure 14-6   Scatter plots.

how closely the data points approximate a straight line. In a positive correlation, the higher the score on one variable, the higher the score on the other. Temperature and pulse are positively correlated; that is, a rise in temperature generally is associated with a rise in the pulse rate. In a negative correlation, the higher the score on one measure, the lower the score on the other measure. A decrease in blood volume is generally associated with a rise in the pulse rate.

CRITIQUING DESCRIPTIVE STATISTICS

Many students who have not had a course in statistics feel that they cannot critique descriptive statistics. However, students should be able to critically analyze the use of statistics even if they do not understand the derivation of the numbers presented. What is most important in critiquing this aspect of a research study is that the procedures for summarizing the data make sense in light of the purpose of the study (Critiquing Criteria box).

Before a decision can be made as to whether the statistics employed make sense, it is important to return to the beginning of the paper and determine the purpose of the study. Although all studies use descriptive statistics to summarize the data obtained, many studies go on to use identical statistics to test specific hypotheses (see Chapter 15). If a study is an exploratory one, it is possible that only descriptive statistics will be presented, because their purpose is to describe the characteristics of a population.

Just as the hypotheses should flow from the problem and purpose of a study, so should the hypotheses suggest the type of analysis that will follow. The hypotheses should indicate the major variables that are expected to be presented in summary form. Each of the variables in the hypotheses should be followed in the *Results* section with appropriate descriptive information.

After studying the hypotheses, the reader should proceed to the *Methods* section. Using the operational definition provided, the level of measurement employed to measure each of the variables that were listed in the hypotheses need to be identified. From this information it should be possible to determine the measures of central tendency and variability that should be employed to summarize the data. For example, you would not expect to see a mean used

CRITIQUING CRITERIA

1. Were appropriate descriptive statistics used?
2. What level of measurement is used to measure each of the major variables?
3. Is the sample size large enough to prevent one extreme score from affecting the summary statistics used?
4. What descriptive statistics are reported?
5. Were these descriptive statistics appropriate to the level of measurement for each variable?
6. Are there appropriate summary statistics for each major variable?
7. Is there enough information present to judge the results?
8. Are the results clearly and completely stated?
9. If tables and graphs are used, do they agree with the text and extend it, or do they merely repeat it?

as a summary statistic for the nominal variable of gender. In all likelihood, gender would be reported as a frequency distribution. The means and SDs should be provided for measurements performed at the interval level. The sample size is another aspect of the methods section that is important when evaluating the researcher's use of descriptive statistics. The larger the sample, the less chance that one outlying score will affect the summary statistics.

Only after these aspects of the study have been examined should the results presented by the researcher be considered. Each important variable should have an appropriate measure of central tendency and variability presented. If tables or graphs are used, they should agree with the information presented in the text. The tables and the charts should be clearly and completely labeled. If the researcher presents grouped frequency data, the groups should be logical and mutually exclusive. The size of the interval in grouped data should not obscure the pattern of the data, nor should it create an artificial pattern. Each table and chart should be referred to in the text, but each should add to the text—not merely repeat it. Each table or graph should have an obvious connection to the study being reported. For example, one table may describe the sample and another may present data relevant to the hypotheses being studied. Table 14-4 illustrates a clearly presented table; each group is mutually exclusive, and the data in the table agree with the data in the text.

The results should be written so that they are understandable to the intended audience. The audience for nursing research is the average practicing nurse. Thus the descriptive information presented should be clear enough that the reader can determine the usefulness of the study in the individual practice situation.

Descriptive statistics cannot be critiqued apart from the study as a whole. Each part of the research paper must make sense in relation to the entire paper. Therefore each portion of the paper should be evaluated in relation to what has preceded it. As such, the evaluation of the descriptive statistics must precede the evaluation of the inferential statistics.

The following is a partial critique of Rudy et al's (1995) study comparing outcomes for chronically critically ill cared for in two different units; only one option is chosen at each step:

Purpose of study:	To compare the effects of a low-technology environment of care and a nurse case management case delivery system with a traditional high-technology environment and primary nursing care delivery system
Hypothesis:	Null hypothesis (no difference in effects of care environment)
Dependent variable:	Length of stay
Conceptual definition:	Time individual remained in hospital
Operational definition:	Number of days individual remained in hospital
Level of measurement:	Ratio

Summary statistics:	Expected	Reported
	Number of days in hospital mean and standard deviation	In table 2—number of days in hospital by site of stay with mean and standard deviation

Sample size:	220 chronically critically ill individuals
Conclusion:	Reported statistics are appropriate for the problem, hypothesis, and level of measurement; sample size is large enough to prevent one score from having a large effect on the mean

KEY POINTS

- Descriptive statistics are a means of describing and organizing data gathered in research.
- The four levels of measurement are nominal, ordinal, interval, and ratio. Each has appropriate descriptive techniques associated with it.
- Measures of central tendency describe the average member of a sample. The mode is the most frequent score, the median is the middle score, and the mean is the arithmetrical average of the scores. The mean in the most stable and useful of the measures of central tendency, and with the standard deviation it forms the basis for many of the inferential statistics described in Chapter 15.
- The frequency distribution presents data in tabular or graphic form and allows for the calculation or observations of characteristics of the distribution of the data, including skewness, symmetry, modality, and kurtosis.
- In nonsymmetrical distributions the degree and direction of the pull of the peak off center are described in terms of skew.
- In speaking of modality the number of peaks is described as unimodal, bimodal, or multimodal.
- The relative spread of the data is described by kurtosis.
- Each characteristic of the frequency distribution is independent.
- Measures of variability reflect the spread of the data.
- The modal percentage is the percent of the cases in the mode.
- The ranges reflect differences between high and low scores.
- The standard deviation is the most stable and useful measure of variability. It is derived from the concept of the normal curve. In the normal curve, sample scores and the means of large numbers of samples group themselves around the midpoint in the distribution, with a fixed percentage of the scores falling within given distances of the mean. This tendency of means to approximate the normal curve is called the sampling distributions of the means. A Z score is the standard deviation converted to standard units.
- The scatter plot shows a measure of correlation.
- When critiquing published research reports, special emphasis should be given to the relationship of levels of measurement and appropriate descriptive techniques.

CRITICAL THINKING CHALLENGES

Barbara Krainovich-Miller

- Discuss the ways a researcher might use the computer in analyzing data and presenting descriptive statistical results of a study.
- What is the relationship between the level of measurement a researcher uses and the choice of a statistical procedure?
- What type of visual representation can be used to demonstrate the use of correlations? Use examples from clinical practice to illustrate the difference between positive and negative correlations.
- A classmate from research class tells you that she thinks it is ridiculous for the instructor to ask the students to critique the descriptive statistics used in a study when none of the students have taken a statistics course. Would you agree or disagree with her claim? Defend your position.

REFERENCES

Badger TA: Family members' experiences living with members with depression, *West J Nurs Res* 18(2):149-171, 1996.

Knapp TR: Treating ordinal scales as interval scales: an attempt to resolve the controversy, *Nurs Res* 39(2):121-123, 1990.

Knapp TR: Treating ordinal scales as ordinal scales, *Nurs Res* 42(3):184-186, 1993.

Pedhazur E, Schmelkin L: *Measurement, design and analysis: an integrated approach,* Hillsdale, NJ, 1991, Lawrence Erlbaum Associates.

Rudy EB et al: Patient outcomes for the chronically critically ill: special care unit versus intensive care unit, *Nurs Res* 44(8):324-331, 1995.

Ward SE, Berry PE, Misiewicz H: Concerns about analgesics among patients and family caregivers in a hospice setting, *Res Nurs Health* 19:205-211, 1996.

ADDITIONAL READINGS

Bluman AG: *Elementary statistics,* ed 2, Dubuque, 1995, WC Brown.

Iverson G: *Elementary statistics,* St Louis, 1995, Mosby.

Lund D: *Elementary statistics,* ed 3, Redwood City, Calif, 1996, Addison-Wesley.

Waltz CF, Strickland OL, Lenz ER: *Measurement in nursing research,* ed 2, Philadelphia, 1991, FA Davis.

Inferential Data Analysis

Margaret Grey

Key Terms

analysis of
  covariance
  (ANCOVA)
analysis of
  variance
  (ANOVA)
chi-square (χ^2)
correlation
degrees of
  freedom
factor analysis
Fisher's exact
  probability test
inferential
  statistics
level of
  significance
  (alpha level)

linear structural
  relationships
  (LISREL)
multiple analysis of
  variance
  (MANOVA)
multiple
  regression
nonparametric
  statistics
nonparametric
  tests of
  significance
null hypothesis
parameter
parametric
  statistics
path analysis

Pearson
  correlation
  coefficient
  (Pearson r;
  Pearson product
  moment
  correlation
  coefficient)
probability
sampling error
scientific
  hypothesis
standard error of
  the mean
t statistic
type I error
type II error

Learning Outcomes

After reading this chapter the student should be able to do
the following:

- Identify the purpose of inferential statistics.
- Distinguish between a parameter and a statistic.
- Explain the concept of probability as it applies to the
  analysis of sample data.
- Distinguish between type I and type II error and its
  effect on a study's outcome.
- Distinguish between parametric and nonparametric tests.
- List the commonly used statistical tests and their
  purposes.
- Critically analyze the statistics used in published research
  studies.

Inferential statistics are used to analyze the data collected in a research study. The reader of research studies needs to understand the purpose and application of statistics. Although it may be useful also to understand how statistical procedures are conducted, such knowledge is not critical to understanding published research findings. The purpose of this chapter is to demonstrate how researchers use inferential statistics to make conclusions about larger groups (the population of interest) from sample data. Basic concepts and terminology are presented in the sections that follow so that the reader can begin to make sense of the statistics used in research papers. Those readers who desire a more advanced discussion should refer to the "Additional Readings" section at the end of this chapter.

DESCRIPTIVE AND INFERENTIAL STATISTICS

Chapter 14 discussed descriptive statistics, which are the statistics used when the researcher needs to summarize the data. In this chapter our attention turns to the use of inferential statistics. **Inferential statistics** combine mathematical processes and logic that allows researchers to test hypotheses about a population using data obtained from probability samples. Statistical inference is generally used for two purposes—to estimate the probability that statistics found in the sample accurately reflect the population parameter and to test hypotheses about a population. In the first purpose, a **parameter** is a characteristic of a population, whereas a *statistic* is a characteristic of a sample. We use statistics to estimate population parameters. Suppose we randomly sample 100 people with chronic lung disease and use an interval scale to study their knowledge of the disease. If the mean score for these subjects is 65, the mean represents the *sample statistic.* If we were able to study every subject with chronic lung disease, we also could calculate an average knowledge score and that score would be the *parameter for the population.* As you know, a researcher rarely is able to study an entire population, so inferential statistics allow the researcher to make statements about the larger population from studying the sample.

The example given alludes to two important qualifications of how a study must be conducted so that inferential statistics may be used. First, it was stated that the sample was selected using probability methods (see Chapter 10). Because you already are familiar with the advantages of probability sampling, it should be clear that if we wish to make statements about a population from a sample, that sample must be representative. All procedures for inferential statistics are based on the assumption that the sample was drawn with a known probability. Second, it was stated that the scale had to reach the interval level of measurement. This is because the mathematical operations involved in doing inferential statistics require this level of measurement. The Critical Thinking Decision Path provides a matrix that researchers use for statistical decision making.

HYPOTHESIS TESTING

The second and most commonly used purpose of inferential statistics is hypothesis testing. Statistical hypothesis testing allows researchers to make objective decisions about the outcome of their study. The use of statistical hypothesis testing allows researchers to answer such questions as "How much of this effect is a result of chance?" or "How strongly are these two variables associated with each other?"

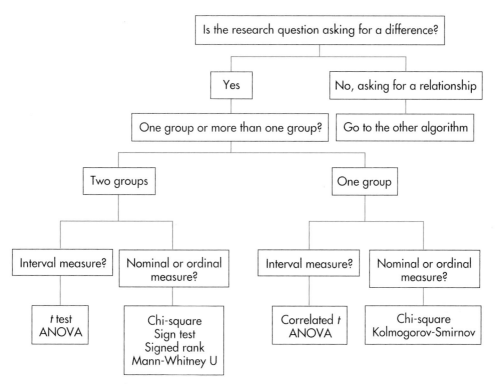

Critical Thinking Decision Path   Inferential statistics.

The procedures used when making inferences are based on principles of negative inference. In other words, if a researcher studied the effect of a new educational program for patients with chronic lung disease, the researcher would actually have two hypotheses—the scientific hypothesis and the null hypothesis. The research or **scientific hypothesis** is that which the researcher believes will be the outcome of the study. In our example the scientific hypothesis would be that the educational intervention would have a marked impact on the outcome in the experimental group beyond that in the control group. The **null hypothesis**, which is the hypothesis that actually can be tested by statistical methods, would state that there is *no* difference between the groups. Inferential statistics use the null hypothesis for testing the validity of a scientific hypothesis in sample data. The null hypothesis states that there is no actual relationship between the variables and that any observed relationship or difference is merely a function of chance fluctuations in sampling.

The concept of the null hypothesis is often confusing. An example may help to clarify this concept. The study by Rudy et al (1995; see Appendix C) provides a good example. The authors were interested in determining whether patients who were cared for in a special care unit had better outcomes than those cared for in a traditional critical care unit. The scientific hypothesis was the patients in the special care unit would have shorter length of stay and lower costs than those in the traditional unit. This hypothesis was based on clinical knowledge and previous findings in the literature. On the basis of this hypothesis, the authors then determined whether the differences found on the various outcome variables differed significantly between the two groups. The researchers used the null hypothesis—that there were no differences between the groups of patients—to test this scientific hypothesis. The authors found that the patients in the special care unit had no differences in length of stay, mortality, or complications when compared to the traditional care unit, but that there were differences in costs. In other words, the investigators found that the differences in the scores between the groups were large enough that they were unlikely to be caused by chance, and the null hypothesis was rejected. Note that the researcher would reject the null hypothesis. All statistical hypothesis testing is a process of disproof or rejection. It is impossible to prove that a scientific hypothesis is true, but it is possible to demonstrate that the null hypothesis has a high probability of being incorrect. To reject the null hypothesis, then, is considered to show support for the scientific hypothesis and is the desired outcome of most studies that use inferential statistics.

HELPFUL HINT

Remember that most samples used in clinical research are samples of convenience, but most researchers use inferential statistics. Although such use violates one of the assumptions of such tests, the tests are robust enough so as to not seriously affect the results unless the data are skewed in unknown ways.

PROBABILITY

The researcher can never prove the scientific hypothesis but can show support for it by rejecting the null hypothesis; that is, show that the null hypothesis has a high probability of being incorrect. We have now introduced the theory underlying all of the procedures discussed in this chapter—probability theory. **Probability** is a concept that we talk about all the time, such as the chance of rain today, but we have a difficult time defining it. The probability of an event is the event's long-run relative frequency in repeated trials under similar conditions. In other words, the statistician does not think of the probability of obtaining a single result from a single study but rather of the chances of obtaining the same result from an idealized study that can be carried out many times under identical conditions. It is the notion of repeated trials that allows researchers to use probability to test hypotheses.

Statistical probability is based on the concept of **sampling error.** Remember that the use of inferential statistics is based on random sampling. However, even when samples are randomly selected, there is always the possibility of some errors in sampling. Therefore the characteristics of any given sample may be different from those of the entire population. Suppose a group of researchers has at their disposal a large group of patients with decubitus ulcers and they wish to study the average length of time for ulcers to heal with the usual nursing care. If the researchers studied the entire population, they might obtain an average healing time of 50 days, with a standard deviation (SD) of 10 days. Now suppose that the researchers did not have the money necessary to study all of the patients but wished instead to do several consecutive studies of these patients. For this study they first draw a sample of 25 patients, calculate the mean and SD, and replace the subjects in the population before drawing the next sample. The researchers repeat this process many times so that they might end up with 50 different means. If the researchers then placed the means in a frequency distribution, it might appear as in Figure 15-1. This frequency distribution is a sampling distribution of the means. It illustrates that

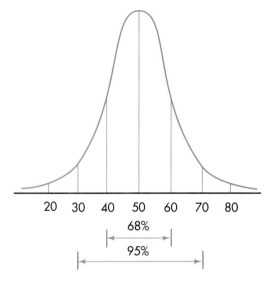

20   30   40   50   60   70   80

68%

95%

Figure 15-1   Sampling distribution of the means.

the researchers might find that one sample's mean might be 50.5, the next 47.5, the next 62.5, and so on. The tendency for statistics to fluctuate from one sample to another is known as *sampling* error.

Sampling distributions are theoretical. In practice, researchers do not routinely draw consecutive samples from the same population; usually they compute statistics and make inferences based on one sample. However, the knowledge of the properties of the sampling distribution—if these repeated samples are hypothetically obtained—permits the researcher to draw a conclusion based on one sample. This is possible because the sampling distribution of the means has certain known properties.

The sampling distribution of the means follows a normal curve, and the mean of the sampling distribution will be the mean of the population. As is discussed in the previous chapter, the fact that the sampling distribution of the means is normal tells us several other important things. When scores are normally distributed, we know that 68% of the cases will fall between +1 SD and −1 SD or that the probability is 68 out of 100 that any one randomly drawn sample mean will lie within the range of values between ±1 SD. In the example given, if we drew only one sample, we would have a 68% chance of finding a sample mean that fell between 40 and 60. The SD of a theoretical distribution of sample means is called the *standard error of the mean.* The word *error* is used because the various means that make up the distribution contain some error in their estimates of the population mean. The error is considered to be standard because it implies the magnitude of the average error, just as a standard deviation implies the average variation from one mean. The smaller the standard error, the less variable are the sample means and the more accurate are those means as estimates of the population value.

Although researchers rarely construct sampling distributions, standard error can be estimated because it bears a systematic relationship to the sample SD and the size of the sample.

This tells us that increasing the size of the sample will increase the accuracy of our estimates of population parameters. It should make intuitive sense that to increase the size of a sample will decrease the likelihood that one outlying score will dramatically affect the sample mean (see Chapter 14). The other reason that the sampling distribution is so important is that there are sampling distributions for all statistics. Researchers consult these distributions when making determinations about rejecting the null hypothesis.

TYPE I AND TYPE II ERRORS

The researcher's decision to accept or reject the null hypothesis is based on a consideration of how probable it is that the observed differences are a result of chance alone. Because data on the entire population are not available, the researcher can never flatly assert that the null hypothesis is or is not true. Thus statistical inference is always based on incomplete information about a population and it is possible for errors to occur when making this decision. There are two types of error in statistical inference—type I error and type II error.

Let us return to the example of the study by Rudy et al (1995; see Appendix C) of chronically critically ill patients in either special care or traditional critical care. Remember that the null hypothesis of the study was that there would be no differences in outcomes and costs between the two groups of patients. There were 145 patients in the special care group and 75 in the critical care unit. The authors found that there were not significant differences in length of stay, complications, or mortality, but that there were differences in costs. If the differences in cost that were found were truly a function of chance (e.g., because this group of patients was unusual in some way) and if the number studied was too small, a type I error would occur. A **type I error** is the researchers' rejection of the null hypothesis when it is actually true. If on the other hand, the researchers had found that the groups did not differ but they had studied only a few patients, a type II error might occur. A **type II error** is the researchers' acceptance of a null hypothesis that is actually false. The relationship of the two types of error is shown in Figure 15-2. In a practice discipline, type I errors are usually considered more serious. This is because if a researcher declares that differences exist where none are present, the potential exists for patient care to be affected adversely.

	REALITY	
Conclusion of test of significance	Null hypothesis is true	Null hypothesis is not true
Not statistically significant	Correct conclusion	Type II error
Statistically significant	Type I error	Correct conclusion

Figure 15-2   Outcome of statistical decision making.

HELPFUL HINT

Decreasing the alpha level acceptable for a study increases the chance that a type II error will occur. Remember that when a researcher is doing many statistical tests, the probability of some of the tests being significant increases as the number of tests increases. Therefore, when a number of tests are being conducted, the researcher will often decrease the alpha level to 0.01.

Level of Significance

The researcher does not know when an error in statistical decision making has occurred. It is possible to know only that the null hypothesis is indeed true or false if data from the total population are available. However, the researcher can control the risk of making type I errors by setting the level of significance before the study begins. The importance of setting the level of significance before the study is conducted is explained in detail by Slakter, Wu, and Suzuki-Slakter (1991). The **level of significance (alpha level)** is the probability of making a type I error, or the probability of rejecting a true null hypothesis. The minimum level of significance acceptable for nursing research is 0.05. If the researcher sets alpha, or the level of significance, at 0.05, the researcher is willing to accept the fact that if the study were done 100 times, the decision to reject the null hypothesis would be wrong 5 times out of those 100 trials. If as is sometimes done, the researcher wants to have a smaller risk of rejecting a true null hypothesis, the level of significance may be set at 0.01. In this case the researcher is willing to be wrong only once in 100 trials. The decision as to how strictly the alpha level should be set depends on how important it is to not make an error. For example, if the results of a study are to be used to determine whether a great deal of money should be spent in an area of nursing care, the researcher may decide that the accuracy of the results is so important that an alpha level of 0.01 is chosen. In most studies, however, alpha is set at 0.05.

Perhaps you are thinking that researchers should always use the lowest alpha level possible, because it makes sense that researchers would like to keep the risk of both types of errors at a minimum. Unfortunately, decreasing the risk of making a type I error increases the risk of making a type II error. What this means is that the stricter the researcher is in preventing the rejection of a true null hypothesis, the more likely is the possibility that a false null hypothesis will be accepted. Therefore the researcher always has to accept more of a risk of one type of error when setting the alpha level.

Practical Versus Statistical Significance

The reader should realize that there is a difference between statistical significance and practical significance. When a researcher tests a hypothesis and finds that it is statistically significant, this means that the finding is unlikely to have happened by chance. In other words, if the level of significance has been set at 0.05, the odds are 19 to 1 that the conclusion the researcher makes on the basis of the statistical test performed on sample data is correct. The researcher would reach the wrong conclusion only 5 times in 100. In other words, the researcher would obtain this result by chance alone only 5 times in 100.

Suppose a researcher is interested in the effect of loud rock music on the behavior of laboratory mice. The researcher could design an experiment to study this question and find that loud music makes the mice act strangely. A statistical test suggests that this finding is not the result of chance. However, such a finding may or may not have practical significance, even though the finding has statistical significance. Although some would argue that this study might have relevance to understanding the behavior of teenagers, some would argue also that the study has no practical value. Thus the findings of a study may have statistical significance, but they may have no practical value or significance. Although researchers should consider the practicality of a problem in the early stages of a research project (see Chapter 3), a distinction between the statistical and practical significance of the findings should also be made when discussing the results of a study. Some people believe that if findings are not statistically significant, they have no practical value. Consider the study by Rudy et al (1995; see Appendix C), who studied the outcomes in patients in two types of patient care systems. In this study some of the scientific hypotheses were also the null hypothesis and the researchers indeed confirmed the null hypothesis that outcomes in the special care unit would not be worse than those of patients in traditional critical care units. These findings have practical importance because they reject common practice on the basis of scientific findings.

TESTS OF STATISTICAL SIGNIFICANCE

Tests of significance may be *parametric* or *nonparametric*. Most of the studies in nursing research literature use parametric tests that have the following three attributes:

1. They involve the estimation of at least one parameter
2. They require measurement on at least an interval scale
3. They involve certain assumptions about the variables being studied

These assumptions usually include that the variable is normally distributed in the overall population. In contrast to parametric tests, **nonparametric tests of significance** are not based on the estimation of population parameters, so they involve less restrictive assumptions about the underlying distribution. Nonparametric tests usually are applied when the variables have been measured on a nominal or ordinal scale.

There has been some debate about the relative merits of the two types of statistical tests. The moderate position taken by most researchers and statisticians is that nonparametric statistics are best used when the data cannot be assumed to be at the interval level of measurement or when the sample is small and the normality of the underlying distribution cannot be inferred. However, if these assumptions can be made, most researchers prefer to use **parametric statistics** because they are more powerful and more flexible than **nonparametric statistics**.

There are many different statistical tests of significance that researchers use to test hypotheses. The procedure and the rationale for their use are similar from test to test. Once the researcher has chosen a significance level and collected the data, the data are used to compute the appropriate test statistic. For each test there is a related theoretical distribution that shows the probable and improbable values for that statistic. On the basis of the statistical result and the values in the distribution, the researcher either accepts or rejects the null hypothesis and then reports both the statistical result and its probability. Thus a researcher may perform a statistical test called a *t test*, obtain a value of 8.98, and report that it is statistically significant at the $P < 0.05$ level. This means that the researcher had 5 chances out of 100 to be wrong in concluding that this result could not have been obtained by chance. In addition, the likelihood of finding a statistic that is high enough to be statistically significant is increased as the sample size

Table 15-1

Tests of Differences Between Means

LEVEL OF MEASUREMENT	ONE GROUP	TWO GROUPS RELATED	TWO GROUPS INDEPENDENT	MORE THAN TWO GROUPS
Nonparametric				
Nominal	Chi-square	Chi-square Fisher exact probability	Chi-square	Chi-square
Ordinal	Kolmogorov-Smirnov	Sign test Wilcoxon matched pairs Signed rank	Chi-square Median test Mann-Whitney U	Chi-square
Parametric				
Interval or ratio	Correlated t ANOVA (repeated measures)	Correlated t	Independent t ANOVA	ANOVA ANCOVA MANCOVA

increases. This likelihood is indicated by the **degrees of freedom** that are often reported with the statistic and the probability value. Degrees of freedom is usually abbreviated as df.

Tables 15-1 and 15-2 show the most commonly used inferential statistics. The test that is used depends on the level of the measurement of the variables in question and the type of hypothesis being studied. Basically these statistics test two types of hypotheses—that there is a difference between groups (Table 15-1) or that there is a relationship between two or more variables (Table 15-2).

HELPFUL HINT

Just because a researcher has used nonparametric statistics does not mean that the study is not useful. The use of nonparametric statistics is appropriate when measurements are not made at the interval level or the variable under study is not normally distributed.

Tests of Difference

Suppose a researcher has done an experimental study using an after-only design (see Chapter 7). What the researcher hopes to determine is that the two randomly assigned groups are different after the introduction of the experimental treatment. If the measurements taken are at the interval level, the researcher would use the t test to analyze the data. If the t statistic were found to be high enough as to be unlikely to have occurred by chance, the researcher would reject the null hypothesis and conclude that the two groups were indeed more different than would have been expected on the basis of chance alone. In other words, the researcher would conclude that the experimental treatment had the desired effect.

A study by Caudell and Gallucci (1995) illustrates the use of the t statistic. The authors were studying the neuroendocrine and immunological responses of women to stress. They

Table 15-2		

Tests of Association

LEVEL OF MEASUREMENT	TWO VARIABLES	MORE THAN TWO VARIABLES
Nonparametric		
Nominal	Phi coefficient	Contingency coefficient
	Point-biserial	
Ordinal	Kendall's tau	Discriminant function analysis
	Spearman rho	
Parametric		
Interval or ratio	Pearson r	Multiple regression
		Path analysis
		Canonical correlation

used the t test for paired samples to determine how the various measures changed from before the stress test to after the stress test. They found that heart rate, skin conductance, peripheral skin temperature, and blood pressure increased, but neuroendocrine measures did not change. These differences were determined using the t statistic.

Parametric Tests

The t statistic is commonly used in nursing research. This statistic tests whether two group means are different. Thus this statistic is used when the researcher has two groups, and the question is whether the mean scores on some measure are more different than would be expected by chance. To use this test the variables must have been measured at the interval or ratio level, and the two groups must be independent. By *independent* we mean that nothing in one group helps to determine who is in the other group. If the groups are related, as when samples are matched (see Chapter 10), and the researcher also wants to determine differences between the two groups, a *paired* or *correlated* t test would be used.

The t statistic illustrates one of the major purposes of research in nursing—to demonstrate that there are differences among groups. Groups may be naturally occurring collections, such as age groups, or they may be experimentally created. The type of test that is used for any particular study depends primarily on whether the researcher is examining differences in one, two, or more groups and whether the data to be analyzed are nominal, ordinal, or interval (see Table 15-1).

Sometimes a researcher has more than two groups, or measurements are taken more than once, as in the study in Appendix C (Rudy et al, 1995). In Table 2 of the study (see Appendix C), the researchers report data about differences between the intensive care patients and the special care unit patients. Because some of the data are at the interval level, the researchers used the statistic known as the **analysis of variance (ANOVA)** for some of the variables. In the table, these variables are the ones in the "STAT" column with an "F." Analysis of variance, like the t statistic, tests whether group means differ, but rather than testing each pair of means separately, ANOVA considers the variation among all groups. In other studies the researchers are interested in differences that occur before and after something occurs. This is the case in the study referred to earlier by Caudell and Gallucci (1995). The appropriate statistic is the repeated measures analysis of variance, because this statistic takes into account the fact that multiple measures affect the potential range of scores.

HELPFUL HINT

A research report may not always contain the test that was done. The reader can find this information by looking at the tables. For example, a table with t statistics will contain a column for "t" values, and an ANOVA table will contain "F" values.

In other cases, particularly in experimental work, the researchers use t tests or ANOVA to determine whether random assignment to groups was effective in creating groups that are equivalent before introduction of the experimental treatment. In this case the researcher wants to show that there is no difference among the groups. In a study by O'Sullivan and Jacobson (1992) of the effects of a special treatment program for teen mothers, the authors report, "There were no statistically significant differences between the experimental group, the control group, and the refusals (nonparticipants) in maternal age, length of prenatal care, whether or not the adolescent had a previous pregnancy, and complications of the mother or infant at delivery." Suppose, however, that these groups had differed on length of prenatal care. For the researchers to conclude that their experimental program was effective, they would need to control statistically for length of prenatal care. This is done by using the technique of **analysis of covariance (ANCOVA)**. ANCOVA also measures differences among group means, and it uses a statistical technique to equate the groups under study on an important variable. Another expansion of the notion of analysis of variance is **multiple analysis of variance (MANOVA)**, which is used also to determine differences in group means, but it used when there is more than one dependent variable.

Nonparametric Tests

In the example from O'Sullivan and Jacobson (1992), we noted that the researchers tested whether the subjects in the experimental or treatment group were similar in the number of complications of pregnancy. The number of complications of pregnancy is not interval level data, so the researchers could not test this difference with any of the tests discussed thus far. When data are at the nominal level and the researcher wants to determine whether groups are different, the researcher uses another commonly used statistic, the **chi-square (χ^2)**. Chi-square is a nonparametric statistic that is used to determine whether the frequency in each category is different from what would be expected by chance. As with the t test and ANOVA, if the calculated chi-square is high enough, the researcher would conclude that the frequencies found would not be expected on the basis of chance alone and the null hypothesis would be rejected. Although this test is quite robust and can be used in many different situations, it cannot be used to compare frequencies when samples are small and expected frequencies are less than 6 in each cell. In these instances the **Fisher's exact probability test** is used. An example of the use of chi-square to determine differences among groups can be found in Rudy et al's (1995) paper reprinted in Appendix C. Refer again to Table 2, and note that some variables, such as mortality, discharge status, and readmission status, are measured at the nominal level. To determine if outcomes were different between the intensive care and special care groups, the researchers used the chi-square statistic.

When the data are ranks, or at the ordinal level, researchers have several other nonparametric tests at their disposal. These include the Kolmogorov-Smirnov test, the sign test, the Wilcoxon matched pairs test, the signed rank test for related groups, and the median test and the Mann-Whitney U test for independent groups. Explanation of these tests is beyond the scope of this chapter; those readers who desire further information are referred to the "Additional Readings" section at the end of the chapter.

A randomized clinical trial by Naylor (1990) of the effects of a comprehensive discharge planning protocol implemented by a gerontological nurse specialist illustrates the use of several of these statistical tests. The researcher was interested in comparing the new method of discharge planning with usual discharge planning. Although the patients were randomly assigned to experimental and treatment groups, it was important to determine whether the random assignment procedure succeeded in creating equivalent groups, especially because the sample was small. For data measured at the nominal level, such as gender and race, the chi-square statistic was used. For data measured at the interval level, such as age, the *t* test was used. Finally, to test the effect of the intervention, either ANOVA or chi-square was used, depending on the level of measurement.

Tests of Relationships

Researchers often are interested in exploring the relationship between two or more variables. Such studies use statistics that determine the **correlation,** or the degree of association, between two or more variables. Tests of the relationships between variables are sometimes considered to be descriptive statistics when they are used to describe the magnitude and direction of a relationship of two variables in a sample and the researcher does not wish to make statements about the larger population. Such statistics can also be inferential when they are used to test hypotheses about the correlations that exist in the target population.

Null hypothesis tests of the relationships between variables assume that there is no relationship between the variables. Thus when a researcher rejects this type of null hypothesis, the conclusion is that the variables are in fact related. Suppose a researcher is interested in the relationship between the age of patients and the length of time it takes them to recover from surgery. As with other statistics discussed, the researcher would design a study to collect the appropriate data and then analyze the data using measures of association. In the example, age and length of time until recovery can be considered to be interval level measurements. The researcher would use a test called the **Pearson correlation coefficient, Pearson *r*,** or **Pearson product moment correlation coefficient.** Once the Pearson *r* is calculated, the researcher consults the distribution for this test to determine whether the value obtained is likely to have occurred by chance. Again the research reports both the value of the correlation and its probability of occurring by chance.

The interpretation of correlation coefficients often is difficult for students who are learning statistics. Correlation coefficients can range in value from −1.0 to +1.0 and also can be zero. A zero coefficient means that there is no relationship between the variables. A perfect positive correlation is indicated by a +1.0 coefficient, and a perfect negative correlation by a −1.0 coefficient. We can illustrate the meaning of these coefficients by using the example from the previous paragraph. If there were no relationship between the age of the patient and the time he or she required to recover from surgery, the researcher would find a correlation of zero. However, if the correlation were +1.0, this would mean that the older the patient, the longer it took him or her to recover. A negative coefficient would imply that the younger the patient, the longer it would take him or her to recover. Of course, relationships are rarely perfect. The magnitude of the relationship is indicated by how close the correlation comes to the absolute value of 1. Thus a correlation of −0.76 is just as strong as a correlation of +0.76, but the direction of the relationship is opposite. In addition, a correlation of 0.76 is stronger than a correlation of 0.32. When a researcher tests hypotheses about the relationships between two variables, the test considers whether the magnitude of the correlation is large enough not to have occurred by chance. This is the meaning of the probability value or the P value reported with correlation coefficients. As with other statistical tests of significance, the larger the sample, the greater the likelihood of finding a significant correlation. Therefore researchers also report the degrees of freedom associated with the test performed.

McCain and Cella (1995) conducted a cross-sectional study to examine the relationships among psychological distress, quality of life, uncertainty, coping patterns, stress, and CD4+ T-lymphocyte levels. The authors found that increased negative stress was correlated significantly with lower quality of life, with a correlation coefficient of 0.64, suggesting that as human immunodeficiency virus–positive (HIV+) patients experienced more negative stressors, they had lower quality of life. This reflects a moderately high correlation, and it indicates that approximately 41.94% (0.64 × 0.64) of the variability in quality of life is explained by negative stressful experiences.

Nominal and ordinal data also can be tested for relationships by nonparametric statistics. When two variables being tested have only two levels (e.g., male/female; yes/no), the phi coefficient can be used to express relationships. When the researcher is interested in the relationship between a nominal variable and an interval variable, the point-biserial correlation is used. Spearman rho is used to determine the degree of association between two sets of ranks, as is Kendall's tau. All of these correlation coefficients may range in value from −1.0 to +1.0. These tests are shown in Table 15-2. Naylor (1990) used the phi coefficient to determine the relationship of type of discharge planning and length of time since discharge.

Nursing problems rarely are so simple that they can be explained by only two variables. When researchers are interested in studying complex relationships among more than two variables, they use techniques other than those we have discussed thus far. When researchers are interested in understanding more about a problem than just the relationship between two variables, they often use a technique called **multiple regression,** which measures the relationship between one interval level dependent variable and several independent variables. Multiple regression is the expansion of correlation to include more than two variables, and it is used when the researcher wants to determine what variables contribute to the explanation of the dependent variable and to what degree. For example, a researcher may be interested in determining what factors help women decide to breastfeed their infants. A number of variables, such as the mother's age, previous experience with breastfeeding, number of other children, and knowledge of the advantages of breastfeeding, might be measured and then analyzed to see whether they, separately and together, predict the length of breastfeeding. Such a study would require the use of multiple regression. The results of a study such as this might help nurses to know that a younger mother with only one other child might be more likely to benefit from a teaching program about breastfeeding than an older mother with several other children.

The reader of research reports often will see multiple regression techniques described as forward solution, backward solution, or stepwise solution. These are techniques that are used in multiple regression to find the smallest group of variables that will account for the greatest proportion of variance in the dependent variable. In the *forward solution* the independent variable with the highest correlation with the dependent variables is entered first, and the next variable is the one that will increase the explained variance the most. In the *backward solution* all variables are entered into the solution and each variable is deleted to see whether the explained variance drops significantly. The stepwise solution is a combination of the two approaches. In general, all of the approaches give similar, although not identical, results (Bryk and Raudenbush, 1992).

Suppose the individual who was researching breastfeeding was interested in not just breastfeeding but also maternal satisfaction. *Canonical correlation* is used when there is more than one dependent variable. If the data are nominal or ordinal, the contingency coefficient or discriminant function analyses are used. These last tests are beyond the scope of this text; further information can be found in the "Additional Readings" section.

In the study by McCain and Cella (1995), the authors were interested in furthering the understanding of the stress-adaptation model of coping with chronic illness. To do so, they needed to go beyond the analysis of relationships between two variables. In a diagram, they describe the interrelationships among the variables as determined by stepwise multiple regression analysis. The authors found that higher levels of negative stress and more frequent use of emotion-focused coping were associated with lower quality of life, higher psychosocial distress, and more uncertainty.

Advanced Statistics

Sometimes researchers are interested in even more complex problems. For example, Hall et al (1996) examined the role of self-esteem as a mediator of the effects of stressors and social resources on mother's postpartum depressive symptoms. On the basis of a theoretical model, the author postulated that self-esteem would be affected by stressors and life events, as well as social resources, and that self-esteem would, in turn, affect depressive symptoms. To test this mediating effect requires a type of advanced statistics called *path analysis*. In **path analysis** the researcher hypothesizes the ways variables are related and in what order and then tests how strong those relationships or paths are. In this study, the authors did find that self-esteem mediated depressive symptoms.

This notion of testing specific relationships in a specific order can be extended further to test hypothesized variables that are made up of several measures. A technique called the analysis of **linear structural relationships (LISREL)** tests path models made up of variables that are not actually measured. For example, a researcher might study the concept of self-esteem and use three different measures to determine subjects' levels of self-esteem. The researcher would test how carefully these three measures actually measure self-esteem by testing a measurement model using LISREL. Because many of the variables of interest to nursing are not easily defined and measured and because we are ultimately interested in causal models, LISREL is becoming more commonly used in nursing studies; for examples, see Mishel et al (1991) and DilOrio, Hennessy, and Mantueffel (1996). In both examples the researchers were testing theories about complex problems, and the LISREL technique allowed them the opportunity to study complex interactions among variables simultaneously.

Another advanced technique often used in nursing research is factor analysis. **Factor analysis** helps us to understand concepts more fully and contributes to our ability to measure concepts reliably and validly (see Chapter 13). Factor analysis takes a large number of variables and groups them into a smaller number of factors. It is used to reduce a set of data so that it may be easily described and used. In addition, factor analysis is used for instrument development and theory development. In instrument development, factor analysis is used to group individual items on a scale into meaningful factors or subscales. Smyth and Yarandi (1996), for example, were interested in testing the reliability and validity of the Ways of Coping Questionnaire in African-American women. Factor analysis was used to determine whether the scale actually measured the concepts that they intended the instrument to measure.

Many other statistical techniques are available to nurse researchers. Consult any of the statistics sources listed in the "Additional Readings" section if further information is desired or if a test not discussed is included in a study of interest to you.

CRITIQUING INFERENTIAL STATISTICAL RESULTS

Many students find that critiquing inferential statistics is difficult or even impossible if they have not taken a course in statistics. Although there is some merit to this feeling, there are aspects of the statistical analysis that should be possible to critique without the benefit of years of statistics course work. Important questions to consider when critiquing the use of inferential statistics are listed in the Critiquing Criteria box.

The first place to begin critiquing the statistical analysis of a research report is with the hypothesis. The hypothesis should indicate to you what type of statistics will be used. If the hypothesis indicates that a relationship will be found, you should expect to find indexes of cor-

CRITIQUING CRITERIA

1. Does the hypothesis indicate that the researcher is interested in testing for differences between groups or in testing for relationships?
2. What is the level of measurement chosen for the independent and dependent variables?
3. Does the level of measurement permit the use of parametric statistics?
4. Is the size of the sample large enough to permit the use of parametric statistics?
5. Has the researcher provided enough information to decide whether the appropriate statistics were used?
6. Are the statistics used appropriate to the problem, the hypothesis, the method, the sample, and the level of measurement?
7. Are the results for each of the hypotheses presented appropriately?
8. Do the tables and the text agree?
9. Are the results understandable?
10. Is a distinction made between practical significance and statistical significance? How?
11. What is the level of significance set for the study? Is it applied throughout the paper?

relation. If the study is experimental or quasiexperimental, the hypothesis would indicate that the author is looking for differences between the groups studied, and you would expect to find statistical tests of differences between means.

Then as you read the *Methods* section of the paper, consider what level of measurement the author has used to measure the important variables. If the level of measurement is interval or ratio, the statistics most likely will be parametric statistics. On the other hand, if the variables are measured at the nominal or ordinal level, the statistics used should be nonparametric. Also consider the size of the sample, and remember that samples have to be large enough to permit the assumption of normality. If the sample is quite small, for example, 5 to 10 subjects, the researcher may have violated the assumptions necessary for inferential statistics to be used. Thus the important question is whether the researcher has provided enough justification to use the statistics presented.

Finally, consider the results as they are presented. There should be enough data presented for each hypothesis studied to determine whether the researcher actually examined each hypothesis. The tables should accurately reflect the procedure performed and be in harmony with the text. For example, the text should not indicate that a test reached statistical significance, while the tables indicate that the probability value of the test was above 0.05. If the researcher has used analyses that are not discussed in this text, you may want to refer to a statistics text to decide whether the analysis was appropriate to the hypothesis and the level of measurement.

There are two other aspects of the data analysis section that the reader should critique. The paper should not read as if it were a statistical textbook. The results of the study in the text of the paper should be clear enough to the average reader so that the reader can determine what was done and what the results were. In addition, the author should attempt to make a distinction between practical and statistical significance. Some results may be statistically significant, but their practical importance may be doubtful. If this is so, the author should note it. Alternatively, you may find yourself reading a research report that is elegantly presented, but you come away with a "so what?" feeling. Such a feeling may indicate that the practical significance of the study and its findings have not been adequately explained in the report.

Note that the critical analysis of a research paper's statistical analysis is not done in a vacuum. It is possible to judge the adequacy of the analysis only in relationship to the other important aspects of the paper: the problem, the hypotheses, the design, the data collection methods, and the sample. Without consideration of these aspects of the research process, the statistics themselves have very little meaning. Statistics can lie; thus it is most important that the researcher use the appropriate statistic for the problem. For example, a researcher may sometimes use a nonparametric statistic when it appears that a parametric statistic is appropriate. Because parametric statistics are more powerful than nonparametric, the result of the parametric analysis may not have been what the researcher expected. However, the nonparametric result might be in the expected direction, so the researcher reports only that result.

EXAMPLE OF THE USE AND CRITIQUE OF INFERENTIAL STATISTICS

Earlier in this chapter reference was made to the study by Rudy et al (1995; see Appendix C) comparing patient outcomes for chronically critically ill patients cared for in a traditional critical care environment versus a special care unit. The statement of purpose implies that the authors were interested in looking at differences among groups. Therefore the reader should expect that the analysis will consist of statistical tests that examine differences between means, such as ANOVA or the *t* test.

Some of the major variables, such as mortality and discharge status, were measured at the nominal level, so nonparametric statistics are used for this comparison. Other major variables, such as length of hospital stay and numbers of complications, were measured at the interval level, and differences between the two groups were determined using ANOVA. The researchers used ANOVA and chi-square to determine that the two groups had equivalent demographic and illness characteristics before determining if the care outcomes differed.

The hypotheses were tested using ANOVA or chi-square, depending on the level of measurement of the variable. These tests are appropriate to the problem, because the researchers were interested in differences between the two types of care systems. Results for each of the hypotheses are presented, and they suggest that there is no difference in many outcomes between the two groups. Tables agree with the text, and the results are understandable to the reader. The discussion points out limitations to the study. Clear implications for practice are found, and they support the practical significance of the study. The statistical level of significance was set at 0.05 and is consistent throughout the paper. Therefore the researchers' statistics were appropriate to the study's purpose, method, sample, and levels of measurement.

KEY POINTS

- Inferential statistics are a tool to test hypotheses about populations from sample data.
- Because the sampling distribution of the means follows a normal curve, researchers are able to estimate the probability that a certain sample will have the same properties as the total population of interest. Sampling distributions provide the basis for all inferential statistics.
- Inferential statistics allow researchers to estimate population parameters and to test hypotheses. The use of these statistics allows researchers to make objective decisions about the outcome of the study. Such decisions are based on the rejection or acceptance of the null hypothesis, which states there is no relationship between the variables.
- If the null hypothesis is accepted, this result indicates that the findings are likely to have occurred by chance. If the null hypothesis is rejected, the researcher accepts the scientific hypothesis of a relationship being present between the variables and that this relationship is unlikely to have been found by chance.
- Statistical hypothesis testing is subject to two types of error—type I and type II.
- Type I error occurs when the researcher rejects a null hypothesis that is actually true.
- Type II error occurs when the researcher accepts a null hypothesis that is actually false.
- The researcher controls the risk of making a type I error by setting the alpha level, or level of significance. Unfortunately, reducing the risk of a type I error by reducing the level of significance increases the risk of making a type II error.
- The results of statistical tests are reported to be significant or nonsignificant. Statistically significant results are those whose probability of occurring is less than 0.05 or 0.01, depending on the level of significance set by the researcher.

- Commonly used parametric and nonparametric statistical tests include those that test for differences between means, such as the *t* test and ANOVA, and those that test for differences in proportions, such as the chi-square test.
- Tests that examine data for the presence of relationships include the Pearson *r*, the sign test, the Wilcoxon matched-pairs, signed ranks test, and multiple regression.
- Advanced statistical procedures include path analysis, LISREL, and factor analysis.
- The most important aspect of critiquing statistical analyses is the relationship of the statistics employed to the problem, design, and method used in the study. Clues to the appropriate statistical test to be used by the researcher should stem from the researcher's hypotheses. The reader also should determine if all of the hypotheses have been presented in the paper.

CRITICAL THINKING CHALLENGES

Barbara Krainovich-Miller

? What assumption(s) is violated when a clinical research study uses a convenience sample and applies inferential statistics?

? What are the advantages and disadvantages of decreasing the alpha level for a study? What is the relationship between setting an alpha level and type I and type II errors?

? Discuss the parameters for using nonparametric statistics in a study and its impact on the usefulness of the findings.

? Discuss the way a reader of a research report can use the Internet to determine if the appropriate inferential statistic was used.

REFERENCES

Bryk AS, Raudenbush SW: *Hierarchical linear models,* Newbury Park, Calif, 1992, Sage.

Caudell KA, Gallucci BB: Neuroendocrine and immunological responses of women to stress, *West J Nurs Res* 17:672-692, 1995.

DilOrio C, Hennessy M, Manteuffel B: Epilepsy self-management: a test of a theoretical model, *Nurs Res* 45:211-217, 1996.

Hall LA et al: Self-esteem as a mediator of the effects of stressors and social resources on depressive symptoms in postpartum mothers, *Nurs Res* 45:231-238, 1996.

McCain NL, Cella DF: Correlates of stress in HIV disease, *West J Nurs Res* 17:141-155, 1995.

Mishel MH et al. Uncertainty in illness theory: a replication of the mediating effects of mastery and coping, *Nurs Res* 40:236-240, 1991.

Naylor MD: Comprehensive discharge planning for hospitalized elderly: a pilot study, *Nurs Res* 39:156-161, 1990.

O'Sullivan AL, Jacobson BS: A randomized trial of a health care program for first-time adolescent mothers and their infants, *Nurs Res* 41:210-215, 1992.

Rudy EB et al: Patient outcomes for the chronically critically ill: special care unit versus intensive care unit, *Nurs Res* 44:324-331, 1995.

Slakter MJ, Wu YWB, Suzuki-Slakter NS: *, **, and ***: statistical nonsense at the .00000 level, *Nurs Res* 40:248-249, 1991.

Smyth K, Yarandi HN: Factor analysis of the Ways of Coping Questionnaire for African American women, *Nurs Res* 45:25-29, 1996.

ADDITIONAL READINGS

Blaloch HM: *Causal inferences in nonexperimental research,* New York, 1972, WW Norton.

Ferketich S, Muller M: Factor analysis revisited, *Nurs Res* 39:59-62, 1990.

Jacobson BS, Tulman L, Lowery BJ: Three sides of the same coin: the analysis of paired data from dyads, *Nurs Res* 40:359-363, 1991.

Joreskog KG, Sorbom D: *Advances in factor analysis and structural equation models,* Cambridge, Ma, 1979, Clark Abt.

Kerlinger FN, Pedhazur EJ: *Foundations of behavioral research,* ed 2, New York, 1986, Holt, Rinehart, & Winston.

Knapp TR: Treating ordinal scales as interval scales: an attempt to resolve the controversy, *Nurs Res* 39:121-125, 1990.

Knapp TR: Regression analysis: what to report, *Nurs Res* 43:187-189, 1994.

Lucke JF: Testing the homogeneity of correlated variances from a bivariate normal distribution, *Nurs Res* 43:314-315, 1994.

Nield M, Gocka I: To correlate or not to correlate: what is the question? *Nurs Res* 42:294-296, 1993.

Pedhazur EJ: *Multiple regression in behavioral research,* ed 2, New York, 1982, Holt, Rinehart, & Winston.

Sidani S, Lynn MR: Examining amount and pattern of change: comparing repeated measures ANOVA and individual regression analysis, *Nurs Res* 42:283-286, 1993.

Analysis of the Findings

Geri LoBiondo-Wood

Key Terms

findings
generalizability
limitations
recommendations

Learning Outcomes

After reading this chapter the student should be able to do the following:

- Discuss the difference between the *Results* section of a study and the discussion of the results.
- Identify the format of the *Results* section.
- Determine if both statistically supported and statistically nonsupported findings are discussed.
- Determine whether the results are objectively reported.
- Describe how tables and figures are used in a research report.
- List the criteria of a meaningful table.
- Identify the format and components of the discussion of the results.
- Determine the purpose of the *Discussion* section.
- Discuss the importance of including generalizations and limitations of a study in the report.
- Determine the purpose of including recommendations in the study report.

The ultimate goals of nursing research are to develop nursing theory and knowledge and to substantiate and improve nursing practice, thereby widening the scientific basis of the nursing profession. From the viewpoint of the research consumer, the analysis of the results, interpretations, and generalizations that a researcher generates from a study becomes a highly important piece of the research project. It is after the analysis of the data that the researcher puts the final pieces of the jigsaw puzzle together to view the total picture with a critical eye. This process is analogous to *evaluation,* the last step in the nursing process. The consumer of research may view these last sections as an easier step for the investigator, but it is here that a most critical and creative process comes into use. It is in these final sections of the report, after the statistical procedures have been applied, that the researcher will interrelate the statistical or numerical findings to the theoretical framework, literature, methods, hypotheses, and problem statements.

The final sections of published research reports generally are titled *Results* and *Discussion,* but other topics, such as limitations of findings, implications for future research, and nursing practice, recommendations, and conclusions may be separately addressed or subsumed within these sections. The presentational format of these areas is a function of the author's and the journal's stylistic considerations. The function of these final sections is then to interrelate all aspects of the research process and to discuss, interpret, and identify the limitations and generalizations relevant to the investigation and thereby further nursing research. The process that both an investigator and the consumer of research use to assess the results of a study is depicted in the Critical Thinking Decision Path. The goal of this chapter is to introduce the purpose and content of the final sections of a research investigation where data are presented, interpreted, discussed, and generalized. An understanding of what an investigator presents in these sections will assist the research consumer to critically analyze an investigator's findings.

FINDINGS

The **findings** of a study are the results, conclusions, interpretations, recommendations, generalizations, implications for future research, and nursing practice, which will be addressed by separating the presentation into two major areas. These two areas are the results and the discussion of the results. The *Results* section will focus on the results or statistical findings of the study, and the *Discussion of the Results* section will focus on the remaining topics. For both sections the rule applies, as it does to all other sections of a report, that the content needs to be presented clearly, concisely, and logically.

Results

The *Results* section of a research report is considered to be the data-bound section of the report. It is here that the researcher presents the quantitative data or numbers generated by the descriptive and inferential statistical tests. The results of the data analysis set the stage for the *Interpretations* or *Discussion* section that follows the results. The *Results* section should then reflect the problem and hypothesis tested. The information from each hypothesis or research question should be sequentially presented. The tests used to analyze the data should be mentioned. If the exact test that was used is not explicitly stated, then the values obtained should be noted. This is done by providing the numerical values of the

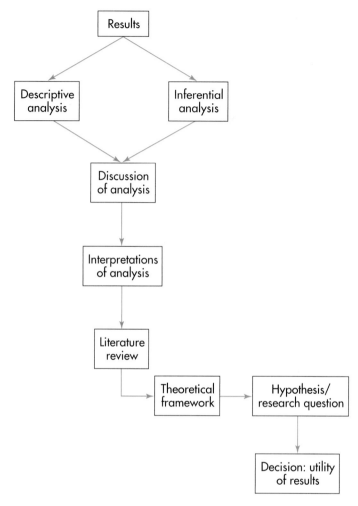

Critical Thinking Decision Path   Assessing study results.

statistics and stating the specific correlation and probability level, or t value (see Chapters 14 and 15). Examples of these can be found in Table 16-1. These numbers and their signs should not frighten the novice. These numbers are important, but there is much more to the research process than the numbers. They are one piece of the whole. Chapters 14 and 15 conceptually present the meanings of the numbers found in studies. Whether the consumer only superficially understands statistics or has an in-depth knowledge of statistics, it should be obvious to the reader that the results are clearly stated, and the presence or lack of statistically significant results should be noted. The "Additional Readings" list at the end of this chapter also provides further detail for those interested in the application of statistics.

Table 16-1

Examples of Reported Statistical Results

STATISTICAL TEST	EXAMPLES OF REPORTED RESULTS
Mean	$m = 118.28$
Standard deviation	$SD = 62.5$
Pearson correlation	$r = 0.39, P < 0.01$
Analysis of variance	$F = 3.59, df = 2, 48, P < 0.05$
t test	$t = 2.65, P < 0.01$
Chi-square	$\chi^2 = 2.52, df = 1, P < 0.05$

HELPFUL HINT

In the *Results* section of a research report the descriptive statistics results are generally presented first, then the results of each of the hypotheses or research questions that were tested.

The researcher is bound to present the data for all of the hypotheses posed, such as whether the hypotheses were accepted, rejected, supported, or not supported. If the data supported the hypotheses, it may be assumed that the hypotheses were proved, but this is not true. It does not necessarily mean that the hypotheses were proved; it means only that the hypotheses were supported and that the results suggest that the relationships or differences tested, which were derived from the theoretical framework, were probably logical. The beginning research consumer may think that if a researcher's results were not supported statistically or only partially supported, the study is irrelevant or possibly should not have been published, but this also is not true. If the data are not supported, the critiquer should not expect the researcher to bury the work in a file. It is as important for a critiquer of research to review and understand nonsupported studies as it is for the researcher. Information obtained from nonsupported studies often can be as useful as data obtained from supported studies. Nonsupported studies can be used to suggest **limitations** of particular aspects of a study's design and procedures. Data from nonsupported studies may suggest that current modes of practice or current theory in an area may not be supported by research and therefore need to be reexamined and researched further. Data then assist a profession to generate new knowledge, as well as prevent stagnation of knowledge. Generally it has been noted that an investigator will interpret the results in a separate section of the report. At times the reader may find that the *Results* section contains the results and the researcher's interpretations, which generally fall into the *Discussion* section. Integrating the results with the discussion in a report becomes the decision of the author or journal editor. Integration of both sections may be used when a study contains several segments that may be viewed as fairly separate subproblems of a major overall problem.

The investigator should also demonstrate objectivity in the presentation of the results. A quote such as: "For women with no barriers, anxiety was related negatively to adherence ($r = -.31, P < .01; n = 79$). For women with barriers, anxiety was not related to adherence ($r = -.05, P < .30; n = 87$)" (Lauver et al, 1997) is the appropriate means to express results. The investigators would be accused of lacking objectivity if they had stated the results in the fol-

Box 16-1   Examples of Results Section

Quantitative Studies

"Significant main effects over time were found in overall quality of life, F (4, 160) = 19.30, $P <$ .001; and in the domains of health functioning, F (4, 160) = 14.30, $P <$ .001; and psychological/spiritual, F (4, 160) = 14.01, $P <$ .001." (LoBiondo-Wood et al, 1997)

"There was no difference between the groups in the number of life-threatening complications, with an average of about one life-threatening complication per patient. However, the SCU patients had significantly more documented episodes of bradycardia (pulse < 40 BPM), 14.5% vs. 3% in the ICUs ($P <$ .006), and more episodes of a decrease in neurological status (SCU 13% vs. ICUs 4%, $P <$ .033) were obtained." (Rudy et al, 1995)

"Patients' and caregivers' total BQ scores were not significantly correlated. Fatalism was the only one of the eight subscales for which the correlation was statistically significant [see Table 16-2]. Even in this instance, the magnitude of the association was not large (R^2 = .24) and the subscale involved (fatalism) is the one with the most questionable reliability." (Ward, Berry, and Misiewicz, 1996)

Qualitative Studies

"Participants emphasized the break from the dungeon and the journey to freedom resulted in lives very different from those experienced before healing. The men indicated that as they began to emerge from their confinement, they felt alive. They came to believe they belonged on earth and had reclaimed their right to live free." (Draucker and Petrovic, 1996) (The researchers detail the meaning of this and provide examples of subjects' responses.)

"Most of the participant discussion concerned antecedent conditions needed before collaboration could occur. Two major processes were required to get to the point where the core of the process, working together, could take place: being available and being receptive. Both nurse and resident participants reported only beneficial outcomes from the process of collaboration." (Baggs and Schmitt, 1997) (The researchers provide further examples of the concepts and a model of the process.)

lowing manner: "The results surprisingly showed that there was a significant relationship between women with no barriers and anxiety." Opinions or reactionary statements to the data in the *Results* section therefore are inappropriate. Box 16-1 provides examples of objectively stated results from both quantitative and qualitative studies. The critiquer of a study should consider the following points when reading a *Results* section:

- The investigators responded objectively to the results in the discussion of the results.
- In the discussion of the results the investigator interpreted the results, with a careful reflection on all aspects of the study that preceded the results.
- The data presented are summarized. A great deal of data are generated, but only the critical numbers for each test are presented. An example of summarized data are the

means and standard deviations of age, education, and income. Including all data is too cumbersome. The results can be viewed as a summation section.

- The condensation of data is done both in the written text and through the use of tables and figures. Tables and figures facilitate the presentation of large amounts of data.
- Results for the descriptive and inferential statistics for each hypothesis or research question are presented. No data should be omitted even if not significant.

In the study by Ward, Berry, and Misiewicz (1996; see Appendix D), the researchers developed tables to present the results visually. Table 16-2 provides demographic descriptive results about the patient and caregivers. Table 16-3 provides the results of testing for a relationship between patients' and caregivers' concerns about barriers to reporting pain and taking analgesics, using Pearson correlation. The tables allow the researchers to provide a more thorough explanation and discussion of the results. If tables and figures are used, they need to be concise. Although the text is the major mode of communicating the results, the tables and figures serve a supplementary but independent role. The role of tables and figures is to report results with some detail that the investigator does not enter into the text. This does not mean that tables and figures should not be mentioned in the text. The amount of detail that the author uses in the text to describe the specific tabled data varies with the needs of the researcher. A good table is one that meets the following criteria:

- Supplements and economizes the text
- Has precise titles and headings
- Does not repeat the text

Table 16-2

Demographic Information About the Patients and the Caregivers

	PATIENTS		CAREGIVERS	
	n	%	*n*	%
Marital status				
Married	21	60%	28	80%
Not married	14	40%	7	20%
Education				
< HS	7	20%	1	3%
HS grad	19	54%	16	46%
> HS grad	8	23%	17	48%
Missing data	1	3%	1	3%
Income				
< $29,000/year	25	71%	18	52%
> $30,000/year	6	17%	17	48%
Missing data	4	12%	—	—

Another example of a table that meets these criteria can be found in the study by Rudy et al (1995; see Appendix C). The research team wanted to report the comparisons of patient outcomes between intensive care unit patients and special care unit patients on a number of variables. Because of the number of variables, it is much clearer for the reader to have a table that easily and clearly summarizes the results as this table does. To describe each one of these in the text of the article would not have economized space and would have been difficult to visualize. The table developed by the researchers (Table 16-4) allows the readers not only to visualize the variables quickly but also to assess the results.

HELPFUL HINT

A well-written *Results* section is systematic, logical, concise, and drawn from all of the analyzed data. All that is written in the *Results* section should be geared to letting the data reflect the testing of the problems and hypotheses. The length of this section depends on the scope and breadth of the analysis.

Discussion of the Results

In the final section of the report the investigator interpretively discusses the results of the study. It is in this section that a skilled researcher makes the data come alive. The researcher gives the numbers in quantitative studies or the concepts in qualitative studies meaning and interpretation. The reviewer may ask where the investigator extracted the meaning that is applied in this section. If the researcher does the job properly, you will find a return to the beginning of the study. The researcher returns to the earlier points in the study where a problem statement was identified and independent and dependent variables were related on the basis

---

Table 16-3

Internal Consistency (Alpha) for BQ Subscale and Total Scores for Patients and Caregivers and Correlation Between Patient and Caregiver BQ Scores

| | ALPHA | | CORRELATION |
SUBSCALE	PATIENT	CAREGIVER	PATIENT/CAREGIVER
Fear of addiction	0.69	0.75	0.36
Fatalism about pain relief	0.57	0.37	0.49*
Concern about drug tolerance	0.76	0.81	0.07
Desires to be a good patient	0.82	0.80	0.26
Concern about side effects	0.58	0.71	0.15
Fear of injections	0.82	0.69	0.28
Concern about distracting MD	0.74	0.70	0.03
Concern pain signifies disease progress	0.91	0.89	0.27
BQ total score	0.82	0.90	0.13

*$P < 0.01$.

Table 16-4

Comparison of Patient Outcomes Between ICU Patients and SCU Patients*

VARIABLE	SPECIAL CARE UNIT $n = 145$	INTENSIVE CARE UNIT $n = 75$	STAT	P VALUE	EFFECT SIZE	POWER
Mortality						
Died	44 (30.3%)	31 (41.3%)	$\chi^2 = 0.66$	0.103	0.05	0.36
Lived	101 (69.7%)	44 (58.7%)				
Discharge disposition from hospital						
Died	44 (30.3%)	31 (41.3%)				
Other hospital	3 (2.1%)	0 (0%)	$\chi^2 = 4.55$	0.473	0.14	0.33
Long-term care	31 (21.4%)	14 (18.7%)				
Rehabilitation	21 (14.5%)	11 (14.7%)				
Home	45 (31.0%)	19 (25.3%)				
Home ventilator	1 (0.7%)	0				
Length of hospital stay (days)	48.6 ± 29.5 (9 to 160)	50.6 ± 33.4 (8 to 176)	$F = 0.20$	0.655	0.03	0.07
Readmit†						
Yes	8 (8%)	9 (20%)	$\chi^2 = 4.65$	0.031	0.18	0.48
No	93 (92%)	35 (80%)				
Total number of infections	1.6 ± 2.3 (0 to 10)	1.7 ± 2.3 (0 to 10)	$F = 0.27$	0.870	0.02	0.05
Total number of respiratory complications	2.14 ± 1.9 (0 to 7)	2.25 ± 1.9 (0 to 7)	$F = 0.10$	0.688	0.03	0.06
Life-threatening complications	1.12 ± 1.4 (0 to 8)	0.88 ± 1.2 (0 to 5)	$F = 2.16$	0.1917	0.09	0.26

*Continuous variables reported as $m \pm SD$, with range noted below.
†The n used for this calculation included only patients who survived to discharge ($n = 145$).

of a theoretical framework and literature review. It is in this section that the researcher discusses the following:

- Both the supported and nonsupported data
- The limitations or weaknesses of a study in light of the design and the sample or data collection procedures
- How the theoretical framework was supported
- How the data may suggest additional or previously unrealized relationships

Even if the data are supported, the reviewer should not believe it to be the final word.

Downs (1984) cautions that the research critiquer should not be overwhelmed by small P values, because they are not indicative of research breakthroughs. To the critiquer of a research study this means that statistical significance in a research study does not always mean that the results of a study are clinically significant. As the body of nursing research grows, so does the profession's ability to critically analyze beyond the tests of significance and assess a research study's applicability to practice. Chapter 19 reviews methods used to analyze the usefulness of research findings. Also, within the nursing literature, discussion about clinical significance has emerged (Becker, 1993; Bergstrom, 1991; LeFort, 1993; Polit and Sherman, 1990; Titler et al, 1994). As indicated throughout this text, many important pieces in the research puzzle need to fit together for a study to be evaluated as a well-done project. Therefore researchers and reviewers should accept statistical significance with prudence. Statistically significant findings are not the sole means of establishing the study's merit. Other aspects, such as theory, sample, instrumentation, and methods, also should be considered.

When the results are not statistically supported, the researcher also returns to the theoretical framework and analyzes the earlier thinking process. Results of nonsupported hypotheses do not require the investigator to go on a fault-finding tour of each piece of the project. Such a course can then become an overdone process. All research has weaknesses. This analysis is an attempt to identify the weaknesses and to suggest what the possible problem or problems were in the study. At times the theoretical thinking is correct, but the researcher finds problems or limitations that could be attributed to the tools (see Chapters 12 and 13), the sampling methods (see Chapter 10), the design (see Chapters 6 through 9), or the analysis (see Chapters 14 and 15). Therefore when results are not supported, the investigator attempts to go on a *fact*-finding tour rather than a *fault*-finding one. The purpose of the discussion then is not to show humility or one's technical competence but rather to enable the reviewer to judge the validity of the interpretations drawn from the data and the general worth of the study (Kerlinger, 1986).

It is in the *Discussion* section of the report that the researcher ties together all the loose ends of the study. It is from this point that reviewers of research can begin to think about clinical relevance, the need for replication, or the germination of a new idea for a prospective research study. Finally, the reviewer of a research project should find this section either in separate sections or subsumed within the *Discussion* section, and it should include generalizability and recommendations for future research, as well as a summary or a conclusion.

Generalizations (**generalizability**) are inferences that the data are representative of similar phenomena in a population beyond the study's sample. Reviewers of research are cautioned not to generalize beyond the population on which a study is based. Beware of research studies that may overgeneralize. Generalizations that draw conclusions and make inferences within a particular situation and at a particular time are appropriate. An example of such a generalization is drawn from the study conducted by Alexy et al (1997) that was designed to determine whether predictors of birth outcomes differ for women in rural versus urban areas. The researchers, when discussing the sample in light of the results, appropriately noted:

To increase the generalizability of this epidemiological study, a larger sample size from multiple sites must be obtained. However, the findings support the contention that rural and urban women are different in both demographic and behavioral factors that potentially influence birth weight.

This type of statement is important for reviewers of research. It helps to guide thinking in terms of a study's clinical relevance, and it also suggests areas for further research (see Chapter 19). One study does not provide all of the answers, nor should it. The final steps of evaluation are critical links to the refinement of practice and the generation of future research. Evaluation of research, like evaluation of the nursing process, is not the last link in the chain but a connection between findings that may serve to improve nursing theory and nursing practice.

HELPFUL HINT
It has been said that a good study is one that raises more questions than it answers. So the research consumer should not view an investigator's review of limitations, generalizations, and implications of the findings for practice as lack of research skills.

The final area that the investigator integrates into the *Discussion* section is the recommendations. The **recommendations** are the investigator's suggestions for the study's application to practice, theory, and further research. This requires the investigator to reflect on the question "What contribution to nursing does this study make?" Box 16-2 provides examples of recommendations for future research and implications for nursing practice. This evaluation places the study into the realm of what is known and what needs to be known before being utilized. Fawcett (1982) noted, "It is through future exploration of the dissemination and utilization of research in nursing practice that the science of nursing will become an entity with which to be reckoned." This thought is critical and has been reaffirmed by many nurse researchers in the past decade, such as Bower (1994), Downs (1996), Gennaro and Vessey (1991), Gortner (1990), and Schmitt (1994).

CRITIQUING THE RESULTS AND DISCUSSION

The results and the discussion of the results are the researcher's opportunity to examine the logic of the hypothesis(es) posed, the theoretical framework, the methods, and the analysis (Critiquing Criteria box). This final section requires as much logic, conciseness, and specificity as was employed in the preceding steps of the research process. The consumer should be able to identify statements of the type of analysis that was used and whether the data statistically supported the hypothesis(es). These statements should be straightforward and not reflect bias (see Table 16-2). Auxiliary data or serendipitous findings also may be presented. If such auxiliary findings are presented, they should be as dispassionately presented as were the hypothesis data. The statistical tests used also should be noted. The numerical value of the obtained data also should be presented (see Table 16-1). The presentation of the tests, the numerical values found, and the statements of support or nonsupport should be clear, concise, and systematically reported. For illustrative purposes that facilitate readability the researchers should present extensive findings in tables.

Box 16-2	Examples of Research Recommendations and Practice Implications

Research Recommendations

"Further research is needed to determine whether patient and caregiver concerns change over the course of the illness and whether one versus the other person's concerns have greater impact on the adequacy with which the patient's pain is managed." (Ward, Berry, and Misiewicz, 1996)

"Longitudinal study of both recipients and their families is necessary for addressing the issues of quality of life. Though recipients' quality of life improves, a question remains regarding family members' view of the recipients' changes." (LoBiondo-Wood et al, 1997)

Practice Implications

"The results of this study demonstrate that carefully selected patients can be cared for outside of the ICU setting under the care of well-trained nurse case managers, with no threat to patient outcomes and with significant cost savings. This finding has major implications for the care of long-term critically ill patients." (Rudy et al, 1995)

"Homophobia was inversely related to intention to provide care. Therefore, interventions should be used that decrease levels of homophobia in student nurses in order to promote care. Workshops and faculty role modeling, as previously mentioned, as well as panel discussions by individuals who are homosexual should prove beneficial." (Cole, 1996)

 CRITIQUING CRITERIA

1. Are all of the results of each hypothesis presented?
2. Is the information regarding the results concisely and sequentially presented?
3. Are the tests that were used to analyze the data presented?
4. Are the results presented objectively?
5. If tables or figures are used, do they meet the following standards?
   a. They supplement and economize the text.
   b. They have precise titles and headings.
   c. They are not repetitious of the text.
6. Are the results interpreted in light of the hypotheses and theoretical framework and all of the other sections that preceded the results?
7. If the data are supported, does the investigator provide a discussion of how the theoretical framework was supported?
8. If the data are not supported, does the investigator attempt to identify the weaknesses and suggest what the possible problems were in the study?
9. Does the investigator discuss the study's clinical relevance?
10. Are any generalizations made?
11. Are the generalizations within the scope of the findings or beyond the findings?
12. Are any recommendations for future research stated or implied?

The *Discussion* section should interpret the data, the gaps, the limitations of the study, and the conclusions, as well as give recommendations for further research. Drawing these aspects into the study should give the consumer a sense of the relationship of the findings to the theoretical framework. Statements reflecting the underlying theory are necessary, whether or not the hypotheses were supported.

If the findings were not supported, the consumer should, as the researcher did, attempt to identify, without fault finding, possible methodological problems. Finally, a concise presentation of the study's generalizability and the implications of the findings for practice and research should be evident. The last presentation can help the research consumer to begin to rethink clinical practice, provoke discussion in clinical settings (see Chapter 19), and find similar studies that may support or refute the phenomena being studied to more fully understand the problem.

KEY POINTS

- The analysis of the findings is the final step of a research investigation. It is in this section that the consumer will find the results printed in a straightforward manner.
- All results should be reported whether or not they support the hypothesis. Tables and figure may be used to illustrate and condense data for presentation.
- Once the results are reported, the researcher interprets the results. In this presentation, usually titled *Discussion,* the consumer should be able to identify the key topics being discussed. The key topics, which include an interpretation of the results, are the limitations, generalizations, implications, and recommendations for future research.
- The section on interpretation of the results is where the researcher draws together the theoretical framework and makes interpretations based on the findings and theory. Both statistically supported and nonsupported results should be interpreted. If the results are not supported, the researcher should discuss the results reflecting on the theory, as well as possible problems with the methods, procedures, design, and analysis.
- The researcher should present limitations or weaknesses of the study. This presentation is important, because it affects the study's generalizability. The generalizations or inferences about similar findings in other samples also are presented in light of the findings.
- The research consumer should be alert for sweeping claims or overgeneralizations that a researcher may state. An overextension of the data can alert one to possible researcher bias.
- The recommendations provide the consumer with suggestions regarding the study's application to practice, theory, and future research. These recommendations furnish the critiquer with a final perspective of the researcher on the utility of the investigation.

CRITICAL THINKING CHALLENGES

Barbara Krainovich-Miller

❓ Defend or refute the following statement: "All results should be reported and interpreted whether or not they support the hypothesis(es)."

❓ What type of knowledge does the researcher draw on to interpret the results of a study? Is the same type of knowledge used when the results of a study are not statistically significant?

? Do you agree or disagree with the statement that a good study is one that raises more
  questions than it answers. Support your view with examples.

? How is it possible for consumers of research to critique the findings and recommendations
  of a reported study? How could you use the Internet for critiquing the findings of a study?

REFERENCES

Alexy B et al: Prenatal factors and birth outcomes in the Public Health Service: a rural/urban
  comparison, *Res Nurs Health* 20:61-70, 1997.

Baggs JG, Schmitt MH: Nurses' and resident physicians' perceptions of the process of collaboration in an MICU, *Res Nurs Health* 20:71-80, 1997.

Becker PT: A lingering identity crisis, *Res Nurs Health* 16:87-88, 1993.

Bergstrom N: Scientific base for nursing practice is a goal of ANA, *Council Nurs Res* 18(2):1,
  7, 1991.

Bower F: Research: outcomes must be the focus, *Image* 26:4, 1994.

Cole FL: Factors associated with student nurses' intent to provide physical and psychosocial
  care to persons with acquired immunodeficiency syndrome, *J Prof Nurs* 12:217-224, 1996.

Downs FS: *A sourcebook of nursing research,* ed 3, Philadelphia, 1984, FA Davis.

Downs FS: Research as a survival technique, *Nurs Res* 45:323, 1996.

Draucker CB, Petrovic K: Healing of adult male survivors of childhood sexual abuse, *Image*
  28:325-330, 1996.

Fawcett J: Utilization of nursing research findings, *Image* 14:57-59, 1982.

Gennaro S, Vessey J: Making practice perfect, *Nurs Res* 40:529, 1991.

Gortner S: Nursing values and science: toward a science philosophy, *Image* 22:101-105, 1990.

Kerlinger FN: *Foundations of behavioral research,* ed 2, New York, 1986, Holt, Rinehart &
  Winston.

Lauver D et al: Testing theoretical explanations of mammography use, *Nurs Res* 46:32-39,
  1997.

LeFort SM: The statistical versus clinical significance debate, *Image* 25:57-62, 1993.

LoBiondo-Wood G et al: The impact of transplantation on quality of life: a longitudinal perspective, *Appl Nurs Res* 10:26-31, 1997.

Polit DF, Sherman RE: Statistical power in nursing research, *Nurs Res* 39:365-369, 1990.

Rudy EB et al: Patient outcomes for the chronically critically ill: special care unit versus intensive care unit, *Nurs Res* 44:324-331, 1995.

Schmitt MH: The connectedness of nursing research: revisiting an old issue, *Res Nurs Health*
  17:319-320, 1994.

Titler M et al: Infusing research into practice to promote quality care, *Nurs Res* 43:307-313,
  1994.

Ward SE, Berry PE, Misiewicz H: Concerns about analgesics among patients and family caregivers in a hospice setting, *Res Nurs Health* 19:205-211, 1996.

ADDITIONAL READINGS

Kirk RE: *Experimental design procedures for the behavioral sciences,* Pacific Grove, Calif, 1995,
  Brooks/Cole.

Munro BH, Page EB: *Statistical methods for health care research,* ed 2, Philadelphia, 1993, JB Lippincott.

Myers JL, Well AD: *Research design and statistical analysis,* Hillsdale, NJ, 1995, Lawrence Erlbaum.

Pedhazer EJ: *Multiple regression in behavioral research,* ed 2, New York, 1986, Holt, Rinehart & Winston.

Critique and Application

Research Vignette
**Intangible Benefits
of Nursing Research**

Chapter 17
**Evaluating Quantitative
Research Studies**

Chapter 18
**Evaluating the Qualitative
Research Report**

Chapter 19
**Use of Research
in Practice**

Research Vignette

INTANGIBLE BENEFITS OF NURSING RESEARCH

Seventeen years of conducting clinical research provides many examples of the value of research for practice and education. Some examples provide an unforgettable window on the intangible human yield from clinical research. Tanya's experience was such an example.

From 1982 to 1986, a group of colleagues and I conducted a classic study on early discharge of very-low-birth-weight (VLBW) infants. In this randomized clinical trial, one group of VLBW infants was discharged earlier than usual and received home visits, telephone outreach, and daily telephone availability of a master's prepared advanced practice nurse (APN) who had specialized in neonatal care. A control group of infants received usual hospital discharge and no home follow-up, which was routine at the time of the study. Both groups of infants were followed from birth to 18 months post discharge.

Tanya, a 17-year-old mother of three other young children, had delivered a fourth child, a premature little boy. His birth weight was almost 3 pounds. As a mother in the intervention group, Tanya was followed by Susan, the APN, from shortly after she gave birth until her son was a year and a half. Over the course of the study, Susan visited Tanya while she was in the hospital, made a total of six home visits, and was with Tanya at many of her son's routine pediatric follow-up visits.

During one home visit, Tanya's mother took Susan aside and shared her frustration over Tanya's repeated pregnancies. Tanya's mother shared that she had raised four children on her own after the death of her husband and that she had done so without the assistance of welfare. Tanya's mother blamed the availability of welfare for her daughter's repeated pregnancies. Susan listened patiently, then continued her counseling of Tanya regarding family planning and how to pursue completion of her high school diploma. On a later visit, Susan brought the application forms to begin enrollment. Tanya seemed interested.

The follow-up of Tanya's son ended some months later and so did contact between Susan and Tanya. The study also ended about a year later with Susan returning to work in the high-risk follow-up clinic of the hospital where the study was conducted.

Almost 2 years later Susan was completing her last day in the clinic before returning full time to school to finish her PhD. That afternoon she felt a tap on her shoulder. As she turned around, there was Tanya. After pleasant exchanges, Tanya told Susan she was completing her GED and was planning to become a nurse. The baby and other children were fine. Susan, although pleased, received Tanya's news with some skepticism. This goal represented a significant change from Tanya's previously undisciplined behavior.

Four years later Susan began collecting follow-up data from infants and families in both the original experimental and control groups for her dissertation. Tanya was among the mothers Susan was able to contact. Tanya was now in her second year of a baccalaureate nursing program at a local university. While Susan was excited to learn this, what Tanya subsequently shared provided a window on the intangible benefits and lasting yield of that study on this young woman's life and likely on the lives of her young children.

"Susan," said Tanya, "you have really made a difference in my life. I heard what you told me about making something of myself, and you helped me begin. But what you may not know is that you were the first successful young woman I had ever had much contact with. Watching and listening to you and having you interested in me and telling me I could do something with my life made the difference. Thank you so much."

The main findings from the research study were published, as were many important secondary analyses. These publications changed clinical practice and were important to nursing education. Yet Tanya's experience serves as one of a number of examples of the intangible, positive, and powerful differences clinical research can and does make. And the difference it made for Tanya may last through generations.

Dorothy Brooten, PhD, FAAN
Associate Dean for Research and Graduate Studies
John Burry Jr. Professor
Case Western Reserve University
Frances Payne Bolton School of Nursing

Evaluating Quantitative Research Studies

Judith A. Heermann ■ Betty J. Craft

Key Terms

replication
research base
scientific merit

Learning Outcomes

After reading this chapter the student should be able to do the following:

- Identify the purpose of the critiquing process.
- Describe the criteria of each step of the critiquing process.
- Evaluate the strengths and weaknesses of a research report.
- Discuss the implications of the findings of a research report for nursing practice.
- Construct a critique of a research report.

Each component of a research study is examined to determine the merit of a research report. Criteria designed to assist the consumer in judging the relative value of a research report are found in previous chapters. An abbreviated set of questions summarizing the more detailed criteria, found at the end of each chapter, is used in this chapter as a framework for two sample research critiques (Table 17-1). These critiques are included to exemplify the process of evaluating reported research for potential application to practice and thus extending the research base for nursing. For clarification, readers are encouraged to refer to the earlier chapters for the detailed presentation of the critiquing criteria and explanations of the research process. The criteria and examples in this chapter apply to quantitative studies.

STYLISTIC CONSIDERATIONS

The evaluator should realize several important aspects related to the world of publishing before beginning to critique research studies. First, different journals have different publication goals and target specific professional markets. For example, *Nursing Research* is a journal that publishes articles on the conduct or results of research in nursing. Although *The Journal of Obstetric, Gynecologic, and Neonatal Nursing* also publishes research articles, it also includes articles related to the knowledge, experience, trends, and policies in obstetrical, gynecological, and neonatal nursing. The emphasis in this latter journal is broader in that it contains clinical and theoretical articles, as well as research articles. Consequently the style and content of the manuscript vary according to the type of journal to which it is being submitted.

Second, the author of a research article prepares the manuscript using both personal judgment and specific guidelines. *Personal judgment* refers to the researcher's expertise developed in the course of designing, executing, and analyzing the study. As a result of this expertise, the researcher is in the position to judge which content is most important to communicate to the profession. The decision is a function of the following:

- The research design: experimental or nonexperimental
- The focus of the study: basic or clinical
- The audience to which the results will be most appropriately communicated

Guidelines are provided by each journal for preparing research manuscripts for publication. The following major headings are essential sections in the research report:

- Introduction
- Methodology
- Results
- Discussion

Depending on stylistic considerations related to authors' preferences and the publishing journal's requirements, specific content is included in each section of the research report. Stylistic variations as factors influencing the presentation of the research study are distinct from the focus of evaluating the reported research for scientific merit. Constructive evaluation is based on objective, unbiased, and impartial appraisal of the study's strengths and limitations. This is a step that precedes consideration of the relative worth of the findings for clinical application to nursing practice. Such judgments are the hallmark of promoting a sound theory base for quality nursing practice.

Table 17-1

Major Content Sections of a Research Report and Related Critiquing Guidelines

SECTION	QUESTIONS TO GUIDE EVALUATION
Problem statement and purpose (see Chapter 3)	1. What is the problem and/or purpose of the research study? Is it appropriately stated? 2. Does the problem or purpose statement express a relationship between two or more variables (e.g., between an independent and a dependent variable)? If so, what is/are the relationship(s)? Are they testable? 3. Does the problem statement and/or purpose specify the nature of the population being studied? What is it? 4. What significance of the problem has been identified, if any, by the investigator?
Review of literature and theoretical framework (see Chapters 4 and 5)	1. What concepts are included in the review? Of particular importance, note those concepts that are the independent and dependent variables and how they are conceptually defined. 2. Does the literature review make explicit the relationships among the variables or place the variables within a theoretical/conceptual framework? What are the relationships? 3. What gaps or conflicts in knowledge about the problem are identified? How does this study intend to fill those gaps or resolve those conflicts? 4. Are the references cited by the author mostly primary or mostly secondary sources? Give an example of each. 5. What are the operational definitions of the independent and dependent variables? Do they reflect the conceptual definitions?
Hypotheses or research question(s) (see Chapter 3)	1. What hypothesis(es) or research questions are stated in the study? Are they appropriately stated? 2. If research questions are stated, are they used in addition to hypotheses or to guide an exploratory study? 3. What are the independent and dependent variables in the statement of each hypothesis/research question? 4. If hypotheses are stated, is the form of the statement statistical (null) or research? 5. What is the direction of the relationship in each hypothesis, if indicated? 6. Are the hypotheses testable?

Continued

Table 17-1—cont'd	
Major Content Sections of a Research Report and Related Critiquing Guidelines	
SECTION	QUESTIONS TO GUIDE EVALUATION
Sample (see Chapter 10)	1. How was the sample selected? 2. What type of sampling method is used in the study? Is it appropriate to the design? 3. To what population may the findings be generalized? What are the limitations in generalizability? 4. Does the sample reflect the population as identified in the problem or purpose statement? 5. Is the sample size appropriate? How is it substantiated?
Research design (see Chapters 6 to 8)	1. What type of design is used in the study? 2. What is the rationale for the design classification? 3. Does the design seem to flow from the proposed problem statement, theoretical framework, literature review, and hypothesis?
Internal validity (see Chapter 6)	1. Discuss each of the threats to the internal validity of the study. 2. Does the design have controls at an acceptable level for the threats to internal validity?
External validity (see Chapter 6) Research approach (see Chapters 11, 12, and 13)	1. What are the limits to generalizability in terms of external validity?
Methods (see Chapter 12)	1. What type(s) of data collection method(s) is/are used in the study? 2. Are the data collection procedures similar for all subjects?
Legal-ethical issues (see Chapter 11)	1. How have the rights of subjects been protected? 2. What indications are given that informed consent of the subjects has been ensured?
Instruments (see Chapter 12)	1. Physiological measurement a. Is a rationale given for why a particular instrument/method was selected? If so, what is it? b. What provision is made for maintaining the accuracy of the instrument and its use, if any? 2. Observational methods a. Who did the observing? b. How were the observers trained to minimize bias? c. Was there an observational guide?

Table 17-1—cont'd

Major Content Sections of a Research Report and Related Critiquing Guidelines

SECTION	QUESTIONS TO GUIDE EVALUATION
	d. Were the observers required to make inferences about what they saw?
	e. Is there any reason to believe that the presence of the observers affected the behavior of the subjects?
	3. Interviews
	a. Who were the interviewers? How were they trained to minimize bias?
	b. Is there evidence of any interview bias? If so, what is it?
	4. Questionnaires
	a. What is the type and/or format of the questionnaire (e.g., Likert, open-ended)?
	5. Available data and records
	a. Are the records that were used appropriate to the problem being studied?
	b. Are these data being used to describe the sample or for hypothesis testing?
Reliability and validity (see Chapter 13)	1. What type of reliability is reported for each instrument?
	2. What level of reliability is reported? Is it acceptable?
	3. What type of validity is reported for each instrument?
	4. Does the validity of each instrument seem adequate? Why?
Analysis of data (see Chapters 14 and 15)	1. What level of measurement is used to measure each of the major variables?
	2. What descriptive or inferential statistics are reported?
	3. Were these descriptive or inferential statistics appropriate to the level of measurement for each variable?
	4. Are the inferential statistics used appropriate to the intent of the hypothesis(es)?
	5. Does the author report the level of significance set for the study? If so, what is it?
	6. If tables or figures are used, do they meet the following standards?
	a. They supplement and economize the text.
	b. They have precise titles and headings.
	c. They are not repetitious of the text.
Conclusions, implications, and recommendations (see Chapter 16)	1. If hypothesis(es) testing was done, was/were the hypothesis(es) supported or not supported?
	2. Are the results interpreted in the context of the problem/purpose, hypothesis, and theoretical framework/literature reviewed?

Continued

Table 17-1—cont'd	
Major Content Sections of a Research Report and Related Critiquing Guidelines	
SECTION	QUESTIONS TO GUIDE EVALUATION
	3. What does the investigator identify as possible limitations and/or problems in the study related to the design, methods, and sample?
	4. What relevance for nursing practice does the investigator identify, if any?
	5. What generalizations are made?
	6. Are the generalizations within the scope of the findings or beyond the findings?
	7. What recommendations for future research are stated or implied?
Application and utilization for nursing practice (see Chapter 19)	1. Does the study appear valid? That is, do its strengths outweigh its weaknesses?
	2. Are there other studies with similar findings?
	3. What risks/benefits are involved for patients if the research findings would be used in practice?
	4. Is direct application of the research findings feasible in terms of time, effort, money, and legal/ethical risks?
	5. How and under what circumstances are the findings applicable to nursing practice?
	6. Should these results be applied to nursing practice?
	7. Would it be possible to replicate this study in another clinical practice setting?

CRITIQUE OF A RESEARCH STUDY: SAMPLE NO. I

The study *A Comparison of the Effects of Jaw Relaxation and Music on Postoperative Pain* by Marion Good, PhD, RN, published in *Nursing Research* (1995), is critiqued. The article is presented in its entirety and is followed by the critique on p. 423.

A COMPARISON OF THE EFFECTS OF JAW RELAXATION AND MUSIC ON POSTOPERATIVE PAIN*

Marion Good

This experimental study compared the effects of jaw relaxation and music, individually and combined, on sensory and affective pain following surgery. Abdominal surgical patients (N = 84) were randomly assigned to four groups: relaxation, music, a combination of relaxation and music, and control. Interventions were taught preoperatively and used by subjects during the first ambulation after surgery. Indicators of the sensory component of pain were sensation and 24-hour narcotic intake. Indicators of the affective component of pain were distress and anxiety of pain. With preambulatory sensation; distress, narcotic intake, and preoperative anxiety as covariates, the four groups were compared using orthogonal a priori contrasts and analysis of covariance. The interventions were neither effective nor significantly different from one another during ambulation. However, after keeping the taped interventions for 2 postoperative days, 89% of experimental subjects reported them helpful for sensation and distress of pain.

Pain following abdominal surgery is an unpleasant sensory and affective experience that can contribute to postoperative complications, prolonging hospitalization and recovery. Pain is not always controlled by prescribed analgesics. To augment medication, patients may use self-care methods such as simple relaxation and soothing music (Acute Pain Management Guideline Panel, 1992). Although a few studies have shown that both relaxation and music reduce postoperative pain, others have not, and none have compared these interventions to a combination of relaxation and music. The purposes of this study were: (a) to conduct a controlled experiment to compare the individual and combined effects of jaw relaxation and music on the sensory and affective components of pain after the first postoperative ambulation, and (b) to describe self-care use and helpfulness of these interventions during the next 48 hours.

Relaxation reduced self-reported sensation of pain (Madden, Singer, Peck, & Nayman, 1978), narcotic intake (Egbert, Battit, Welch, & Bartlett, 1964; Voshall, 1980; Wilson, 1981), and affective pain (Aiken, 1972; Egbert et al., 1964; Field, 1974; Johnson, 1966) in a few postoperative studies, but had no effect in others on sensation (Levin, Malloy, & Hyman, 1987; Voshall, 1980; Wells, 1982; Zeimer, 1983) or affective pain (Levin et al., 1987; Woshall, 1980). These differing outcomes may be due to lack of control of pretreatment pain and narcotic intake, inconsistent definitions of the distress of pain as emotional or physical, and use of a variety of relaxation techniques.

None of these effectiveness studies replicated the same relaxation technique. The jaw relaxation technique, however, has been replicated four times and tested after initial ambulation, or, in the case of hip surgery, after initial turning. There was, however, insufficient control of pretreatment pain and narcotic intake in these replications. Jaw relaxation reduced sensation, distress of pain, and narcotic intake in patients after ambulation in cholecystectomy and herniorrhaphy patients (Flaherty & Fitzpatrick, 1978) and in hip surgery patients after turning (Ceccio, 1984). However, it failed to decrease any of these outcomes following ambulation in

---

*This section, from pp. 413 to 423, is taken from Good M: A comparison of the effects of jaw relaxation and music on postoperative pain, *Nurs Res* 44:52-57, 1995.

cardiac surgery patients (Horowitz, Fitzpatrick, & Flaherty, 1984) or abdominal surgery patients (Mogan, Wells, & Robertson 1985), possibly because oral treatment implementation varied within and among investigations.

Preliminary results of studies of the effect of music on postoperative pain were also conflicting. Pretest pain was not usually controlled, and differences in types of surgery, postoperative day, setting, measures of pain, and types of music may have contributed to the mixed results. None of the studies tested music during ambulation. Preferred music reduced behavioral responses to postoperative pain (Locsin, 1981); classical or contemporary music reduced descriptive reports of emotional and physical pain in the ICU (Updyke, 1990); and easy-listening music reduced visual analogue measures of postoperative pain and anxiety of patients in bed (Mullooly, Levin, & Feldman, 1988). However, precategorized stimulating or sedative music did not reduce reports of pain or morphine requirements of patients in a postanesthesia recovery unit (Heitz, Symreng, & Scamman, 1992). It is not known whether patients in most of these studies liked the music. No studies comparing music to relaxation for relief of postoperative pain were found. The combination of relaxation and music has been used effectively with Lamaze training (Standley, 1986), but results were mixed when combined with imagery for postoperative pain (Gaffam & Johnson, 1987; Swinford, 1987).

The conceptual framework for the study, based on Orem's (1991) self-care deficit theory of nursing and the gate-control theory of pain (Melzak, 1982; Wall, 1979), proposed that self-care action for pain relief could improve well-being by reducing the sensory and affective components of pain. One of Orem's three related theoretical constructs, the theory of self-care, states in part that nurses assist patients in using self-care activities to regulate health and well-being. Nurses instruct and support patients in the use of self-care interventions, such as relaxation and music, to improve well-being during pain.

The gate-control theory posits that pain is the result of an integrated sensory, affective, and motivational system that modulates noxious input, attenuates the perception of pain, and stimulates action to relieve it. Patient reaction to pain includes muscular and mental tension that increases sympathetic outflow and its effect on the integrated modulation centers. Use of relaxation and music may reduce tension and pain by reducing sympathetic influences on the centers, thereby modulating input and perception of both components of pain.

The nurse's role is to adjust the dose and interval of prescribed medication until there is satisfactory pain relief. If relief is unsatisfactory or if side effects are unacceptable, adding an adjuvant self-care intervention is one option to be considered (Acute Pain Management Guideline Panel, 1992). This study is an investigation of the effectiveness of three such techniques.

This experimental study was designed to investigate differences in sensory and affective pain for three self-care actions: relaxation, music, and the combination of relaxation and music. The sensory component of pain was measured by sensation of pain and narcotic intake; the affective component by distress and anxiety of pain. The treatments were chosen because they are easily learned, efficient, and safe, but have uncertain effectiveness. Because of equivocal results in quasi-experimental studies and lack of data about the relative strength of these interventions, a controlled experiment was needed to determine single and combined effectiveness. Three hypotheses were posed:

I. Controlling for preambulatory sensation, distress, narcotic intake, and preoperative anxiety, there will be a difference between the individual groups (relaxation and music) in sensation, distress, and anxiety of pain after the first postoperative ambulation and in narcotic intake during the next 24 hours.

II. Controlling for preambulatory sensation, distress, narcotic intake, and preoperative anxiety, there will be a difference between the relaxation and music groups taken together and compared to the combination group in sensation, distress, and anxiety of pain after the first postoperative ambulation and in narcotic intake during the next 24 hours.

III. Controlling for preambulatory sensation, distress, narcotic intake, and preoperative anxiety, the relaxation, music, and combination groups taken together will have less sensation, distress, and anxiety of pain after the first postoperative ambulation and less narcotic intake during the next 24 hours than the control group.

METHOD

Sample

The sampling frame included every eligible patient listed for elective abdominal surgery in two teaching and two community hospitals during a 7-month period. Patients were identified daily by the investigator from surgery lists, and eligibility was decided in consultation with office nurses. Inclusion criteria were: (a) aged 21 to 65 years, (b) scheduled for major abdominal surgery, (c) receiving intramuscular (IM) PRN or intravenous (IV) PRN analgesia, and (d) hospitalized 2 or more days postoperatively. Patients who had laparoscopic surgeries or psychosis or retardation were excluded. All eligible patients ($N = 126$) were contacted in the nursing unit, holding area, clinic, or by telephone. Of the 102 patients who consented and were assigned, 2 patients later withdrew and 16 were excluded from the analysis because of cancelled surgery ($n = 4$), inability to ambulate after surgery ($n = 2$), unforeseen patient-controlled analgesia ($n = 9$), or treatment error ($n = 1$).

Thus, the sample consisted of 84 subjects, 25 men and 59 women aged 23 to 64 years ($M = 46$ years, $SD = 12.54$) in four treatment groups of 21 each: relaxation (4 males), music (6 males), combination (8 males), or control (7 males). Most subjects were white ($n = 70$, 83%), married ($n = 54$, 64%), and high school graduates ($n = 52$, 62%). Almost half were employed ($n = 41$, 49%), and most had undergone previous surgery ($n = 75$, 89%), $M = 3.51$ surgeries, $SD = 2.74$).

Subjects spent an average of 3.5 ($SD = 2.2$) hours in surgery, and 18 (21%) spent from 1 to 5 days in surgical intensive care units. Most ($n = 79$, 94%) ambulated by the first postoperative day. Surgical procedures involved upper ($n = 35$, 42%), lower ($n = 34$, 41%), and combined abdominal incisions ($n = 15$, 18%). Nearly half the subjects received IM PRN narcotics ($n = 37$, 44%), a fourth received IV PRN ($n = 20$, 24%), and a third received both ($n = 27$, 32%).

Measures

The sensory component of pain was defined as the unpleasant, physical perception of hurt associated with tissue damage following surgery. It was measured by the Sensation of Pain Scale (Johnson, 1973) and 24-hour narcotic use. The affective component of pain is the presence of general bodily feelings (Flaherty & Fitzpatrick, 1978) and emotions (Johnson, 1973) concurrent with the sensory component. It was measured by the Distress of Pain Scale (Johnson, 1973) and the State Anxiety Inventory (Spielberger, 1983).

The Sensation of Pain and the Distress of Pain scales each consist of a horizontal line numbered from 0 to 10 with three verbal anchors: no sensation, medium sensation, and most sensation, and no distress, moderate distress, and extremely distressing. Subjects marked the sensation scale to indicate the amount of physical pain felt at the area of the operation. They marked the distress scale to indicate how much the sensations bothered them and the rest of their body. There were no vertical lines corresponding with the numbers on the scales. Later, a transparent overlay with markings for each number and four markings between numbers was used to estimate scores to the nearest 20% of each interval. Validity of the scales was supported by Johnson (1973), who found that subjects could differentiate between pain and distress during induced ischemic pain. However, reliability of these single-item measures of changeable states was not addressed. The presence of verbal anchors was expected to enhance accuracy in surgical patients.

The State Anxiety Inventory (STAI) was used twice: preoperatively, to measure anxiety in relation to approaching surgery, and, after the first ambulation following surgery, to measure the emotional factor of affective pain. As a factor in pain, it augmented the concept of distress, which has been used in a more physical sense as the affective component of pain. Anxiety is an emotion consisting of feelings of apprehension, tension, and worry in relation to a situation. The STAI has been used to study anxiety of approaching surgery and of postoperative pain. Subjects were asked how they felt in relation to the situation of interest, that is, the approaching surgery or pain following ambulation. The STAI consists of 20 statements on a 4-point Likert scale, with responses ranging from 1 (not at all) to 4 (very much so). Construct and divergent validity and test-retest reliability of the STAI are described by Spielberger (1983). Patients with higher preoperative anxiety report greater pain (Johnson, Leventhal, & Dabbs, 1971); therefore, in this study, preoperative anxiety was measured to control this extraneous influence. Internal consistency reliability using Cronbach's alpha was .89 for preoperative anxiety and .90 for postambulatory anxiety of pain, with a correlation of $r = .37, p < .001$ between the two measures.

The amount of postambulatory narcotic intake was measured during the 24 hours after ambulation. To control for the extraneous influence of analgesic action at the time of the intervention, narcotic intake within 2.5 hours before ambulation was also measured. Both measures of narcotic intake were obtained by record review and converted to milligrams of morphine equivalent. Because the possibility exists that incisional strain in heavy persons will affect pain when ambulating, body mass was calculated with the Quetelet Index (weight/height^2) (Jequier, 1987).

Pain was also measured after ambulation with the Pain Rating Index (PRI-R) of the McGill Pain Questionnaire (MPQ) to evaluate the validity of the single-item sensation and distress scales. The PRI-R contains 78 descriptors of pain, presented in 20 groups of two to six words that have been ranked by patients and physicians according to severity. Subjects chose one word from each group if there was one that described their pain. The rank assigned to that descriptor was the score for that group of words. The PRI-R has demonstrated construct and concurrent validity and test-retest reliability (Melzak, 1975). In the present study, the internal consistency reliability of the PRI-R, using Cronbach's alpha, was marginal (.60). Nevertheless, postambulatory scores of the PRI-R were positively and strongly correlated with those of the sensation ($r = .44, p < .001$) and distress ($r = .55$,

$p < .001$) scales. Correlations in this range support the concurrent validity of the sensation and distress scales, especially in light of the weakness of the alpha for the PRI-R (Zeller & Carmines, 1980).

Procedure

At the first visit, preoperatively, the data collector obtained informed written consent and randomly assigned subjects to one of the four treatment groups: relaxation, music, combination, or control. Random assignment without replacement to a discrete pool of experimental conditions ensured an equal number of subjects per group. The data collector then conducted a structured interview to obtain demographic data, measured preoperative anxiety, and explained the Sensation and Distress scales. An introductory tape was used to describe the purpose, effects, and technique of each intervention. Repetition of the technique on the tape provided for practice, coaching by the data collector, and mastery. Instruction and experimenter contact took 20 minutes in each treatment group. Controls were engaged in casual conversation for 10 minutes in place of the tape. The data collector observed the experimental subjects during instruction and ambulation and rated them on five criteria for mastery of the technique: no tension around the mouth, no grimace or frown, not talking, slow respirations, face relaxed. During the preoperative visit, most subjects (95%) were observed to achieve mastery (4/5) using the tape ($M = 4.68$, $SD = .56$), with no difference in mastery among treatment groups, $F(2, 60) = .34$, $p > .05$.

After surgery, the data collector brought the tape recorder, earphones, and the assigned 60-minute intervention tape to the bedside and measured preambulatory sensation and distress. Experimental subjects used the technique for 2 minutes before ambulation. As a check on manipulation, the data collector rated mastery of the technique during ambulation. Most of the subjects (89%) achieved mastery (4/5) at ambulation ($M = 4.44$, $SD = .78$), indicating that subjects had indeed used the assigned technique and used it effectively. There was no difference among groups, $F(2, 60) = 2.86$, $p > .05$.

After subjects returned to bed following their first ambulation, the data collector measured postambulatory sensation, distress, and anxiety. Pain was then measured with the McGill Pain Questionnaire to assess the validity of the sensation and distress scales. Subjects kept the tape for 2 days to use for treatment of pain. The data collector visited subjects 48 hours after ambulation and asked if any other self-care methods were used for pain management. Experimental subjects were asked about the amount of use and helpfulness of the assigned technique. Tape recorders were returned.

Three comparisons were made: (a) between the individual treatment groups, (b) between the individual and combination treatment groups, and (c) between the three treatment groups and the no-treatment control group. The first two comparisons were exploratory. However, based on studies reviewed, the third comparison was expected to show that persons who used the treatments would have less pain compared to the controls who did not use them.

Experimental Interventions

The type of self-care intervention for pain management consisted of four levels: (a) jaw relaxation, (b) music, (c) a combination of relaxation and music, and (d) control.

Jaw relaxation was used to manage pain through reducing muscle and mental tension. The procedure described by Flaherty and Fitzpatrick (1978) was replicated. This involved lowering the jaw and making the lips soft, the tongue quiet, breathing slow, and thoughts absent. Instructions on its use were recorded on audiotape for consistent presentation to all subjects.

Listening to music was used to reduce pain through distraction and/or relaxation. Subjects chose one of five types of taped sedative music: synthesizer, harp, piano, orchestral, or slow jazz music. The music, without lyrics, was recorded from compact discs, with control of variations in volume and pitch.

The combination of relaxation and music involved use of the jaw relaxation technique while listening to the chosen music in the background. Nearly all subjects in the music and the combination groups ($n = 41$, 98%) liked their chosen music. The control group received routine care.

Data Analysis

To determine whether differences in sensation, distress, anxiety, and 24-hour narcotic intake existed between the individual and combined groups, three orthogonal a priori contrasts or comparisons were used. Because of differences in preambulatory distress and preoperative anxiety, analysis of covariance was used to assess the significance of the comparisons. Since these were orthogonal a priori contrasts, the alpha level of significance remained at .05 (Kirk, 1982). Use of comparisons is consistent with Kirk (1982) and Winer, Brown, and Michels (1991). First, individual treatment group differences following ambulation were examined by comparing the means of the relaxation and music groups. Second, differences between the individual and combination groups were explored. The mean of the combination group was compared to the average of the means of the relaxation and music groups. Third, differences between the treatment groups and the group that did not receive a self-care intervention were compared. The mean of the control group was compared to the average of the means of the three treatment groups. These comparisons were done with ANCOVA to control for covariates.

When postambulatory sensation and distress were tested, preambulatory sensation and distress were used as covariates. For postambulatory anxiety of pain, covariates were preoperative anxiety and preambulatory sensation and distress. Covariates for 24-hour narcotic intake were preambulatory sensation and narcotic intake. Correlations of covariates with dependent variables ranged from $r = .29$ to .63, all p values $< .01$. Body mass was not significantly correlated with the dependent variables and was not used as a covariate.

RESULTS

Means for each group, with F statistics for each comparison, are shown in Table 1. Comparisons were made before and after the first ambulation. The relaxation group scored significantly lower on preambulatory distress than the music group. The mean of the relaxation and music groups taken together was lower than the score of the combination group on presurgical anxiety. No other significant presurgical or preambulatory differences were found.

To check the randomization procedure, subjects in the four groups were compared and found equivalent on demographic and surgical variables. Using analysis of variance, no significant differences were found in age, number of previous surgeries, hours in surgery, days in in-

Table I

Means, Standard Deviations, and F Tests of Comparisons on Four Indicants of Pain

	INDICANTS OF PAIN											
	SENSATION			DISTRESS			ANXIETY			NARCOTIC INTAKE		
COMPARISONS	M	SD	F	M	SD	F	M	SD	F	M	SD	F
Pretest using												
ANOVA												
Relaxation	5.01	(2.86)		4.20	(2.95)		37.40	(9.44)		6.87	(4.50)	
Music	6.56	(2.35)	3.91	5.92	(2.59)	4.00*	34.81	(6.78)	.81	4.73	(5.02)	1.88
Relaxation and Music	5.79			5.07			36.11			5.80		
Combination	5.79	(2.32)	.00	5.23	(2.51)	.05	44.76	(9.80)	12.10**	6.62	(5.12)	.37
Relaxation, Music, and Combination	5.79			5.12			38.99			6.07		
Control	5.69	(2.59)	.03	5.37	(3.08)	.13	37.14	(10.76)	.62	4.83	(5.57)	.96
Posttest using												
ANCOVA												
Hypothesis I												
Relaxation	5.28	(2.62)		4.53	(2.54)		38.40	(8.66)		34.78	(24.11)	
Music	6.58	(2.26)	.54	5.74	(2.52)	.41	40.00	(12.72)	.00	33.81	(20.68)	.01
Hypothesis II												
Relaxation and Music	5.93			5.14			39.20			34.30		
Combination	5.94	(2.15)	.00	5.61	(2.06)	.57	45.10	(7.12)	1.76	28.91	(23.41)	1.51
Hypothesis III												
Relaxation, Music, and Combination	5.93			5.29			41.16			32.50		
Control	5.23	(2.52)	1.63	5.34	(2.73)	.01	41.67	(10.42)	.09	34.67	(26.52)	.78

$*p < .05$; $**p = .001$.

tensive care, days until ambulation, or body mass. Using chi-square, no significant differences were found in sex, employment, ethnic group, marital status, education, mastery of the technique, use of other self-care methods of pain management, or route of medication administration.

None of the hypotheses were supported. With statistical control of extraneous influences, no significant differences were found in sensation, distress, anxiety, or narcotic intake between (a) relaxation and music, (b) the individual treatments and the combination of relaxation and music, or (c) the three treatment groups and the controls. Analysis of the 66 subjects who did not go to the ICU after surgery produced the same results. Controlling for preambulatory sensation and distress, no significant differences were found in pain measured by the McGill Pain Questionnaire (PRI-R).

Subjects kept their taped intervention to use whenever they wished for 48 hours after the first ambulation. In retrospect, the relaxation group reported listening to the tape from 15 to 180 minutes ($M = 74$, $SD = 41.33$) during the 2 days, while the music group listened from 15 to 480 minutes ($M = 156$, $SD = 92.06$), and the combination group listened from 30 to 300 minutes ($M = 108$, $SD = 61.63$). The relaxation tape was used the least, perhaps because it was less interesting than the music and combination tapes. Subjects reported their tape moderately or very helpful ($n = 48$, 76%). It reduced sensation and distress ($n = 56$, 89%). However, subjects preferred to use it in bed ($n = 56$, 89%), would use it again for surgery ($n = 58$, 92%), and would recommend it to others ($n = 60$, 95%). There were no differences between the treatment groups.

DISCUSSION

Contrary to expectations and the conceptual framework for the study, patient use of tape-recorded relaxation and music, alone or in combination, was neither effective nor differentiated in reducing four measures of the sensory and affective components of pain: sensation, distress, anxiety after ambulation, and narcotic intake during the next 24 hours. This finding, which refutes deductions from both Orem's theory of self-care and the gate-control theory, suggests that these particular self-care actions, taken by patients to relieve pain, did not improve well-being by modulating perception of pain during the activity of initial ambulation. Because reports after 48 hours of self-care use were favorable, however, future support for these relationships may be found by modifying the type, context, and timing of the self-care activities.

The lack of findings at ambulation is consistent with some previous studies that did not find relaxation and music effective for pain, but is in contrast to others that did. The disparities among previous studies may have been related to methodological problems rectified in the present study by using a taped intervention, replication of measures, a randomized and adequate sample, and control of extraneous variables. Even with methodological refinements, however, the interventions were not effective at ambulation.

The findings may have been related to a number of factors that provide direction for practice and future research. First, the difficulty of demonstrating an effect might have been due to higher and more variable pain scores than in previous studies. Future studies could compare effects of interventions on pain during the first versus the second ambulation. Second, providing patients with taped relaxation instructions rather than verbal instructions by the nurse may have reduced the effectiveness of the relaxation and combination interventions (Snyder, 1992). Comparisons of taped and live relaxation instructions would demonstrate their relative usefulness. Comparisons also need to be made between different ambulation directives given by the nurse and with different patient characteristics.

Use of relaxation or distraction techniques during initial ambulation may have been difficult for some patients. If interventions were not strong enough for the complex activity of ambulation, they might be more effective during simple rest in bed. Patient reports at the final visit indicated that most preferred to use the tapes in bed and reported them to be moderately to very helpful. Mullooly et al. (1988), in a randomized study with control for pretest pain, found that easy-listening music decreased pain and anxiety of patients in bed.

Other relaxation techniques may be more effective. To augment medication for surgical pain, the Acute Pain Management Guideline Panel (1992) has suggested several relaxation techniques. Jaw relaxation and slow rhythmic breathing could be compared during activity. Clenching the fists, going limp, and yawning might be appropriate during rest. Progressive relaxation techniques of tensing and relaxing oral and jaw muscles may be added to the teaching of jaw relaxation to increase awareness of tension and relaxation in muscles (Snyder, 1992). Other techniques were found in the literature. Patients who were taught to allow the abdominal wall to relax were found to have lower narcotic intake and greater observed comfort (Egbert et al., 1964). Horowitz et al. (1984) found that Benson's relaxation response reduced distress of pain during ambulation while jaw relaxation had no effect on either sensation or distress. Levin et al. (1987) found in a small sample that Benson's technique resulted in less combined sensation and distress than the attention control group, but not the usual-care control group. The most appropriate and effective types of relaxation technique for postoperative activity and rest have not yet been identified.

The music selections used in this study should be compared to others. Effectiveness of music on physiological variables has been reported to be related to patients' liking the selection (Standley, 1986). Although 33 (79%) of subjects who received music liked the selections, only 8 (19%) loved them. The study tapes could be compared to self-selected music and to other types, tempos, and cultural preferences for music.

Future research should be focused on exploring appropriate interventions in relation to contextual and personal variables, and then determining effectiveness using a controlled experiment. This study provided support for the concurrent validity of the sensation and distress scales using the MPQ as a criterion. In the past, single-item measures have been said to lack the validity and sensitivity of multiple-item measures, but recent research indicates that single-item scales may be psychometrically acceptable measures of global patient ratings (Youngblut & Casper, 1993). Increasing support for these simple and direct scales means that they can be used with more confidence in the future.

Because relaxation and music interventions pose a low risk to patients and may reduce pain and side effects of medication in some people, their usefulness should continue to be explored in practice and research. Nurses may try them in interested, capable, and adequately medicated patients who need additional analgesia or wish to reduce side effects. Patients should be asked about their pain intensity before and after use, and whether they think the intervention is helpful.

REFERENCES

Acute Pain Management Guideline Panel. (1992). *Acute pain management: operative or medical procedures and trauma. Clinical practice guideline.* AHCPR Pub. No. 92-0032, Rockville, MD: Agency for Health Care Policy and Research, Public Health Service, U.S. Department of Health and Human Services.

Aiken, L.H. (1972, June). Systemic relaxation to reduce preoperative stress. *Canadian Nurse, 38-42.*

Ceccio, C.M. (1984). Postoperative pain relief through relaxation in elderly patients with fractured hips. *Orthopaedic Nursing, 3,* 11-14.

Egbert, L.D., Battit, G.E., Welch, C.E., & Bartlett, M.K. (1964). Reduction of postoperative pain by encouragement and instruction of patients. *New England Journal of Medicine, 270,* 825-827.

Field, P.B. (1974). Effects of tape recorded hypnotic preparation for surgery. *The International Journal of Clinical and Experimental Hypnosis, 22* (1), 54-61.

Flaherty, G.G., & Fitzpatrick, J.J. (1978). Relaxation technique to increase comfort level of postoperative patients: A preliminary study. *Nursing Research, 27,* 352-355.

Gaffam, S., & Johnson, R. (1987). A comparison of two relaxation strategies for the relief of pain and its distress. *Journal of Pain and Symptom Management, 2,* 229-231.

Heitz, L., Symreng, T., & Scamman, F.L. (1992). Effect of music therapy in the postanesthesia care unit: A nursing intervention. *Journal of Post Anesthesia Nursing, 7* (1), 22-31.

Horowitz, B., Fitzpatrick, J.J., & Flaherty, G.G. (1984). Relaxation techniques for pain relief after open heart surgery. *Dimensions of Critical Care Nursing, 3,* 364–371.

Jequier, E. (1987). Energy, obesity and body weight standards, *American Journal of Clinical Nutrition, 45,* 1035-1036.

Johnson, J.E. (1966). The influence of a purposeful nurse patient interaction on the patients' postoperative course. In *Exploring progress in medical-surgical nursing practice* (pp. 16-22). New York: American Nurses Association.

Johnson, J.E. (1973). Effects of accurate expectations about sensations on the sensory and distress components of pain. *Journal of Personality and Social Psychology, 27,* 261-275.

Johnson, J.E., Leventhal, H., & Dabbs, J.M. (1971). Contribution of emotional and instrumental response processes in adaptation to surgery. *Journal of Personality and Social Psychology, 20,* 55-64.

Kirk, R.E. (1982). *Experimental design: procedure for the behavioral sciences* (2nd ed.). Belmont, CA: Brooks Cole.

Levin, R.F., Malloy, G.B., & Hyman, R.B. (1987). Nursing management of postoperative pain: Use of relaxation techniques with female cholecystectomy patients. *Journal of Advanced Nursing, 12,* 463-472.

Locsin, R. (1981). The effect of music on the pain of selected post-operative patients. *Journal of Advanced Nursing, 6,* 19-25.

Madden, C., Singer, G., Peck, C., & Nayman, J. (1978). The effect of EMG biofeedback on postoperative pain following abdominal surgery. *Anesthesia Intensive Care, 6,* 333-336.

Melzak, R. (1975). The McGill Pain Questionnaire: Major properties and scoring methods. *Pain, 1* (3), 277-299.

Melzak, R. (1982). Recent concepts of pain. *Journal of Medicine, 13,* 147-160.

Mogan, J., Wells, N., & Robertson, E. (1985). Effects of preoperative teaching on postoperative pain: A replication and expansion. *International Journal of Nursing Studies, 22,* 267-280.

Mullooly, V.M., Levin, R.F., & Feldman, H.R. (1988). Music for postoperative pain and anxiety. *Journal of the New York State Nurses Association, 19* (3), 4-7.

Orem, D. (1991). *Nursing: Concepts of practice.* New York: McGraw Hill.

Snyder, M. (1992). Progressive relaxation. In M. Snyder (Ed.), *Independent nursing interventions* (2nd ed., pp. 47-62). Albany: Delmar Publications.

Spielberger, C.D. (1983). *Manual for the State-Trait Inventory, STAI (Form Y).* Palo Alto, CA: Consulting Psychologists Press.

Standley, J.M. (1986). Music research in medical/dental treatment: Meta-analysis and clinical applications. *Journal of Music Therapy, 23,* 56-122.

Swinford, P. (1987). Relaxation and positive imagery for the surgical patient: A research study. Perioperative Nursing Quarterly, 3 *(3), 9-16.*

Updyke, P.A. (1990). Music therapy results for ICU patients. *Dimensions of Critical Care Nursing,* 9(1), 39-45.

Voshall, B. (1980). The effects of preoperative teaching on postoperative pain. *Topics of Clinical Nursing: Pain Management,* 2,(1), 39-43.

Wall, P.D. (1979). On the relation of injury to pain. The John J. Bonica lecture, *Pain, 6,* 253-264.

Wells, N. (1982). The effect of relaxation on postoperative muscle tension and pain. *Nursing Research, 31,* 236-238.

Wilson, J.F. (1981). Behavioral preparation for surgery: benefit or harm? *Journal of Behavioral Medicine,* 4 (1), 79-102.

Winer, B.J., Brown, D.R., & Michels, K.M. (1991). *Statistical principles in experimental design* (3rd ed.). New York: McGraw-Hill.

Youngblut, J.M., & Casper, G.R. (1993). Focus on psychometrics: Single-item indicators in nursing research. *Research in Nursing and Health,* 16, 459-465.

Zeimer, M.M. (1983). Effects of information on postsurgical coping. *Nursing Research, 32,* 282-287.

Zeller, R.A., & Carmines, E.G. (1980). *Measurement in the social sciences: The link between theory and data.* New York: Cambridge University Press.

INTRODUCTION TO CRITIQUE NO. I

The article *A Comparison of the Effects of Jaw Relaxation and Music on Postoperative Pain* by Good (1995) is critically examined in terms of its quality and the potential usefulness of the findings for application to nursing practice.

Problem and Purpose

The author states that the purposes of this study were "(a) to conduct a controlled experiment to compare the individual and combined effects of jaw relaxation and music on the sensory and affective components of pain after the first postoperative ambulation, and (b) to describe self-care use and helpfulness of these interventions during the next 48 hours." In the first purpose, jaw relaxation and music are the independent variables affecting the dependent variable of sensory and affective components of pain. In the second purpose, the goal is to describe the self-care variables of jaw relaxation and music in terms of usefulness over the next 48 hours. The purpose specifies a postoperative population. The purposes are appropriately stated and provide direction for statistical analyses.

Good (1995) identifies the significance of the problem as improved control of pain after abdominal surgery. Failure to control pain by prescribed analgesics contributes to complications along with lengthened recovery and hospital stay.

Review of Literature and Definitions

The conceptual framework for this study is based on Orem's self-care deficit theory of nursing and the gate-control theory of pain. The concepts that are discussed include noxious stimuli, self-care action, and pain perception. The conceptual definition of noxious stimuli is abdominal surgery; self-care action is use of jaw relaxation, music or both; and perceptions of pain include sensory and affective components. Good (1995) identifies tissue damage associated with abdominal pain as the stimulus causing pain. Self-care actions are introduced as adjuncts to analgesics to assist in relieving pain perceptions.

Gaps justifying the research include inconsistent findings relative to the effectiveness of the use of relaxation and music in ameliorating postoperative pain and no comparisons of these individual interventions with the combined use of relaxation and music. This study uses a controlled experimental design to determine single and combined effectiveness of the interventions.

An appropriate theoretical base is derived from predominantly primary sources. The reference to Flaherty and Fitzpatrick (cited by Good, 1995) is an example of a primary source, because it is identified as a preliminary study using jaw relaxation technique that is being replicated in this study. The reference selected to illustrate the use of a secondary source is the AHCPR Publication by the Acute Pain Management Guideline Panel, which presents guidelines based on the review of relevant research studies (cited by Good, 1995).

The independent variable of jaw relaxation was operationalized by replicating the procedure described by Flaherty and Fitzpatrick to reduce muscle and mental tension. The use of music to reduce pain was operationalized through subject's choice from one of five types of sedative music taped without lyrics. The combined intervention was operationalized as practicing jaw relaxation while listening to subject selected music. The control was operationalized as routine care.

The dependent variables were the sensory and affective components of pain. Sensory component of pain was measured by the Sensation of Pain Scale and 24-hour narcotic use. Affective component of pain was measured by the Distress of Pain Scale and the State Anxiety Inventory. All operational definitions reflect the conceptualization of the respective independent and dependent variables.

Hypotheses and/or Research Questions

Hypotheses rather than research questions are used appropriately in this study. The hypotheses are the following:

1. Controlling for preambulatory sensation, distress, narcotic intake, and preoperative anxiety, there will be a difference between the individual groups (relaxation and

music) in sensation, distress, and anxiety of pain after the first postoperative ambulation and in narcotic intake during the next 24 hours.

2. Controlling for preambulatory sensation, distress, narcotic intake, and preoperative anxiety, there will be a difference between the relaxation and music groups taken together and compared to the combination group in sensation, distress, and anxiety of pain after the first postoperative ambulation and in narcotic intake during the next 24 hours.

3. Controlling for preambulatory sensation, distress, narcotic intake, and preoperative anxiety, the relaxation, music, and combination groups taken together will have less sensation, distress, and anxiety of pain after the first postoperative ambulation and less narcotic intake during the next 24 hours than the control group.

The independent variables in the three hypotheses are (1) relaxation and music; (2) relaxation, music, and combined relaxation and music; and (3) relaxation, music, combined relaxation and music, and control. The dependent variables in the three hypotheses are sensation, distress, anxiety of pain, and narcotic use. All hypotheses are stated in research form and are testable. The first two hypotheses are nondirectional, and the third is directional. The third hypothesis predicts that relaxation, music, and combination groups will have less sensation, distress, and anxiety of pain after the first postoperative ambulation and less narcotic intake during the next 24 hours than the control group.

Sample

The convenience sample was recruited from a sampling frame comprised of all eligible patients scheduled for elective abdominal surgery in four hospitals over a 7-month period. The investigator determined eligibility from surgery lists in consultation with office nurses. Each eligible patient was contacted and invited to participate. The use of a nonprobability sample limits generalization to the sample itself. The sample selected for inclusion in the research project matches the population proposed in the purpose statement, because data collection occurred during the postoperative period. The 84 subjects who agreed to participate were randomly assigned to four groups of 21 each. The adequacy of sample size would be questionable given the criteria of a minimum of 20 and a preference for 30 per group. There is no report of power analysis to support the desired sample size.

Research Design

The three criteria for a true experiment are met in the design of this study. The patients who signed informed consent were randomly assigned to four groups, one of which was a control group, thus meeting the criteria of randomization and control. Manipulation was met by three groups receiving different interventions (i.e., jaw relaxation, music, and combined jaw relaxation and music). The choice of an experimental design is congruent with (1) the purpose of comparing individual and combined effects of the designated interventions on pain relief postoperatively; (2) the conceptual framework (as presented in the literature review), which supports the efficacy of enhancing patient self-care actions on decreasing pain perceptions; and (3) the hypotheses, which predict differences in sensation, distress, and anxiety of pain between groups with less in the treatment groups than in the control group.

Internal Validity

Examination of threats to internal validity reveals no indication of difficulty associated with history or maturation with this adult population over a brief time span. Selection bias is controlled by specific selection criteria used to identify subjects who are randomly assigned to groups. Mortality is probably not a threat, because the number of subjects per group was maintained despite the subject loss of 18 of the 102 patients who initially consented. Of the 18, 15 no longer met inclusion criteria, leaving only 3 who remained eligible but were lost to the study. Good (1995) reports that subjects in the four groups when compared were equivalent on demographic and surgical variables. Potential threat due to instrumentation appears controlled through use of a standardized procedure to ensure consistency in observation and measurement of variables. Repeated use of measures may contribute to threat due to testing. The State Anxiety Scale was administered after obtaining consent and after first ambulation. The measures of sensation and distress were taken before and after first ambulation postoperatively. The threats identified seem minimal, but it is difficult to discern whether these are contributing to the nonsignificant findings.

External Validity

Generalizability of findings is limited by the use of a nonprobability sampling technique. The findings may be generalized only to the sample.

Research Approach

Methods

Data collection methods include interview, questionnaires, observation, and use of available records. Data collection procedures as described are consistent and systematic for both the experimental and control groups. Written informed consent was obtained at the first visit, and those who consented were assigned to groups.

Instruments

Structured interviews and observations were completed by the data gatherer or interviewer who first contacted the patient preoperatively. Training of the data gatherers is not reported. Observation was used during instruction and ambulation to validate mastery of the intervention technique. The subjects were rated on five criteria: "no tension around the mouth, no grimace or frown, not talking, slow respirations, face relaxed" (Good, 1995). Inferences appear to be necessary, because these descriptors might be interpreted differently by different observers. There is a possibility of modification of responses due to the presence of an observer. Demographic data and a measure of preoperative anxiety were obtained by the interviewer. The potential for interviewer bias does exist, although there is no discussion of evidence of such bias in the research report.

Questionnaires used included the Sensation of Pain scale, the Distress of Pain scale, and the State Anxiety Inventory. Both pain scales are a horizontal line numbered from 0 to 10 with three verbal anchors. The State Anxiety Inventory is made up of 20 statements on a 4-point Likert scale.

Good (1995) justifies the use of recorded narcotic intake in the $2\frac{1}{2}$ hours before ambulation as a control for the extraneous influence of analgesic action at the time of intervention.

The postambulatory narcotic intake for 24 hours was used as an indication of pain and pain management. The recorded data are used for hypotheses testing.

Reliability and Validity

The single-item measures, the Sensation of Pain and the Distress of Pain scales, lack established reliability. Good (1995) acknowledges this limitation and states, however, that "the presence of verbal anchors was expected to enhance accuracy in surgical patients." The adequacy of the reliability for these measures is questionable.

Good (1995) reports that test-retest reliability of the State Anxiety Inventory has been described. In this study, a correlation of $r = 0.37$, $p < 0.001$ is reported between the two measurement times. Internal consistency reliability using Cronbach's alpha was 0.89 for preoperative anxiety, and 0.90 for postambulatory anxiety. The reliability of 0.89 and 0.90 in this study exceeds the standard of 0.80 and would be considered adequate for this instrument.

The reliability for the measure of 24-hour narcotic use is not discussed. Reliability cannot be determined.

Construct validity of the Sensation of Pain and the Distress of Pain scales was supported by subjects being able to differentiate between pain and distress during induced ischemic pain in earlier research by Johnson (cited in Good, 1995). Concurrent validity was demonstrated in this study using the Pain Rating Index (PRI-R) of the McGill Pain Questionnaire (MPQ) as a criterion. "Postambulatory scores of the PRI-R were positively and strongly correlated with those of the sensation ($r = .44$, $p < .001$) and distress ($r = .55$, $p < .001$) scales. Correlations in this range support the concurrent validity of the sensation and distress scales" (Good, 1995). Validity of these measures is adequate.

Construct and divergent validity of the State Anxiety Inventory are said to be described by Speilberger. Information from previous studies is not available in this report, and thus adequacy of the validity cannot be judged based on the information presented. The State Anxiety Inventory generally is accepted as an established instrument and considered a valid measure of anxiety.

The validity of the measure of 24-hour narcotic use is not discussed, but its use appears obvious.

Analysis of Data

Both the Sensation of Pain and Distress of Pain scales consist of one item with "a horizontal line numbered from 0 to 10 with three verbal anchors" and produce data at what is commonly accepted as interval level of measurement. The State Anxiety Inventory score is a sum of 20 statements rated on a 4-point Likert scale and also produces data at an interval level of measurement. The measure of narcotic intake was converted to milligrams of morphine equivalent, which would be a ratio level of measurement.

Good (1995) reports results of data analyses using descriptive and inferential statistics. Descriptive statistics reported are means, standard deviations, frequencies, percents, and ranges. Inferential tests used include ANOVA, ANCOVA, chi-square, and correlations. The statistics are appropriate to the variables' respective levels of measurement. The use of ANCOVA to test the hypothesized differences between groups on the specified variables while controlling for preoperative and preambulatory measures is appropriate. The level of significance set for preoperative and preambulatory measures is appropriate. The level of significance set for the study is specified as 0.05.

One table is used to present additional information. This table is precisely titled and headed, and it supplements the content on data analyses presented in the narrative. Unnecessary repetition is avoided.

Conclusions, Implications, and Recommendations

None of the hypothesis were supported. The author appropriately interprets the findings in relation to the study's purpose: that of comparing the effects of jaw relaxation and music on the sensory and affective components of pain after first postoperative ambulation, and notes that the findings are contradictory to the expectations articulated in the hypotheses and to the conceptual framework used for the study. Good (1995) implies limitations in the discussion of factors for modification in future research, including strengthening interventions in relation to personal and contextual variables.

Good's (1995) implications for practice are in the summary statement, "because relaxation and music interventions pose a low risk to patients and may reduce pain and side effects of medication in some people, their usefulness should continue to be explored." Within the qualifying limits stated for implications for practice, Good elaborates, "Nurses may try them in interested, capable, and adequately medicated patients who need additional analgesia or wish to reduce side effects." The use of the term explored (above) reflects recognition of nonsignificance of findings, continued support of potential benefits, and continued examination of possible use of these interventions (already being used in nursing practice) rather than direct application. Thus the generalization is within the scope of the study.

Application to Nursing Practice

Strengths are evident in the design and conduct of this research. However, the lack of significant findings is consistent with some earlier studies that fail to support the effectiveness of relaxation and music for pain control at ambulation. Thus direct application to nursing practice is not supported. This study should be replicated in another clinical setting using Good's (1995) suggestions for strengthening the intervention and validating adequacy of sample size through power analysis.

CRITIQUE OF A RESEARCH STUDY: SAMPLE NO. 2

The study *Problem-Focused Coping in HIV-Infected Mothers in Relation to Self-Efficacy, Uncertainty, Social Support, and Psychological Distress* by Nancy C. Sharts-Hopko, RN, PhD, FAAN; Mary Jo Regan-Kubinski, RN, PhD; Patricia S. Lincoln, RN, BSN; and Mary Ann Heverly, PhD, published in *IMAGE: Journal of Nursing Scholarship* (1996), is critiqued. The article is presented first and is followed by the critique on p. 438.

PROBLEM-FOCUSED COPING IN HIV-INFECTED MOTHERS IN RELATION TO SELF-EFFICACY, UNCERTAINTY, SOCIAL SUPPORT, AND PSYCHOLOGICAL DISTRESS*

Nancy C. Sharts-Hopko, Mary Jo Regan-Kubinski, Patricia S. Lincoln, Mary Ann Heverly

A preliminary investigation of relationships among perceived self-efficacy, uncertainty, social support, psychological distress, and problem-focused coping was conducted in a convenience sample of 41 HIV-infected mothers. The mothers represented 93% of the clients in a large HIV clinic in 1992 who met the study criteria. Support was found for using Lazarus and Folkman's stress, appraisal, and coping framework to understand the health-related needs of HIV-infected mothers. Maternal coping was related to living with one's children and their HIV-status. The feasibility of studying this population of women was demonstrated. Findings suggest the need for exploration of family-focused interventions.

Women constitute the fastest growing segment of people infected with human immunodeficiency virus (HIV) in the United States (Sabo & Carwein, 1994). The gender difference in incidence of newly infected individuals is expected to disappear soon (Jemmott & Jemmott, 1994). In nine American cities, HIV/AIDS is now the number one killer of young women. In Newark, New Jersey for example, deaths among young women from HIV/AIDS is as high as 43% (Selik, Chu, & Buehler, 1993).

About 30% of the infected women who are pregnant transmit HIV to their infants (Wilfert, 1991). HIV-infected women who are mothers have an especially heavy burden—to prepare for the care of their children who will be left motherless or orphaned. Often, they must also care for children and other family members who are HIV-infected, generally in impoverished circumstances (Michaels, 1992; Rosser, 1991). Given current trends, it is estimated that by the year 2000, over 80,000 American children age 17 and younger will have been left motherless because of HIV/AIDS.

Current understanding of the way people experience HIV/AIDS has been gained primarily through the study of gay men (Rosser, 1991). This population tends to be better educated and more affluent, and face different family obligations than do HIV-infected women. Knowledge of how women experience other life-threatening illnesses fails to explain the experience of HIV-infection because of the stigma of HIV/AIDS, the demographics of the women most likely to get the disease, and the erratic course of the disease (Nichols, 1985). To date, there is little research about how infected women experience or cope with HIV/AIDS. Growing evidence among diverse study populations supports the importance of self-efficacy to effective coping. Therefore, this study was undertaken to explore relationships among perceived self-efficacy, uncertainty, social support, psychological distress, and problem-focused coping in HIV-infected mothers. This report is from a larger project that also included qualitative exploration of illness cognition and illness-related decision-making (Regan-Kubinski & Sharts-Hopko, 1995).

*This section, from pp. 429 to 438, is taken from Sharts-Hopko NC et al: Problem-focused coping in HIV-infected mothers in relation to self-efficacy, uncertainty, social support, and psychological distress, *Image J Nurs Sch* 28:107-111, 1996. Reprinted with permission of Sigma Theta Tau.

REVIEW OF LITERATURE

Until recently, symptoms typical of HIV-infection in women were not included in diagnostic criteria for AIDS that were established by the Centers for Disease Control and Prevention (CDC). These omissions led to failures in diagnosis and treatment of HIV infection in women. Further, women have been systematically excluded from research on HIV therapies because of concerns about compliance related to their socioeconomic deprivation and about fetotoxic effects if women on experimental therapies were to become pregnant (Rosser, 1991). Over 70% of HIV-infected women are persons of color (CDC, 1993). They tend to be poor and over 70% have contracted the disease through drug use or having sexual relations with drug users. The sociodemographic characteristics of HIV-infected women make access to them difficult. This plus the tendency for health care workers to protect the privacy of AIDS patients create formidable barriers for investigators (Fetter & Larson, 1990; Gaskins, Sowell & Gueldner, 1991).

Research on HIV-infected women tends to focus on prevalence (Morse, Lessner, Medvesky, Glebatis, & Novick, 1991), women's knowledge of HIV/AIDS and of risk of avoidance (Hale, Char, Nagy, & Stockert, 1993; Harrison et al., 1991), and the capacity of women to infect men (Rosser, 1991; Smeltzer & Whipple, 1991). Researchers have also explored the effect of maternal HIV/AIDS on children (Ehrnst et al., 1991; Michaels, 1992; Van de Perre et al., 1993; Wilfert, 1991).

Of the few studies that exist regarding the effect of HIV illness on women, most have used extremely small samples. Hutchinson and Kurth (1991) interviewed 11 HIV-infected women about their pregnancy-related decision-making. Three chose to terminate their pregnancies, while eight did not. Factors influencing the women's decision-making included their degree of child-centeredness, their desire for a child, the influence of family dynamics and religious faith, assessment of risk, attitude toward abortion, degree of optimism, prior experience with pregnancy, death of a child, fears related to childbearing pain, and their ability to care for the child. Hutchinson and Kurth also identified a sense of isolation among these women as important.

Andrews, Williams, and Neil (1993) analyzed interview data from 80 HIV-infected women about their social support. The positive value of relationships with their children was emphasized. However the burden of child care responsibilities, the guilt associated with exposing children to HIV as well as eventually abandoning their children, and the pain associated with sharing the stigma of HIV/AIDS with their children also emerged as important facets of women's experience of HIV/AIDS. Additional research about how women cope with HIV-infection, including assessment of women's perceptions of their ability to cope effectively, is needed.

FRAMEWORK FOR THE STUDY

The theoretical basis for this study was derived from the stress, appraisal, and coping framework of Lazarus and Folkman (1984). Stress is defined in this framework as a response to an interaction between a person and an event in the environment that taxes and potentially exceeds a person's resources, resulting in endangerment to well-being. Appraisal is the perception, assessment, and evaluation of threat. One's ability to cope with stress and deal with problems that emerge from a stressful situation depends on one's appraisal of the situation.

Antecedent or stress-induced psychopathology impedes a person's ability to appraise a stressful situation and to cope effectively with it.

Within this framework, coping is the process of managing the demands imposed by a stressor and the related feelings that arise. Coping with stress can be problem-focused or emotion-focused. Problem-focused coping is analyzing alternative solutions and selecting an action. Emotion-focused coping involves use of cognitive processes directed at lessening emotional distress (Lazarus & Folkman, 1984, pp. 150-152). While emotion-focused coping can be a helpful outlet for individuals, problem-focused coping is associated with actions that lead to positive change.

Successful problem-focused coping depends on the availability and mobilization of resources, balanced by constraints. Making use of resources is contingent on a person's appraisal of a stressful situation (Cohen & Lazarus, 1983). Uncertainty is associated with unfamiliar stressors such as a diagnosis of HIV infection and is stressful in itself. A high degree of uncertainty may foster avoidance behaviors and impede problem-directed action, i.e., problem-focused coping (Christman, 1990; Lazarus & Folkman, 1984, pp. 101-102; Mishel, 1981; Mishel & Braden, 1988). Internal and external resources, such as perceived ability to cope, or self-efficacy, and social support, can buffer stress and facilitate problem-focused coping (Lazarus & Folkman, 1984, pp. 69-70, 243-250).

This study explored relationships among perceived self-efficacy; uncertainty associated with HIV infection; the availability of such resources as perceived social support and advantageous socioeconomic status; psychological distress associated with the experience of HIV infection; and problem-focused coping in a sample of HIV-infected mothers. In addition, the influence of illness factors was examined.

METHODOLOGY

Subjects

Participants were recruited in a large, federally funded HIV community program at an infectious disease clinic in a Mid-Atlantic medical center. The study was approved by appropriate human subjects review committees. Over a 6 month data collection period in 1992, a nurse clinical specialist at the site recruited women who met the study criteria. Of about 125 women in the clinic, 44 who met the criteria for inclusion had clinic visits during the data collection period, and 41 (93%) participated. Informed consent was obtained. The women were paid $25 for participating.

Most personal data obtained about the study participants are summarized in Table 1. All women were mothers. No woman had left school before completion of eighth grade, and one had attained a master's degree. Seven (17%) stated they had no family income. Living arrangements of some women could not be identified with precision, and homelessness was common. While data on how women became HIV-infected are imprecise, two were known to have been transfused with infected blood, and several were able to identify the sexual partner who infected them. Most were at risk because of a lifestyle involving sex with many partners, and drugs.

Among the women, 28 pregnancies had occurred since diagnosis with HIV: 13 had one pregnancy since diagnosis, 6 had been pregnant twice, and 1 had had three pregnancies. Three of the 28 pregnancies had been terminated. Among offspring, 3 children were HIV-infected

Table I

Study Participants

CONTINUOUS VARIABLES	MEAN	SD
Age (years)	31.71	7.29
Time since last employment (months)	13.76	17.38
Years of schooling (years)	11.83	.27
Annual family income	$9311.12	$10,005.88
Time since diagnosis (months)	30.17	15.26
Gravidity	3.32	2.35
Parity	2.20	1.57
Children at home	1.27	1.34
Number prescribed medications	3.32	3.62

CATEGORICAL VARIABLES	FREQUENCY	PERCENT
Ethnic/racial background		
African American	28	68
Caucasian	8	20
Native American	3	7
Latina/Hispanic	2	5
Church affiliation		
Yes	38	92
No	3	8
Marital status		
Divorced or single	28	68
Married	7	17
Cohabiting	4	10
Widowed	2	5
Work status		
Unemployed	27	66
Employed	13	32
Student	1	2
Previously employed	40	98
Never employed	1	2

and 10 were being evaluated at the time of data collection. Within 9 months of the completion of data collection, over 10% of the women in the sample had died.

Measures

Six questionnaires were administered. According to Bandura (1977, 1986), who advanced the construct of perceived self-efficacy (PSE), the expectation of self-efficacy is subjective and situation specific (Alden, 1986; Beck & Lund, 1982). PSE was measured by asking subjects to rate themselves on visual analog scales scored from 1 (Most negative) to 100 (Most affirmative) for two dimensions: Their perceived capability of meeting challenges associated with their HIV infection (PSE-1), and their confidence that they would succeed in meeting those challenges (PSE-2). The potential range was 1 to 100 on each scale (2 to 200 for the total).

Uncertainty was measured using the Mishel Uncertainty in Illness Scale (MUIS) (Mishel, 1981; Mishel & Braden, 1988). The MUIS is a 33-item Likert-type scale with a potential range of 33 to 165. Internal consistency using Cronbach's alpha was .78 for this sample. Factor analysis has supported construct validity and the MUIS has been shown to discriminate among medical, surgical, and diagnostic populations.

Perceived social support was assessed using the short form of the Interpersonal Relationship Inventory (IPRI) (Tilden, 1991). The IPRI has 26 five-point Likert-type items, with a potential range of 13 to 65 for each of two subscales: (a) social support and (b) conflict, or cost of support. This view of social support is consistent with that of Lazarus and Folkman (1984, pp. 243-250). Development of the instrument included subjects in a range of stressful life situations such as being homeless and having cancer. Test-retest correlations of up to .91 have been reported and for this sample, Cronbach's alpha coefficients were .87 on the social support subscale, .82 on the conflict subscale, and .83 for the total. Validation strategies have included factor analysis, criterion referencing, and use of known groups.

The Brief Symptom Inventory (BSI) was used to measure perceived psychological distress (Derogatis & Spencer, 1982). This is a self-report measure of current psychological status that consists of 53 five-point Likert-type items measuring an individual's level of psychopathology in terms of number as well as severity of symptoms. It has a potential range of scores of 0 to 212. For this sample, a Cronbach's alpha coefficient of .96 was calculated, surpassing the authors' reported test-retest reliabilities of up to .91. Derogatis and Spencer have documented a high degree of convergent and discriminate as well as known group validity using psychiatric and nonpsychiatric populations. The BSI is sensitive to changes in psychological status arising from mental illness, treatment, life stress, and chronic pain.

Problem-focused coping (PFC) was measured using a subscale of the Ways of Coping Revised Checklist (Folkman & Lazarus, 1980, 1985). This measure includes six items rated on four-point Likert-type scales, with a possible range of scores of 0 to 18. Internal consistency as assessed using Cronbach's alpha statistic was .71. Construct validity in stress research has been demonstrated on populations experiencing stress in health, work, family, and school. Other subscales of the Ways of Coping Revised Checklist were omitted in this study because of the human subjects review committee's concerns about subjects' fatiguability.

A personal data questionnaire was used to elicit information about sociodemographic factors, reproductive history, HIV status of children, and current medications. Number of prescribed medications serves as one indicator of severity of illness.

Procedure

One investigator collected all data in private examining rooms in the clinic. An open-ended interview was tape recorded. The six questionnaires were administered with the researcher reading each item and recording the participant's oral response. Data collection took about 1-hour per subject. (One exceptional interview lasted nearly 4-hours because the subject shared so much detail and insight about her long, downhill course of illness; she died soon after.)

RESULTS

The scores are summarized in Table 2. Despite the degree of unemployment, lack of income, and uncertain housing arrangements, means were located in the middle ranges or better of possible ranges. A significance level of .01 was established to ensure that unimportant relationships would not be deemed significant when many correlations were examined. Table 3 shows inter-correlations among those variables for which relationships significant at the .01 level were observed.

While a larger sample would have supported examination of multiple correlations, the size of this sample ($N = 41$) guided the decision to report Pearson product-moment correlations. Categorical data were dichotomized. For example, ethnicity was coded as "Caucasian/women of color" and work status was "currently employed/currently unemployed," allowing for computation of point-biserial correlations.

Perceived self-efficacy was inversely associated with psychological distress and duration of an HIV-infected child's illness, and was positively associated with problem-focused coping. Problem-focused coping was inversely related to duration of an HIV-infected child's illness; and psychological distress was inversely related to number of children residing with the participant.

Perceived social support was inversely associated with length of time since last employment, while the perceived cost of social support was inversely associated with psychological distress. Caucasian women were more likely to have greater family income and, not surprisingly, current employment was positively associated with household income.

DISCUSSION

While this sample of HIV-infected mothers reflects the population of HIV-infected women in the United States in terms of race, income level, and lifestyle factors that may have contributed to their HIV status, it did not mirror the general population's experience of HIV/AIDS in terms of access to and quality of health care and social services. Rather, this data reflects the experience of women who had access to comprehensive, multiservice care through a coordinated effort of the community programs and various private, religious, municipal, state, and federal programs. All of these women were able to identify active supportive relationships. However, even in view of these relatively good circumstances, the day-to-day experience of the women was extremely difficult.

Interpretation of these results requires caution because of the limited sample size. Despite the study's limitations, there appears to be some degree of interrelatedness among correlates of coping, including perceived self-efficacy, perceived social support, psychological distress, and problem-focused coping. These observations are congruent with Lazarus and Folkman's

Table 2

Mean Scores, Standard Deviations, and Ranges of Scores on Measures of Study Variables Administered to 41 HIV-Infected Mothers

TESTS*	MEAN	SD	RANGE
PSE-1	70.34	20.27	24-100
PSE-2	78.98	20.23	24-100
PSE-Total	149.32	37.40	50-200
MUIS	89.80	18.99	45-127
IPRI	97.07	28.93	19-193
IPRI-Support	58.68	4.94	40-65
IPRI-Conflict	35.93	12.56	16-61
BSI	65.78	43.18	6-187
PFC	13.78	3.85	1-18

*PSE, Perceived Self-Efficacy; MUIS, Mischel Uncertainty in Illness Scale; IPRI, Interpersonal Relationship Inventory; BSI, Brief Symptom Inventory; PFC, Problem-Focused Coping.

Table 3

Intercorrelations Among Study Variables, Demographic, and Illness Factors (N = 41)

	BSI	PSE	IPRI-S	IPRI-C	PFC	ETHNIC	EMPL
BSI		−.40*	.10	−.56†	.12	−.05	−.16
PFC	.12	.44*	−.06	−.28		−.15	−.09
CHLDILL	.05	−.43*	.06	.14	−.46*	.02	−.01
CHLDHM	−.42*	−.04	.20	−.08	−.09	−.36	.20
TIMEMP	.20	−.00	−.37*	−.19	.05	−.15	−.58†
INCOME	.20	.01	−.02	.28	−.18	.47*	.44*

*p < .01.
† p < .001.

BSI, Brief Symptom Inventory; PSE, Perceived Self-Efficacy; IPRI-S, Interpersonal Relationship Inventory-Support; IPRI-C, Interpersonal Inventory-Conflict; PFC, Problem-Focused Coping; ETHNIC, Ethnicity; EMPL, Employment status; CHLDILL, Duration of HIV-infected child's illness; CHLDHM, Number of children in the home; TIMEMP, Months since last employed; INCOME, Annual family income.

(1984) conceptual framework. For example, social support is a coping resource. Among women in this sample, social support was less likely to be available with increasing length of time unemployed. This finding is not surprising in the context of Lazarus and Folkman's (1984) observations that stressors often lead to more stressors or that individuals are unable to mobilize beyond a certain person-specific stress level.

Tilden's (1991) assumption that social support may come at a personal cost made her Interpersonal Relationship Inventory consistent with Lazarus and Folkman's (1984) view of the impact of social support on individual coping. In this group of unusually stressed women, greater acknowledgement of the cost of social support came with decreased psychological distress. The ability to recognize the costs of social support may be an indicator of coping or at least of a lesser degree of neediness. Ethnicity, employment status, and household income were clustered. It is not unexpected that Caucasian women have social advantages over women of color even in the circumstances of HIV/AIDS illness.

Most mothers continued their pregnancies after HIV diagnosis, a finding consistent with the report by Hutchinson and Kurth (1991). This decision warrants further study. In addition, the number of children in the home was inversely related to psychological distress. The lifestyles of some of these women resulted in their loss of custody of their children. Women who experience better mental health are more likely to maintain a home for their children, though the sequence of cause and effect is not known. Interviews with these women strongly suggested that assuming responsibility for one's children forces one to be more competent and capable. The children of the women in the study were tremendously motivating to them in making lifestyle changes that would enhance their health status, a finding that warrants further study.

Duration of an HIV-infected child's illness was inversely related to perceived self-efficacy and problem-focused coping. While caution must be exercised in interpreting this finding, because of the limited number of women whose children were known to be HIV-infected, the relationship to measures of maternal well-being of children's residence with their mothers and the children's health status is consistent with nursing's emphasis on the family as client. This finding suggests the need for exploration of family-care strategies for families affected by HIV/AIDS.

Statistically significant relationships are not to be confused with clinical significance. But these findings suggest the need to examine the relationships among those variables in a larger random sample, which would allow for use of multivariate techniques and determination of unique contributions to variance in problem-focused coping.

An important observation was the strong desire of the HIV-infected women to participate in this study. The modest cash honorarium for participation was important; also many of the women stated during the interview that they valued being able to make a personal contribution to understanding the effect of HIV/AIDS on individuals and families. Staff and volunteers reported that participants often stated during clinic visits or support group sessions that the interviews had been helpful to them.

CONCLUSION

Findings of this preliminary study suggest that the experience of HIV-infected mothers can be studied within a stress, appraisal, and coping framework. Correlates or indicators of effective coping, psychological distress, perceived self-efficacy, and problem-focused coping are interrelated, as are measures of social advantage. Indicators of resources such as social support are relevant to indicators of positive coping in this group and indicators of positive coping are related to residence with and the HIV-status of one's children.

Relationships between mothers' coping and the HIV-status of and residence with their children underscore the need for nurses to approach HIV/AIDS as a disease affecting whole families. The unique role of women in relation to their families that prompted this investigation of coping during HIV-infection was affirmed by the findings.

REFERENCES

Alden, L. (1986). Self-efficacy and causal attributions of social feedback. Journal of Research in Personality, 20, 460-473.

Andrews, A., Williams, A.B., & Neil, K. (1993). The mother-child relationship in the HIV-1 positive family. Image: Journal of Nursing Scholarship, 25, 193-198.

Bandura, A. (1977). Self-efficacy: Toward a unifying theory of behavioral change. Psychology Review, 84, 191-215.

Bandura, A. (1986). Fearful expectations and avoidant actions as coefficients of perceived self-efficacy. American Psychologist, 41, 1389-1391.

Beck, K.H., & Lund, A.K. (1982). The effects of health threat seriousness and personal efficacy upon intentions and behavior. Journal of Applied Social Psychology, 11(5), 401-415.

Centers for Disease Control and Prevention (1993). Facts about women and HIV/AIDS. CDC HIV/AIDS Prevention (February), 1-2.

Christman, N.J. (1990). Uncertainty and adjustment during radiotherapy. Nursing Research, 39, 17-20.

Cohen, F., & Lazarus, R.S. (1983). Coping and adaptation in health and illness. In D. Mechanic (Ed.), Handbook of health, health care, and the health professions (pp. 608-635). New York: Free Press.,

Derogatis, L., & Spencer, P.M. (1982). The brief symptom inventory (BSI) administration, scoring & procedures manual-I. Towson, MD: Clinical Psychometric Research.

Ehrnst, A., Lindgren, S., Dictor, M., Johansson, B. Sonnerborg, A., Czajkowski, J., Sundin, G., & Bohlin, A-B. (1991, July 17). HIV in pregnant women and their offspring: Evidence for later transmission. Lancet, 338, 203-207.

Fetter, M.S., & Larson, E. (1990). Preventing and treating human immunodeficiency virus infection in the homeless. Archives of Psychiatric Nursing, 4 (6), 379-383.

Folkman, S., & Lazarus, R. (1980). An analysis of coping in a middle-aged community sample. Journal of Health and Social Behavior, 21, 219-239.

Folkman, S., & Lazarus, R. (1985). If it changes it must be a process: Study of emotion and coping during three stages of a college examination. Journal of Personality and Social Psychology, 48, 150-170.

Gaskins, S., Sowell, R., & Gueldner, S. (1991). Overcoming methodological barriers to HIV/AIDS nursing research. Journal of Nurses in AIDS Care, 2 (4), 33-37.

Hale, R.W., Char, D.F.B., Nagy, K., & Stockert, N. (1993). Seventeen-year review of sexual and contraceptive behavior on a college campus. American Journal of Obstetrics & Gynecology, 168 (6), 1833-1838.

Harrison, D.F., Wambach, K.G., Byers, J.B., Imershein, A.W., Levine, P., Maddox, K., Quadagno, D.M., Fordyce, M.L., & Jones, M.A. (1991). AIDS knowledge and risk behaviors among culturally diverse women. AIDS Education and Prevention, 3 (2), 79-89.

Hutchinson, M., & Kurth, A. (1991, Feb.) I need to know that I have a choice . . . A study of women, HIV, and reproductive decision-making. AIDS Patient Care, 5, 17-25.

Jemmott, L.S., & Jemmott, J.B. (1994). Health promotion and disease prevention: New strategies targeting HIV/AIDS. In W.L. Holzemer & C.J. Portillo (Eds.), HIV/AIDS nursing care summit proceedings (pp. 58-74). Washington, DC: American Academy of Nursing.

Lazarus, S., & Folkman, R.S. (1984). Stress, appraisal and coping. New York: Springer.

Michaels, D. (1992). Estimates of the number of motherless youth orphaned by AIDS in the United States. Journal of the American Medical Association, 268, 3456-3461.

Mishel, M. (1981). The measurement of uncertainty in illness. Nursing Research, 30, 258-263.

Mishel, M., & Braden, C.J. (1988). Finding meaning: Antecedents of uncertainty in illness. Nursing Research, 37, 98-103.

Morse, D.L., Lessner, L., Medvesky, M.G., Glebatis, D.M., & Novick, L.F. (1991). Geographic distribution of newborn HIV seroprevalence in relation to four sociodemographic variables. American Journal of Public Health, 81(May Supp.), 25-29.

Nichols, S.E. (1985). Psychosocial reactions of persons with the acquired immunodeficiency syndrome. Annals of Internal Medicine, 103, 765-767.

Regan-Kubinski, M.J., & Sharts-Hopko, N. (1995). Illness cognition of HIV-infected mothers. Issues in Mental Health Nursing, 16, 327-344.

Rosser, S.V. (1991). AIDS and women. AIDS Education and Prevention, 3 (3), 230-240.

Sabo, C.E., & Carwein, V.L. (1994). Women and HIV/AIDS. Journal of Nurses in AIDS Care, 5 (3):15-21.

Selik, R.M., Chu, S.Y., & Buehler, J.W. (1993). HIV infection as leading cause of death among young adults in US cities and states. Journal of the American Medical Association, 269, 2991-2994.

Smeltzer, S.C., & Whipple, B. (1991). Women with HIV infection: The unrecognized population. Health Values, 15 (6), 41-48.

Tilden, V.P. (1991). The Tilden interpersonal relationship inventory (IPRI) instrument development summary. Portland, OR: Oregon Health Sciences University School of Nursing.

Van de Perre, P., Simonon, A., Hitimana, D.G., Dabis, F., Msellati, P., Mukamabano, B., Butera, J.B., Van Goethem, C., Karita, E., & Lapage, P. (1993). Infective and anti-infective properties of breast milk from HIV-1 infected women. Lancet, 341 (8850), 914-918.

Wilfert, C.M. (1991, May 15). HIV infection in maternal and pediatric patients. Hospital Practice, 26, 55-57.

INTRODUCTION TO CRITIQUE NO. 2

This critique examines the research reported by Sharts-Hopko et al (1996) that explored "the relationships among perceived self-efficacy, uncertainty, social support, psychological distress, and problem-focused coping in HIV-infected mothers." The purpose of this critique is to determine the quality of the research on the basis of the information provided in the report, as well as its potential usefulness for nursing practice.

Problem and Purpose

The identified purpose is "to explore relationships among perceived self-efficacy, uncertainty, social support, psychological distress, and problem-focused coping in HIV-infected mothers." The statement suggests the use of correlations to test the relationships among the identified variables in a population of human immunodeficiency virus (HIV) infected mothers. The authors appropriately identify the significance of the problem of HIV in women through documentation of this group as the fastest-growing population segment infected with HIV and the lack of information related to their experiences, coping, and decision making.

Review of Literature and Definitions

The concepts included in the literature review are congruent with those of the theoretical framework: appraisal, coping, uncertainty, perceived ability to cope, and resources. Appraisal is conceptually defined as "the perception, assessment, and evaluation of threat"; coping as the "process of managing the demands imposed by a stressor and the related feelings that arise"; problem-focused coping (PFC) as "analyzing alternative solutions and selecting an action"; internal and external resources as including "perceived ability to cope or self-efficacy, and social support" (Sharts-Hopko et al, 1996). The relationship of these variables is based on Lazarus and Folkman's theory of stress, appraisal, and coping. Problem-focused or emotion-focused coping depends on the appraisal of a situation. Problem-focused coping involves use of resources responsive to the appraisal, with unfamiliar stressors such as HIV diagnosis contributing to uncertainty. Uncertainty may contribute to avoidance rather than action based on problem solving. Resources such as perceived ability to cope and social support may serve to buffer stress and "facilitate problem-focused coping."

The authors identify a gap in the literature as the limited study on how women cope with HIV infection and their own perception of their ability to cope. The majority of the sources cited by these authors are primary. The reference by Christman, in which the author reports her research, constitutes a primary source (cited in Sharts-Hopko et al, 1996). The article by Wilfert, who draws on a variety of sources in describing infection in maternal and pediatric patients (cited in Sharts-Hopko et al, 1996), provides an example of a secondary source.

Adequate measurement or operationalization of the variables is accomplished as follows: the subjects' perceived self-efficacy (PSE) by use of the two visual analog scales, one on perceived ability to meet challenges associated with their HIV infection (PSE-1) and the other on confidence of succeeding in meeting challenges associated with their HIV infection (PSE-2); uncertainty through use of the Mishel Uncertainty in Illness Scale (MUIS); perceived social support through use of the short form of the Interpersonal Relationship Inventory (IPRI); perceived psychological distress through use of the Brief Symptom Inventory (BSI); and problem-focused coping (PFC) through use of a subscale of the Ways of Coping Revised Checklist. Sociodemographic variables, reproductive history, HIV status of children, and current medications are measured via the personal data questionnaire.

Hypotheses and/or Research Questions

No research questions or research hypotheses are stated. The inferred question is: How are "perceived self-efficacy, uncertainty, social support, psychological distress, and problem-focused coping related to HIV-infected mothers" (Sharts-Hopko et al, 1996)? This question is stated in the form of a purpose and is used to guide the study.

Sample

The sample was selected from a large HIV program at an infectious disease clinic. Forty one out of 44 women who met the study criteria during a 6-month data collection period participated. A nurse clinical specialist at the site recruited subjects. This is a nonprobability convenience sample and necessitates caution in generalizing beyond the sample. The sample includes mothers who are infected with HIV and thus is consistent with the population identified in the purpose. No justification is provided for the sample size. The sample size is small, considering the number of variables being studied. The authors do identify limitations in the analysis due to the limited sample size in the statement that "a larger sample would have supported examination of multiple correlations" (Sharts-Hopko et al, 1996). However, the size may be considered adequate for the early stage of studying the identified problem.

Research Design

Sharts-Hopko et al (1996) use a nonexperimental design, specifically a correlational design. Correlational designs are nonexperimental, because there is no manipulation of an independent variable. This type of design permits the determination of whether two or more variables are related, as well as the direction and strength of the relationships. The design is consistent with the purpose of examining relationships among self-efficacy, uncertainty, social support, psychological distress, and problem-focused coping. The correlational design allows testing the relationships proposed in the theoretical framework, literature review, and inferred research question.

Internal Validity

Although the threats to internal validity are most clearly applicable to experimental research designs, attention to the relationships among the identified variables and rival interpretations that might potentially compromise the study is necessary for correlational designs as well. Possible threats of history, maturation, instrumentation, and mortality are not identified for this study. Testing is not a problem, because measures are taken only one time. Selection bias is noted as the major threat to internal validity because of the use of a small convenience sample. The lack of random selection negates control for such variables as differences in subjects' life experiences and differences in length of time since diagnosis and types of difficulties experienced associated with HIV. There are few threats to internal validity that would decrease confidence in the results.

External Validity

Generalizability is limited to the sample because of the effect of sample selection.

Research Approach

Methods

One researcher collected all data using six questionnaires. Data collection procedures are described as the same for all subjects: the investigator read each item from the questionnaires to the participants and recorded their oral responses in a private examining room. This process required about 1 hour per subject. Evidence of meeting ethical standards is indicated by Sharts-Hopko et al's (1996) report that "informed consent was obtained."

Instruments

Six questionnaires are used as interview guides, considering that the items were read to the subjects and their responses recorded. One investigator is reported as collecting all the data with no description of training before conducting the interviews. No evidence is provided to indicate any interviewer bias. It is not known whether any inflections in the voice or clarification of items occurred that might have influenced responses.

The six questionnaires used are PSE, MUIS, short form of the IPRI, the BSI, the PFC subscale of the Ways of Coping Revised Checklist, and a personal data questionnaire. The PSE consists of two visual analog scales on which the subjects rate themselves from 1 (most negative) to 100 (most affirmative) in terms of their perceived capability of meeting HIV-related challenges and in terms of their confidence in actually succeeding in meeting those challenges. The MUIS measuring uncertainty consists of 33 items rated on a five-point Likert-type scale. The IPRI consists of two subscales, one measuring social support and the second conflict, or cost of support, with a total of 26 items rated on a five-point Likert scale. The BSI, measuring perceived psychological distress, has 53 five-point Likert-type items. The PFC consists of six items using a four-point Likert-type rating scale. The format of the personal data questionnaire is not described but is assumed to have some open-ended questions to gather information on sociodemographics, history of reproduction, HIV status of children, and current medications.

Reliability and Validity

Sharts-Hopko et al (1996) assessed internal consistency reliability using Cronbach's alpha for their sample and reported coefficients of 0.78 for the MUIS; 0.82 to 0.87 for the IPRI; 0.96 for the BSI; and 0.71 for the PFC, which is only a six-item scale. Test-retest reliabilities of 0.91 from previous studies are reported for both the IPRI and the BSI. These all exceed the desired 0.70 level and indicate acceptable reliability. No reliability information is provided for the PSE or the personal data questionnaire.

Validity is not reported for either the PSE or the personal data questionnaire. Support for construct validity is alluded to for the other four instruments, as is criterion validity for the IPRI. The construct validity for the MUIS reportedly is supported by factor analysis and its ability "to discriminate among medical, surgical, and diagnostic populations" (Sharts-Hopko et al, 1996). The construct validity for the IPRI is reportedly established through strategies of factor analysis and use of known groups in previous studies. Criterion referencing strategies were used to support the instrument's criterion validity in past research, but no further elaboration is provided. The construct validity of the BSI is documented by Derogatis and Spencer (cited in Sharts-Hopko et al, 1996), who report a high degree of convergent, discriminant, and known group validity. The PFC is reported as having construct validity demonstrated through use in research of stress experienced by populations in the areas of health, work, family, and school. The validity reported appears adequate assuming the authors critiqued the validation strategies reported from previous works and determined that these were sound studies. Without this assumption, the information provided in the article is insufficient to judge the adequacy of the validity of the measurement instruments.

Analysis of Data

The scores derived from the six questionnaires used to measure the major variables are considered interval levels of measurement in this study. The PSE has two items rated on visual analog scales of 1 to 100 and the investigators appear to assume these to be equal intervals, which is a common assumption in behavioral research. The analysis uses these items separately as two individual scores (PSE-1 and PSE-2), as well as summing them for a total score (PSE-Total). The MUIS, IPRI, BSI, and PFC all have scores determined by summing the Likert ratings for a series of items. Scores such as these are commonly accepted as interval levels of measurement and are treated as such by these investigators. From the personal data questionnaire, ethnicity, church affiliation, marital status, and work status are categorical variables at a nominal level of measurement. Variables measured in months and years such as age and schooling, number of children in the home and medications, annual family income, gravidity, and parity are ratio levels of measurement.

Descriptive statistics reported are frequency counts, percentages, means, standard deviations, and ranges. Pearson product-moment correlations and point-biserial correlations are the inferential statistics used in this study. The descriptive and inferential statistical procedures are applied appropriately considering the levels of measurement identified for the variables. The use of correlations is appropriate to the intent of the study as ascertained from the purpose statement, which is to explore relationships among self-efficacy, uncertainty, social support, psychological distress, and problem-focused coping. Significance was set at 0.01, a conservative level, to avoid identifying unimportant relationships as being significant, because a large number of correlations were being examined.

Three tables are used to present detailed information. The tables are clearly titled and headed and supplement the content on data analyses presented in the narrative, thus preventing unnecessary repetition. Table 1 clarifies what information was collected via the personal data questionnaire and is useful for determining the levels of measurement of variables when evaluating the appropriateness of the statistical analysis.

Conclusions, Implications, and Recommendations

The purpose of the study was to explore the relationships among the identified variables, but no explicit hypotheses were tested. Rather, the researchers explored a large number of correlations among the study variables, demographic, and illness factors. Statistical testing was done to determine which of the correlations were significantly different from zero at the 0.01 level of significance. The investigators identify the small sample size ($n = 41$) as a limitation of their study and the rationale for using only correlations in the analysis rather than multivariate techniques, as well as for exercising caution in interpreting their findings. The significant relationships and their directions are discussed and interpreted within the context of Lazarus and Folkman's conceptual framework with the conclusion that HIV-infected mothers' experiences can be appropriately studied from a stress, appraisal, and coping perspective.

The relevance for nursing practice from this study is the affirmation of the importance of nurses approaching HIV/AIDS as a disease that affects whole families. This seems to be an appropriate conclusion that is supported by findings such as the positive relationship between mother's coping and the number of children residing with her and the inverse relationship between mother's coping and the duration of her child's HIV illness. No generalizations are made beyond this, and even this suggestion was couched in terms of caution due to the small sample size and the population studied. The investigators clearly note that while this sample "reflects the population of HIV-infected women in the United States in terms of race, income level, and lifestyle factors that may have contributed to their HIV status, it did not mirror the general population's experience of HIV/AIDS in terms of access to and quality of health care and social services" (Sharts-Hopko et al, 1996). Their sample consisted of women who had access to comprehensive, multiservice care, which is not usually the case for women experiencing HIV/AIDS.

Recommendations for further study include (1) exploring mothers' decision making regarding continuing their pregnancies after HIV diagnosis, (2) examining the influence of children in motivating mothers in making life-style changes to enhance their health status, (3) exploring family-care strategies for use with families affected by HIV/AIDS, and (4) replicating the examination of the relationships among the study variables using a larger randomly selected sample.

Application to Nursing Practice

The study has merit, given the stage of the research program. The strengths include identification of a problem for which Sharts-Hopko et al (1996) establish significance and an appropriate conceptual framework for studying the variables of interest. Instruments are identified with established reliability and validity, with the exception of the measures for perceived self-efficacy. However, this study's results provide beginning support for the validity of the PSE, because the significant associations found for the PSE, such as being positively related with problem-focused coping, are what would be expected within the theoretical framework. Results consistent with other studies are identified. For example, the finding that most mothers decided to continue with their pregnancies in spite of an HIV diagnosis is consistent with a report by Hutchinson and Kurth (cited in Sharts-Hopko et al, 1996). The major limitation of a small sample size is acknowledged by the investigators and serves to direct the need for future research.

No risks are apparent in nurses approaching HIV/AIDS as a disease that affects whole families. Benefits of this approach would be supporting HIV-infected mothers by recognizing their unique role in the family and developing interventions to strengthen their coping resources. This approach to HIV-infected mothers would be an appropriate conceptual or cognitive application of the results from this correlational study to clinical practice from the perspective of Stetler's (1994) model of research utilization. Replication of the study is feasible and necessary using a larger random sample.

CRITICAL THINKING CHALLENGES

Barbara Krainovich-Miller

? Discuss the ways stylistic considerations of a journal impact on the researcher's ability to present research findings of a quantitative study.

? Are critiques of quantitative studies by consumers of research, either in the role of student or practicing nurse, valid? What level quantitative study is best for consumers of research to critique? What assumptions did you use to make this determination?

? What is essential for the consumer of research to use when critiquing a quantitative research study? Discuss the ways you might use Internet resources now or in the future when critiquing studies.

? Discuss your agreement or disagreement with Heermann and Craft's critique that Good's findings should not be directly applied to practice. Before defending your position consider Good's statement that "because relaxation and music interventions pose a low risk to patients and may reduce pain and side effect of medication in some people, their usefulness should continue to be explored in practice and research." Decide whether you agree or disagree with their evaluation of these researchers' application of the findings to practice.

REFERENCES

Good M: A comparison of the effects of jaw relaxation and music on postoperative pain, *Nurs Res* 44:52-57, 1995.

Sharts-Hopko NC et al: Problem-focused coping in HIV-infected mothers in relation to self-efficacy, uncertainty, social support, and psychological distress, *Image J Nurs Sch* 28:107-111, 1996.

Stetler CM: Refinement of the Stetler/Marram model for application of research findings to practice, *Nurs Outlook* 42:15-25, 1994.

ADDITIONAL READINGS

American Psychological Association: *Publication manual of the American Psychological Association,* ed 4, Washington, DC, 1994, APA.

Funk SG, Tornquist EM, Champagne MT: A model for improving the dissemination of nursing research, *West J Nurs Res* 11:361-367, 1989.

Larson E: Using the CURN project to teach research utilization in a baccalaureate program, *West J Nurs Res* 11:593-599, 1989.

Nolan MT et al: A review of approaches to integrating research and practice, *Appl Nurs Res* 7:199-207, 1994.

Titler MG, Goode CJ, eds: Research utilization, *Nurs Clin North Am* 30(3), 1995.

Evaluating the Qualitative Research Report

Helen J. Streubert

Key Terms

auditability
credibility
fittingness

Learning Outcomes

After reading this chapter the student should be able to do the following:

- Identify the influence of stylistic considerations on the presentation of a qualitative research report.
- Identify the criteria for critiquing a qualitative research report.
- Evaluate the strengths and weaknesses of a qualitative research report.
- Describe the applicability of the findings of a qualitative research report.
- Construct a critique of a qualitative research report.

Nursing research is focused on the generation of new knowledge. The information discovered through rigorous research methods assists nurses in the development, implementation, and evaluation of nursing interventions. For most of the early history of nursing research, nurse researchers have directed their endeavors toward objective, empirical research. The use of empiricism has contributed significantly to nursing. The compatibility and applicability of this approach to the human phenomena, which is of paramount interest to nursing, has been limited at times because of the focus on objectivity. In general, it is difficult to make the human experience objective.

Qualitative research is another means of generating nursing knowledge that provides opportunity for studying phenomena that are not able to be made objective. Because qualitative researchers are making important contributions to nursing, nurses should know how to evaluate qualitative research reports. In this chapter the reader is offered the criteria used to evaluate qualitative research studies. In addition, a published research report is presented to demonstrate the application of the criteria.

STYLISTIC CONSIDERATIONS

Qualitative research reports are presented in a manner different from quantitative research reports. In a qualitative research report, the reader will not find hypotheses, dependent and independent variables, large or randomized samples, statistical analyses, conceptual frameworks, or scaled instruments. Because the intent of the research is to describe or explain phenomena or culture, the report is generally written in a way that allows the researcher to convey the richness of the research. Narrative is essential to conveying the depth and richness of the data. This is significantly different from a quantitative research report.

The goal of an empirical research report is to convey in an abbreviated manner the most critical aspects of the research findings. Numerical data that make up the findings section of a quantitative research article are reportable in an abbreviated format. In contrast, the qualitative research critique will include direct quotes from the participants that highlight the findings of the study, which are generally reported as themes. An example of this type of reporting can be found in Hall's (1996) study of childhood sexual abuse. In describing the life histories of women who experienced childhood sexual abuse, Hall identifies "scapegoating" as one of the major themes. In reporting this theme, she uses the following participant quote to illustrate the theme: "My mother always said my hair was too kinky, that I was skinny and ugly. She favored my sister. One Christmas she got my sister her own princess phone, her own line. The only thing she got me was a comb and brush. It was like a baby brush, real soft. I was too old for that. I have black people's hair. It wasn't the kind of comb I could use. She said I looked like a porcupine so that's what I deserved."

The ability of the qualitative researcher to convey the richness of the data and to do so within the publication guidelines of particular nursing journals is a challenge. Nursing journals are committed to publishing qualitative research studies. This is evident in the ever-increasing numbers of qualitative studies found in leading nursing journals. In addition, qualitative researchers can find journals that are committed to publication of qualitative research exclusively. An example is *Qualitative Health Research*. In addition, examples of journals that demonstrate strong support for publication of qualitative research studies include *Image: Journal of Nursing Scholarship, Western Journal of Nursing Research,*

Advances in Nursing Science, Research in Nursing and Health, and *Nursing Science Quarterly.*

Guidelines for the publication of research reports generally are listed in nursing publications. However, criteria for publication of research based on a specific type of research method—that is, quantitative versus qualitative—are not stated. The primary goal of journal editors is to provide articles that are informative, timely, and interesting to their readers. To meet this goal, regardless of the type of research report, editors prefer to publish articles that have scientific merit, present new knowledge, and will engage their readers. The challenge for the qualitative researcher, like the quantitative researcher, is to demonstrate the significance of the work and its scientific merit within the page limitations imposed by the journal of interest.

The qualitative researcher also must be aware of the traditional evaluation framework used by most researchers to evaluate the merits of studies published in journals. Generally speaking, reviewer's guidelines are framed within the context of empirical research. Therefore the qualitative researcher has the challenge of presenting his or her findings within the framework of quantitative approaches while maintaining the integrity of the qualitative study by presenting the richness of data within the page limits specified by the journal. In Table 18-1 the reader is provided with general criteria to be used in evaluating the scientific merit and significance of qualitative research. You are directed to Chapter 9 for additional information on the specifics of qualitative research design.

APPLICATION OF QUALITATIVE RESEARCH FINDINGS IN PRACTICE

The purpose of qualitative research is to describe or explain a phenomenon or culture. Because the goal is not to predict or control, the findings of qualitative research are used differently from findings of quantitative research. For example, the results of qualitative research are not generalizable to larger groups. The individual who plans to use the findings of qualitative research has the responsibility of validating whether the findings accurately reflect the phenomenon in another setting. For instance, LeMone (1993), in describing the process that insulin-dependent diabetic adults move through in reestablishing their sexuality, defines a substantive theory of transformation. The theory she describes is grounded in human experiences of both men and women who are insulin-dependent diabetics. If her theory accurately reflects the process these individuals move through, her ideas are applicable to other adult diabetics who are insulin dependent. However, nurses who wish to apply her findings must validate through their own practice whether the process is applicable to patients with whom they work. Validation of her findings through empirical research adds further support to the results and subsequently adds to the progression of nursing research knowledge.

Similar to the findings of qualitative studies that describe particular processes or phenomena, the findings from qualitative studies of culture also must be viewed within a context. In other words, the descriptions of culture documented through ethnographic study are specific to the culture studied. In the case of ethnographic research, the information collected on cultural norms, values, and mores can be applied only to the group studied. A nurse who is interested in the cultural values of senior citizens living in an apartment complex in New York could not use the results generated from a study of this group and apply it to senior citizens living in a nursing home in Louisiana. The findings of all qualitative research studies are context bound.

Table 18-1

Critiquing Guidelines for Qualitative Research

SECTION	QUESTIONS TO GUIDE EVALUATION
Statement of the phenomenon of interest	1. Is the phenomenon of interest clearly identified? 2. Has the researcher identified why the phenomenon requires a qualitative design for study? 3. Are the philosophical underpinnings of the research described?
Purpose	1. Is the purpose of conducting the research made explicit? 2. Does the researcher describe the projected significance of the work to nursing?
Method	1. Is the method used to collect data compatible with the purpose of the research? 2. Is the method adequate to address the phenomenon of interest? 3. If a particular approach is used to guide the inquiry, does the researcher complete the study according to the processes described?
Sampling	1. Does the researcher describe the selection of participants? Is purposive sampling used? 2. Are the informants who were chosen appropriate to inform the research?
Data collection	1. Is data collection focused on human experience? 2. Does the researcher describe data collection strategies (i.e., interview, observation, field notes)? 3. Is protection of human subjects addressed? 4. Is saturation of the data described? 5. Are the procedures for collecting data made explicit?
Data analysis	1. Does the researcher describe the strategies used to analyze the data? 2. Has the researcher remained true to the data? 3. Does the reader understand the procedures used to analyze the data? 4. Does the researcher address the credibility, auditability, and fittingness of the data?
Credibility	a. Do the participants recognize the experience as their own?
Auditability	a. Can the reader follow the thinking of the researcher? b. Does the researcher document the research process?
Fittingness	a. Are the findings applicable outside the study situation? b. Are the results meaningful to individuals not involved in the research? 5. Is the strategy used for analysis compatible with the purpose of the study?

Table 18-1—cont'd	

Critiquing Guidelines for Qualitative Research

SECTION	QUESTIONS TO GUIDE EVALUATION
Findings	1. Are the findings presented within a context?
	2. Is the reader able to apprehend the essence of the experience from the report of the findings?
	3. Are the researcher's conceptualizations true to the data?
	4. Does the researcher place the report in the context of what is already known about the phenomenon?
Conclusions, implications, and recommendations	1. Do the conclusions, implications, and recommendations give the reader a context in which to use the findings?
	2. Do the conclusions reflect the findings of the study?
	3. Are recommendations for future study offered?
	4. Is the significance of the study to nursing made explicit?

Nurses who wish to use the findings of qualitative research in their practice must validate, either through their own observations or through interaction with groups similar to the study participants, whether the findings accurately reflect their practice experience.

Another use of qualitative research findings is to initiate examination of important concepts in nursing practice, education, or administration. For example, in a study conducted by Beck (1996), the researcher used phenomenology to examine the concept of postpartum depression. The focus of the study was to examine the "meaning of postpartum depressed mothers' interactions with their infants and older children." This study adds to the existing body of knowledge on the concept of postpartum depression and offers the reader direction for future research related to this concept. Similarly, in a study by Grigsby and Megel (1995), these authors examine the concept of caring. Specifically Grigsby and Megel wanted to know how nurse educators experience caring. In this study the authors offered an exhaustive description of caring experienced by nurse educators in their work environment. This study not only provides information to nurse educators but also builds on the work of other nurse researchers who are committed to the study of caring. Caring is a concept that has been identified as an integral one for nursing practice.

Finally, qualitative research can be used to discover information about a phenomenon of interest that can lead to development of research instruments. When qualitative methods are used to direct the development of a structured research instrument, it is usually part of a larger empirical research project. Instruments developed from qualitative research are useful to practicing nurses because they are grounded in the reality of human experience with a particular phenomenon.

CRITIQUE OF A QUALITATIVE RESEARCH STUDY

The study *The Lived Experience of Women Military Nurses in Vietnam during the Vietnam War* by Elizabeth A. Scannell-Desch, RN, MSN, PhD, published in *Image: The Journal of Nursing Scholarship* (1996), is critiqued. The article is presented in its entirety and followed by the critique on p. 461.

THE LIVED EXPERIENCE OF WOMEN MILITARY NURSES IN VIETNAM DURING THE VIETNAM WAR*

Elizabeth A. Scannell-Desch

The lived experience of 24 military nurses during the Vietnam War is described in addition to common elements of their lives after returning from Vietnam. In-depth interviews generated data about personal and professional aspects of the lives of women nurses in the war zone. Data analysis incorporated the qualitative methods of Colaizzi, Lincoln and Guba, and Van Manen. Findings revealed that the nurses struggled with moral and ethical dilemmas of wartime nursing, felt out-of-place, and lacked privacy. The nurses described a deep and special bonding, and many found serving in Vietnam to be the most rewarding experience in their careers. The Vietnam War continues to have an effect on the lives of the nurses who served there. They balance their personal and professional growth gleaned from this experience with the physical and emotional stresses experienced during the war and since the war. The findings of this study have implications for further research about nurses in Vietnam and nurses who have served in other wars.

The longest war to affect the United States was the Vietnam War. Active U.S. involvement began in 1961 and lasted until early 1973 (Santoli, 1985). Humanitarian aeromedical evacuation missions were flown until 1975 (Schimmenti & Darmoody, 1986). A total of 2.6 million U.S. personnel served in Vietnam (Frye & Stockton, 1982), more than 250,000 were seriously wounded (Cook, 1988) and 58,132 were killed (Jones & Janello, 1987).

According to the US Department of Defense about 7,500 military women served in Vietnam (Walker, 1985). About 80 percent were members of the military Nurse Corps (Marshall, 1988). Among the names carved on the Vietnam Veterans Wall, are those of eight female nurses who died in Vietnam. Although nurses are represented in official records, little is written about the women who served. Only three studies (Norman, 1986; Paul & O'Neill, 1983; Schnaier, 1982) and a few anecdotal accounts (Freedman & Rhoads, 1987; Marshall, 1988; McVicker, 1985; Schwartz, 1987; Van Devanter & Morgan, 1983; Walker, 1985) have explored nurses' experience. In comparison to what has been written about men veterans, much of the women's experience has gone untold. Women's experience in and following Vietnam has not been explored from a phenomenological perspective.

The purpose of this study was to explore common components of the lived experience of women military nurses who served in Vietnam and common elements of life after returning from Vietnam. Study of the lived experience of nurses during a war is timely, relevant, and significant to nursing today.

Much of nursing's history is rooted in caring for the wounded in war (Donahue, 1985). Florence Nightingale and Clara Barton, two of the world's most famous nurses, won recognition for their heroic and steadfast efforts to organize nurses to treat wartime casualties. Additionally, our recent Persian Gulf War, Kurdish relief efforts, and humanitarian missions in Somalia, Cuba, Haiti, and Rwanda vividly demonstrate that military nurses remain on duty around the globe caring for people in need. Furthermore, study of the lived experience of mil-

*This section, from pp. 450 to 461, is taken from Scannell-Desch EA: The lived experience of women military nurses in Vietnam during the Vietnam War, *Image J Nurs Sch* 28(2):119-124, 1996.

itary nurses in Vietnam significantly contributes to the developing body of knowledge about women, nurses, and war, and may help future generations of nurses.

RESEARCH APPROACH

This study was a phenomenological inquiry with emphasis on description of women's Vietnam experience and its aftermath. The researcher did not attempt to support or validate any preselected model or framework (Omery, 1983), but rather to embrace the phenomena as they unfolded from the perspective of the people experiencing them. This approach attempts to understand the structure and meaning of human experience as it is lived.

The population consisted of women nurses who served in the Army, Navy, or Air Force in Vietnam, including nurses on hospital ships, in hospitals, and in air transport vehicles. A list of Vietnam nurses did not exist in the defense department or veteran's agencies, therefore the sample was obtained using "snowball" sampling (Polit & Hungler, 1995, p. 232). The sample included 24 women nurses who served in Vietnam between 1965 and 1973. Nine nurses served in the Army, eight were in the Navy, and seven were in the Air Force. They served the standard 12-month tour with four exceptions: one Army nurse returned early because of pregnancy; one Navy nurse left early when her ship was taken out of service; one Army nurse served two non-consecutive tours; and one Air Force nurse served in Vietnam for 3 years.

All Army nurses were assigned to hospitals, five Navy nurses worked on hospital ships, two Navy nurses worked at a Vietnamese provincial hospital and one was assigned to a Navy hospital. Three Air Force nurses served as flight nurses and four served in hospitals. Eight nurses left active duty after Vietnam, seven remained in the military until retirement, one joined the Reserves and eight were on active duty at the time of this study. Mean respondent age on arrival in Vietnam was 26.5 years, with a range from 21 to 44 years. Mean respondent age at the time of this study was 47.5 years, with a range from 42 to 66 years.

DATA COLLECTION

In-depth interviewers were audiotaped for transcription and analysis. Four data generating questions guided the interviews: How would you describe the circumstances surrounding your assignment to Vietnam? What word, image or words, come to mind when you hear the word "Vietnam"? What was the essence of your Vietnam experience for you? What advice or guidance would you give the next generation of military nurses who may have to go to war? Follow-up questions were asked to clarify ideas, thoughts, and feelings—and to gain a fuller understanding. Reflective questions were asked; suggestive questions were avoided.

DATA ANALYSIS

Data were analyzed using procedures adapted from Colaizzi (1978), Lincoln & Guba (1985), and Van Manen (1990). Significant statements were extracted from transcriptions. Each unit of information was compared to previous units. As analysis progressed, theme categories emerged. Seven broad theme categories were identified (Table 1). As analysis continued, previous units of information were compared to new units in the same and in different categories.

Table I

Describing the Lived Experience of Nurses in Vietnam—Categories and Theme Clusters

CHARACTERISTICS OF THE SITUATION IN VIETNAM	COPING WITH VIETNAM
Assignment to Vietnam	Maintaining a perspective
Arrival in Vietnam	Use of support systems
Living conditions	Inner strength
Description of perceived danger	Diversional activities
Description of hospital facility	Use of alcohol and drugs
Schedules, duties, equipment	Humor
Patient trauma	Emotioal hardships
Cultural differences/endemic diseases	Stress reactions
Social life	Talking about Vietnam
Problems with men	Not talking about Vietnam
	Attempts to talk about Vietnam
	Delayed talking about Vietnam
RELATIONSHIPS	Feelings of futility and frustration
	Feelings of uncertainty and unreality
American GI	
Camaraderie	
Professionalism	
Friendships	ADVICE TO NEXT GENERATION
Remembrance of special patients	Advice about training
	Advice about journaling
LIFE AFTER VIETNAM	Advice about support systems
	Advice about caring for self
Homecoming	Understanding the mission
Family reaction to homecoming	Lack of preparation for war
Life transitions	
Transition in nursing practice	
	METATHEMES
GROWTH EXPERIENCE AS ESSENCE	Facing moral and ethical dilemmas
	Giving of oneself
Personal growth as essence	Improvising
Professional growth as essence	Feeling out of place
	Lacking privacy
	Re-creating home
IMAGES OF VIETNAM	Bonding
Visions of Vietnam	
Thoughts of Vietnam	
Sounds of Vietnam	
Smells of Vietnam	

Repetitious units of information were retained. As data were compared within and across categories, information was synthesized into theme clusters. For example, in the category "Images of Vietnam," four theme clusters emerged: (a) visions of Vietnam, (b) thoughts of Vietnam, (c) sounds of Vietnam, and (d) smells of Vietnam.

Theme clusters were further synthesized into metathemes. Findings were integrated into an exhaustive, or "thick" description of the lived experience. All significant statements, categories, clusters, metathemes, and exhaustive description were validated by three doctorally prepared reviewers. This helped prevent any unwarranted jump beyond the data. Lastly, credibility of data, categories, clusters, metathemes, and final conclusions were validated by four respondents.

FINDINGS

Characteristics of the Situation

The majority of the nurses studied volunteered for duty in Vietnam. They volunteered for reasons of patriotism, adventure, or combating feelings of professional stagnation. A few described themselves as "non-volunteers," but reluctantly and fearfully answered their country's call. Some vividly described their arrival as an experience they would never forget. Descriptions included airfield attacks, the sight of caskets being loaded on departing aircraft, and fatigue. One nurse recalled, "I was the only female on the plane. We had to go around a typhoon. When we finally went into the Danang area, we couldn't land because the airport was under rocket attack. It was a scary beginning!"

Hospital and flight nurses usually lived in metal Quonset huts or plywood structures, called "hooches." These dwellings were primitive and cramped. Sea nurses shared a tiny room with metal bunks. Although sea nurses' quarters were air-conditioned, nurses assigned to hospitals did not have such conveniences.

Nurses perceived their environment as dangerous, especially if they ventured outside the base. One flight nurse said:

I never thought about the danger until it was all over. I think it was blind faith or just being young and naive. We had air evac planes come back with holes in them. We would land, and you could see some of the fire in certain areas, but you just didn't dwell on it.

Sometimes it did not seem any safer in hospitals. Nurses described intermittent rocket and mortar attacks during which they had to don flak vests and helmets, transport patients to bunkers, and pad immobile patients with extra bedding for protection. Army, Navy, and Air Force nurses were assigned to hospitals varying from 50 to over 1,000 beds. The Repose and Sanctuary were the only hospital ships in Vietnam and each could accommodate 700 patients. Most nurses worked 12-hour shifts, 6 days a week; they described their patient load as heavy and found the work exhausting. "You just work, sleep, and go back to work. I honestly don't know how I did it, being the only nurse on nights with 18 ICU patients and having to mix all my own IVs."

In retrospect, some nurses questioned the morality of saving patients with multiple amputations, severe brain damage, and quadriplegia, but acknowledged this was not their decision. One nurse stated, "It's hard to picture in your mind or prepare yourself for the kinds of injuries we saw." Most cared for American GIs, but some cared for enemy POWs and Vietnamese nationals. Not all patients had traumatic injuries; nurses graphically described the physical sequelae of malaria, typhoid, parasitic diseases, and plague.

An Army nurse stated:

Having intestinal worms was like something you've never seen in your life. There were jars of worms that were just unbelievable in length and width. That was such a surprise to me, to see them coming through the N.G. tube. At night, I would get a flashlight, and I'd look and I'd think, what is this? And then, it would be a worm.

The social life was "anything you wanted it to be." Parties, sporting events, USO shows, alcohol, and drugs were all available. Nurses described life as intense. "You worked hard and you played hard." Some discussed the problems that accompanied the disproportionate ratio of men to women. Others described being the target of sexual remarks and being treated like objects. Although they were warned about involvement with married men, two nurses had relationships with married men and another—an unmarried nurse became pregnant.

Images of Vietnam

Visions of Vietnam contrasted the beauty of the countryside and white sandy beaches with the stark realities of war: limbless soldiers, aircraft ferrying patients, flares lighting up the sky, and the blood and death of young men. One nurse recalled:

My image is of a young boy that died in my arms. There were eight of them that came in one day, everybody was peppered with frag. This one young boy, blonde hair, blue eyes, came in with just one—just one wound in his chest and died. As I gave him death care, his wallet fell out and opened to a picture of a girl, probably his high school sweetheart.

When the nurses heard the word "Vietnam," they thought of people struggling to survive and the waste of human life. One said, "I think of dying and pain, but also a feeling of closeness to people that I had never felt before." The sound of Vietnam was the universal whine of helicopters and dull concussion of artillery in the distance. One comment was: "Anytime I hear a chopper, it takes me back instantly to Vietnam." The smell of Vietnam was a mixture of war smells: Blood, burning flesh, pseudomonas-infected tissue, and burning human waste.

Personal Relationships in Vietnam

Many nurses described their colleagues as "family." There was a strong sense of teamwork characterized by people working together in the face of danger and uncertainty. One nurse stated, "There was a type of camaraderie that you just can't explain." Another added:

I have never been in a situation so professionally satisfying, even though you have to separate out that we never got used to seeing men blown apart. The people were always willing to help their colleagues. I've never seen this happen to that degree since Vietnam. It was professionalism at its best.

The nurses also described friendships that continue today. "These are deep friendships, lasting friendships, friendships that you might not correspond for 10 years, and then you can pick up like it was yesterday." Another relationship each nurse would never forget was a special patient. Even after some 20 years, each nurse vividly recalled her encounter with one particular patient, what he looked like, what he said, what happened to him, and how his presence touched her life. One said:

The patient I remember best was a Marine who stepped on a land mine. It caused him to have a bilateral flail chest. The only thing that saved his life was his foot in his boot splinted his chest. It came off and embedded into his chest wall. So they wrapped the boot and foot in his chest because it splinted the chest and allowed him to breathe. I took care of him the whole time he was at the 85th. He was really adjusting. He went through the grieving process. He used humor to help him cope. He was really a nice boy from Pennsylvania. He was evacuated to Japan after he was stabilized. I thought he was going to make it but he didn't. I found his name on the Wall. He showed me the strength that you need to survive. He loved life. I think he knew he was dying, but he never hinted at it.

Coping With the Vietnam Experience

The nurses identified methods they used to cope: maintaining a perspective, using support systems, inner strength, diversional activities, alcohol, drugs, and humor. To maintain a perspective, nurses developed DEROS (Date of Expected Return from Overseas) calendars to mark the passage of time. They tackled the challenges by facing one day at a time and said this perspective kept them from becoming overwhelmed. Support systems were primarily other nurses and medical personnel. Some felt only those sharing the same experience could truly understand and provide support. Nurses defined inner strength as either a belief in God or as an internal toughness. One nurse stated: "I came to believe it was God's will that I went over there and since he sent me, I didn't worry. Faith! Some people call it denial but it worked!" Some found that sports activities reduced stress. Others used alcohol and marijuana. "There was a lot of drinking, I did it but it made talking easier," one nurse commented. Another nurse described humorous situations:

They sometimes had swim call on the ship. They would have one side of the ship, down low, where they'd put out some type of platform and people could dive into the water. All of the heads were to have been secured on that side of the ship. Well, someone didn't get the word, and you could see somebody flushed a toilet. The sewage came out that side, so people swam away from that pretty quick.

Nurses identified their emotional hardships: the overwhelming volume of wounded, clinical inexperience, sending recovered soldiers back to battle, the youth of patients and severity of injuries, alcohol abuse by others, demanding physicians, the morality of saving the severely injured, and the politics of a "limited war." One nurse recalled:

I was just 21 when I went to Vietnam, terrified of making mistakes. I would see other people who seemed to be functioning so well and it just made me feel very insecure. You had to make life and death decisions. Sometimes, I just felt so stressed out and insecure—plus caring for patients that were so severely burned or had limbs blown off was so hard for me.

Life After Vietnam

Most nurses described homecoming as a happy event; many were greeted by family and friends. Some delayed their trip to decompress alone or with friends. They were not emotionally ready to face their families and needed time to get reoriented. Some identified a withdrawal period of about a year following return. Many were shocked by instructions to shed uniforms before traveling in the United States, and some were enraged by anti-war protesters. The uniform, for many, had become their identity, a source of pride and commitment. Lastly, some felt guilty about leaving. One nurse summarized the thoughts of many:

Going home was very hard. I was ready to go home, it was time to go home, but it was so hard leaving. It was like leaving a family or before our job was done. I got home, there was no hoopla, no nothing. I felt like I was incognito because I could not wear the uniform I was so proud of.

The 24 nurses described a variety of life transitions after returning from Vietnam. One said her outlook on life changed because of feminism. Others reported valuing freedom and people more after Vietnam. A few reported a "numbness," others sought isolation and privacy. One nurse said, "I spent a lot of time by myself when I got home. I wanted to be alone. I didn't get close to anyone for a long time, but eventually I worked out some solutions. Now, I value people more than I ever did before Vietnam."

Some nurses found the transition to stateside nursing difficult. They missed the excitement and challenge of Vietnam. Many felt underutilized, devalued, and unappreciated in peacetime nursing. One said:

My skills weren't welcome. In my ICU, I can remember asking doctors questions and being told you're the nurse, shut up, this is the way I want to do it. They told me my main job was to get coffee. I was so disgusted with stateside nursing, I volunteered for another tour in Vietnam.

Advice to the Next Generation of Military Nurse

Nurses advised keeping a journal of activities, thoughts, and feelings. "My journal helped me remember people, what I was thinking in those days, and how I reacted to situations. I look back on it now and it was very useful in helping me put Vietnam in perspective." Additionally, nurses emphasized that training needs to be intensive, realistic, and must focus on trauma care without use of sophisticated equipment. They emphasized that support systems are very important; so is confiding in others and maintaining a link with home. Furthermore, nurses believed it is vitally important to understand the mission and role military nurses play. One nurse said:

I think when you join the military, you must join with full knowledge that it is a 24 hour-a-day job and if there is a war, you can be called for that. We didn't join because we wanted a nice 7-to-3 job, and, of course, it may involve making the ultimate sacrifice, your life.

Growth as Essence

The nurses described personal and professional growth as an essence of their experience. Personal growth was characterized as a process of maturation whereby they gained increased awareness of the value of life, a self-realization of their capabilities and limitations, an appreciation for what was given them, a less judgmental attitude toward others, a deeper feeling of pride and patriotism toward their country, and a self-determination to do whatever they chose in life after Vietnam. Professional growth was characterized not only in terms of gaining advanced clinical knowledge and skills, but also by gaining tremendous satisfaction, respect, and value as a team member. Many described their tour in Vietnam as the most rewarding experience in their careers:

I was doing what I came in the Navy to do. It was the ultimate challenge for me. It certainly broadened my perspective on nursing care. It showed me that all I learned in nursing school was not all there was to being a nurse. I came out of Vietnam a much better nurse and a much better person.

The Metathemes

From a thorough review of data within and across theme clusters and categories, seven metathemes emerged to further describe the lived experience: facing moral and ethical dilemmas; giving of oneself; improvising; feeling out of place; lacking privacy; recreating home; and bonding (Table 1).

Facing Moral and Ethical Dilemmas

The nurses expressed difficulty accepting the politics of war, which included returning physically recovered soldiers to combat, participating in triage where some patients were placed in the "expectant" area to die, fighting the war in a piecemeal manner, and saving the lives of patients whose future quality of life was expected to be very poor. A nurse recalled:

Sometimes I look back and wonder if these guys have cursed us for saving them because they have handicaps, like the spinal cord injuries or the one that lost several limbs. It bothered me that some of the policies and politics would not allow the fighting to be conducted in a way it was supposed to be.

Giving of Oneself

The dedication, devotion, and selflessness identified the nurses as people who gave of themselves to patients, colleagues, and the mission. A nurse summarized:

It was a difficult time because of the types of patients we cared for . . . the distance from home, but there was more to it than that. You were a mother, you were a girlfriend, you were a sister, you were a nurse. We had the feeling that every GI who came throught that door—they were our neighbors and brothers, and we had to save them.

Improvising

The nurses didn't have the modern equipment and supplies they were accustomed to in the U.S., nor did they have many conveniences of daily living, but they learned to "make do." A nurse from Phu Bai recalled, "I could make pizza in a frying pan, in fact, I could cook a full-course dinner in a frying pan."

Feeling Out-of-Place

The nurses described being outnumbered by men, feeling uneasy and out-of-place in the dirty, unsafe, male-dominated world of the military. Some found that no advanced preparation had been made for their arrival and that living in a foreign land with strange customs and language contributed to their ill-at-ease. An Army nurse said: "They didn't sell much in the way of female supplies in the PX at Long Binh post. We mostly had to rely on family to send us tampons, hair spray, and stuff like that."

Lacking Privacy

Nurses described a lack of, and a yearning for, privacy. One recalled: I remember one night, a nurse came down and asked if she could use my room. I asked her what she had in mind, and she said she was looking for a place to cry. There just wasn't any place to be alone.

Re-creating Home

Within the nurses' description of life in Vietnam, a desire for the normalcy, safety, comforts, activities, and familiarity of home emerged. The nurses missed and attempted to re-create home through decorating their hooches, celebrating holidays, and participating in activities such as ball games to mirror life in the United States. A Navy nurse recalled, "We had Thanksgiving dinner at our place. We had everything we would ordinarily have. We sent someone to Saigon to get everything and it worked. We did have a turkey, mashed potatoes, and cranberry sauce and some vegetables."

Bonding

Bonding was characterized as a unity of purpose in providing care, a sense of equality and kinship among military personnel and a sense of loyalty to each other, the medical mission, and their country. A nurse recalled:

I think that I probably have never felt the same way about a group of people as I did about that group; they were the best! There was a bond I had never felt before. We each had a role to play and each one was as distinctly important as the next.

Exhaustive Description of the Lived Experience

According to Patton (1990), an exhaustive description goes beyond mere fact or surface appearances, but stops short of becoming trivial and mundane. In exhaustive description, "the voices, feelings, actions, and meanings of interacting individuals are heard" (Denzin, 1989, p. 83). Van Manen (1990) found that four existentials proved to be useful tools in the process of examining and describing the lived experience. These existentials are lived space (spatiality), lived time (temporality), lived body (corporeality), and lived human relation (relationality or communality) (Van Manen, 1990, p. 101). From the metathemes of this study, an exhaustive description was derived. Van Manen's (1990) four existential life themes were used in formulating this description.

Lived Space

The nurses experienced their lived space as foreign, dangerous, frightening yet challenging, and lacking privacy. Rocket and mortar attacks occurred intermittently while a stream of young soldiers with mutilating injuries ebbed and flowed, and sometimes gushed, into their space. The nurses experienced their space as shared because of others—more urgent needs. They could not put boundaries on their personal space; their space was merged with the space of patients and colleagues. From the moment they left the United States, they felt out-of-place amidst hordes of men in combat gear. They used diverse strategies to cope with the strangeness. They improvised and creatively altered their space to re-create home. They succeeded to a degree in adding a sense of normalcy and "home" to their space.

Lived Time

The nurses experienced time as moving too fast and in short supply during mass casualty situations and as almost standing still when the end of their tour drew close. Time was measured by a DEROS calendar; by letters from home; by formed and lost relationships; by events in Vietnam and back in the "World;" and by the dawn and darkness of each day, since most of the heavy fighting occurred at night. Time was something busy nurses and dying soldiers had too little of and bed-ridden patients had too much of.

Lived Body

The nurses experienced their lived body as a tangle of thoughts, emotions, and physical sensations. They experienced a heightened sensory awareness, contrasting the visions of a beautiful countryside with the blackened, bomb-crater pocked, defoliated terrain of war. Their visions were of the many limbless, mindless, paralyzed, burned and maimed soldiers and peasants. They carry with them forever images of standing ankle-deep in blood, of young men with their faces blown-off, of holding a young Marine as he died and accompanying his body to "graves registration," but never letting go of the memory. To this day, the pungent odor of pseudomonas, burned flesh, and a mixture of blood, sweat, mud, and burning human waste is "Vietnam." The "whap-whap" of helicopter blades pounding overhead instantly transports some nurses back to Vietnam. Like the sound of the bell for Pavlov's dogs, the helicopter signaled an onslaught of casualties, another night without sleep, and a cascade of emotions and psychological responses within the lived body. Futility, frustration, anger, and then sadness surfaced as they faced the moral and ethical dilemmas of who could be saved and who was beyond saving.

Lived Relationships

The nurses experienced lived relationships as intense, significant, and long lasting. They were characterized by an intense bonding with patients and colleagues. They experienced a closeness different from any other experience. There was a cohesion, a oneness against all odds, a professionalism, and a camaraderie that many admitted as difficult to describe. Over 20 years later, nurses proclaimed that their strongest and most highly valued relationships were those formed in Vietnam. Within this bonding, the nurses gave of themselves in a selfless, caring, and relentless manner. The intensity of feeling was clearly apparent as nurses tearfully recalled visits to the "Wall" to find names of patients and colleagues and to remember a period of time that changed their lives forever.

DISCUSSION

The nurses' lived experience was one of personal and professional challenge and growth, heart-breaking and rewarding clinical situations, physical danger and exhaustion, and professional and personal insecurity in an environment that was unstable, austere, and lacked privacy. The nurses struggled with the moral and ethical dilemmas of wartime nursing and with problems associated with being outnumbered by men, far away from home, and in a foreign culture. This study supported previous research (Norman, 1986; Schnaier, 1982) and anecdotal accounts (Freedman & Rhoads, 1987; Marshall, 1988) that found it virtually impossible to separate professional from personal experiences in Vietnam. The nurses lived, worked, and played in the same environment. The current study also supported previous findings (Norman, 1986; Paul & O'Neill, 1983; Schnaier, 1982; Stretch, Vail, & Maloney, 1985) by demonstrating that caring for young, severely injured soldiers was a significant stressor. However, the current study exposed the very fiber of the experience through the process of phenomenological inquiry, a new method to describe the experience of nurses in war.

This study illuminated the need for nurses to be clinically prepared with solid medical-surgical and trauma nursing skills before being deployed in a war zone. Additionally, the findings demonstrated that nursing education programs should emphasize that the emotional sequelae of catastrophic events such as serving in a war zone, last a long time after the event and that memories of the event may be extremely painful and disruptive for years after the event is over. Afterwards, methods of caring for the emotional needs of caregivers in such events should be as important as taking care of victims during the event itself. Lastly, the findings of this study have implications for further research about women nurses in Vietnam and other groups of people who have served in war and disaster situations.

In her poem, "Our War," Evans (1983) wrote:

I don't go off to war so they say, I'm a woman. Who then has worn my boots? And whose memories are these of youth suffering? Of blood and burns, of their tears and their cries? (p. 1)

This poem seems to mirror the traditional view in our society that war is strictly a man's business. However, as this study describes, war experiences and memories are not limited to the male gender alone. Women nurses have experienced the trauma of war since before the founding of our nation; however, little has been written or studied about their experiences.

The Vietnam war continues to have an effect on the lives of the nurses who served there. They balance their personal and professional growth and self-knowledge gleaned through their experience with the physical and emotional stresses experienced during and since the war. The war, with its personal and professional triumphs and tragedies, was a unique and special experience.

REFERENCES

Colaizzi, P.F. (1978). Psychological research as the phenomenologist views it. In R.S. Valle & M. King (Eds.), Existential-phenomenological alternatives for psychology (pp. 48-71). New York: Oxford University Press.

Cook, J.L. (1988). Dust off: The Vietnam war. New York: Bantam Books

Denzin, N.K. (1989). Interpretive interactionism. Newbury Park, CA: Sage.

Donahue, P. (1985). Nursing: The finest art. St. Louis, MO: C.V. Mosby.

Evans, D.C. (1983). Our war. In Vietnam women's memorial project: A legacy of healing and hope. Washington, DC: IDS Financial Services.

Freedman, D. & Rhoads, J. (Eds.) (1987). Nurses in Vietnam: The forgotten veterans. Austin, TX: Texas Monthly Press.

Frye, J., & Stockton, R. (1982). Discriminant analysis of PTSD in a group of Vietnam veterans. American Journal of Psychiatry, 139, 52-56.

Jones, B., & Janello, A. (1987). The wall: Images and offerings from the Vietnam veterans memorial. New York: Collins.

Lincoln, Y., & Guba, E. (1985). Naturalistic inquiry. Beverly Hills, CA: Sage.

Marshall, K. (1988). In the combat zone: An oral history of American women in Vietnam. Boston: Little, Brown, & Co.

McVicker, S.J. (1985). Invisible veterans: The women who served in Vietnam. Journal of Psychosocial Nursing, 23(1), 13-19.

Norman, E. (1986). Nurses in war: A study of female military nurses who served in Vietnam during the war years 1965-1973. Unpublished doctoral dissertation, New York University.

Omery, A. (1983). Phenomenology: A method for nursing research. Advances in Nursing Science, 5(2), 49-63.

Patton, M.Q. (1990). Qualitative evaluation and research methods. Newbury Park, CA: Sage.

Paul, E., & O'Neill, J. (1983). The psychosocial milieu of nursing in Vietnam and its effects on Vietnam nurse veterans. Unpublished research report, Northwestern State University of Louisiana.

Polit, D., & Hungler, B. (1995). Nursing research: Principles and methods (5th ed.). Philadelphia: J.B. Lippincott.

Santoli, A. (1985). To bear any burden: The Vietnam war and its aftermath. New York: E.P. Dutton.

Schimmenti, C., & Darmoody, M. (1986). Taking flight. American Journal of Nursing, 86, 1420-1423.

Schnaier, J.A. (1982). Women Vietnam veterans and mental health adjustment: A study of their experiences and post-traumatic stress. Unpublished master's thesis, University of Maryland, College Park.

Schwartz, L. (1987). Women and the Vietnam experience. Image: Journal of Nursing Scholarship, 19, 168-175.

Stretch, R., Vail, J., & Maloney, J. (1985). PTSD among Army Nurse Corps Vietnam veterans. Journal of Consulting and Clinical Psychology, 53, 704-708.

Van Devanter, L., & Morgan, C. (1983). Home before morning. New York: Warner Communications.

Van Manen, M. (1990). Researching lived experience. New York: State University of New York Press.

Walker, K. (1985). A piece of my heart. New York: Ballentine Books.

INTRODUCTION TO THE CRITIQUE

The research report *The Lived Experience of Women Military Nurses in Vietnam During the Vietnam War* (Scannell-Desch, 1996) is critically examined for its rigor in qualitative method, its contribution to nursing, and its utility in practice. The criteria identified in Table 18-1 are used to guide the evaluation.

Statement of the Phenomenon of Interest

Scannell-Desch clearly states that she is interested in studying women military nurses who were in Vietnam during the Vietnam War. She describes the importance of studying women's experiences related to the Vietnam War by illustrating the impact the war had on U.S. service personnel, specifically those who were wounded or died as a result of the war. She further addresses the subject of women who served—military nurses in particular. Finally in the introduction, Scannell-Desch tells the reader that little has been written about women nurses' experiences in Vietnam and that their perspective of the war has not been documented using a phenomenological research approach. Other than to describe her data analysis strategy, which does not explore the philosophical underpinnings of the research method used, no reference is made to the philosophical framework that creates the basis for the research approach utilized. Full disclosure of the philosophical position of the researcher enhances the reader's ability to determine the rigor of the approach used.

Purpose

The purpose of the study is "to explore common components of the lived experience of women military nurses who served in Vietnam and the common elements of life after returning from Vietnam." Scannell-Desch (1996) demonstrates the significance of the study to nursing by describing nurses' contributions during times of military crisis. Finally, she explains that this research "contributes to the developing body of knowledge about women, nurses, and war." She believes that exploring this topic will help further generations of nurses.

Method

Scannell-Desch (1996) does not report a particular research method. Rather, in the *Data Analysis* section of the report, she speaks about the research methods used to analyze data. This can be viewed as a weakness in this study. Although the reader could infer from the title of the study, her use of the term "lived experience," and the authors/researchers cited in her *Data Analysis* section of the report that the method used is a phenomenology, Scannell-Desch (1996) does not explicitly identify the approach as such until the *Discussion* section of the study, at which time she only states "the current study exposed the very fiber of the experience through the process of phenomenological inquiry, a new method to describe the experience of nurses in war." By not identifying a method early and not sharing with her readers exactly which phenomenological approach she is using, Scannell-Desch limits the reader's ability to determine whether or not the method was adequate to address the topic and whether she followed the processes identified as part of the method.

Sampling

Scannell-Desch (1996) reports that she used "snowball" sampling. She does not explain how she obtained her first participant to begin the "snowball" sampling technique. She does report the number of nurses in the study, the branches of the service in which they served, the term of their service, and their ages. Based on her description, the reader can infer that those she chose to participate were knowledgeable about the phenomenon under study. From her description of the participants, it can be inferred that a purposive sample was used. Specifically, nurses were chosen for the purpose of being able to describe their lived experience as military health care personnel during the Vietnam War.

Data Collection

Data collection is described by telling the reader that in-depth interviews were audiotaped. Scannell-Desch (1996) further identifies the four guide questions that were used to initiate description of the experience. There is no mention of protection of human subjects. Scannell-Desch (1996) also does not report whether data were saturated. In the analysis section of the report, she does tell the reader that themes were maintained based on repeating appearance. The researcher is clear in describing what strategies she used in eliciting information. For example, she reports, "follow-up questions were asked to clarify ideas, thoughts, and feelings— to gain a fuller understanding. Reflective questions were asked; suggestive questions were avoided." These sentences give the research consumer a clear picture of how she collected data during the interviews.

An important component of qualitative research is to conduct the study from an atheoretical position. In Scannell-Desch's (1996) report, she clearly states that she did not attempt to validate a particular model or framework. This is a strength of the study and demonstrates her understanding of qualitative research's philosophical underpinnings.

Data Analysis

Data were analyzed by "using procedures adapted from Colaizzi (1978), Lincoln and Guba (1985) and Van Manen (1990)." Scannell-Desch (1996) tells the reader the procedures she used to arrive at the seven broad themes. In addition, she uses a table to further illustrate categories and theme clusters (see Table 1 in research article, p. 452). From these categories and theme clusters, she derives what she labels *metathemes*. The use of the term *metatheme* is not discussed and may cause some degree of confusion for the reader. The research consumer would be enlightened by an explanation of how she used this term. It is not clear from her exhaustive description how these are different from or the same as those items she labels as categories and theme clusters.

Table 1 in the research article (p. 452) serves as an outline of major categories of data found under each heading. However, it does not clearly demonstrate how the researcher moved from categories and theme clusters to metathemes. The reader could infer that the metathemes actually are the major theme categories that create meaning from the raw data ultimately leading to development of the exhaustive description. However, without the researcher's explicit direction, the reader may be making an incorrect inference. As stated earlier, the reader is unable to differentiate the categories, themes, and metathemes in the exhaustive description.

Qualitative researchers generally use three criteria to judge the validity and reliability (more commonly known as trustworthiness) of qualitative data. These include credibility, auditability, and fittingness. **Credibility** refers to whether the research informants recognize the description of the experience as their own. In this study, Scannell-Desch (1996) reports that four respondents did review her categories, clusters, metathemes, and conclusions. She does not, however, explain why only four of her 24 participants reviewed the data.

Auditability refers "to the ability of another researcher to follow the thinking, decisions and methods used by the original researcher" (Yonge and Stewin, 1988). Table 1 in the research article (p. 452) is offered as an example of Scannell-Desch's (1996) thinking process regarding themes. As stated earlier, how she arrived at her conclusions is not entirely clear. She does report using three doctorally prepared reviewers to validate her "significant statements, category clusters, metathemes and exhaustive description." This certainly can be viewed as one way the reader can determine that the data analysis procedures used by the researcher were carried out appropriately.

Fittingness of the research refers to how well the findings fit outside the study situation. To demonstrate the fittingness of the findings, Scannell-Desch (1996) places the study in context by providing the reader with examples of other research studies that have found similar perceptions reported by nurses who were in Vietnam during the Vietnam War. It is difficult to determine whether the findings of the study have meaning for others who have experienced this phenomenon based on the research report. However, the rich description provided by the researcher certainly provides the framework for another individual to determine whether his or her experience was similar to those who informed this study.

Findings

The findings of Scannell-Desch's (1996) research are presented in the context of the group that she studied: women military nurses in Vietnam during the Vietnam War. The data are presented using both the informants' words and Scannell-Desch's interpretations. Table 1 in the research article, (p. 452) is used to demonstrate the categories, theme clusters, and metathemes Scannell-Desch found based on her analysis of data. When reading this report, the reader is able to get an idea of what military nurses in Vietnam observed and felt during their tour of duty. Rich descriptions such as those presented in her report provide the interested reader with a personal view of the intensity of this experience. In the discussion portion of the report, Scannell-Desch provides a context for this study based on what is already known about women who were part of the military nurse corps in Vietnam during the war. In the case of a few categories and theme clusters, Scannell-Desch's interpretations and insights are presented more than the actual commentaries by the informants. The findings would be enhanced by inclusion of informants' remarks rather than the author's interpretation of their conversations.

The use of van Manen's (199) four existential life themes assists Scannell-Desch in developing her description of the experience. The concepts of lived space, lived time, lived body, and lived relationships help to organize the exhaustive description. However, it is not essential that this framework be used by other phenomenologists.

Conclusions, Implications, and Recommendations

The conclusions of this study are related to the literature on the topic of nurses' experiences in Vietnam. The reader would be enlightened by knowing whether the experiences in Vietnam are similar to those of nurses who have served in other wartime active-duty situations. Scannell-Desch concludes that based on this study, it is important for military nurses to be prepared in medical-surgical and trauma nursing skills before being sent to war. She further shares with her audience that the scars of war last for a long time after military conflicts are resolved.

Discussion of appropriate training for the wartime nursing and the prolonged personal effects of caring for casualties during wartime experience are significant to nursing. Knowing how to educate nurses to meet the expectations of wartime nursing will better prepare those who are called to serve and thus hopefully lead to a realistic perception of what will be expected. Further, information related to the long-term effects of wartime nursing on those who have served can enlighten both military and civilian personnel who hope to prepare nurses to provide care in disaster/casualty situations.

Finally, Scannell-Desch reports that her study provides implications for further research. She states that additional research is needed on "women nurses in Vietnam and other groups of people who have served in war and disaster situations." The reader would have benefitted greatly if the researcher had reported in what context the findings of this study could be used.

CRITICAL THINKING CHALLENGES
Barbara Krainovich-Miller

? Discuss the similarities and differences between the stylistic considerations of reporting a qualitative versus a quantitative study in a professional journal.
? Are critiques of qualitative studies by consumers of research, either in the role of student or practicing nurse, valid? Which type of qualitative study is the most difficult for consumers of research to critique? Discuss what assumptions you made to make this determination.
? What is essential for the consumer of research to use when critiquing a qualitative research study? Discuss the ways you might use Internet resources now or in the future when critiquing studies.
? Streubert concludes her critique of Scannell-Desch's study in this chapter with the following statement: "The reader would have benefitted greatly if the researcher had reported in what context the findings of this study could be used." Discuss what Streubert meant by this criticism and whether or not you agree or disagree with her evaluation.

REFERENCES

Beck CT: Postpartum depressed mothers' experiences interacting with their children, *Nurs Res* 45(2):98-104, 1996.

Colaizzi PF: Psychological research as the phenomenologist views it. In Valle, RS, King M, eds: *Existential-phenomenological alternatives for psychology,* New York, 1978, Oxford University Press.

Grigsby KA, Megel ME: Caring experiences of nurse educators, *J Nurs Educ* 34(9):411-418, 1995.

Hall JM: Geography of childhood sexual abuse. Women's narratives of their childhood environments, *Adv Nurs Sci* 18(4):29-47, 1996.

LeMone P: Human sexuality in adults with insulin-dependent diabetes mellitus, *Image J Nurs Sch* 25(2):101-105, 1993.

Lincoln Y, Guba E: *Naturalistic inquiry,* Beverly Hills, Calif, 1985, Sage.

Scannell-Desch EA: The lived experience of women military nurses in Vietnam during the Vietnam War, *Image J Nurs Sch* 28(2):119-124, 1996.

Van Manen M: *Researching lived experience,* New York, 1990, State University of New York Press.

Yonge O, Stewin L: Reliability and validity: misnomers for qualitative research, *Can J Nurs Res* 20(2):61-67, 1988.

Use of Research in Practice

Marita G. Titler

Key Terms

conduct of research
diffusion
dissemination
integrative research review
research-based practice
research-based protocols
research utilization

Learning Outcomes

After reading this chapter, the student should be able to do the following:

- Differentiate between conduct and use of nursing research.
- Cite examples of research utilization projects that have improved quality of care and contained costs.
- Identify examples of an individual model and an organizational model of research utilization.
- List key steps and decision points when undertaking research utilization.
- Identify three barriers to research utilization and strategies to address each.
- Use research findings to improve the quality of care.

The conduct of research is of little value if findings are not used in practice to improve patient care. Contributions of nursing to improve patient outcomes can be optimized by the use of **research-based protocols** (practice standards that are formulated from findings of several studies). Several studies have demonstrated that use of research-based interventions is more likely to result in better outcomes than ritual-based nursing care (Goode and Bulechek, 1992; Heater, Becker, and Olson, 1988; Titler, 1997; Titler, Goode, and Mathis, 1992). Incorporation of research findings into practice, however, is a difficult and challenging process. Experts in the field of research utilization note that, in many ways, utilization presents more challenges to overcome than does the conduct of research (Prevost, 1994). Influencing behavior of multiple caregivers to let go of ritual-based practices is not an easy task (Titler, 1997). The benefits for nurses and patients by use of research in practice, however, make the challenges worthwhile. This chapter presents an overview of research utilization and its relationship to conduct and dissemination of research, describes the steps of research utilization with a special emphasis on evaluation, discusses implementation of a research utilization program, and sets forth future directions for nursing with regard to research utilization.

OVERVIEW OF RESEARCH UTILIZATION

Defined in various ways by experts, **research utilization** is essentially a process of using research findings as a basis for nursing practice (Gift, 1994). It encompasses dissemination of new scientific knowledge, applying that knowledge in practice, and evaluating use of research-based practice with respect to staff, patients and cost/resource utilization (Goode and Bulechek, 1992; Stetler et al, 1995; Titler et al, 1994a). In comparison with research utilization, the **conduct of research** is the analysis of data collected from a homogenous group of subjects who meet study inclusion and exclusion criteria for the purpose of answering specific research questions or testing specified hypotheses. Research design, methods, and statistical analyses are guided by the state of the science in the area of investigation. Traditionally, conduct of research has included dissemination of findings via research reports in journals and at scientific conferences. Research utilization begins when nurses are exposed to this new knowledge. The relationships among conduct, dissemination, and utilization of research are illustrated in Figure 19-1.

Research utilization can be undertaken from an individual and/or organizational perspective. Specifically, a nurse can read and synthesize research and use the information in practice. In contrast, an organization (e.g., hospital) or health care system (e.g., Columbia HCA) can make an institutional commitment to incorporate research into their agency, resulting in practice policies and procedures that are research based (Goode and Titler, 1996).

Cronenwett (1995) describes two forms of research utilization: conceptual and decision driven. Conceptual driven forms of research utilization influence thinking, not necessarily action. Exposure to new scientific knowledge occurs, but the new knowledge may not be used to change or guide practice. An integrative review of the literature, formulation of a new theory, or generating new hypotheses may be the result. This type of research utilization is referred to as *knowledge creep* or *cognitive application*. It is often used by individuals who read and incorporate research into their critical thinking (Stetler, 1994; Weiss, 1980). Decision-driven forms of research utilization encompass application of scientific knowledge as part of a new practice, policy,

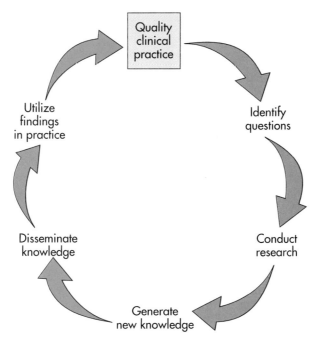

Figure 19-1   The model of the relationship among conduct, dissemination, and use of research. (Redrawn from Weiler K, Buckwalter K, Titler M: Debate: is nursing research used in practice? In McCloskey J, Grace H, eds: *Current issues in nursing,* ed 4, St Louis, 1994, Mosby.)

procedure, or intervention. In this type of research utilization, a critical decision is reached to change or endorse current practice based on review and critique of studies applicable to that practice. Examples of decision-driven models of research utilization are the Iowa Model of Research Based Practice to Promote Quality Care (Critical Thinking Decision Path, p. 470), the Stetler model (Critical Thinking Decision Path, p. 471) (Stetler, 1994), and the Conduct and Utilization of Research in Nursing (CURN) project (Haller, Reynolds, and Horsley, 1979).

Historical Perspective of Research Utilization

Use of research in practice was not an issue for Nightingale, who used data to change practices that contributed to high mortality rates in hospitals and communities (Nightingale, 1858, 1863). In the early 1900s, however, few nurses built on the solid foundation of research utilization exemplified by Nightingale. Separation of conduct and use of research is rooted in the 1930s and 1940s, a period in nursing when there were few educationally qualified nurse researchers, most nursing research was done by nonnurses, and hospitals were used as the primary setting for nursing education. During the mid-1900s, nurses were being prepared as researchers in fields other than nursing and most research focused on nurses rather than patients (Titler, 1993). Today more nurses are being prepared as researchers in nursing, and the scientific body of nursing knowledge is growing. It is now every nurse's responsibility to facilitate the use of that knowledge in practice (Titler, 1997).

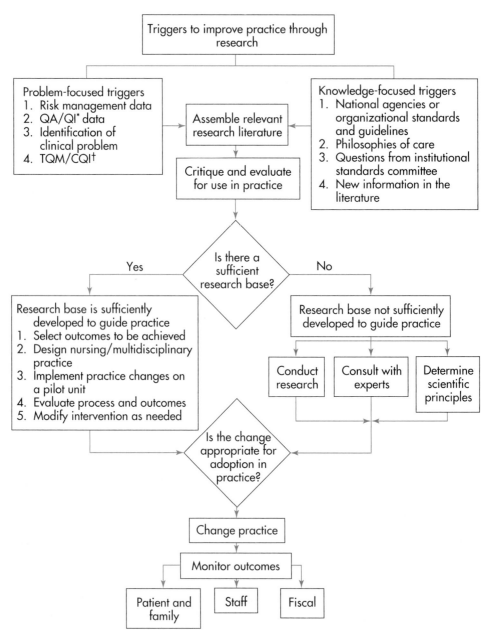

*QA/QI, quality assessment/quality improvement.
† TQM/CQI, total quality management/continuous quality improvement.
◇ = a decision point.

Critical Thinking Decision Path   The Iowa model for research-based practice to promote quality care.   (Redrawn from Titler M et al: Infusing research into practice to promote quality care, *Nurs Res* 43(5):307-313, 1994b.)

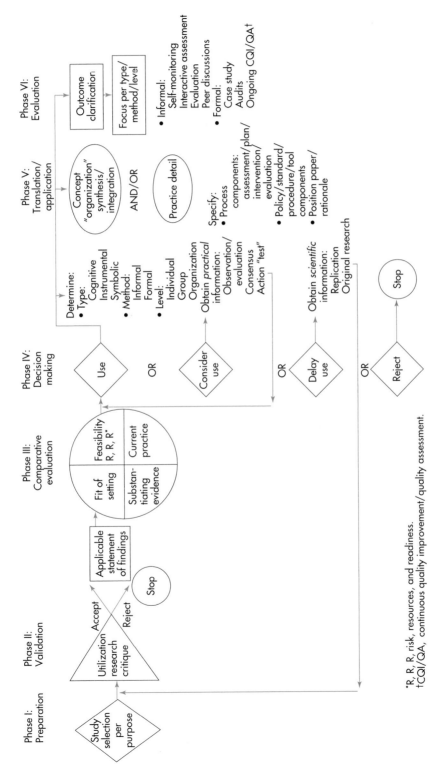

Critical Thinking Decision Path The Stetler model for research utilization. (Redrawn from Stetler C: Refinement of the Stetler/Marram model for application of research findings to practice, *Nurs Outlook* 42:15-25, 1994.)

*R, R, R, risk, resources, and readiness.
†CQI/QA, continuous quality improvement/quality assessment.

Demonstration Projects of Research Utilization

Use of research findings in clinical practice has been the focus of nursing leaders since the mid-1970s. This has resulted in several research utilization demonstration projects. Three federally funded projects in the mid-1970s and early 1980s focused on educating nurses to integrate research into clinical practice. These projects include the Western Interstate Commission for Higher Education in Nursing (WICHEN) regional program on nursing research development, the CURN project, and the Nursing Child Assessment Satellite Training project (NCAST).

The WICHEN project was the earliest research utilization project. Through a series of workshops and the linker model, pairs of clinical nurses and nurse researchers from education learned methods of planned change and research utilization. Participants were challenged to implement changes in patient care based on research by identifying a specific nursing care problem in their agency and reviewing research literature pertaining to the problem. Each dyad developed plans for implementing and evaluating the research based change. The major challenges encountered were finding studies addressing the identified clinical problem (Krueger, 1978; Krueger, Nelson, and Wolanin, 1978; Lindeman and Krueger, 1977). Although three reports from this project were published (Axford and Cutchen, 1977; Dracup and Breu, 1978; Wichita, 1977), it was difficult to identify programs of clinical research that were ready for use in practice.

The CURN project, directed by the Michigan Nurses Association, produced 10 research-based clinical protocols and demonstrated that 1 year after the implementation in an acute care hospital, experimental settings used more research findings than the control settings (Haller, Reynolds, and Horsley, 1979; Horsley et al, 1983). Another result of the CURN project is a written guide that describes, from an organizational perspective, how to advance nursing practice via research utilization (Horsley et al, 1983). The CURN project and resulting written materials have served as a framework for other nurses committed to research utilization.

The NCAST was a 10-year project carried out over three phases. Phase I focused on testing the use of a communication satellite for **dissemination** (communicating information) of research results that focused on health assessment techniques for children; phase II added the use of videotaped parent-child interactions and written materials; and during phase III, public health nurses were taught the use of a protocol in the follow-up care of preterm infants and their families (King, Barnard, and Hoehn, 1981).

Other demonstration projects in the early to mid-1990s were continuing education programs and conferences that focused on integration of research findings and dissemination to nurses in practice. Various methods of dissemination were used, such as linking nurses' work areas with locally and nationally maintained scientific information systems and annual research conferences that brought together clinicians and nurse researchers for the purpose of bridging the gap between research and practice (Cronenwett, 1995; Funk et al, 1995; Rutledge and Donaldson, 1995; White, Leske, and Pearcy, 1995). The federally funded Moving New Knowledge into Practice project of Funk, Tornquist, and Champagne (1989) brought together nurse scientists and clinicians in a series of five conferences for the purpose of disseminating research findings for application in practice. Each conference had a specific conceptual theme (e.g., Key Aspects of Chronic Illness: Hospital and Home Care), and the focus of the conference was to examine the state of the science, share the latest research findings, and discuss together the implications for practice. The link among researchers and nurses in practice was maintained through the use of newsletters and consultation services. A series of five conference monograph texts was published from each of the conferences to share the information with the broader nursing community (Funk et al, 1995). Their work also resulted in development of the Barriers to Research Utilization scale and an identification of barriers to using research in practice (Funk et al, 1991a, 1991b, 1995).

The Orange County Research Utilization in Nursing Project created a regional network of 20 hospitals and home health nursing service organizations (NSOs) and 6 schools of nursing. The purpose was to provide research utilization networking and continuing education to registered nurses (RNs) employed by participating NSOs and to influence the strategic commitment of NSOs to research-driven clinical practice. During the project, all participating NSOs completed at least one research utilization project, and many reported beginning to implement innovations based on the Agency for Health Care Policy and Research (AHCPR) guidelines (e.g., acute pain management). Nurse executives of the NSOs reported that the department became more research oriented over the life of the project and used a more scientific approach with clinical data (Rutledge and Donaldson, 1995).

An annual conference entitled *Toward Research-Based Nursing Practice,* sponsored by Dartmouth-Hitchcock Medical Center and St. Aslem College, focuses on integrative research in which the presenter describes a practice problem, integrates findings from the relevant research **(integrative research review)**, and describes the meaning for practice (Cronenwett, 1995). An annotated bibliography of the most relevant research is distributed to conference participants. The Retrieval and Application of Research in Nursing project at Stanford University Hospital provides hospital-based computer terminals linked to the Internet for access to national databases and retrieval of key studies that may be applicable for practice. This provides staff on clinical units with direct access to computer database searches such as CINAHL and MEDLine (Bostrom and Wise, 1994).

Models of Research Utilization

Several models of research dissemination and utilization have been explicated over the past several years. Many of these are an outgrowth or extension of the demonstration projects. Although a thorough discussion of each model is beyond the scope of this text, a brief discussion is provided.

The Stetler model emphasizes use of research from the *individual clinician perspective* (Stetler, 1994). The model shown in the Critical Thinking Decision Path on p. 471 has six phases. The tool that facilitates the use of this model is in Box 19-1. The first phase, preparation, focuses on the purpose and context for which the reviewed research will be used (e.g., for changing practice, for summarizing the state of the science). The second phase, validation, encompasses critique of the study (scientific validity) for purposes of utilization rather than replication. Phase III is comparative evaluation, which focuses on applicability of the reviewed findings with regard to the following:

1. Significant, substantiating evidence from the critiqued study
2. Appropriateness of study findings for the targeted practice situation
3. Feasibility of using the study findings in practice
4. State of the current practice.

Box 19-1	Refinement of the "Stetler/Marram Tool for Evaluation of Applicability of Research Findings"

Phase I: Preparation (Purpose and Context of Research Utilization)

A. What initiated review of this article/topic?
   1. _____ general interest
   2. _____ a problem
   3. _____ task assignment
   4. _____ knowledge update
   5. _____ other
B. If relevant, what is the desired *outcome* of this or multiple related reviews? In particular, for option 2, how will you evaluate if the problem is "solved" or, for option 3, if the task has been effectively completed?
C. What intervening factors, if any (environmental/personal characteristics), might influence your decision making?
   _____ tight deadline
   _____ need for consultation in the topical area
   _____ committee approval
   _____ other

Phase II: Validation (Scientific Soundness and Potential for Application)

A. What are the methodological strengths of this study?
B. What are the major methodological weaknesses and the limitations of this study relative to acceptability for potential application?
C. Given A and B above, rate scientific soundness in terms of the degree to which the findings are acceptable for *potential* application in practice:
   Nonacceptable/low degree   High degree
   _____ _____ _____ _____ _____ _____

Applicable Statement of Findings

In your own words, write a brief statement specifying the findings of the study: use operational definitions; state results in day-to-day terms; indicate qualifiers and limiting conditions of application.

Phase III: Comparative Evaluation (Criteria of Applicability)

A. Fit of setting:
   1. How similar are the characteristics of the sample to those of the population with which you work?
      STUDY SAMPLE =
      YOUR CLIENTS =
   Level of similarity: _____ acceptable _____ unacceptable
   2. How similar is the study's environment to the one in which you work?
      STUDY SETTING =
      YOUR SETTING =
   Level of similarity: _____ acceptable _____ unacceptable

From Stetler C: A strategy for teaching research utilization, *Nurs Educ* 13:17-20, 1989; modified by Stetler C et al: Enhancing research utilization by clinical nurse specialists, *Nurs Clin North Am* 30(3):457-473, 1995.

Box 19-1	Refinement of the "Stetler/Marram Tool for Evaluation of Applicability of Research Findings"—cont'd

B. Current practice:
   1. Do you have a theoretical/scientific basis for your current practice behavior?
      _____ No _____ Yes (Describe)
      Is it congruent with the basis for this study? _____ No _____ Yes
   2. How *effective* is your current method of practice in this area?
      Not at all effective _____ _____ _____ _____ _____ Highly effective
      How do you know? What are your source/s of evaluative data?
      Or: _____ don't know
      Do you need evaluative data before proceeding?

C. Feasibility (risk, resource, and readiness):
   1. What degree of potential risk could be associated with implementation of these findings? (Consider patients and staff)
      No risk _____ _____ _____ _____ _____ High risk
   2. Readiness
      a. What level/s of the organization would need to be involved in this change in practice? Check all that apply.
         _____ only you as an individual practitioner
         _____ other nurses on a single unit
         _____ interdisciplinary health care team
         _____ collaborative management team
         _____ nurse managers
         _____ upper nursing administration
         _____ private attendings
         _____ other departments
         _____ others =
      b. Given the level/s involved, what is the degree of readiness of each for such a change in practice?
         Not at all ready _____ _____ _____ _____ _____ Highly ready
         (Specify level _____)
         Not at all ready _____ _____ _____ _____ _____ Highly ready
         (Specify level _____)
         Not at all ready _____ _____ _____ _____ _____ Highly ready
         (Specify level _____)
         Not at all ready _____ _____ _____ _____ _____ Highly ready
         (Specify level _____)
   3. What amount of resources would be needed to implement such a change?
      No resources _____ _____ _____ _____ _____ Great resources
   4. What is the risk/benefit ratio involved?

Continued

D. Substantiating evidence (Is there an integrated review; should there be one?):
   1. What other research has been conducted that examined a similar question/hypothesis?
   2. Were the findings the same, similar or conflicting? (Specify)
   3. What other nonresearch-information/knowledge is available regarding this topic?
   4. Overall, to what degree are the findings substantiated?
      Low degree _____ _____ _____ _____ _____ High degree

Phase IV: Decision Making (Use or Non-Use; Nature of Use)

A. Given all of the above factors, do you believe these research findings are:
   _____ Not applicable at this time (Reject)
   _____ May be used in the future in light of additional, scientific information (Delay)
   _____ Can be considered for use in light of additional, practical information (see B, below)
   _____ Can be used *now* to validate, discontinue, or change practice (see C, below)
B. Consider use: [Then return to start of Phase IV, Decision making]
   1. How can such practical information be obtained?
      _____ through day-to-day observation
      _____ through routine evaluation
      _____ through discussion/input of others
      _____ through an action test or other formal pilot/evaluation of the innovation
      _____ other
   2. Who would be involved?
      _____ self
      _____ peers/other professionals
      _____ committee/task force
      _____ experts/consultant
      _____ other
C. Use now: [Then go to Phase V below]
   1. What type(s) of use?
      _____ cognitive
      _____ instrumental
      _____ symbolic
   2. What method?
      _____ informal
      _____ formal
   3. What level?
      _____ by an individual
      _____ by a group
      _____ by an organization

From Stetler C: A strategy for teaching research utilization, *Nurs Educ* 13:17-20, 1989; modified by Stetler C et al: Enhancing research utilization by clinical nurse specialists, *Nurs Clin North Am* 30(3):457-473, 1995.

Box 19-1	Refinement of the "Stetler/Marram Tool for Evaluation of Applicability of Research Findings"—cont'd

4. Potentially, how to use?
_____ for validation
_____ for discontinuation
_____ modification/change

Phase V: Translation/Application (Synthesis and Specification)

A. Organize and synthesize the separate findings, and state results in terms of meaningful concepts and generalization(s) about the identified issue/area.
B. In practical terms, specify exactly how you will use these findings:
_____ as orientation/background/reference information
_____ as part of a set of principles or guiding framework
_____ as part of routine nursing process or practice [specify]
_____ for a policy/standard/critical path/etc. [specify]
_____ for persuasive purposes [describe]
_____ for identification of QM indicators
_____ for routine measurement
_____ others [describe]
C. List any caveats/qualifiers/special circumstances of the above use
D. Have you "applied" too far beyond the knowledge base?
_____ No _____ Yes/Maybe [re-review or recognize that the application is *not* research based]
E. Will "planned change" be required? If yes, proceed to related project management planning/dissemination/etc. Refer back to readiness assessment.

Phase VI: Evaluation (Results of Utilization)

A. Reaffirm/state the outcomes you expected/needed to achieve; make sure they are measurable [refer back to Phase I].
B. Given the type/method/level/nature of application, indicate exactly the how, what, who, where, and when of evaluation.

Phase IV is the decision making, that is, selecting the type and nature of use or nonuse of the research findings from the critiqued study. Translation/application is phase V and requires that findings from multiple studies are synthesized and integrated into some conclusive sort of research-based statements. This synthesis is then used to guide or frame the development of a research-based practice, which may take the form of a state of the science or position paper; a practice standard, procedure, or policy; or a research-based plan of care (e.g., clinical practice guideline, nursing care plan). The last phase (VI) is evaluation. Decisions are made about the type of outcomes to be measured based on the original purpose delineated during phase I. (Stetler, 1994; Stetler et al, 1995). The unique perspective of this model is viewing research utilization from an individual clinician perspective rather than an organizational perspective.

Several other methods of research utilization have an *organizational* perspective. These include the Horn and Goode models, the Children's Hospital of Philadelphia (CHOP) model, and the Iowa Model. These models evolved from an integration of demonstration project findings, the CURN project, and Rogers' seminal work on innovation diffusion (Rogers, 1983). Rogers defines **diffusion** as the "process by which 1) an innovation 2) is communicated through certain channels, 3) over time, 4) among the members of a social system" (Rogers, 1983). Studies and models of research utilization are replete with Rogers' language of innovation adoption.

The Horn model focuses on use of research in practice from an organizational perspective. Research utilization is viewed as an organizational process that is operationalized through the building blocks of developing organizational commitment, identifying and empowering change agents, and instituting a planned change process (Goode et al, 1996). This model has been recently refined to include the health care system, because many organizations are part of a health care system with linkages to primary care providers, specialty providers, other hospitals, and other health care agencies (Goode and Titler, 1996). Strategies for developing organizational commitment to research utilization include articulating the value of research utilization in strategic plans and organizational documents, mission statements, and job descriptions. Establishing expectations that research utilization activities are integrated into the fabric of the organization necessitates leadership behaviors from administrators and nurse executives that clearly communicate the value of research utilization activities. Such behaviors include allocation of resources, communicating the importance of research utilization in written and verbal communication, and incorporating and using research utilization activities in pay for performance criteria. Change agents, an important part of this model, are needed at all levels of the organization. Some individuals serve as clinical change agents as they focus on achieving clinical standards through research utilization. An example of clinical change agents are staff nurses who act as "change champions" when implementing research-based visiting practices in the intensive care unit (ICU) through the following:

- Educating staff about the research base for the practice
- Influencing practice behavior of their peers to be congruent with less restricted visiting
- Providing leadership for solving problems when they occur

Organizational change champions are individuals within the organization who advance creative research-based changes in practice beyond bureaucratic obstacles and thus unfreeze some key stakeholders. The third building block is the planned change process, a process that is often underestimated in terms of its complexity and time commitment (Goode and Titler, 1996; Goode et al, 1996). Complimentary to this model is the Goode model of research utilization, which is based on systems theory and was developed inductively from 6 years experience of using research in a community hospital (Goode et al, 1987).

The CHOP Department of Nursing views research as the foundation of practice (Barnsteiner, Ford, and Howe, 1995). Six Department of Nursing committees are responsible for professional nursing practice from an organizational perspective. Clinical leadership and staff nurses from each nursing area are represented on each of the committees. In addition to research activities undertaken by the research committee, research-based practice information is disseminated by integrating the information into the work of the standards, procedures, and patient/family education committees. Results of a research synthesis project undertaken by members of the Research Committee are sent to the Nursing Practice Committee to integrate into written materials that guide practice. Generally, the work of research utilization is done around clinical topics, such as enteral feeding or pain management, and information appropriate for each committee is disseminated to it. The goal of this model is to integrate efforts so that the entire continuum of activities is coordinated from review of the research to quality improvement monitoring (Barnsteiner, Ford, and Howe, 1995).

The Iowa Model of Research in Practice incorporates both conduct and utilization of research (see the Critical Thinking Decision Path on p. 470) (Titler et al, 1994b). It is an organizational, collaborative model developed by the University of Iowa Hospitals and Clinics and the University of Iowa College of Nursing. In this model, knowledge- and problem-focused "trigger(s)" create questioning by staff of current nursing practice and whether patient care can be improved through the use of research findings. If through the process of literature review and critique of studies it is found that there is not a sufficient number of scientifically sound studies to use as a base for practice, consideration is given to conducting a study, consulting with experts, and/or using scientific principles to guide practice. Nurses in practice collaborate with scientists in nursing and other disciplines to conduct clinical research that addresses practice problems encountered in the care of patients. Findings from such studies can then be combined with findings from existing scientific knowledge to develop and implement **research-based practice** protocols.

If there are a sufficient number of studies available, the studies are critiqued and synthesized, and a research-based practice is developed. The recommended research-based practice is compared to current practice, and a decision is made about the necessity for a practice change. If a research-based practice is warranted, practice changes are implemented using a process of planned change. The practice is first implemented with a small group of patients, and an evaluation is carried out. The research-based practice is then refined based on evaluation data, and the change is implemented with additional patient populations for which it is appropriate. Patient/family, staff, and fiscal outcomes are monitored. Organizational and administrative support facilitates the success of using this model in acute care settings. This model has not been trialed in nonacute care settings.

STEPS OF RESEARCH UTILIZATION

The Iowa Model of Research Based Practice to Promote the Quality of Care serves as the organizing framework for discussing the steps of research utilization as illustrated on the left side of the model in the Critical Thinking Decision Path on p. 470. It is our experience that for all steps of the research utilization process to be carried out, a group approach is most helpful with one person in the group providing the leadership for the project. The group may be an existing committee such as the quality improvement committee, the practice council, or the research committee. A task force approach may also be used, in which a group is appointed to address a specific practice issue and use research findings to resolve the issue or improve practice.

Selection of a Topic

The first step in carrying out a research utilization project is to select a topic. Ideas for research utilization come from several sources categorized as problem- and knowledge-focused triggers. Problem-focused triggers are those identified by staff through quality improvement, risk surveillance, or recurrent clinical problems. An example of a problem-focused trigger is increased incidence of deep venous thrombosis and pulmonary emboli in trauma and neurosurgical patients (Blondin and Titler, 1996; Stenger, 1994). Knowledge-focused triggers are ideas generated when staff read research, listen to scientific papers at research conferences, or encounter clinical practice guidelines published by federal agencies or specialty organizations. Examples of research utilization initiated from knowledge-focused triggers include pain management, prevention of skin breakdown, assessing placement of nasogastric and nasointestinal tubes, and use of saline to maintain patency of arterial lines. Sometimes topics arise from a combination of problem- and knowledge-focused triggers such as the length of bedrest time after femoral artery catheterization (Lundin, Sargent, and Burke, 1997). Criteria to consider when selecting a topic for research utilization are outlined in Box 19-2. Figure 19-2 shows a helpful chart for selecting a topic for a research utilization project.

The individuals responsible for the research utilization project should work collectively to achieve consensus in topic selection. Working in groups to brainstorm about ideas and to achieve consensus about the final selection is helpful. For example, a unit staff meeting may be used to discuss ideas for research utilization; quality improvement committees may identify three to four practice areas that are in need of attention (e.g., urinary tract infections in elderly, restraint reduction, preventing constipation in the elderly) and forward them to the appropriate committees for a final selection; a research utilization task force may be appointed to select and address a clinical practice issue (e.g., pain management); or a Delphi survey technique may be used to prioritize areas for research utilization.

HELPFUL HINT

No matter what method is used to select a research utilization topic, it is critical that staff who will implement the potential practice changes are involved in selecting the topic and view it as contributing significantly to the quality of care (Cole and Gawlinski, 1995).

Box 19-2   Criteria to Consider for Research Utilization Topic Selection

1. The priority of this topic for nursing and for the organization
2. The magnitude of the problem (small, medium, large)
3. Applicability to several or few clinical areas
4. Likelihood of the change to decrease length of stay, contain costs, and improve patient satisfaction
5. Potential "landmines" associated with the topic and capability to diffuse them
6. Availability of baseline quality improvement or risk data that will be helpful during evaluation
7. Multidisciplinary nature of the topic and ability to create collaborative relationships to effect the needed changes
8. Interest and committment of staff to the potential topic

Literature Retrieval and Critique of Studies

Once a topic is selected, relevant literature needs to be retrieved, particularly clinical studies, metaanalyses, and integrative literature reviews on the selected topic. Before reading and critiquing the research, it is useful to read theoretical and clinical articles to have a broad view of the nature of the topic and related concepts.

In addition to using traditional methods of finding published literature (e.g., card catalogs, health indexes), other sources of information include bibliographies of integrative reviews, abstracts published as part of conference proceedings, master's theses and doctoral dissertations, direct written or verbal communication with scientists who are investigating a particular topic but have not yet published the results, and others who may have completed a research utilization project on the same topic. A number of health care indexes, such as the Cumulative Index to Nursing and Allied Health Literature (CINAHL), have electronic databases available

Selection of a Topic for Research Utilization

Topic ideas	Priority for		Magnitude of the problem (small = 1; large = 5)	Applicability (narrow = 1; broad = 5)	Likelihood to		
	Nursing (1 = low; 5 = high)	Organization (1 = low; 5 = high)			Decrease length of stay (1 = low; 5 = high)	Contain cost (1 = low; 5 = high)	Improve satisfaction (1 = low; 5 = high)
Chest physiotherapy							
Diarrhea intube-fed patients							
Clogged small-bore feeding tubes							
Treatment of pressure ulcers							

Figure 19-2   Tool to use in selecting a topic for research utilization. Each topic should be rated by using the scoring criteria and a 1-to-5 scale. The topic(s) receiving the higher score(s) should be considered for selection.

to assist with the search process. Electronic journals such as the *On-Line Journal of Knowledge Synthesis for Nursing* are particularly helpful for research utilization projects, because each article provides a synthesis of the research and an annotated bibliography for selected references. In using all of these sources, it is important to identify key search terms and to use the expertise of health science librarians in locating publications relevant to the project. Further information regarding location of publications is in Chapter 4.

Once the literature is located, it is helpful to classify the articles as clinical (nonresearch), integrative research reviews, theory articles, and research articles. It is also helpful to read articles in the following order:

1. Integrative review articles to understand the state of the science
2. Clinical articles to understand the state of the practice
3. Theory articles to understand the various theoretical perspectives and concepts that may be encountered in critiquing studies
4. Research articles including the metaanalyses

Critiques of the research articles are undertaken next. Integrative review articles such as *Drawing Coagulation Studies from Arterial Lines* (Laxson and Titler, 1994) and *Nasogastric and Nasointestinal Feeding Tube Placement* (Rakel et al, 1994) provide a good foundation for critique of research published subsequent to the integrative review article (Alpen and Titler, 1994). The original research, cited in the integrative review, may warrant a critique with a forward look toward application of findings in practice (Pettit and Kraus, 1995).

Critique of each study should use the same methodology, and the critique process should be a shared responsibility. It is helpful, however, to have one individual provide leadership for the research utilization project and design strategies for completing critiques. For research utilization, a group approach to critiques is recommended because it distributes the workload, helps those responsible for implementing the changes to understand the scientific base for the change in practice, arms nurses with citations and research-based sound bites to use in effecting practice changes with peers and other disciplines, and provides novices an environment to learn how to critique and apply research findings in practice. Methods to make the critique process fun and interesting include the following:

- Using a journal club to discuss critiques done by each member of the group
- Pairing a novice and expert to do critiques
- Eliciting assistance from students who may be interested in the topic and want experience doing critiques
- Assigning the critique process to graduate students interested in the topic
- Making a class project of the critique and synthesis of research for a given topic

Several resources available to assist with the critique process include the following:

- *Research Utilization: A Study Guide* (Goode et al, 1996)
- *Reading Research: A User-Friendly Guide for Nurses and Other Health Professionals* (Davies and Logan, 1993)
- A video entitled *Reading and Critiquing a Research Report* (Goode, Cipperly, and Wellendorf, 1991)
- A CD-ROM entitled *Critiquing Research for Use in Nursing Practice* (Horn Video Productions, 1997)

HELPFUL HINT
Keep critique processes simple, and encourage participation by staff who are providing direct patient care.

Synthesis of Research Findings

Once studies are critiqued, a decision is made regarding use of each study in the synthesis of research findings for application in clncal practice. Factors that should be considered for inclusion of studies in the synthesis of findings process are overall scientific merit of the study, type (e.g., age, gender, pathology) of subjects enrolled in the study and the similarity to the patient population to which the findings will be applied, and relevance of the study to the topic of question. For example, if the research utilization topic is prevention of deep venous thrombosis in postoperative patients, a descriptive study using a heterogenous population of medical patients is not appropriate for inclusion in the synthesis of findings.

To synthesize the findings from research critiques, it is helpful to use a summary table (see also summary tables in Chapters 17 and 18), in which critical information from studies can be documented. Essential information to include in such summaries is the following:

- Study purpose
- Research questions/hypotheses
- The variables studied
- A description of the study sample and setting
- The type of research design
- The methods used to measure each variable
- Detailed description of the independent variable/intervention tested
- The study findings

An example of a summary form is illustrated in Figure 19-3.

HELPFUL HINT
Use of a summary form helps identify commonalities across several studies with regard to study findings and the types of patients to which study findings can be applied.

Decision to Change Practice

When the studies are critiqued and synthesized, the next step is to decide if findings are appropriate for use in practice. Some criteria that should be considered in making these decisions include the following:

- Relevance of findings for practice
- Consistency in findings across studies
- A significant number of studies with sample characteristics similar to those to which the findings will be used
- Feasibility for use in practice
- The risk/benefit ratio

It is best to make practice changes based on several studies with similar findings.

Summary Table for
Synthesis of Research Critiques

Citation	Purpose/research question	Sample size	Variable and measures		Statistical tests	Significance level	Results	Implications
			Independent	Dependent				

Figure 19-3   Example of a summary table for synthesis of research critiques.

Synthesis of study findings may result in supporting current practice, making minor practice modifications, undertaking major practice changes, or developing a new area of practice. For example, a research utilization project on gauze versus transparent dressings did not result in a practice change because the studies reviewed substantiated current practice (Pettit and Kraus, 1995). In comparison, a Pediatric Intravenous (IV) Infiltration Guideline was developed from a combination of research findings and expert consultation because few studies used pediatric subjects, sample sizes were small, and research results were inconclusive (Montgomery and Budreau, 1996). This research utilization project resulted in a new practice for treatment of IV infiltrations, resulting in a significant reduction in tissue damage.

Development of Research-Based Practice

The next step is to put in writing the research base of the practice (Haber et al, 1994). When results of the critique and synthesis support current practice or suggest a change in practice, a written research-based practice protocol is warranted so that individuals know that the practices are based on research. Several different formats can be used to document research-based practice changes. The format chosen is influenced by what and how the document will be used. Written research-based practices should be part of the organizational policy and procedure manual and should include detailed references to the parts of the policy and procedure that are research based. An example of a written research-based procedure is in Box 19-3.

Box 19-3   Protocol

Subject
Intravenous flush (peripheral) for adults

Purpose
To utilize normal saline* to maintain a patent peripheral intravenous access for intermittent use without the aid of an anticoagulant.

Equipment
IV catheter
IV catheter plug, Luer-Lok (H5361) or IV reflux valve with cap (H6904)
IV extension tube, 7-inch minibore Luer-Lok (H6437) or IV (SANSERIF)T port injec-
  tion site, Luer-Lok (H4897)
IV reflux valve cap replacement (H6903) or stopcock cover, disposable port cap
  (H3981)
Normal saline vial or normal saline IV solution
3-cc syringe and needle
Gloves, clean disposable

Procedure
1. Assemble equipment.
2. Wash hands thoroughly. Put on gloves.
3. Set up intravenous lock with infusion plug or Luer-Lok extension set.
   a. Infusion plug (IV catheter plug or IV reflux valve)
      (1) Draw up 1 cc of normal saline* in the syringe.
      (2) Insert IV catheter plug or IV reflux valve into IV catheter.
      (3) When utilizing an IV catheter plug, wipe rubber diaphragm of infusion plug
          with an alcohol swab and allow to dry. Inject 1 cc of the normal saline* solu-
          tion through the infusion plug.
      (4) When utilizing an IV reflux valve, remove needle from syringe of normal
          saline and attach hub of syringe to reflux valve. Inject 1 cc of the normal
          saline* solution.
      (5) Inject 1 cc of the normal saline solution through the infusion plug. Inject
          saline slowly to minimize discomfort (burning) at the site.
   b. Luer-Lok extension set (IV extension tube or IV T port injection site)
      (1) Draw up 2 cc of normal saline solution in the syringe.
      (2) Flush Luer-Lok extension set with normal saline to prime tubing (1 cc).
      (3) Attach Luer-Lok extension set to the IV catheter.
      (4) Slowly inject 0.8 cc of the normal saline* solution through the Luer-Lok ex-
          tension set, close slide clamp, and attach cap.
4. Normal saline flush* is necessary after each medication administration or at least
   every 12 hours unless ordered otherwise.
5. After intermittent IV medication administration via the minibag system, flush a
   small amount of normal saline solution (flush line) through the catheter (1 cc), then
   close the roller clamp on the IV line and disconnect. For further information refer
   to procedure for "Administration of Intravenous Medication."

Continued

Box 19-3   Protocol—cont'd

6. Wash hands thoroughly
7. Record normal saline flush on the "Medication Kardex" (A-1-a-5).

Precautions, Considerations, and Observations

1. If the IV cannula becomes clotted, do not flush lock with heparin or irrigate with fluid to dislodge clot.
2. Strict aseptic technique must be maintained at all times to prevent contamination of IV equipment.
3. A sterile needle must be used for each injection through the rubber diaphragm of the IV catheter plug or IV T port injection site.
4. Change cap on IV reflux valve, IV extension tube, and IV T port injection site each time the cap is removed.
5. Change infusion plug or Luer-Lok extension set at least every 72 hours.
6. The IV insertion site should be changed every 72 hours.
7. Insertion site care should be given every 72 hours. Refer to procedure for "Intravenous Site Care."
8. The 30-cc vial of bacteriostatic 0.9% sodium chloride must be discarded every 24 hours and the vial may only be used for a multiple patients.

Research References

*Goode CJ et al: A meta-analysis of effects of heparin flush and saline flush: quality and cost implications, *Nurs Res* 40:324-330, 1991.

Related References

Infection Control Manual, Policy #235: *Assignment of Drug Expiration Dates and Control for Length of Time Drugs are on Patient Care Units.*

HELPFUL HINT
Use a consistent approach to writing research-based practice standards and referencing the research literature.

Implementing the Practice Change

If a practice change is warranted, the next steps are to make the research-based changes in practice. Hersey and Blanchard (1988) offer two approaches for change—directive and participative. Participative change is more likely to be effective when implementing changes in practice related to research. Developing a positive attitude and a commitment among clinicians to become involved in research is an important first step. This goes beyond making new knowledge available to staff and encompasses attitudinal changes in which staff are encouraged to think critically about their current practice and to question if perhaps there is a more scientific approach to a certain aspect of care. Involvement of staff in selecting a research utilization topic and helping to determine the methods by which the research will be reviewed, critiqued, and translated into practice is particularly effective and is analogous to group participation in problem solving (Weiler, Buckwalter, and Titler, 1994).

Staff nurses and other health care providers within an organization may become barriers to using research in practice if they perceive that the aspect of care is not important, do not understand the reasons for the practice change, do not perceive that they have the authority to make practice changes, or feel powerless in effecting change in their clinical setting (Funk et al, 1995). Incorporation of research utilization behaviors, job descriptions, and performance appraisals is an important strategy for facilitating use of research findings in practice. Examples of research utilization behaviors include identifying potential topics for research utilization; participating in the critique of research; and serving on the research utilization committee.

Making a research-based change in practice involves a planned change process incorporating the following steps:

- Unfreezing old behaviors or attitudes
- Adopting new behaviors or practices
- Refreezing or integrating the change into the work role of the unit or practice setting

The new practice must be continually reinforced and sustained or the practice change will be intermittent and soon fade. More traditional methods of care will return.

The role of the nurse manager is critical in making a research-based practice change a reality for staff at the bedside. Nurse managers must expect that staff will participate in research utilization activities, role model the change in their practice, and provide written and verbal support for the practice change. When selecting a potential topic for research utilization, it is important that the nurse manager values the idea and will support the potential changes.

Advanced practice nurses (APNs) are critical to helping staff retrieve and critique the studies on the selected topic. Although staff nurses are often willing to participate, the APN provides significant leadership in the research utilization process by facilitating synthesis of the research, critically analyzing what practices should be changed, assisting staff to communicate these changes to their peers, and role modeling the changes in his or her practice.

For potential research-based changes in practice to reach the bedside, it is imperative that one or two "change champions" be identified for each patient care unit or service where the change is being made (Scott and Rantz, 1994). It is our experience that staff nurses are among some of the best change champions available for research utilization. The following are characteristics of successful staff nurse change champions:

1. Expert clinicians
2. Viewed as informal leaders by their peers
3. Positive working relationship with other nurses and health professionals
4. Committed to providing quality patient care

One effective method for implementing the practice change is the "core group" approach that was used in a critical care unit to change pain management practices (Titler et al, 1994). The change champion in each unit identified several staff to assist with effecting the practice. This core group became knowledgeable about the scientific basis for pain management, assisted with disseminating the research-based information to other staff, and reinforced the practice change on a daily basis. The change champion concentrated on educating staff regarding pain management and assisted the core group of staff in changing their pain management practices. Each of the core group staff, in turn, took the responsibility for effecting the change in two to three of their peers. Core group members provided positive feedback to their assigned staff who were changing their pain management practices and encouragement to those who were more reluctant to change. Core group members were also able to provide assistance to the change champion in identifying the best way to teach staff about the practice change and to proactively solve issues that arose (Titler et al, 1994).

It is important that staff are educated about changes in practice with regard to the knowledge and skills needed to make the practice changes. Staff need to know the scientific basis for the changes in practice and improvements in quality of care that are anticipated by the change. Disseminating this information to staff needs to be done creatively using various strategies. A staff inservice may not be the most effective method nor reach the majority of the staff. Although it is unrealistic for all staff to have participated in the critique process or to have read all studies used to develop the research-based practice, it is important that they know the myths and realities of the practice. One method of communicating this information to staff is through use of colorful posters that identify myths and realities or describe the essence of the change in practice (Titler et al, 1994).

Staff also need the skills to carry out the practice change. For example, if using pH to check placement of nasogastric and nasointestinal tubes is to be used rather than auscultation, staff knowledge and skill to obtain aspirate from small-bore feeding tubes is essential (Rakel et al, 1994).

Visibly identifying those who have learned the information and are using the research-based practice protocol (e.g., buttons, ribbons, pins) stimulates interest in others who may not have internalized the change. As a result, the "new" learner may begin asking questions about the practice and be more open to learning the research-based practice.

Implementing the change will take several weeks, depending on the nature of the practice change. It is important that those leading the research utilization project are aware of change as a process and continue to encourage and teach peers about the change in practice.

Evaluation

Evaluation provides an opportunity to collect and analyze data with regard to use of a new research-based practice and then to modify the practice as necessary. It is important that the research-based change is evaluated, both on the pilot area and when the practice is changed in additional patient care areas. The importance of the evaluative component cannot be overemphasized.

A desired outcome achieved in a more controlled environment, when a researcher is implementing a study protocol to a homogeneous group of patients (conduct of research), may not result in the same outcome when the practice is implemented in the natural clinical setting, by several caregivers, to a more heterogeneous patient population. Steps of the evaluation process are summarized in Box 19-4.

Evaluation should include both process and outcome measures (Goode, 1995). The process component focuses on how the research-based practice change is being implemented. It is important to know if staff are using the practice in care delivery and if they are implementing the practice as noted in the written research-based practice standard. Evaluation of the process

Box 19-4　Steps of Evaluation for Research Utilization Projects

1. Identify process and outcome variables of interest.
   Example: Process variable—Patients > 65 years of age will have a Braden scale completed upon admission
   > Outcome variable—Presence/absence of nosocomial pressure ulcer; if present—stage I, II, III, IV
2. Determine methods and frequency of data collection.
   Example: Process variable—Chart audit of all patients > 65 years old, 1 day a month
   > Outcome variable—Patient assessment of all patients > 65 years old, 1 day a month
3. Determine baseline and follow-up sample sizes.
4. Design data collection forms.
   Example: Process chart audit abstraction form
   > Outcome variable—pressure ulcer assessment form
5. Establish content validity of data collection forms.
6. Train data collectors.
7. Assess interrater reliability of data collectors.
8. Collect data at specified intervals.
9. Provide "on-sight" feedback to staff regarding the progress in achieving the practice change.
10. Assist change champions and other staff to problem solve issues.
11. Provide feedback of analyzed data staff.
12. Use data to assist staff in modifying or integrating the research-based practice change.

should also note any barriers that staff encounter in carrying out the practice such as lack of information, skills, or necessary equipment; differences in opinions among health care providers; and difficulty in carrying out the steps of the practice as originally designed (e.g., shutting off tube feedings 1 hour before aspirating contents for checking placement of nasointestinal tubes). Process data can be collected from staff and/or patient self-reports, medical record audits, or observation of clinical practice. Examples of process questions are shown in Box 19-5.

Outcome data are an equally important part of evaluation. The purpose of outcome evaluation is to assess whether the patient, staff, and/or fiscal outcomes expected are achieved. Therefore it is important that baseline data be used for a pre/post comparison. The outcome variables measured should be those that are projected to change as a result of changing practice (Goode, 1995). For example, research demonstrates that less restricted family visiting practices in critical care units result in improved satisfaction with care. Thus patient and family member satisfaction should be an outcome measure that is evaluated as part of changing visiting practices in adult critical care units. Outcome measures should be available or measured before the change in practice is implemented and then after implementation. It is our experience that outcome measures should be evaluated for 6 to 12 months after implementation, and data should be provided to clinicians to reinforce the impact of the change in practice. Outcome measures can be incorporated into quality improvement programs. For example, an organizational task force to

Box 19-5	Evaluation of Research Utilization Example Process Questions

Nurses	SD	D	NA/D	A	SA
1. I feel well prepared to use the Braden Scale with older patients.	1	2	3	4	5
2. Malnutrition increases patient risk for pressure ulcer development.	1	2	3	4	5

SD, strongly disagree; *D*, disagree; *NA/D*, neither agree nor disagree; *A*, agree; *SA*, strongly agree.

Patient	Example Outcome Question
1. On a scale of 0 to 10, how much pain have you experienced over the past 24 hours?	0 1 2 3 4 5 6 7 8 9 10

institute AHCPR guidelines for pain management included members from the Department of Nursing Quality Improvement Committee. Data collection focused on adequacy of pain control and patient satisfaction with pain management. Representatives from nursing divisional quality improvement committees were responsible for collecting data from at least 20 patients per unit or clinical area. Results of the quality improvement monitor were distributed to each nursing unit, and staff were encouraged to use this information in identifying ways to improve pain management practices (Schmidt, Alpen, and Rakel, 1996).

When collecting process and outcome data for evaluation of research-based practice change, it is important that the data collection tools are user friendly, short, concise, easy to complete, and have content validity. Focus must be on collecting the most essential data. Those responsible for collecting evaluative data must be trained on the methods of data collection and be assessed for interrater reliability (see Chapter 13). It is our experience that those individuals who have participated in implementing the protocol can be very helpful in evaluation by collecting data, providing timely feedback to staff, and assisting staff to overcome barriers encountered when implementing the changes in practice.

The question that often arises is how much data are needed to evaluate this change. The preferred number of patients *(n)* is somewhat dependent on the size of the patient population affected by the practice change. For example, if the practice change is for families of critically ill adult patients and the organization has 1000 adult critical care patients annually, then 50 to 100 satisfaction responses preimplementation, and 25 to 50 responses postimplementation, at 3 and 6 months should be adequate to look for trends in satisfaction and possible areas that need to be addressed in continuing this practice (e.g., more bedside chairs in patient rooms). The rule

---

Box 19-6 Use of Saline to Flush Peripheral Intravenous Devices: Cost and Quality

- Use of saline flush is an effective method for maintaining patency, decreasing incidence of phlebitis, and increasing duration of peripheral IV catheter placement.
- By using saline flush rather than heparin for peripheral IV catheters, risks related to heparin use are reduced.
- Use of saline flush saves $20,000 to $40,000 per hospital per year.
- Patients report that saline does not burn as much as heparin flush.
- Use of saline flush for peripheral intermittent infusion devices improves quality of care and contains cost (Goode et al, 1991, 1993).

---

of thumb is to keep the evaluation simple, because data are often collected by busy clinicians who may lose interest if the data collection, analysis, and feedback are too long and tedious.

The evaluation process should include planned feedback to staff who are making the change. The feedback needs to include verbal and/or written appreciation for the work and visual demonstration of progress in implementation and improvement in patient outcomes. The key to effective evaluation is to ensure that the research-based change in practice is warranted (e.g., will improve quality of care) and that the intervention does not bring harm to patients (Goode, 1995; Lepper and Titler, 1997). For example, when instituting a research-based protocol for using saline flush rather than heparin flush for peripheral intravenous locks (Box 19-6), it was important to inform staff that the use of saline did not result in increased loss of patency, saved the organization $38,000 annually, and resulted in fewer complaints of pain and burning while flushing the lock (Goode et al, 1991, 1993).

 HELPFUL HINT
Include patient outcome measures (e.g., pressure ulcer prevalence) and cost (e.g., cost savings, cost avoidance) in evaluation of research utilization projects.

IMPLEMENTING A RESEARCH UTILIZATION PROGRAM

Implementing a research utilization program in health care agencies requires an organizational commitment, as well as commitment of nurses employed in the setting. This is an interactive process, because the expectations of the organization are a reflection of the individuals employed in the setting.

For research utilization to be a reality in health care, organizations must make a commitment to providing the infrastructure for research utilization (Goode and Bulechek, 1992; Horsley, Crane, and Bingle, 1978; Kirchhoff and Titler, 1994; Titler, Goode, and Mathis, 1992). Three essential ingredients of this infrastructure are (1) access to information, (2) access to individuals who have skills necessary for research utilization, and (3) verbal and written commitment to research as part of the organization's operations in provision of patient care. Research utilization projects improve patient outcomes, may contain costs, and assist in meeting requirements of the Joint Commission on Accreditation of Healthcare Organizations (JCAHO).

Information

Access to information includes computer access to research publications and research utilization projects and access to quality data for the evaluation component of research utilization. Use of research list servers and computerized literature databases are two examples of increasing access by nurses to research information. Journals that emphasize reporting research in a manner that facilitates use in practice are available. These include *Applied Nursing Research, Clinical Nursing Research,* and specialty journals such as the *American Journal of Critical Care.* Research columns are also printed in many clinical journals and provide a starting point for research utilization activities. The *Annual Review of Nursing Research* publishes integrative research reviews that are helpful in understanding the state of the science in an area and the components of the science that may be ready for practice.

We need to make better use of the electronic superhighway to share research-based information and to minimize current duplicative efforts of critiquing and synthesizing research (Crane, 1995; Cronenwett, 1995). A central clearinghouse for dissemination of written research-based practices would be helpful.

Human Resources

Access to people with expertise in critique and synthesis of research and translating research findings into practice is also important. Such experts can be employed within the organization, shared with a nearby collegiate setting, or contracted on an "as needed" basis. Nurses with master's degrees often have the skill set to lead a research utilization project and can seek consultation from doctorally prepared researchers employed outside the organization, when necessary. Master's-prepared nurses are now, however, substitutes for doctorally prepared researchers. Nurse executives should not expect the same type of outcomes as can be achieved with employment of a doctorally prepared clinical nurse researcher who has more extensive research knowledge and skill and who can serve as a consultant to address practice-based research issues (Kirchhoff and Titler, 1994).

Organizational Climate

An organizational climate conductive to research utilization will reflect the value of research and data-based decision making in the mission, philosophy, goals, and organizational performance standards. The type of research activities that nurse executives can integrate into the practice setting are influenced by the implicit and explicit value statements found in these documents. Nurse executives (NEs) set the climate for nursing practice, and if they are not supportive of research utilization it more than likely will not occur (Goode and Bulechek, 1992). Thus NEs have a responsibility to influence the nature of the organizational documents to encompass value statements regarding research (Kirchhoff and Titler, 1994).

Research behaviors must also be built into job descriptions so that research-based practice is the expectation rather than the exception. Such behaviors should be used in performance appraisals of staff.

Nurse executives communicate the value of research by legitimizing research activities. This includes instituting recognition programs for participating in research, encouraging staff to participate in research courses, providing verbal and written feedback to staff who carry out research utilization projects, encouraging staff to attend regional and national meetings to present conduct and utilization of research, and nominating staff for regional and national research awards.

An important responsibility of nurse executives is exploring the options for integration of research into practice. Practice-based research can be enacted at various levels using different strategies as outlined in Box 19-7 (Kirchhoff and Titler, 1994).

Individuals within the organization can influence the organizational climate by reading professional journals, questioning tradition-based practices, serving as change champions, and disseminating research-based information to their peers. For example, a nurse reads a study on accuracy of coagulation profiles drawn from heparinized arterial lines (Laxson and Titler, 1994). She approaches the nurse manager and medical director about this issue, and questions if perhaps this is an area of practice where improvements might occur. Having received the preliminary support of the nurse manager and medical director, she proceeds to discuss this issue with her co-workers and seeks additional studies that have been done on this topic. Finding several studies, she seeks the consultation of an APN to assist with the critique and synthesis of the research findings. The nurse continues to provide leadership in making the prac-

---

Box 19-7   Options for Integrating Research Into a Nursing Department

Listed in order from limited enactment to fuller enactment:
1. Research committees
   a. Ad hoc
   b. Standing
2. Consultation
   a. Contractual agreements
   b. Pooled resources of practice agencies to hire consultative services of a nurse scientist
3. Use of existing personnel
   a. Clinical nurse specialist
   b. Nurse managers
   c. Education specialist
4. Collaboration
   a. Doctorally prepared clinical nurse specialist
   b. Consortium arrangements
   c. Joint appointment
5. Doctorally prepared research specialist
   a. Part-time
   b. Full-time
6. Research department
   a. Budgeted staff positions
   b. Supply budget
   c. Travel budget

Modified from Kirchhoff K, Titler MG: Responsibilities of nurse executives for research in practice. In Spitzer-Layman R, ed: *Nursing management desk reference*, Philadelphia, 1994, Saunders.

tice change and serves as the change champion in her unit. This nurse, by her individual interest in research and commitment to research-based practice, will have a ripple effect on the organization and use of research to improve the quality of care.

Criteria for evaluating the success of a research utilization program include a combination of traditional scientific criteria, effect on the organizational climate, and improvements in providing cost-effective quality care. These criteria are summarized in Box 19-8. Research utilization projects such as use of saline to flush peripheral IV devices in adults and appropriate use of sequential compression devices for prevention of deep vein thrombosis (DVT) have resulted in improved quality of care while containing costs (Stenger, 1994).

FUTURE DIRECTIONS

Use of research across health care systems for improving quality of care is essential. As systems of health care become the reality, the challenge of the future is to weave research utilization activities beyond the acute care setting into long-term care, community health agencies, and home care. The processes used to translate research findings into practice in acute care may not be the type of processes needed in other parts of the health care system. Methods for using research in nonacute care practice settings need to be tested.

For organizations to take full advantage of research utilization projects undertaken at various sites throughout the country, a National Center for Research Utilization is needed. Such a center would encompass a computerized database of research-based pro-

---

Box 19-8 Outcomes of an Effective Research Utilization Program

Scientific Criteria
1. The number of research utilization projects
2. The number of research utilization publications
3. The number of grants submitted and funded in which staff are investigators

Organizational Climate Criteria
1. Number of research-based practice protocols used by staff
2. Number of staff participating in research activities
3. Climate of inquiry whereby staff question their practice
4. Increased number of professional nurses recruited and retained
5. Return of nurses to school for baccalaureate or higher degrees
6. National reputation, consultations, and visits to the organization

Cost and Quality of Care
1. Decreased length of stay
2. Cost avoidance
3. Cost savings
4. Improved quality of care (e.g., decreased nosocomial urinary tract infections, improved pain management, decrease in nosocomial pressure ulcer development, increased satisfaction of families of critically ill patients)

tocols that include the relevant policy and procedure, the population to which it applies, the quality improvement indicators and data collection forms used in evaluation, a list of references, suggested strategies for change, the type of institutions where the protocol has been implemented, contact people at each agency, and the protocol content expert. Ideally this information should be available on-line through electronic communications such as a dedicated list serve, the Virtual Hospital System, or some other form of electronic media. Such a center could facilitate networking among health care professionals working on similar research utilization projects and provide lists of consultants and educational materials that may be helpful to those beginning to use research findings in their practice (Titler, 1997).

CRITICAL THINKING CHALLENGES

Barbara Krainovich-Miller

? Discuss the three types of validity that must be established before a reviewer invests a high level of confidence in the tool. Include examples of each type of validity.

? What are the major tests of reliability? Is it necessary to establish more than one measure of reliability for each instrument used in a study? Which do you think is the most essential measure of reliability? Include examples in your answer.

? Is it possible to have a valid instrument that is not reliable? Is the reverse possible? Support your answer from instruments you might use in the clinical setting with your patients/clients.

? The researchers, in an article you are critiquing, state that the validity and reliability of the several instruments used in the study were established at an acceptable level. Their study was published in a refereed journal. You are unfamiliar with these instruments. You believe that to critique this section of the report is it necessary to find out how the validity and reliability of these instruments were determined or the criteria used to determine acceptability. How would you proceed? Include in your discussion how technology might help you; support your position with examples.

REFERENCES

Alpen MA, Titler MG: Pain management in the critically ill: what do we know and how can we improve? *AACN Clin Iss* 5(2):159-168, 1994.

Axford R, Cutchen L: Using nursing research to improve preoperative care, *J Nurs Admin* 7(10):16-20, 1977.

Barnsteiner JH, Ford N, Howe C: Research utilization in a metropolitan children's hospital, *Nurs Clin North Am* 30(3):447-455, 1995.

Blondin MM, Titler MG: Deep vein thrombosis and pulmonary embolism prevention: what roles do nurses play? *Medsurg Nurs* 5(3):205-208, 1996.

Bostrom J, Wise L: Closing the gap between research and practice, *J Nurs Admin* 24(5):22-27, 1994.

Cole KM, Gawlinski A: Animal-assisted therapy in the intensive care unit, *Nurs Clin North Am* 30(3):529-537, 1995.

Crane J: The future of research utilization, *Nurs Clin North Am* 30(3):565-577, 1995.

Cronenwett LR: Effective methods for disseminating research findings to nurses in practice, *Nurs Clin North Am* 30(3):429-438, 1995.

Davies B, Logan J: *Reading research: a user-friendly guide for nurses and other health professionals,* Ottawa, Ontario, Canada, 1993, Canadian Nurses Association.

Dracup KA, Breu CS: Using nursing research findings to meet the needs of grieving spouses, *Nurs Res* 27(4):212-216, 1978.

Funk SG, Tornquist EM, Champagne MT: A model for improving the dissemination of nursing research, *West J Nurs Res* 11:361-367, 1989.

Funk SG et al: Barriers: the barriers to research utilization scale, *Appl Nurs Res* 4:39-45, 1991a.

Funk SG et al: Barriers to using research findings in practice: the clinician's perspective, *Appl Nurs Res* 4:90-95, 1991b.

Funk SG et al: Administrators' views on barriers to research utilization, *Appl Nurs Res* 8:44-49, 1995.

Gift A: Nursing research utilization, *Clin Nurs Spec* 8(6):306, 1994.

Goode CJ: Evaluation of research-based nursing interventions. In Titler MG, Goode CJ, eds: *Nurs Clin North Am* 30(3), Philadelphia, 1995, WB Saunders.

Goode C, Bulechek G: Research utilization: an organization process that enhances quality of care, *J Nurs Care Qual* 27-35, 1992 (special report).

Goode CJ, Cipperley JA, Wellendorf SA: *Reading and critiquing a research report,* Ida Grove, Iowa, 1991, Horn Video Productions.

Goode CJ, Titler MG: Moving research-based practice throughout the health care system, *Medsurg Nurs* 5(5):380-383, 1996.

Goode CJ et al: Use of research based knowledge in clinical practice, *J Nurs Admin* 17(12):11-17, 1987.

Goode CJ et al: A meta-analysis of effects of heparin flush and saline flush: quality and cost implications, *Nurs Res* 40(6):324-330, 1991.

Goode CJ et al: Improving practice through research: the case of heparin vs. saline for peripheral intermittent infusion devices, *Medsurg Nurs* 2(1):23-27, 1993.

Goode CJ et al: *Research utilization: a study guide,* ed 2, Ida Grove, Iowa, 1996, Horn Video Productions.

Haber J et al: Shaping nursing practice through research-based protocols, *J NY State Nurs Assoc* 25(3):3-8, 1994.

Haller KB, Reynolds MA, Horsley JA: Developing research-based innovation protocols: process, criteria, and issues, *Res Nurs Health* 2:45-51, 1979.

Heater BS, Becker AM, Olson RK: Nursing interventions and patient outcomes: a meta-analysis of studies, *Nurs Res* 37(5):303-307, 1988.

Hersey P, Blanchard KH: *Management of organizational behavior,* ed 5, Englewood Cliffs, NJ, 1988, Prentice-Hall.

Horn Video Productions: Critiquing research for use in nursing practice, *Research utilization* (1997 catalogue), Ida Grove, Iowa, 1997, Horn Video Productions.

Horsley J, Crane J, Bingle JD: Research utilization as an organizational process, *J Nurs Admin* 8(7):4-6, 1978.

Horsley J et al: *Using research to improve nursing practice: a guide,* Philadelphia, 1983, WB Saunders.

King D, Barnard KE, Hoehn R: Disseminating the results of nursing research, *Nurs Outlook* 29:164-169, 1981.

Kirchhoff K, Titler MG: Responsibilities of nurse executives for research in practice. In Spitzer-Layman R, ed: *Nursing management desk reference,* Philadelphia, 1994, Saunders.

Kreuger JC: Utilization of nursing research: the planning process, *J Nurs Admin* 8:6-9, 1978.

Kreuger JC, Nelson AH, Wolanin MO: *Nursing research: development, collaboration, and utilization,* Germantown, Md, 1978, Aspen.

Laxson CJ, Titler MG: Drawing coagulation studies from arterial lines: an integrative literature review, *Am J Crit Care* 3(1):16-22, 1994.

Lepper H, Titler MG: Program evaluation. In Mateo M, Kirchhoff K, eds: *Conducting and using nursing research in the clinical setting,* ed 2, Baltimore, 1997, Williams & Wilkins (in press).

Lindeman CA, Krueger JC: Increasing the quality, quantity, and use of nursing research, *Nurs Outlook* 25(7):450-454, 1977.

Lundin L, Sargent T, Burke LJ: Length of bed rest time following femoral artery cardiac catheterization. Paper presented at conference sponsored by Aurora Health Care Department of Nursing, Building Bridges to Research Based Practice: Enhancing Outcomes to Nursing Practice, Brookfield, Wisconsin, 1997.

Montgomery LA, Budreau GK: Implementing a clinical practice guideline to improve pediatric intravenous infiltration outcomes, *AACN Clin Iss* 7(3):411-424, 1996.

Nightingale F: *Notes on matters affecting the health, efficiency, and hospital administration of the British Army,* London, 1958, Harrison & Sons.

Nightingale F: *Observation on the evidence contained in the statistical reports submitted by her to the Royal Commission on the Sanitary State of the Army in India,* London, 1863, Edward Stanford.

Pettit DM, Kraus V: The use of gauze versus transparent dressing for peripheral intravenous catheter sites, *Nurs Clin North Am* 30(3):495-506, 1995.

Prevost SS: Research-based practice in critical care, *AACN Clin Iss Crit Care Nurs* 5(2):101, 1994.

Rakel BA et al: Nasogastric and nasointestinal feeding tube placement: an integrative review of research, *AACN Clin Iss* 5(2):194-206, 1994.

Rogers EM: *Diffusion of innovations,* New York, 1983, The Free Press.

Rutledge DN, Donaldson NE: Building organizational capacity to engage in research utilization, *J Nurs Admin* 25(10):12-16, 1995.

Schmidt KL, Alpen MA, Rakel BA: Implementation of the agency for health care policy and research pain guidelines, *AACN Clin Iss* 7(3):425-435, 1996.

Scott J, Rantz M: Change champions at the grassroots level: practice innovation using team process, *Nurs Admin Q* 18(3):7-17, 1994.

Stenger K: Putting research to good use, *Am J Nurs* Suppl:30-38, 1994.

Stetler C: A strategy for teaching research utilization, *Nurs Educ* 13:17-20, 1989.

Stetler CB: Refinement of the Stetler/Marram model for application of research findings to practice, *Nurs Outlook* 42:15-25, 1994.

Stetler C et al: Enhancing research utilization by clinical nurse specialists, *Nurs Clin North Am* 30(3):457-473, 1995.

Titler MG: Critical analysis of research utilization (RU): an historical perspective, *Am J Crit Care* 2(3):264, 1993.

Titler MG: Research utilization: necessity or luxury. In McCloskey JC, Grace H, eds: *Current issues in nursing,* ed 5, St Louis, 1997, Mosby.

Titler M, Goode C, Mathis S: Nursing research in times of economic cutbacks: implications for nurse administrators, *Series Nurs Admin* 4:167-182, 1992.

Titler MG et al: Research utilization in critical care: an exemplar, *AACN Clin Iss* 5(2):124-132, 1994a.

Titler M et al: Infusing research into practice to promote quality care, *Nurs Res* 43(5):307-313, 1994b.

Weiler K, Buckwalter K, Titler M: Debate: is nursing research used in practice? In McCloskey J, Grace H, eds: *Current issues in nursing,* ed 4, St Louis, 1994, Mosby.

Weiss CH: Knowledge creep and decision accretion, *Knowledge Creation Diffusion Utilization* 1:381-404, 1980.

White J, Leske J, Pearcy J: Models and processes of research utilization, *Nurs Clin North Am* 30(3):409-415, 1995.

Wichita C: Treating and preventing constipation in nursing home residents, *J Gerontol Nurs* 3(6):35-39, 1977.

A Comparison of Three Wound Dressings in Patients Undergoing Heart Surgery

Karin Wikblad ■ Beth Anderson

Two hundred fifty patients undergoing heart surgery were randomized in a prospective comparative study of a semiocclusive hydroactive wound dressing, an occlusive hydrocolloid dressing, and a conventional absorbent dressing. The wounds were evaluated during the 4 weeks after surgery. Color photographs were used for a blind evaluation of wound healing. The conventional absorbent dressing was more effective in wound healing, compared with the hydroactive dressing. Further, there were fewer skin changes and less redness in the wounds with the conventional dressing than with the hydroactive dressing; the differences were not significant with the hydrocolloid dressing. The conventional dressing was less painful to remove than the hydroactive and hydrocolloid dressings. More frequent dressing changes, however, were needed when using the conventional dressing. Despite this, it was the least expensive alternative.

Appendix A Reprinted with permission from *Nurs Res* 44(4):312-316, 1995.

Many demands are put on a wound dressing used after heart surgery. The dressing has to promote rapid reepithelialization and provide protection against infections. It must absorb large amounts of blood and tissue fluids and, ideally, allow ongoing evaluation of the incision. The adhesive ability must be good because the sternum incision is quite difficult to protect, for example, during daily showers. In addition, the dressing should be comfortable for its wearer and inexpensive.

In two review articles on wound dressings, the authors stressed the necessity of a systematic approach to wound assessment because of the complexity of wound care products (Bolton & van Rijswijk, 1991; Cuzzell, 1990). The objective of the present study was to assess clinical aspects of a semiocclusive hydroactive dressing and an occlusive hydrocolloid dressing in comparison with a conventional absorbent nonocclusive wound dressing. The evaluation included effectiveness (wound healing), safety (presence of infections and skin changes), clinical utility (ability to allow ongoing evaluation of the incision), patient comfort (adhesion, pain at removal), and cost.

RELATED LITERATURE

Many randomized studies have compared surgical wound dressings. In one study in a pediatric setting, the authors compared DuoDERM (an occlusive hydrocolloid dressing) with an absorbent dressing, Cutiplast (Rasmussen, Larsen, & Skeie, 1993). The authors found that DuoDERM required fewer bandage changes, but not significantly less, and was less painful on removal than an absorbent wound dressing. Another advantage of DuoDERM was that its waterproof qualities enabled the patient to bathe the first day after surgery.

Clinical benefits of DuoDERM were also evaluated in a postoperative setting (Hermans & Skillman, 1993). The results showed that the dressing was comfortable for its wearer and could reduce cost through a reduction in dressing changes. Another advantage was the possibility of inspecting the incision through the dressing, since the dressing was reported to be transparent after 12 to 24 hours. In another study (Phillips, Kapoor, Provan, & Ellerin, 1993), Cutinova hydro (a hydroactive dressing) was compared with conventional treatment. The hydroactive dressing provided no advantages over the conventional dressing (Band-Aid), except that the former was more convenient to use.

In a prospective trial on skin graft donor sites, a hydrocolloid dressing (DuoDERM) and a water vapor–permeable dressing (Biobrane) were compared with a fine-mesh gauze dressing (Feldman, Rogers, & Karpinski, 1991). The results showed that DuoDERM was useful for small donor sites in that pain could be reduced with a small increase in cost. The gauze dressing, on the other hand, enabled more rapid healing than DuoDERM or Biobrane and was less expensive to use. The water vapor–permeable dressing was not recommended for routine use as a donor-site dressing, because it was too costly and the infection rate was too high (29%). Studies on surgical wound dressings have shown an infection rate that varies from 2% (Hermans & Skillman, 1993) to 7% (Reinicke, Nowak, & Adler, 1990).

Several studies have also been focused on comfort for the patient and the clinical utility of wound dressings. Rasmussen et al. (1993) reported the advantage of occlusive hydrocolloid dressings over absorbent wound dressings as the ability of patients to bathe before removal of the dressing. The authors also noted less pain and discomfort at removal of the occlusive dressing. Feldman et al. (1991) also found that an occlusive hydrocolloid dressing was more comfortable for the patient than a conventional gauze dressing. Hermans and Skillman (1993) noted that 92% of the patients in their study rated a hydrocolloid dressing as very comfortable. However, the results from controlled studies on wound dressings in postoperative settings are inconsistent, and further controlled clinical studies are required to resolve the ambiguities.

METHOD

Subjects

This study was reviewed and approved by the university hospital Research Ethical Committee. The study included 250 patients undergoing elective coronary bypass or valve replacement surgery. The majority of the subjects, 186 (74%), were males. Ages ranged from 38 to 85 years, with a mean age of 64 years ($SD = 9.3$ years).

The patients were randomly assigned to three groups: Group 1 received absorbent dressings (92 patients; mean age, 63.4 years; $SD = 9.7$), Group 2 received hydrocolloid dressings (77 patients; mean age, 63.3 years; $SD = 9.1$), and Group 3 received hydroactive dressings (81 patients; mean age, 65.5 years; $SD = 9.1$).

Of the 250 patients, 216 (86%) were evaluated during the hospital stay for 5 consecutive days (87 in the absorbent, 63 in the hydrocolloid, and 66 in the hydroactive dressing groups). Of those, 78% ($n = 169$) were followed for another 3 weeks. The reasons for ineligibility were excessive bleeding in 15 patients, reoperation in 7 patients, and postoperative complications (stroke) in 1 patient. Eight patients died during the first week after surgery, and registration for 3 patients was missed. The mean age for the dropout group ($n = 34$, 22 males and 12 females) was 68.1 years (range, 39 to 80 years). At the 4-week evaluation, 22% of the patients did not return their protocols. Most of them ($n = 30$) had forgotten to fill in the protocol. Six patients were still in the hospital, 3 had died, and 8 were unreachable by phone.

Measures

Nurses' Protocol

The protocol was filled in from Day 1 (first day after surgery) to Day 5 (discharge from hospital). On a graded scale from 1 to 3, each nurse rated how well the incision could be seen through the dressing and how much the dressing had loosened. The number of bandage changes and the reasons for these changes were also noted. On the 5th day after surgery, the dressing was removed, and pain at removal was rated on a 3-point scale from "no pain at all" to "very painful." Difficulty in removing the dressing was also noted.

Five nurses from each of the three units were trained to examine the dressings. They rated the above parameters for five patients' dressings, compared their results, and discussed ratings that deviated from each other. This procedure was repeated on five new patients until there was total agreement in their ratings.

Wound Culture

A culture was taken from the incision on Day 5 after surgery in the following way: The dressing was removed, and a sterile cotton bud soaked in salt solution was drawn back and forth over the incision. The culture was then sent to the bacteriological laboratory for identification of bacterial isolates and antibiotic resistance.

Photographs

On Day 5 after surgery, a color picture of the wound was taken by the university hospital photographer at a distance of 90 cm and from a 90° angle. The photographs were evaluated according to redness, degree of wound healing, and skin changes (erythema and blisters). Redness was rated on a 3-point scale: 0 = no redness, 1 = slight redness, 2 = excessive redness. The degree of wound healing was classified into three categories: 1 = well healed (wound edges are well together; a gap of less than 5% of the entire length of the incision is allowed, with no or slight redness), 2 = partially healed (gaps more than 5% but less than 20% of the incision's whole length, with slight to excessive redness), and 3 = poorly healed (gaps greater than 20% of the entire length of the incision, with excessive redness). The evaluation was done by two independent raters, neither of whom was aware of the experimental conditions. The interrater reliability was calculated by use of kappa statistics (Brennan & Hays, 1992). The kappa coefficient for ratings of wound healing was .81, and the agreement between the two raters was 91%. For ratings of redness, the agreement was 85% (kappa coefficient = .73). To examine intrarater reliability, 5% of the photographs were duplicated. Agreement in those ratings reached 100%.

Patient Protocol

The patients filled in a simplified protocol once a week after discharge from the hospital. The protocol included yes/no questions, such as, Is the wound red? Does the wound look swollen? Is the wound running? Does the wound itch? Do you think the wound is well/partially/poorly healed?

Public Health Nurses' Protocol

During the 4th week after surgery, each patient was asked to have a public health nurse assess the incision and fill in the protocol. The public health nurses' assessment included degree of wound healing (rated on a 3-point scale), redness (yes/no), infection, and treatment with antibiotics (yes/no). Finally, they were asked to describe the skin around the incision. Once completed, the protocols were mailed to the clinic.

Procedure

When patients arrived on the units, they were signed in by a secretary who presented written information about the voluntary study. A nurse then informed patients orally about the study and offered them the opportunity for participation. After the patient agreed orally to participate, the secretary randomly selected a number from 1 to 3 (a number for each dressing type) and put the selected number on the anesthesiologist's order sheet (first page in the patient's record). The nurse who assisted during the operation selected the dressing that corresponded to the number on the order sheet.

Wound Dressings

The absorbent wound dressing, serving as a control, is a conventional nonocclusive dressing. It is 10 × 30 cm in size, inexpensive ($0.43/dressing), and routinely used at the clinic.

    The hydrocolloid occlusive wound dressing (DuoDERM, Convatec/Bristol-Myers Squibb) is a sterile dressing measuring 3 × 20 cm. The wound side of the dressing contains hydrocolloids (pectin, gelatin, carboxymethylcellulose) in a polymer matrix, which is self-adhesive to normal skin. The dressing does not allow passage of microbes, water, or oxygen. The price for each dressing is $3.00.

The hydroactive wound dressing (Cutinova hydro, Beiersdorf AG, Hamburg) contains highly absorbent particles embedded in a self-adhesive polyurethane matrix. It is covered by a polyurethane film and is water-resistant and permeable to oxygen and water vapor. The dressing is not available in the size needed for the sternum incisions and was, therefore, cut to the same size as the hydrocolloid dressing (3 × 20 cm) and then resterilized with beta radiation (25 kilo-Gray, kGy). Cost per dressing in the new size was estimated to be $2.78 (the cost for resterilization is not included in the estimated price).

After the operation, the dressings were examined daily and changed only if leaking of exudate was noted. Dressings with no leakage were left in place for 5 days and then removed. On the 5th day, the dressing was removed, a picture of the wound was taken, and a culture was obtained from the incision. Before removal of the dressing, the nurse rated the abilty to inspect the incision through the dressing. Pain at removal and difficulty in removing the dressing were also noted.

On discharge, patients were again informed about the protocol. Thereafter, they followed the instructions in the protocol and answered the questions once a week for 2 weeks. On the fourth week after surgery; they visited the public health nurse for the final evaluation of the wound. The protocol was then mailed to the clinic.

RESULTS

Effectiveness (Wound Healing)

The degree of wound healing was evaluated from photographs of the wound by two independent raters who had no knowledge of the experimental conditions. The degree of healing was rated on a 3-point scale: 1 = well healed, 2 = partially healed, 3 = poorly healed.

Patients in the hydroactive dressing group had significantly poorer wound healing (27% of the wounds were well healed, and 25% were partially healed), compared with patients treated with the absorbent dressing (57% of the wounds were well healed, and 33% were partially healed); χ^2 (2, $n = 153$) = 23.1, $p < .0001$; and with patients in the hydrocolloid dressing group (50% of the wounds were well healed, and 27% were partially healed); χ^2 (2, $n = 129$) = 7.6, $p < .02$. The differences in wound healing between the hydrocolloid and the absorbent dressing groups were not significant; χ^2 (2, $n = 150$) = 5.3, $p > .05$.

Redness in the wounds on the fifth day following surgery showed the same pattern as for wound healing. The hydroactive dressing group had significantly more wounds with excessive redness (48%), compared with the absorbent dressing group (16%); χ^2 (2, $n = 153$) = 17.8, $p < .0001$. Redness in wounds in the hydrocolloid dressing group did not differ significantly from the absorbent dressing group; χ^2 (2, $n = 150$) = 4.1, $p > .05$.

Safety

Ninety-one wounds showed a positive culture. Of those, 35 belonged to the absorbent, 31 to the hydrocolloid, and 25 to the hydroactive dressing groups. The differences between the groups were not significant. The most common microbe isolated from the incisions was *Staphylococcus albus* ($n = 66$), followed by *Propionibacterium* ($n = 10$) and *Escherichia coli* ($n = 6$).

In the public health nurses' reports, 11 patients had been treated with antibiotics because of wound infections. Eight of the 11 infections were found in the sternum incisions. Five of the eight infections were found in the absorbent dressing group. Of the eight infections, only two had had a positive wound culture *(S. albus)* at Day 5 after surgery.

Clinical Utility, Comfort, and Cost

Inspection of the Incision

The possibility of inspecting the incision through the dressing was rated by the nurses on a 3-point scale: 1 = good, 2 = partially, 3 = not at all. None of the wounds covered with the absorbent dressing in place was possible to inspect, and only 3 of the 61 wounds with hydrocolloid dressings enabled partial inspection. The only dressing that enabled large-scale inspection was the hydroactive dressing (17 wounds could be totally inspected, 25 could be inspected partially, and 19 were not possible to inspect).

Removal of the Dressing

According to the nurses' reports, it was significantly easier to remove the absorbent dressings than the other two; hydrocolloid compared with absorbent: χ^2 (1, $n = 145$) = 7.7, $p < .005$; hydroactive compared with absorbent: χ^2 (1, $n = 144$) = 73.6, $p < .0001$. Five of 84 absorbent, 13 of 61 hydrocolloid, and 45 of 60 hydroactive dressings were reported difficult to remove.

Pain at removal of the dressing was rated on a 3-point scale from no pain at all to very painful. Both the hydroactive dressing (14% reported no pain at all at removal) and the hydrocolloid dressing (61% reported no pain at all at removal) were significantly more painful for the patients at removal than the absorbent dressing (76% of the patients reported no pain at all at removal of the dressing); hydroactive versus absorbent: χ^2 (2, $n = 144$) = 55.6, $p < .0001$; hydrocolloid versus absorbent: χ^2 (2, $n = 146$) = 7.6, $p < .02$.

Skin Changes

Skin changes (erythema) at the site of the dressing were reported by 25 patients. Of these, 19 had been treated with hydroactive, 4 with absorbent, and 2 with hydrocolloid dressings; χ^2 (2, $n = 216$) = 29.2, $p < .0001$. Of the 25 patients with skin changes, 16 were female. Two of the patients in the hydroactive group also had blisters on the dressing site.

Dressing Changes and Cost Per Patient

The number of dressing changes and the reason for these changes were noted in the wound protocol during the first 5 days after surgery. The absorbent dressing had the highest number of changes and was changed significantly more often than the two other dressings; χ^2 (6, $n = 213$) = 33.0, $p < .0001$. In the absorbent dressing group, 86 patients used 143 dressings (1.7 dressings/patient) during 5 days; cost per patient (in U.S. dollars) was $0.73. In the hydrocolloid dressing group, 62 patients used 73 dressings (1.2 dressings/patient); cost per patient was $3.60. In the hydroactive dressing group, 65 patients used 80 dressings (1.2 dressings/patient); cost per patient was $3.34 (registration for 3 patients was missed).

The most common reasons for dressing changes were bleeding through the dressing ($n = 51$), followed by necessity to inspect the incision because the patient had a high temperature or other clinical signs of wound infection ($n = 9$). A few changes were necessary because the dressing had loosened ($n = 16$). Some dressings were changed because they were soiled with vomit or spilled food ($n = 5$) or were wet after patients had showered ($n = 2$).

Patients' Ratings 2 and 3 Weeks After Surgery

During the 2nd week after surgery, 104 (61.5%) of the 169 patients reported well-healed wounds (absorbent dressing, 43; hydrocolloid, 31; and hydroactive, 30). During Week 3, 140 patients reported well-healed wounds. Redness in wounds was reported by 45 patients during Week 2 and by 35 during during Week 3. No significant differences were noted among the three dressings. Swollen wounds were reported by 30 patients in Week 2 and 20 patients in Week 3. The number of patients who reported that their wounds were itching was 42 during the second week and 40 during the third week. Skin changes were reported by 36 and 21 patients for Weeks 2 and 3, respectively. The most common skin change was erythema of the skin, surrounding the incision.

Public Health Nurses' Ratings 4 Weeks After Surgery

The public health nurses classified 139 (82%) of the patients' 169 wounds as well healed. No significant differences were noted among the three dressings. Four weeks after surgery, 29 wounds were still erythematous, and 8 wounds were rated as infected (6 of those belonged to the absorbent dressing group). Skin changes around the incision were found in 20 patients. Eleven patients had been treated with antibiotics postoperatively. Eight of these had had infection in the sternum incision.

DISCUSSION

With regard to the effectiveness of the wound dressings, both the conventional absorbent and the occlusive hydrocolloid dressings were sufficient, whereas the hydroactive dressing was not. The hydroactive dressing was difficult to remove and painful for the patient. A plausible explanation could be that the thin reepithelialization that had developed in the incision was damaged when the dressing was removed. Bolton and van Rijswijk (1991) have shown that epithelialization can be delayed by repeated trauma or removal of dressings with aggressive adhesives. The hydroactive dressing, therefore, probably should not be used in this kind of wound without a modification in the adhesive ability.

Feldman et al. (1991) compared DuoDERM with a gauze dressing and found that the latter gave more rapid healing and was less expensive than DuoDERM. Similar findings are reported in the present study. The hydrocolloid dressing had fewer well-healed wounds than the absorbent dressing and was much more expensive to use. Studies on cost-effectiveness in hydrocolloid dressings have usually been done on small wounds. In those studies (e.g., Feldman et al., 1991; Phillips et al., 1993), the dressing was cut to size for several applications, and thereby, the cost was lowered.

The safety of the three dressings was found to be acceptable. Positive wound culture at Day 5 after surgery was found in 39% of the incisions, but only 4.7% of the patients developed wound infections that were necessary to treat with antibiotics 4 weeks after surgery. Bolton and van Rijswijk (1991) also found that wounds healed normally without signs of clinical infection, despite far denser populations of pathogenic bacteria. A total of 5% of the patients had been treated with antibiotics because of infection in the sternum incision. This can be compared with earlier studies, for example, Reinicke et al. (1990), who noted an infection rate of 7%, and Hermans and Skillman (1993), who reported a total incidence of 2%.

Skin changes were found more often around wounds treated with the hydroactive dressing (19 of 25); 16 of the 25 patients with skin changes were women. It is possible that the adhesive ability of the hydroactive dressing is "too good" on surgical wounds. The hydroactive dressing was much more difficult and more painful to remove than the two other dressings. Although it is desirable that the dressing remain firmly in place, it is a disadvantage if it adheres too strongly to be removed without damaging the wound surface or the surrounding skin. The resterilization of the hydroactive dressing might have disturbed the adhesive ability of the dressing and could have contributed to the difficulty in removal. There are, however, no earlier clinical studies on Cutinova hydro used in surgical wound treatment for comparison. The company responsible for Cutinova hydro is aware of the problem and has now modified the adhesiveness in the hydroactive dressing.

Clinical utility, measured in terms of the possibility of inspecting the incision, was good in the hydroactive dressing, less so in the hydrocolloid dressing, and poor in the absorbent dressing. Hermans and Skillman (1993) suggested that DuoDERM became transparent after 12 to 24 hours and allowed wound inspection without removal. This could not be verified in the current study. Only 3 of the 66 wounds covered with the hydrocolloid dressing could be at least partially inspected. The possibility for inspection of the wound without removal of the dressing might result in a less expensive wound treatment. The number of bandage changes was higher in the absorbent dressing group than in the two other groups. Patients treated with the absorbent dressing used 1.7 dressings (mean value) during the 5 days after surgery, and those treated with hydrocolloid or hydroactive dressings used 1.2 dressings. This small reduction in dressing changes in the hydrocolloid and the hydroactive dressings probably does not compensate for the great difference in price ($2.61 to $2.87). The cost of nursing time to make these additional dressing changes when using the absorbent dressing has been calculated by the nurses at the clinic to cost 3 minutes of extra work (in Sweden, approximately $0.50).

In sutured surgical wounds, dressings should provide comfort to the patient and must protect the wound against contamination. According to the findings in this study, the absorbent dressing was safe and comfortable and gave satisfactory wound healing. Although use of the conventional absorbent dressing slightly increases the cost of nursing time, it appears to be the best dressing for this type of surgical wound.

REFERENCES

BOLTON, L., & VAN RIJSWIJK, L. (1991). Wound dressings: Meeting clinical and biological needs. *Dermatology Nursing, 3,* 146-161.

BRENNAN, P. F., & HAYS, B. J. (1992). The kappa statistic for establishing interrater reliability in the secondary analysis of qualitative clincal data. *Research in Nursing and Health, 15,* 153-158.

CUZZELL, J. Z. (1990). Choosing a wound dressing: A systematic approach. *AACN Clinical Issues in Critical Care Nursing, 1,* 566-577.

FELDMAN, D. L., ROGERS, A., & KARPINSKI, R. H. (1991). A prospective trial comparing Biobrane, Duoderm and Xeroform for skin graft donor sites. *Surgery, Gynecology & Obstetrics, 173,* 1-5.

HERMANS, M. H., & SKILLMAN, N. J. (1993). Clinical benefit of a hydrocolloid dressing in closed surgical wounds. *Journal of ET Nursing, 20*(2), 68-72.

PHILLIPS, T. J., KAPOOR, V., PROVAN, A., & ELLERIN, T. (1993). A randomized prospective study of a hydroactive dressing vs conventional treatment after shave biopsy excision. *Archives of Dermatology, 129,* 859-860.

RASMUSSEN, H., LARSEN, M. J., & SKEIE, E. (1993). Surgical wound dressing in outpatient pediatric surgery: A randomized study. *Danish Medical Bulletin, 40,* 252-254.

REINICKE, G., NOWAK, W., & ADLER, K. P. (1990). Does the elastic rapid wound dressing Ankerplast spray modify wound healing? *Zentralblatt für Chirurgie, 115,* 111-116.

Healing of Adult Male Survivors of Childhood Sexual Abuse

Claire Burke Draucker ■ Kathleen Petrovic

Objective: *To generate a framework of healing by male survivors of childhood sexual abuse.*

Design: *Qualitative using grounded theory methodology.*

Population, Sample, Setting, Years: *Population was American men living in the community who have experienced some healing from childhood sexual abuse. Sample was 19 men who were recommended by area therapists or who had publicly identified themselves as survivors. Participants were interviewed in 1993 and 1994.*

Method: *Formal, unstructured interviews using open-ended questions.*

Findings: *The core variable that emerged was "Escaping the dungeon: The journey to freedom." The metaphor of "dungeon" reflects the men's experiences of powerlessness, isolation, silence and darkness, shame, and pain from their abuse. Healing was described as breaking free, living free, and freeing those left behind.*

Conclusions: *Healing involves a struggle against an internal force, emotional pain, and against an external force, the sociocultural prescription that men should not be victims.*

Clinical implications: *Clinicians working with adult male survivors should consider the pervasive effects of some childhood sexual abuse experiences. Therapists can address the intrapsychic wounds of male survivors while acknowledging the context of their healing, a society where the victimization of men is often invalidated.*

Appendix B Reprinted with permission from *Image J Nurs Sch* 28(4):325-330, 1996.

Childhood sexual abuse is a significant problem for many survivors. Much research has been conducted with female survivors of childhood sexual abuse, but few studies focus on adult male survivors. Although, historically, sexual abuse of males was considered rare, researchers now estimate that between 11% and 16% of American men experienced sexual abuse as children (Finkelhor, Hotaling, Lewis, & Smith; 1989; Urquiza & Keating, 1990; Violato & Genuis, 1993). Men who were sexually abused as children are at risk of experiencing long-term negative effects from their abuse (Collings, 1995; Mendel, 1995; Violato & Genuis, 1993) including depression (Urquiza & Crowley, 1986); anxiety and post-traumatic stress symptoms (Briere, Evans, Runtz, & Wall, 1988); low self-esteem (Urquiza & Crowley, 1986); sexual identity confusion (Dimock, 1988); substance abuse (Stein, Golding, Siegel, Burnam, & Sorenson, 1988); compulsive spending, overworking, and overeating (Olson, 1990); and sexual acting out (Olson, 1990).

Although many of the long-term effects reported in the literature are similar for men and women, male survivors are affected by different sociocultural factors (Crowder, 1995; Etherington, 1995; Mendel, 1995). Men in U.S. society are expected to be self-reliant, independent, and productive; protect themselves from violations by others; and internalize emotions (Struve, 1990). Society in general does not recognize the victimization of men. Struve (1990) suggests that some symptoms exhibited by male survivors represent "exaggerated efforts to reassert their masculinity" (p. 37) and attempts to deal with emotions they cannot express.

Sepler (1990) argues the treatment of sexual assault victims has been based primarily on models used for female rape victims, which involve "unequivocal reinforcement of the blamelessness of the victim . . . accompanied by practical assistance and expression of appropriate anger" (p. 75). Because male survivors of sexual assault experience victimization from a different worldview than do female rape victims, they may be alienated by treatment that assumes a universal response to victimization.

Mental health professionals, based on their clinical experiences treating male survivors, have identified activities that seem to facilitate recovery such as disclosing and accepting the reality of the abuse (Bolton, Morris, & MacEachron, 1989), memory retrieval (Bolton et al., 1989; Timms & Connors, 1990), grief resolution (Bolton et al., 1989; Hunter & Gerber, 1990), acceptance and expression of emotion (Bolton et al., 1989; Timms & Connors, 1990), empowerment (Timms & Connors, 1990), and anger management (Bruckner & Johnson, 1987).

Although clinicians have identified several aspects of recovery based on their work with abused men, the healing experiences of male survivors from their own perspectives have not been systematically studied. The purpose of this study was to generate a theoretical framework of the healing process of male survivors based on the perspective of those who had experienced some healing.

METHODS

A qualitative study using grounded-theory methods (Glaser & Strauss, 1967) was conducted. Grounded theory is an inductive method used to generate a theoretical framework based on concepts that emerge from the data. In this study, data consisted of descriptions of life experiences by male survivors who had experienced healing from the trauma of childhood sexual abuse.

Information related to the study was sent to area professionals who specialize in working with men; they were asked to invite men who had been sexually abused and who seemed to have experienced some healing to contact the investigators. Also, individuals who had identified themselves as sexual abuse survivors and who had shared their own healing experiences in some public context were contacted individually by the investigators to request their participation. The study was conducted between 1993 and 1994.

Nineteen men who ranged in age from 23 to 55 participated. Seven were married, four were divorced, and eight were single. Nine had children, 17 were Caucasian, and two were Hispanic. Although sexual preference was not asked on the demographic information sheet, several identified themselves as gay men. Most of the men were abused by family members, acquaintances, or authority figures, although a few were molested by strangers. Duration of abuse experiences ranged from a single incident to many years.

Eight participants were interviewed in person and, because of geographic constraints, two were interviewed by telephone. In addition, interviews were conducted with members of two therapy groups. One group had five members and the other had four members. In two instances, the group interview was followed with an individual interview. Several participants provided additional information throughout the course of the study with letters and phone calls to the investigators.

Before the beginning of the interview, participants were asked to read and sign a consent form and to complete a brief demographic information sheet. Formal, unstructured interviews were conducted and tape recorded. The questions were open-ended to encourage participants to describe experiences from their perspective. For example, one question was, "What does it mean to be healing from childhood sexual abuse?" Another question was: "How are you healing from your experience of childhood sexual abuse?" The interviews lasted from 1 to 3 hours.

Data analysis was based on techniques from grounded-theory method (Corbin, 1986b; Glaser, 1978; Glaser & Strauss, 1967). Substantive coding was done. Facts and incidents were abstracted as concepts and identified by code words. The codes were compared for similarities and differences. Large spread-sheets were used to organize the codes into theoretical groups or categories. The core variable (Glaser, 1978), which explains much variation in the data and links the categories into a descriptive framework, was identified and labeled, "Escaping the dungeon: The journey to freedom." Through constant comparison and reflection on the data, the investigators developed the theoretical framework.

Several strategies (Corbin, 1986a) were simultaneously employed to carry out the analysis and to enhance the credibility of the study. Analytic memos were kept to reflect the investigators' thinking while coding the data, identifying and linking categories, and determining the core variable. Diagrams were constructed showing the categories and the way they were related to one another. Peer debriefing, defined as "exposing oneself to a disinterested peer . . . for the purpose of exploring aspects of inquiry that might otherwise remain only implicit with the inquirer's mind" (Lincoln & Guba, 1985, p. 308), was accomplished through interactions with a research consultant, who is a doctorally prepared nurse with expertise in the grounded-theory method.

Member checks, validing reconstructions with the original informants (Lincoln & Guba, 1985), were conducted. All 19 participants were sent copies of the framework. Of the 12 who were interviewed individually, nine were contacted by phone and asked to respond to the framework. These participants indicated that the final theoretical framework accurately reflected their experiences and was comprehensive. The seven participants who were involved in the group interviews only were not involved in the member checks as the groups were no longer in session.

THEORETICAL FRAMEWORK

The survivors described healing from childhood sexual abuse as a process of breaking free from lives marred by the effects of the abuse to lives characterized by a sense of freedom, belonging, and power (see Table 1). The metaphor of "Escaping the dungeon: The journey to freedom" is used to reflect healing as it was discussed by the men.

Participants indicated their lives, before healing, were marked by powerlessness, isolation, silence and darkness, shame, and pain. The metaphor of a "dungeon" reflects the men's sense of being confined by the effects of their abuse, being alienated from others, and being condemned because of their childhood experiences. The men identified that the healing process involved breaking free from the confines of the "dungeon" to a life of freedom, which included a feeling of vitality, a sense of belonging, and an active commitment to remain free. While breaking free often began as an intense and explosive experience, overall it was described as a journey that was time-consuming, difficult, and painful. Participants emphasized that while

Table 1

Escaping the Dungeon: The Journey to Freedom

I.   Living in the dungeon

    A. Being confined

        1. Being trapped

        2. Being silenced

        3. Being stifled

        4. Being idled

    B. Being alienated

        1. Being abandoned

        2. Being disconnected

        3. Feeling abnormal

    C. Being condemned

        1. Being found guilty

        2. Being punished

II. Breaking free

    A. Preparing for the break

        1. Releasing that which is damaged

        2. Releasing excess baggage

        3. Joining with comrades

    B. Escaping to freedom

        1. Breaking out of the dungeon

        2. Journeying to free soil

III. Living free

    A. Feeling alive

        1. Awakening of the senses

        2. Discovering a voice

    B. Reclaiming a place on earth

        1. Finding a place to fit in

        2. Doing normal things

    C. Affirming the right of freedom

        1. Being vindicated

        2. Regaining power

IV. Freeing those left behind

    A. Exposing the dungeon

    B. Destroying the dungeon

living free is an experience to be savored; it also is an experience that has to be continually protected and shared with those who have not yet broken free.

LIVING IN THE DUNGEON

People who are imprisoned in actual dungeons are not only confined and isolated but also alienated from all those who are free. Participants spoke symbolically of being confined and cut off from resources they needed to sustain their life and health (being buried in a "grave"), feeling isolated from other humans (being an "island"), believing they were being punished for being bad or evil (being in a "prison cell"), and experiencing pain that was pervasive and often intense (being in "hell"). The image of a dungeon reflects these experiences.

Hopkins (1897) wrote *The Dungeons of Old Paris;* many parallels exist between Hopkins' descriptions of life in ancient dungeons and the participants' description of their lives before healing. Hopkins said of life in a dungeon: "Punishment . . . it is quite without system and means only the vengeance of the strong on the week . . . the prison which was intended . . . as a living tomb" (p. 6).

Being Confined

Hopkins (1897) described a dungeon as "The expression in stone and mortar of the power and hatred of the builders," where there was a "sense of suffocation" and where the prisoner is "crushed beneath the weight of society" (p. 8). Participants described being trapped, silenced, stifled, and idled.

The sense of *being trapped,* often buried, by their abuse experiences was described by some men as "having problems snowball on top of me" and "being caught in a spider web." Many indicated that the walls that trapped them were built by themselves as protection from further hurt. One stated:

You know how most people build a wall in front of themselves trying to protect themselves. I didn't build a wall in front of myself. I made myself part of that wall. So you couldn't see me from front or back. I had actually hid myself that much . . . I was somewhere back in the mortar.

Being silenced was frequently described by participants. Not having their voices heard, either as children being abused or as adult male survivors, compounded their suffering. One man said his father had witnessed his abuse by two brothers, but did not intervene. Later when discovering the boy crying in his room, his father said, "Shut up, you're a man, you're not supposed to cry." Another confided his abuse by a priest, but the priest responded by "being very distant, very put off, very cold, very mechanical or academic."

A sense of confinement was also related to the feeling of *being stifled* and deprived of the elements necessary for life. Many of the men referred to living in darkness and several described living without human touch, which had become aversive because of the abuse. Some compared their experience to being ill or diseased and many spoke of a "deadening" of their feelings.

Feeling confined was also related to the participants *being idled.* They indicated that because their lives had become unmanageable or chaotic, they were deprived of being able to fully participate in the activities of everyday life: Working, learning, or playing. Several described not being able to hold a job or go to school and some described being unable to relax and have fun.

Being Alienated

Hopkins (1897) spoke of dungeon prisoners as people "who had never been guilty of crimes, [but who] lay for years in the Bastille, forgotten and uncared for . . ." (p. 203). Just as those imprisoned in a dungeon would have felt acutely separate and different from those who were free, the participants in this study described experiences that extended beyond loneliness to a profound sense of alienation.

For participants, the sense of alienation often stemmed from *being abandoned* and betrayed at the time of the abuse. The experience of abandonment frequently extended into adulthood. The men described how others in their lives denied, minimized, or perpetuated their abuse.

The alienation experienced by participants was also related to a general sense of *being disconnected* from others. For example, one man stated that he had the "Leave me alone syndrome." Several discussed feeling especially distant from other men. One man explained, "I'm like sitting up against the wall [in a bar], all by myself. Trying to ward off everybody in the room. I'm scared to death of everybody." *Feeling abnormal* or inherently different from those who were not abused also contributed to many participants' experience of alienation. They related having felt weird, bizarre, or strange. Two said they felt like "aliens from outer space." Many emphasized that society contributed to their feelings of being abnormal by denying their victimization.

Being Condemned

Just as unfortunate victims were thrown into ancient dungeons for supposed wrong-doings, many participants described believing, at one point, that their suffering was punishment for their sins. Just as dungeon prisoners were condemned to "endure all the horrors, physical and mental" (Hopkins, 1879, p. 28) so too were the men in this study.

The experience of condemnation was related to a sense of *being found guilty*, because others often had told the participants that they were responsible for the abuse. Many of the men believed that they were abused because they were inherently bad. One participant stated that he had believed for 30 years that he was "somehow or other intrinsically evil." Another stated, "When I've been hurt or things have happened to me I kind of sat there and said, 'Well, God is punishing me. I'm such an evil, nasty, rotten person and I deserve these things.'"

For the participants, condemnation resulted in *being punished*. The majority of participants had been physically as well as sexually abused as children. All described some emotional torment, including depression, anxiety, fear, and desperation, that extended into their adult lives. Several spoke of learning to "dissociate" as a way of warding off unbearable pain. Many indicated that they used drugs and alcohol to numb the pain that stemmed from their abuse.

BREAKING FREE

Healing began when the men were able to break free from the "dungeon"—from the confinement, alienation, and condemnation. Breaking free forever changed their lives.

Preparing for the Break

Breaking out of a dungeon involves planning and timing. Participants in this study indicated that breaking free required a period of time or some specific activities. For some, preparation was described as *releasing that which was damaged,* typically letting go of what felt evil, bad, or destructive. One compared the beginning of his healing to an "exorcism" or a "plumbing job." Others used visceral images (e.g., vomiting, blood letting) to describe the letting go of that which was damaged. One man told of a poignant experience in which he and his wife received the "baptism of the holy spirit" following a prayer meeting:

And he [the leader of the prayer meeting] had everyone gather around and lay hands on us and it was just like a real beautiful prayer and it was like he knew everything that happened . . . it was definitely from God that he brought us all there. . . . Then it was like, the only way I can describe it, it felt like my heels came off and all that crap just drained out and something new, warm, and unbelievably good re-placed it.

For others, preparing to break free was described as *releasing excess baggage,* most often leaving behind relationships that were holding them back from healing. For many participants, *joining with other comrades,* often other male survivors, was crucial in preparing to break free. Those who were in the therapy groups emphasized that the support of other men who could truly understand their experiences was extremely helpful in facilitating recovery.

Escaping to Freedom

Breaking free is a monumental life experience. Many participants identified a discrete and intense incident that began their healing, or an initial *breaking out of the dungeon.* These incidents were frequently an initial disclosure of the abuse to someone supportive or an important insight or memory related to the abuse experience. Many of the participants described these incidents as an "explosion" or the "eruption of a volcano" that involved intense anxiety and emotional turmoil followed by relief and a sense of hope.

An actual escape from a dungeon is often followed by a dangerous trip to safe ground with the threat of recapture ever present. Similarly, for many of the participants breaking out was followed by the difficult, tedious, and threatening work of dealing with the abuse: Remembering it, talking about it, and coming to understand its effect. Because this process could be long, painful, and frightening, several of the participants described it as a "bumpy" journey with many "stumbling blocks." *Journeying to free soil,* therefore, while lacking the intensity of the initial breaking out, involved many "small steps" and consistent hard work and persistence. The men described the journey as "eating an elephant," "peeling layer after layer of an onion," "plugging away," "muddling along," and "digging and digging."

LIVING FREE

Participants emphasized the break from the dungeon and the journey to freedom resulted in lives very different from those experienced before healing. The men indicated that as they began to emerge from their confinement, they felt alive. They came to believe they belonged on earth and had reclaimed their right to live free.

Feeling Alive

For many participants, living free began with a sense of being alive and vital or "being able to breath again." One participant stated he had felt "dead inside" and healing allowed him to experience life. Just as a prisoner emerging from a dungeon again sees the light, feels the warmth of the sun, and experiences human touch, the participants frequently associated their early healing with images of an *awakening of the senses* and an appreciation for the environment. One stated, "I sense things better, I smell things better. A sunrise is a joyous thing to me now."

Many spoke of coming out of the darkness. Several described an important insight or new understanding with references to seeing or to light. They spoke of "A light dawning," "Experiencing a real eye opener," "Starting to see things," or "Having a light bulb come on." One participant compared an experience of self-awareness to "taking the lid off a well and seeing this great expansion."

As senses returned, the men took other information from the environment as well. Just as those in captivity are often deprived of news from the outside, several participants indicated that they were hungry for information related to abuse. Two participants pointed out that most survivor literature is geared toward women. Several referred to reading everything about male survivors they could find once they had begun healing.

Several stated that healing involved gaining an appreciation of the sense of touch and an awareness of physical sensations. One spoke of his decision to exercise and receive massage therapy stating, "I think just the awareness of the sensation, or whatever, the energy in my body . . . is just really enlivening for me."

Discovering a voice was identified as a crucial aspect of feeling alive. Several spoke of disclosing their abuse and sharing their feelings and personal lives with others. One participant, who has written and spoken publicly about abuse, addressed the relationship of speaking out, being heard, and healing:

On the one hand, it [speaking publicly] helps in that I feel I'm speaking to my family, who are not listening. So those who are in the audience are listening to me. I'm feeling I'm talking to them, to members of my family. So in that sense its a relief of some of the pain that I have had to deal with by having someone hear it.

Because they were heard by family and society, the men were no longer silenced. Several told of speaking to and being heard by God. One said:

I really didn't see any point [to living]. I said, "Well, God really loves me, I'll think about it [committing suicide]." I prayed and it felt really, really [as though] I had a religious experience. I felt like God really touched me and I felt like I had love in my heart. There was hope. I felt really whole.

Reclaiming a Place on Earth

Dungeon prisoners who break free would then have to return to society. Participants indicated that to live free they also had to reclaim their place on earth.

For many of the men, this typically meant *finding a place to fit in*. Several stated that they were no longer "the outsider." They spoke of "feeling normal," having their "feet on the ground," and "being a part of something." The experience of feeling comfortable and connected to others was exemplified in the following quote:

In fact, I just ordered a brand new one [Harley Davidson] and to do that, I know its macho bull. . . . a lot of it, but to get on that thing, ride out and camp and I have a circle of friends across the country and we get together three or four times a year, who I really appreciate. We sit around and tell war stories and drink beer and that kind of male bonding. . . . Real helpful. Not that it has to be a motorcycle, but finding myself comfortable in an all male environment is very helpful for me.

In addition, *doing normal things,* like working, learning, and playing, validated the men's sense of belonging in society. For example, one man identified the importance of having a job by saying, "I'm actually feeling a part of society." After being back to work only for a short time he had received a significant pay raise, two promotions, and several positive evaluations from his supervisor.

Affirming the Right of Freedom

Living free is not an experience the men take for granted. In fact, most emphasized that ensuring their on-going healing will be a life-long effort. The participants affirmed their right of freedom by vindicating themselves of wrong-doing and regaining the power robbed from them in childhood.

For many, *being vindicated* was identified as an important aspect of healing. Most stated that they no longer blamed themselves for their abuse and could now feel good about themselves, appreciate their worth as individuals, and cease to be overly critical or demanding of themselves. The guilt and shame they had lived with for years had begun to dissipate allowing them to savor their new life experiences.

Regaining power was also seen as essential. By gaining control over their lives and making choices, participants assured their on-going freedom. One stated, "Now [that] I understand why I reacted that way, I can choose not to react that way. And that's been freeing."

FREEING THOSE LEFT BEHIND

The majority indicated that once they had experienced and affirmed their own freedom, they chose to engage in some sort of activity to free those still being victimized and oppressed. They were committed to breaking free those yet imprisoned.

Exposing the Dungeon

Many participants chose to speak out to expose the social problem of the victimization of males. These activities took the form of disclosing their abuse through the news media or other public forums, writing books or music, or being involved in advocacy organizations.

Destroying the Dungeon

In addition to speaking out, many of the men were actively working to destroy dungeons by bringing offenders to justice. Prosecuting their own offenders or exposing offenders who were harming others were two ways participants worked to give the gift of freedom to others who were still suffering. One participant described placing "Wanted" posters of a rapist in local stores. His action was instrumental in leading to an arrest.

The commitment of participants to destroying the dungeon in which they themselves existed is summed up in the following statement:

This [project] is important work. Until children are able to grow in a wholesome, nourishing environment or until we are able to help children escape the effects of a less-than-wholesome environment, I see little hope for achieving peace and justice throughout the nation . . . or our world.

SUMMARY AND CONCLUSIONS

The framework adds to the literature by describing healing as a journey from captivity to freedom. Participants in this study described their prehealing experiences not merely as a sum of negative effects but rather a state of being, marked by a sense of confinement, alienation, and condemnation. Conceptualizing healing as an escape from the dungeon captures the survivors' struggle against internal forces stemming from abuse (e.g., emotional pain) and against external forces that kept them imprisoned (e.g., society).

Although the framework cannot be generalized to all male survivors and more empirical investigation is needed to further develop the theory, the findings suggest some problems that might be important for clinicians to consider when working with male survivors. Because participants in this study described a lifestyle actually defined by the abuse, clinicians working with men should consider the potential pervasiveness of the effect of an experience of childhood sexual abuse. By carefully attending to a client's descriptions of his experiences, clinicians can appreciate the depth and uniqueness of the effect of victimization. Participants in this study did not describe "low self-esteem," rather they spoke of feeling "evil" or "damaged." They did not feel "different," rather they felt "alien." They described not merely being maltreated, but being "silenced," "stifled," and "diseased."

Because the image of an escape reflects the men's battle against society's stereotypes, as well as against internal turmoil, this metaphor can add to our awareness of the nature of healing. Clients who are male survivors of sexual abuse are not only healing internal psychic wounds but they are also struggling against a society that invalidates their trauma, discourages them from seeking help, and sequelches their painful emotions (i.e., "Real men don't cry").

This theoretical framework provides a beginning understanding of the unique healing process of male survivors of childhood sexual abuse. All participants felt that the experience of "living free" was well worth the struggle and the pain of "breaking free." As stated by one participant, "freeing those left behind" was part of bringing peace and justice to the world.

REFERENCES

Bolton, F.G., Morris, L.A., & MacEachron, A.F. (1989). Males at risk: The other side of child sexual abuse. Newbury Park, CA: Sage.

Briere, J., Evans, D., Runtz, M., & Wall, T. (1988). Symptomatology in men who are molested as children: A comparison study. American Journal of Orthopsychiatry, 58, 457-461.

Bruckner, D.F., & Johnson, P.E. (1987). Treatment for adult male victims of childhood sexual abuse. Social Casework: The Journal of Contemporary Social Work, 68, 81-87.

Collings, S.J. (1995). The long-term effects of contact and noncontact forms of child sexual abuse in a sample of university men. Child Abuse & Neglect, 19(1), 1-6.

Corbin, J. (1986a). Coding, writing memos, and diagramming. In W.C. Chenitz & J.M. Swanson (Eds.), From practice to grounded theory, (102-120). Menlo Park, CA: Addison-Wesley.

Corbin, J. (1986b). Qualitative data analysis for grounded theory. In W.C. Chenitz & J.M. Swanson (Eds.), From practice to grounded theory, (91-101). Menlo Park, CA: Addison-Wesley.

Crowder, A. (1995). Opening the door: A treatment model for therapy with male survivors of sexual abuse. New York: Brunner/Mazel.

Dimock, P. (1988). Adult males sexually abused as children. Journal of Interpersonal Violence, 3, 203-221.

Etherington, K. (1995). Adult male survivors of sexual abuse. Counseling Psychology Quarterly, 8, 233-241.

Finkelhor, D., Hotaling, G.T., Lewis, I.A., & Smith, C. (1989). Sexual abuse and its relationship to later sexual satisfaction, marital status, religion, and attitudes. Journal of Interpersonal Violence, 4, 379-399.

Glaser, B.G. (1978). Theoretical sensitivity: Advances in the methodology of grounded theory. Mill Valley, CA: The Sociology Press.

Glaser, B.G., & Strauss, A.L. (1967). The discovery of grounded theory: Strategies for qualitative research. Chicago: Aldine.

Hopkins, T. (1897). The dungeons of old Paris. New York: G.P. Putnam's Sons.

Hunter, M., & Gerber, P.N. (1990). Use of terms victim and survivor in the grief stages commonly seen during recovery from sexual abuse. In M. Hunter (Ed.), The sexually abused male: Vol. 2: Application of treatment strategies, (79-90). Lexington, MA: Lexington Books.

Lincoln, Y.S., & Guba, E.G. (1985). Naturalistic inquiry. Beverly Hills, CA: Sage.

Mendel, M.P. (1995). The male survivor: The impact of sexual abuse. Thousand Oaks, CA: Sage.

Olson, P.E. (1990). The sexual abuse of boys: A study of the long-term psychological effects. In M. Hunter (Ed.), The sexually abused male: Vol. 1: Prevalence, impact, and treatment (137-152). Lexington, MA: Lexington Books.

Sepler, F. (1990) Victim advocacy and young male victims of sexual abuse: An evolutionary model. In M. Hunter (Ed.), The sexually abused male: Vol. 1: Prevalence, impact, and treatment (73-85). Lexington, MA: Lexington Books.

Stein, J.A., Golding, J.M., Seigel, J.M., Burnam, M.A., & Sorenson, S.B. (1988). Long-term psychological sequelae of child sexual abuse. In G.E. Wyatt and G.J. Powell (Eds.), Lasting effects of child sexual abuse. (135-154). Newbury Park, CA: Sage Publications.

Struve, J. (1990). Dancing with the patriarchy: The politics of sexual abuse. In M. Hunter (Ed.). The sexually abused male: Vol. 1: Prevalence, impact, and treatment, (3-16). Lexington, MA: Lexington Books.

Timms, R., & Connors, P. (1990). Integrating psychotherapy and body work for abuse survivors: A psychological model. In M. Hunter (Ed.), The sexually abused male: Vo. 2: Application of treatment strategies, (117-136). Lexington, MA: Lexington Books.

Urquiza, A.J., & Crowley, C. (1986, May). Sex differences in long-term adjustment of child sexual abuse victims. Paper presented at the Third National Conference of the Sexual Victimization of Children, New Orleans, LA.

Urquiza, A.J., & Keating, L.A. (1990). The prevalence of the sexual victimization of males. In M. Hunter (Ed.), The sexually abused male: Vol. 1: Prevalence, impact, and treatment, (89-104). Lexington, MA: Lexington Books.

Violato, C., & Genuis, M. (1993). Problems of research in male child sexual abuse: A review. Journal of Child Sexual Abuse, 2(3), 33-54.

Patient Outcomes for the Chronically Critically Ill: Special Care Unit Versus Intensive Care Unit

Ellen B. Rudy ▪ Barbara J. Daly ▪ Sara Douglas ▪ Hugo D. Montenegro ▪ Rhayun Song ▪ Mary Ann Dyer

The purpose of this study was to compare the effects of a low-technology environment of care and a nurse case management case delivery system (special care unit, SCU) with the traditional high-technology environment (ICU) and primary nursing care delivery system on the patient outcomes of length of stay, mortality, readmission, complications, satisfaction, and cost. A sample of 220 chronically critically ill patients were randomly assigned to either the SCU (n = 145) or the ICU (n = 75). Few significant differences were found between the two groups in length of stay, mortality, or complications. However, the findings showed significant cost savings in the SCU group in the charges accrued during the study period and in the charges and costs to produce a survivor. The average total cost of delivering care was $5,000 less per patient in the SCU than in the traditional ICU. In addition, the cost to produce a survivor was $19,000 less in the SCU. Results from this 4-year clinical trial demonstrate that nurse case managers in a SCU setting can produce patient outcomes equal to or better than those in the traditional ICU care environment for long-term critically ill patients.

Appendix C Reprinted with permission from *Nurs Res* 44(6):324-331, 1995.

The original purpose of intensive care units (ICUs) was to locate groups of patients together who had similar needs for specialized monitoring and care so that highly trained health care personnel would be available to meet these specialized needs. As the success of ICUs has grown and expanded, the assumption that a typical ICU patient will require only a short length of stay in the unit during the most acute phase of an illness has given way to the recognition that stays of more than 1 month are not uncommon (Berenson, 1984; Daly, Rudy, Thompson, & Happ, 1991).

These long-stay ICU patients represent a challenge to the current system, not only because of costs, but also because of concern for patient outcomes. These patients are often elderly, have underlying chronic conditions that complicate or exacerbate their acute illness, and often require sustained ventilatory and nutritional support. A prime example of these types of patients are those referred to as "ventilator dependent," found to varying degrees in nearly every ICU in the country (American Association for Respiratory Care, 1991).

The term "chronically critically ill" has been previously used (Daly et al., 1991) to describe patients who have extended stays in the ICU. These patients have become the most burdensome to nurses and physicians, who see their progress as slow and frustrating, to hospital administrators because of the extended bed occupancy in times of high demand, and to hospital financial officers because of costs that usually exceed the diagnosis-related group (DRG) cost allocation. Patients who have ICU length of stays greater than 21 days account for approximately 3% of the total number of patients admitted to the ICUs, yet they account for approximately 25% to 38% of the patient days (Daly et al.).

While ample evidence confirms that this subpopulation of ICU patients represents a drain on hospital resources, few studies have attempted to evaluate the effects of a care delivery system outside the ICU setting on patient outcomes, costs, and nurse outcomes. The majority of studies that have examined ICU patient outcomes have been limited primarily to mortality and length of stay (Bersenson, 1984; Borlase et al., 1991; Madoff, Sharpe, Fath, Simons, & Cerra, 1985). More recently, attention has been given to cost in terms of risk-adjusted ICU length of stays, cost and utility of diagnostic and laboratory tests, and time on mechanical ventilation (Gundlach & Faulkner, 1991; Kappstein et al., 1992; Roberts et al., 1993; Schapira, Studnicki, Bradhan, Wolff, & Jarrett, 1993; Zimmerman et al., 1993).

In studies limited to mechanically ventilated patients, comparisons on legnth of stay and costs have been examined in "a before-and-after" design following initiation of a ventilatory management team (Cohen et al., 1991), on overall costs for mechanically ventilated patients cared for in an ICU versus a noninvasive respiratory care unit (Elpern, Silver, Rosen, & Bone, 1991), and on hospital charges and life expectancy for elderly mechanically ventilated ICU patients (Cohen, Lambrinos, & Fein, 1993). The lack of randomized trials comparing care delivery systems for these high-cost patients is noteworthy, as well as the limitation of outcome measurements to mortality and cost.

The purpose of the current study was to compare the effects of a low-technology environment of care based on a nurse-managed care delivery system (special care unit [SCU] environment) with the traditional high-technology ICU environment based on a primary nursing care delivery system. The two groups were compared on the outcomes of length of stay, mortality, readmission to the hospital, complications, patient and family satisfaction, and cost. The complications were defined as number and type of infections, number and type of respiratory complications, and number and type of life-threatening complications.

METHOD

Sample

A total of 276 subjects were eligible for the study. Table 1 lists eligibility criteria. Only four refused to participate; of the remaining 272 subjects, 220 (81%) were able to be randomized. Of the 52 subjects who were not randomly assigned to a treatment group, the majority ($n = 37$, 71%) were due to bed availability, with only 13 (25%) due to physician refusal to allow randomization to treatment assignment, and 2 (4%) because of family unwillingness to allow treatment assignment.

The final sample for analysis consisted of 145 subjects cared for in the SCU environment and 75 subjects in the ICU environment. The sample was nearly equally divided between males and females, was predominantly White (70%), with an average age of 64 years (range 16 to 90 years). The groups were equivalent to gender, age, and race, on the prior ICU length of stay ($M = 16$ days, $SD = 13.3$), and on the general medical diagnosis of patients. Significant differences were found in the type of ICU where patients received their care prior to the study and in source of payment for care. A higher percentage of no payment source and private insurance was found in the ICU group, with a higher percentage of public (Medicare and Medicaid) insurance in the SCU group.

To ensure similiarity of acuity of illness between the two groups of subjects, a variety of variables were compared. No significant difference between the groups was noted on the Acute Physiological and Chronic Health Evaluation II (APACHE II) on admission to the ICU or at time of eligibility for the study, the Therapeutic Intervention Scoring System (TSS) at the time of eligibility for the study, and the number of infections prior to admission to the study. In terms of these known risk predictors, then, the experimental and control groups were equivalent. There were, however, significantly ($p \leq .03$) more respiratory complications prior to the study in the patients admitted to the SCU. While statistically significant, in practical terms, the means of the two groups varied by only 0.5, with a very similar range and standard deviation. Furthermore, the higher risk from prior respiratory complications was in the SCU sample, so claims that patients in the ICU were sicker can be refuted.

Table 1

Eligibility Criteria for Patients in the Study

Length of stay (LOS) in ICU > 5 days*
Not currently receiving IV vasopressor (exception; low-level maintenance drip)
No pulmonary artery monitor required
No acute event (arrest, unstable event) in past 3 days
APACHE II 18 or less
TISS class II or III (10 to 39 points)
Unable to be cared for on a general nursing unit

NOTE: APACHE, Acute physiological and chronic health evaluation; TISS, Therapeutic intervention scoring system.
*First 2 years of study LOS in ICU was > 7 days, but with experience the LOS was shortened to ≥ 5 days.

Setting

The environments of care were conceptualized according to the sociotechnical theory of work, which proposes that both the physical environment in which work occurs, the procedures and processes of work, and the way workers interact with one another and with the environment will influence the way in which the work is accomplished and ultimately the output of the work (Happ, 1993; Pasmore, 1988; Pasmore & Sherwood, 1978).

The SCU environment of care was designed to decrease technology and ensure privacy in order to promote sleep and rest, allow for more freedom for interaction with family and friends, ensure continuity of care by nurse case managers working with medical protocols, and create an opportunity for a self-directed governance model. The significant contrasting features of the SCU versus the ICU were the physical environment, the nursing practice model, and the nursing management model.

The SCU environment was a 7-bed unit with only private rooms. Technology was limited to electrocardiographic monitors, ventilators, and occasional arterial pressure monitoring. Family involvement was encouraged through unlimited visiting and overnight accommodations. The care delivery system was case management, with the nurse case manager accountable clinically and financially for each patient's outcomes. Interns and residents were not in the unit. Each patient's plan of care was established, coordinated, and evaluated by the case manager working in close collaboration with the unit's attending physician. Case managers participated in an 8-week training program for the SCU and, with the medical director of the unit, developed protocols that addressed such activities as ventilator weaning, nutrition, pain management, and sedation. In addition, the SCU initiated a shared governance management model, which vested the authority and responsibility for managing the work environment in the staff nurses.

The ICU environments included primarily a 12-bed medical intensive care unit and an 18-bed surgical intensive care unit. A small percentage of subjects (19%) who met the study criteria came from the neurosurgical intensive care unit or the coronary intensive care unit. The majority (80%) of bed spaces were open or curtained off from a central nursing station. Visitor lounges were outside the units, family visiting was controlled, and overnight stays were not accommodated. Technology and physiological monitoring devices were not limited, and lighting and noise from the overall unit was difficult to exclude from the patient bed spaces. A primary nursing model of care was used in all of the ICUs, with total nursing care the responsibility of the primary nurse. Interns and residents delivered most of the medical care, as is the standard practice in academic medical centers. A bureaucratic management model was used with centralized decision making at the head nurse level, and organizational responsibility and authority descending within each unit through a distinct chain of command.

Procedure

Rounds were made every other day in all ICUs to assess patient eligibility. Using a coin toss, eligible patients were assigned to either the experimental or control group. Consent to participate was then obtained from both the primary physician and the patient. If the patient was unable to consent, the next of kin was asked for permission. If the patients and their physicians consented, patients were then enrolled and, if in the experimental group, transferred to the SCU. This procedure for consent and group assignment was approved by the hospital's Institutional Review Board.

Every effort was made to randomize subject assignment to groups, but because of the practical need to keep the 7-bed SCU occupied, a distribution of approximately 2:1 was needed to meet this obligation. Based on various options for randomization of subject assignment in the clinical trials literature (Efron, 1971; Hjelm-Karlsson, 1991; Meinert & Tonasicia, 1986), a biased-coin format was used in which two out of every three eligible subjects were assigned to the experimental group (SCU), and one was assigned to the control (Rudy, Vaska, Daly, Happ, & Shiao, 1993). While this design helped to ensure a more steady occupancy of the SCU, the disadvantage was that at certain times the investigator know ahead of time where the next eligible patient would be assigned. Efforts were made to overcome this bias. First, the date on which a patient became eligible for the study was used to determine who was next in line for assignment, and this was outside the direct control of the investigators. Second, caregivers in both the SCU and ICU were not involved in determining patient eligibility or patient assignments. Furthermore, patients transferred to SCU because of a low census in the SCU rather than through the randomized assignment were not part of the study sample. Even with these disadvantages, this assignment procedure was far superior to a simple comparative design without a randomization procedure, allowing real comparisons to occur within the limitations of a clinical setting.

Following group assignment and transfer of experimental subjects to the SCU, data collection was done prospectively. Patient records were reviewed at least every other day until the patient was discharged from the hospital or died.

Instruments

The Acute Physiological and Chronic Health Evaluation II (APACHE II) was used to establish the similarity of severity of illness between the experimental and control groups and as a measure of severity of illness at entry to the study. This instrument, a refinement of the original APACHE (Knaus, Draper, Wagner, & Zimmerman, 1986), is a severity of disease classification system that predicts risk of death. It is based on the assumption that the severity of disease can be quantified by the degree of abnormality of physiologic variables in combination with age and the presence of chronic disease. The range of possible scores is 0 to 71. Accuracy in predicting death was found to be 86% in a study of 5,815 patients (Knaus et al.). This is consistent with earlier studies in which regression analysis was used to validate mortality prediction using the acute physiology portion of the tool (Wagner, Knaus, & Draper, 1983). In a multihospital study of critically ill patients that used the APACHE classification, an interrater agreement of .95 was maintained (Knaus et al.).

The Therapeutic Intervention Scoring System (TISS) (Keene & Cullen, 1983) was designed to classify intensive care patients according to intensity of resource utilization. The TISS score is obtained by recording the number of weighted interventions actually used on the patient from a list of 76. The range of total scores is 0 to 181. TISS has been used since 1974 in multiple studies to assess severity of illness, outcomes of critical care, and utilization of ICU beds (Byrick, Mindorff, McKee, & Mudge, 1980; Schwartz & Cullen, 1981), and recently to examine the relationship between charges and reimbursement in different patient populations (Bekes, Fleming, & Scott, 1988; Teres et al., 1988). It was used in this study to compare utilization of resources in groups matched for severity of illness by APACHE. Validity is based on the initial study by Cullen, Civetta, Briggs, & Ferrara (1974) who recorded all interventions according to critically ill subjects and subsequently divided these into classes to be used to describe resource utilization: Class I = 0 to 9, Class II = 10 to 19; Class III = 20 to 39, Class IV ≥ 40. Experts in critical care validated the list of interventions as adequately and accurately reflecting critical care patient management (Byrick et al.; Schwartz & Cullen). Four experienced ICU nurses were trained in the use of TISS and 20 critically ill patients were evaluated at the start of this study, each by two nurses within 1 hour of each other. The correlation coefficient for this interrater reliability was $r = .96$.

The LaMonica-Oberst Patient Satisfaction Scale measures satisfaction with care, defined as the degree of congruence between patients' expectations of nursing care and their perceptions of care actually received (LaMonica, Oberst, Madea, & Wolf, 1986). Three dimensions of nursing care are measured: technical-professional, trusting relationships, and education relationship. The scale is based on the Risser scale (1975) and was modified to be appropriate for the acute care setting. Internal consistency of the three subscales in separate studies ranged from .80 to .90. The LaMonica-Oberst instrument consisted of 41 statements about nursing care to which the patient indicated agreement or disagreement using a Likert scale.

After preliminary use in this study, it became apparent that the instrument was too difficult for patients who were recovering from a critical illness to complete. Following a factor analysis, the scale was shortened to 15 items by removing items that demonstrated redundancy. Post-hoc analysis identified three factors. The alpha coefficient for the revised Patient Satisfaction scale has averaged .92 ($n = 93$). Construct validity is supported in that the identified factors are the same as those identified in LaMonica's original work.

A similar analysis was performed on the Family Satisfaction scale. This instrument was developed from the LaMonica-Oberst Patient Satisfaction scale by changing the wording of items to reflect the family member's satisfaction with the care received by the patient. This scale was shortened from the original 41 items to 29 items.

The Respiratory Complications Index (RCI) was developed by the investigators. It is a checklist that is easily administered and scored. It includes the categories of respiratory complications evident in critical care areas. The range of total possible scores is 0 to 10. The criteria used to determine the presence of a pulmonary complication include: radiologic reports of atelectasis, consolidation, or collapse; fever; arterial blood gas results; positive sputum cultures; and clinical signs as documented in progress notes. While this checklist was constructed specifically for the study, these criteria are routinely used by other investigators in studying frequency of pulmonary complications (Ali, Serrette, Wood, & Anthomisen, 1985; Kirilloff, Owens, Rogers, & Mazzocco, 1985; Morran et al., 1983). Some association between occurrences of individual complications can be expected. For example, respiratory infections may commonly be associated with increased likelihood of hypoxia or failure to wean. The construct validity of the instrument is supported by the data obtained from both preliminary studies and the special care unit. Rules for use of the tool were established in these preliminary studies and average interrater reliability of .94 was maintained.

The Infection Complications Index (ICI) is an investigator-developed checklist. It includes the specific sites of infections commonly found in critical care areas, as well as general indicators of infection. The checklist identifies critical indicators from the respiratory and urinary tracks, blood, and wound, as well as general indicators of present infections. The general criteria are considered to be positive critical indicators of infection of unknown source only when other noninfectious causes are absent. While this checklist was constructed specifically for the study, these criteria are routinely used by other investigators studying nosocomial infections (Bartlett, O'Keefe, Tally, Louie, & Gorbach, 1986; Garner & Favero, 1986; Parkhurst, Blaser, Laxson, & Wang, 1985).

Construct validity was established by testing the relationship between the total number of infections and length of hospital stay ($r = .78$) and ICU length of stay ($r = .88$). Interrater reliability was maintained at $\leq 90\%$ throughout the study.

The Life-Threatening Complication Index (LTCI) was developed in the second year of the study when it became evident that the occurrence of such complications as seizures, ventricular fibrillation, and gastrointestinal bleeding were frequent enough that the rate of occurrence could serve as additional outcome measures. The LTCI includes 15 life-threatening events or episodes. To be counted as life threatening, the event must have required medical treatment.

The LTCI is scored by giving one point for each event. Scores range from 0 to 15. Construct validity is supported by the positive correlation between the LTCI and hospital mortality ($r = .24$), hospital length of stay ($r = .32$), and critical care days ($r = .40$). The interrater reliability averaged .97 over the 4 years of the study. Data for the LTCI were obtained retrospectively for those patients who had entered the study prior to the design of the instrument; for all other patients, the data were collected prospectively with the other outcome measures.

Since each instrument is dependent on accurate abstraction of data from the patient record, interrater agreement was carefully monitored. Each member of the research team who participated in data collection was trained by the project director and had to achieve a 90% agreement on each measurement before independent data were collected. In addition, a detailed rule book was kept so that reliability could be maintained. Interrater reliability was checked on a random selection of 10% of records and maintained at 90% agreement between coders. Whenever agreement dropped below 90%, differences in scoring were analyzed and resolved, usually through the construction of additional coding rules.

Cost

Two sources of financial information were used in this study: charge data from actual patient bills and cost data from the hospital's cost management information system (CMIS). The CMIS uses product- or service-specific cost data provided by each hospital department. In most cases, the costs per product or per service delivered were derived by calculating the actual cost of material and labor, such as a CAT scan or physical therapy session, projecting the estimated volume of all services, and then adding a weighted portion of that department's indirect cost to each product or service. Room costs included only direct cost of nursing salaries, including benefits, and unit specific costs such as equipment depreciation and supplies. While questions of accuracy always arise, the method of calculating specific costs at the level of individual products or services delivered is generally acceptable and is as close to "true" costs as possible at this setting. A variety of analyses were performed on these data and a fuller description is provided in another publication (Douglas, Daly, Rudy, Song, & Dyer, in press). The comparisons between DRG weight, total charges for the entire hospitalization, total costs, total payment or reimbursement from any payor, the margin, study period charges, and charges and costs to produce a survivor are described in this report.

DRG weight is the adjustment for variance of complexity used by the federal government for diagnosis-related groups. The margin is the difference between the cost of each patient's care and the reimbursement or payment actually received. Charges accruing after the patient

entered the study were also obtained by subtracting the prestudy period charges from the total hospitalization charges. The cost and charge to produce a survivor in each of the study environments was also calculated by adding the charges (or costs) for every study patient in each
unit and then dividing this total by the number of survivors in that unit.

RESULTS

The results are presented according to each patient outcome that was compared (see Table 2).
When data were in interval level, ANOVA was used with significance set at $p \leq 0.5$. When
nominal level data were compared, a chi-square statistic was used with significance set at
$p \leq .05$.

Mortality

Although a higher percentage of patients cared for in the ICUs died in the hospital (41.3%
versus 30.3% for the SCU), this difference was not statistically significant. While a higher percentage of patients from the SCU were discharged home ($n = 45$; 31%) or to a rehabilitation facility ($n = 21$; 14.5%), these differences were also not significant.

Length of Stay

The hospital length of stay (LOS) for the total sample ranged from 8 to 176 days, with an
overall mean of 49.3 days. There was a large standard deviation in both groups of patients.
While the mean LOS for the SCU patients was 2 days less than the ICU patients, this difference was not significant.

Readmission

A total of 17 patients were readmitted to the hospital after discharge. The SCU percentage at
8% is significantly ($p \leq .03$) lower than the ICU's at 20%.

Infections

The total number of infections ranged from 0 to 10 for both groups with an overall mean of
1.6 ($SD = 2.3$) and with no difference between the groups. Approximately one third of the
patients in both groups had respiratory infections and one third had urinary tract infections.
Only 9% ($n = 13$) of the SCU patients had sepsis (blood infections) compared to 16%
($n = 12$) of ICU patients. None of the differences noted between the groups was significant.

Respiratory Complications

In both groups, the number of respiratory complications ranged from 0 to 7, with an overall
mean of 2.17 ($SD = 1.9$) per patient and with no significant difference between groups. Only
1% ($n = 2$) of SCU patients had adult respiratory distress syndrome (ARDS) versus 5%
($n = 4$) of ICU patients.

Table 2

Comparison of Patient Outcomes Between ICU Patients and SCU Patients*

VARIABLE	SPECIAL CARE UNIT $n = 145$	INTENSIVE CARE UNIT $n = 75$	STAT	p VALUE	EFFECT SIZE	POWER
Mortality						
Died	44 (30.3%)	31 (41.3%)	$\chi^2 = .66$	.103	.05	.36
Lived	101 (69.7%)	44 (58.7%)				
Discharge disposition from hospital:						
Died	44 (30.3%)	31 (41.3%)	$\chi^2 = 4.55$	.473	.14	.33
Other hospital	3 (2.1%)	0 (0%)				
Long-term care	31 (21.4%)	14 (18.7%)				
Rehabilitation	21 (14.5%)	11 (14.7%)				
Home	45 (31.0%)	19 (25.3%)				
Home ventilator	1 (0.7%)	0				
Length of hospital stay (days)	48.6 ± 29.5 (9 to 160)	50.6 ± 33.4 (8 to 176)	$F = 0.20$	.655	.03	.07
Readmit†						
Yes	8 (8%)	9 (20%)	$\chi^2 = 4.65$	.031	.18	.48
No	93 (92%)	35 (80%)				
Total number of infections	1.6 ± 2.3 (0 to 10)	1.7 ± 2.3 (0 to 10)	$F = 0.27$	.870	.02	.05
Total number of respiratory complications	2.14 ± 1.9 (0 to 7)	2.25 ± 1.9 (0 to 7)	$F = 0.10$	.688	.03	.06
Life-threatening complications	1.12 ± 1.4 (0 to 8)	.88 ± 1.2 (0 to 5)	$F = 2.16$	.1917	.09	.26

*Continuous variables reported as $M \pm SD$, with range noted below.
†The n used for this calculation included only patients who survived to discharge ($n = 145$).

Life-Threatening Complications

There was no difference between the groups in the number of life-threatening complications, with an average of about one life-threatening complication per patient. However, the SCU patients had significantly more documented episodes of bradycardia (pulse < 40 BPM), 14.5% vs. 3% in the ICUs ($p \leq .006$), and more episodes of a decrease in neurological status (SCU 13% vs. ICUs 4%, $p \leq .033$).

Patient and Family Satisfaction

No difference was noted between the groups on either patient or family satisfaction. The overall patient satisfaction scores ranged from 43 to 105 ($M = 90.1$), and the family satisfaction scores ranged from 125 to 210 ($M = 186.5$). Satisfaction scores were all skewed to the high end of the scale with minimal variability for nearly all patients and family members. Because of this, data collection on this variable was discontinued after 2 years.

Cost

Comparisons of financial data associated with the two study environments are shown in Table 3. Although the differences in total charges, costs, and margin were not significantly different, both charges and costs were lower for patients in the SCU by 6% to 7%. Combined with the lower mortality rate in the SCU, this resulted in both significantly lower costs and charges to produce a survivor. The actual cost savings were $5,000 less per patient in the SCU, and the cost to produce a survivor was $19,000 less in the SCU versus the ICU. SCU charges were also significantly lower when the prestudy period (prior to the point at which the patient became eligible for the study and experimental patients were transferred into the SCU) was excluded.

DISCUSSION

While the original expectation of the ICUs was for short-term stays during a vulnerable period of an acute illness, patients today may require life-support technology with intensive monitoring and care for extended periods of time. These chronically critically ill represent a subgroup of patients whose outcomes of care have not been carefully examined and whose care may be equally effective outside the traditional ICU setting.

The similarity in outcomes is striking considering the differences in the two environments. The special care unit environment was purposely planned to have less technology, be more open to visitors, have less ambient noise and distraction through the use of private rooms, and patient care managed by nurse case managers. The lack of differences between the groups including mortality and length of stay indicate that chronically critically ill patients can be cared for outside the standard ICU setting when their care is managed by skilled nurse case managers. The study confirms that care managed by nurses working with collaboratively derived medical protocols produces outcomes that are equal to or that exceed those of patients whose care is managed by residents and interns in the routine ICU setting. While a significantly lower percentage of ICU patients required readmission, the effect size and power were low, indicating a need for a larger sample size.

Table 3

Comparison of Finance Data Between ICU Patients and SCU Patients*

VARIABLE	SPECIAL CARE UNIT n = 145	INTENSIVE CARE UNIT n = 70	F	p VALUE	EFFECT SIZE	POWER
Charges	$151,226 ± $92,621 (23,388 to 586,139)	$162,718 ± $107,818 (26,621 to 548,829)	.6792	.4107	.05	.12
Payment	$65,709 ± $46,391 (0 to 212,452)	$66,364 ± $55,452 (0 to 305,362)	.0084	.9272	.01	.04
Cost	$76,077 ± $45,401 (13,853 to 231,125)	$81,212 ± $50,186 (9,436 to 251,000)	.5832	.4459	.05	.11
Margin	$−10,899 ± $39,241 (−153,795 to 103,184)	$−14,694 ± $48,083 (−138,015 to 131,297)	.3806	.5379	.04	.09
DRG weight	8.230 ± 5.708 .454 to 16.986)	8.579 ± 6.039 (.5123 to 16.986)	.1783	.6733	.00	.04
Study period charge	$69,132 ± $53,222 (9,330 to 277,239)	$94,045 ± $85,915 (7,474 to 472,470)	5.3394	.022‡	.17	.69
Charge per survivor	$215,351 ± $85,303 (98,690 to 482,733)	$279,870 ± $110,407 (139,522 to 661,730)	14.5741	.0002‡	.30	.95
Cost per survivor†	$109,220 ± $45,117 (48,007 to 265,279)	$138,434 ± $44,736 (66,467 to 234,619)	12.684	.0005‡	.30	.95

*Continuous variables reported as $M ± SD$, with range noted below.
†The n used in this calculation included only survivors; SCU $n = 101$, ICU $n = 44$.
‡Significant at $p \leq .05$ level.

The average LOS for all patients was extremely long, and therefore costly in terms of intensive care resources. Because of the wide variability in length of stay (8 to 176 days), those patients at the extreme end of the spectrum should be examined. Patients who require intensive care services up to 3 months are obviously a major financial and personnel burden to hospitals. This calls for an examination of such patients beyond simple mortality statistics to questions of functional status, quality of life, and family response to an extended critical illness. Patients such as the chronically critically ill survive one complication only to develop another. Thoughts regarding the futility of care in some cases of elderly patients with multiple complications, setbacks, and prolonged lengths of stay need to be addressed by the entire health care team before health care providers are forced into making decisions solely on the basis of cost. To provide a fuller picture of the differences between the two groups, post-hoc effect size and power were calculated for each of the fiscal variables (Borenstein & Cohen, 1988; SOLO Power Analysis, 1992). The differences in the fiscal aspects of care associated with the SCU environment were marked. It is important to note that these differences do not represent savings associated only with reduced nursing care or lower nurse-patient ratios. In fact, the nurse-patient ratio for each patient was nearly identical to that found in ICUs, with the exception of the night shift when the ratio in the SCU was occasionally 1:3 rather than 1:2 or 1:1 in the ICUs. Use of cost data, rather than charge data, confirms the conclusion that the differences between the study units was not just a reflection of charging different rates for the SCU.

The primary source of savings in the SCU stems from a different philosophy and approach to the care of these very ill patients. Most ICUs, quite appropriately, are founded on the assumption that the goal of care is to preserve life at all costs. Every precaution is taken to identify and prevent complications; the rule of thumb is to err on the side of aggressive intervention. This approach is appropriate for the typical ICU patient who experiences a very brief and very acute episode of a life-threatening, but survivable illness. It is less appropriate and less effective for chronically critically ill patients whose problems are not short-term, whose illness may not be reversible, and whose course is not improved by the use of therapies, each of which carries with it the possibility of iatrogenic harm. By segregating these patients in the current study, it was possible to change the norms underlying the approach to care, to question what gains were to be made by aggressive pursuit of every abnormal diagnostic test, to reduce the use of daily laboratory testing surveillance, and to tailor care to the specific needs and goals of each patient. This resulted directly in reduced use of X rays, blood tests, and some therapies. The management of the patients in the SCU by expert nurses undoubtedly contributed to the success of this conservative approach to care.

The results of this study demonstrate that carefully selected patients can be cared for outside the ICU setting under the care of well-trained nurse case managers, with no threat to patient outcomes and with significant cost savings. This finding has major implications for the care of long-term critically ill patients. It would seem prudent for those institutions that have such patients to explore the potential for creating a special care unit with trained nurse case managers.

To replicate these results, it is necessary to recognize the sociotechnical theory that underpins the SCU environment of care (Daly et al., 1991; Happ, 1993), thereby creating a work environment that encompasses both a carefully designed physical space for these patients, as well as an expanded case management role for nurses who work in and contribute to the environment of care. A medical director of the unit who not only understands the medical care of critically ill patients but who supports the collaborative development of treatment protocols and the need for consistency of care provided by case managers is an essential part of the model. Thus, the evidence strongly suggests that the use of a special environment for chronically critically ill patients headed by nurse case managers, as reported in this study, offers health care facilities a viable, cost-effective alternative to traditional ICU units, without sacrificing quality of care.

REFERENCES

ALI, J., SERRETTE, C., WOOD, L. D. H., & ANTHOMISEN, N. R. (1985). Effect of postoperative intermittent positive pressure breathing on lung function. *Chest, 85,* 192-196.

AMERICAN ASSOCIATION FOR RESPIRATORY CARE. (1991). *A study of chronic ventilator patients in the hospital.* Dallas: Author.

BARTLETT, J. G., O'KEEFE, P., TALLY, F. P., LOUIE, T. J., & GORBACH, S. L. (1986). Bacteriology of hospital-acquired pneumonia. *Archives of Internal Medicine, 146,* 868-871.

BEKES, C., FLEMING, J., & SCOTT, W. E. (1988). Reimbursement for intensive care services under diagnosis-related groups. *Critical Care Medicine, 16,* 470-481.

BERENSON, R. A. (1984). *Intensive care units: Clinical outcomes, costs, and decision making.* Health Technology Case Study 28 (OTA-28). Office of Technology Assessment, Washington, DC: U.S. Government Printing Office.

BORENSTEIN & COHEN, J. (1988). *Statistical power analysis: A computer program.* New Jersey: Lawrence Erlbaum.

BORLASE, B. C., BAXTER, J. T., BENOTTI, P. N., STONE, M., WOOD, E., FORSE, R. A., BLACKBURN, G. L., & STEELE, G. JR. (1991). Surgical intensive care unit resource use in a specialty referral hospital: I. Predictors of early death and cost implications. *Surgery, 109,* 687-693.

BYRICK, R. J., MINDORFF, C., McKEE, L., & MUDGE, B. (1980). Cost-effectiveness of intensive care for respiratory failure patients. *Critical Care Medicine, 8,* 332-337.

COHEN, I. L., BARI, N., STROSBERG, M. A., WEINBERG, P. F., WASKSWAN, R. M., MILLSTEIN, B. H., & FEIN, I. A. (1991). Reduction of duration and cost of mechanical ventilation in an intensive care unit by use of a ventilatory management team. *Critical Care Medicine, 19,* 1278-1284.

COHEN, I. L., LAMBRINOS, J., & FEIN, I. A. (1993). Mechanical ventilation for the elderly patient in intensive care. Incremented changes and benefits. *JAMA,* 269-1029.

CULLEN, D. J., CIVETTA, J. M., BRIGGS, B. A., & FERRARA, L. C. (1974). Therapeutic intervention scoring system: A method for quantitative comparison of patient care. *Critical Care Medicine, 2,* 57-62.

DALY, B. J., RUDY, E. R., THOMPSON, K. S., & HAPP, M. B. (1991). Development of a special care unit for chronically critically ill patients. *Heart and Lung, 20,* 45-51.

DOUGLAS, S., DALY, B., RUDY, E., SONG, R., & DYER, M. A. (in press). Cost effectiveness of a special care unit to care for the chronically critically ill. *Journal of Nursing Administration.*

EPRON, B. (1971). Forcing a sequential experiment to be balanced. *Biometrika, 58,* 403-417.

ELPERN, E. H., SILVER, M. R., ROSEN, R. L., & BONE, R. C. (1991). The non-invasive respiratory care unit. Patterns of use and financial implications. *Chest* 990-208.

GARNER, J. S., & FAVERO, M. S. (1986). CDC guidelines for handwashing and hospital environmental control, 1985. *Infection Control, 7,* 231-243.

GUNDLACH, C. A., & FAULKNER, T. P. (1991). Charge and reimbursement analysis for intensive care unit patients in a large tertiary teaching hospital, *DICP, 25,* 1231-1235.

HAPP, M. B (1993). Sociotechnical systems theory: Analysis and application for nursing administration (tables/charts). *Journal of Nursing Administration, 23/-54.*

HJELM-KARLSON, K. (1991). Using the biased coin design for randomization in health care research. *Western Journal of Nursing Research, 13,* 284-288.

KAPPSTEIN, I., SCHULGEN, G., BEYER, U., GEIGER, K., SCHUMACHER, M., & DASCHNER, F. D. (1992). Prolongation of hospital stay and extra costs due to ventilator-associated pneumonia in an intensive care unit. *European Journal of Clinical Microbiology and Infectious Diseases, 11,* 504-508.

KEENE, A. R., & CULLEN, D. J. (1983). Therapeutic intervention scoring system: Update, 1983. *Critical Care medicine, 11,* 1-4.

KIRILLOFF, L. H., OWENS, G. R., ROGERS, R. M., & MAZZOCCO, M. C. (1985). Does chest physical therapy work: A review. *Chest, 88,* 436-444.

KNAUS, W. A., DRAPER, E. A., WAGNER, D. P., & ZIMMERMAN, J. E. (1986). An evaluation of outcome from intensive care in major medical centers. *Annals of Internal Medicine, 104,* 410-418.

LaMONICA, E. L., OBERST, M. T., MADEA, A. R., & WOLF, R. M. (1986). Development of a patient satisfaction scale. *Research in Nursing and Health, 9,* 43-50.

MADOFF, R. D., SHARPE, S. M., FATH, J. J., SIMONS, R. L., & CERRA, F. B. (1985). Prolonged surgical intensive care. *Archives of Surgery, 120,* 698-702.

MEINERT, C. L., & TONASICIA, S. (1986). *Clinical trials, design, conduct and analysis.* New York: Oxford University Press, pp. 90-112.

MORRAN, C. G., FINLAY, I. G., MATHIESON, M., McKAY, A. J., WILSON, N., & McARDLE, C. S. (1983). Randomized controlled trial of physiotherapy for postoperative pulmonary complications. *British Journal of Anesthesia, 55,* 1113-1116.

PARKHURST, S. M., BLASER, M. J., LAXSON, L., & WANG, W. (1985). Surveillance for the detection of nosocomial infections and the potential for nosocomial outbreaks: Development of a laboratory-based system, part 2. *American Journal of Infection Control, 13*(1), 7-15.

PASMORE, W. (1988). *Designing effective organizations: The sociotechnical systems perspective.* New York: John Wiley.

PASMORE, W., & SHERWOOD, J. (1978). *Sociotechnical systems: A sourcebook.* San Diego, CA: University Associates, Inc.

RISSER, N. (1975). Development of an instrument to measure patient satisfaction with nurses and nursing care in primary care settings. *Nursing Research, 24,* 45-52.

ROBERTS, D. E., BELL, D. D., OSTRYZNIUK, T., DOBSON, K., OPPENHEIMER, L., MARTEN, D., HONCHARIK, N., CRAMP, H., LOEWEN, E., BODNAR, S., GUENTHER, A., PRONGER, L., ROBERTS, E., & McEWEN, T. (1993). Eliminating needless testing in intensive care—an information-based team management approach. *Critical Care Medicine, 21,* 1452-1458.

RUDY, E. B., VASKA, P., DALY, B., HAPP, M. B., & SHIAO, P. (1993). Permuted block design for randomization in a nursing clinical trial. *Nursing Research, 42,* 287-289.

SCHAPIRA, D. V., STUDNICKI, J., BRADHAM, D. D., WOLFF, P., & JARRETT, A. (1993). Intensive care, survival, and expense of treating critically ill cancer patients. *Journal of the American Medical Association, 269,* 783-786.

SCHWARTZ, S., & CULLEN, D. J. (1981). How many intensive care beds does your hospital need? *Critical Care Medicine, 9,* 625-630.

SOLO POWER ANALYSIS (1992). Los Angeles, CA: BMDP Statistical Software.

TERES, D., RAPAPORT, J., LEMESHOW, S., HABER, R., GAGE, R. W., & AVRUNIN, J. S. (1988). Using a severity of illness measurement with critically ill patients to explain cost validity within diagnostic-related groups (abstract). *Critical Care Medicine, 16,* 406.

WAGNER, D. P., KNAUS, W. A., & DRAPER, E. A. (1983). Statistical validation of a severity of illness measure . . . Acute physiology score of APACHE. *American Journal of Public Health, 73,* 878-884.

ZIMMERMAN, J. E. SHORTELL, S. M., KNAUS, W. A., ROUSSEAU, D. M., WAGNER, D. P., GILLES, R. R., DRAPER, E. A., & DEVERS, K. (1993). Value and cost of teaching hospitals: A prospective, multicenter, inception cohort study. *Critical Care Medicine, 21,* 1432-1442.

Concerns about Analgesics Among Patients and Family Caregivers in a Hospice Setting

Sandra E. Ward ■ Patricia Emery Berry ■ Hollis Misiewicz

Patients receiving curative treatment for cancer have concerns about report-ing pain and using analgesics. These concerns are associated with underuti-lization of analgesics. To extend knowledge about such concerns to the con-text of palliative care, the concerns of hospice patients and family caregivers were compared. Within 5 days of admission to hospice, 35 patients with can-cer and their caregivers each completed a measure of eight concerns such as fear of addiction, worry about tolerance, and worry about side effects. There was no correlation between caregiver and patient concerns and means for the two groups were similar, indicating that within a given dyad either the pa-tient or the caregiver may have greater concerns. The findings highlight the need for patient and caregiver education about reporting pain and using analgesics.

Appendix D Reprinted with permission from *Res Nurs Health* 19:205-211, 1996.

Many patients with cancer remain in pain despite the availability of effective therapies (Foley & Arbit, 1989). Patients receiving curative treatment have concerns about reporting pain and using analgesics. These concerns contribute to the problem of inadequate pain control; persons with high levels of concern, compared to those with low levels of concern, use less adequate analgesic medication (Ward et al., 1993). Because of this association with adequacy of analgesic use, these concerns have been called patient-related barriers to pain management. Such barriers have received little attention in the research literature, particularly in the area of palliative care. Nor is much information available about family caregiver perceptions of barriers (Berry & Ward, 1995; Dar, Beach, Barden, & Cleeland, 1992). The purpose of this study was to compare patient and family caregiver concerns about reporting pain and using analgesics in a hospice setting. In the following review of literature, we first describe the current understanding of patient and caregiver concerns and then consider possible relationships between patient and caregiver concerns.

Eight concerns about (barriers to) reporting pain and using analgesics are prevalent in persons with cancer: (a) fear of addiction to analgesics, (b) fatalism about the possibility of achieving pain control, (c) concern about drug tolerance, (d) belief that "good" patients do not complain, (e) belief that side effects from analgesics are even more bothersome than pain, (f) fear of injections, (g) fear of distracting a physician from treating one's disease, and (h) belief that increased pain signifies disease progression (Hodes, 1989; Ward et al., 1993).

Patients often are worried about becoming addicted to opioid analgesics, yet evidence demonstrates that addiction is extremely rare in persons using analgesics for pain (Chapman & Hill, 1989; Perry & Heidrich, 1982; Porter & Jick 1980). Similarly, the fatalistic belief that pain with cancer is inevitable and uncontrollable is a misconception because analgesics prescribed and administered in accord with the WHO analgesic ladder can control cancer pain in most patients (Ventafridda, Tamburini, Caraceni, De Conno, & Naldi, 1987). Concern about tolerance reflects a lack of understanding that those administering the opioid analgesic can escalate safely the dosage in accord with increasing pain. Morphine shows no analgesic ceiling, and patients develop tolerance to most adverse effects of morphine more rapidly than they develop tolerance to analgesia (Bruera, Macmillan, Hanson, & MacDonald, 1989; Twycross, 1994). Therefore, it is erroneous to assume that patients should "save" analgesics "in case the pain gets worse." The preferred route of analgesic administration is oral, but many patients mistakenly believe that injections provide superior pain control; at the same time they may find injections noxious and wish to avoid them.

Three of the identified concerns are not misconceptions, but rather may be related to care provider behavior. Clinicians may, sometimes unintentionally, communicate the exception that "good" patients do not complain about pain. Similarly, if a clinician does not attempt to prevent or alleviate analgesic side effects, a patient may have negative experiences with those side effects and may prefer to live with pain. It is unknown whether patients' complaints of pain distract physicians from focusing on curative treatment, but there is a rationale for patients' thinking this may be the case because of the either–or choice often offered between symptom-focused palliative care and cure-oriented care (Rhymes, 1990).

Finally, increased pain usually signifies disease progression (Collin, Poulain, Gauvain-Piquard, Petit, & Pichard-Leandri, 1993), but patients who are resistant to acknowledging this possibility may be unwilling to report pain. Therefore, although the concern that pain indicates disease progression is medically accurate, it can be a barrier to pain control.

These concerns are important because whether medically accurate or not, patients' beliefs drive their coping efforts (Leventhal, Meyer, & Nerenz, 1980; Ward, 1993). For example, these concerns are linked to patients' hesitancy to report pain (Ward & Gatwood, 1993) and to the adequacy of analgesics patients use (Breitbart et al., 1994; Lin & Ward, 1995; Ward et al., 1993; Ward & Hernandez, 1994). Research in this area, however, has been limited to ambulatory patients and has not addressed family caregivers.

Pain is a major worry for persons involved in caring for a family member who has cancer (Dar et al., 1992; Decker & Young, 1991; Ferrell, Ferrell, Rhiner, & Grant, 1991; Hinds, 1985; Hull, 1989; Longman, Atwood, Sherman, Benedict, & Shang, 1992). In addition to worrying about their family members *experiencing* pain, caregivers have many of the same concerns about reporting pain and using analgesics that patients report. In a study of 40 patient–spouse dyads, Dar et al, found that 43% of the spouses believed that the patient ". . . should not take narcotic medication on a regular basis, but only when the pain is extreme" (Dar et al., 1992, p. 91). Similarly, Ferrell and colleagues described a caregiver who was concerned that ". . . the use of morphine will result in immunity to morphine . . ." (Ferrell et al., 1991, p. s67). Thus, although family caregivers worry about their loved ones experiencing pain, they have misconceptions that may contribute to inadequate pain management.

Attention to caregiver concerns is critical in a hospice setting where patients must identify a primary caregiver at admission and where the patient–caregiver dyad is the unit of care (Rhymes, 1990). Family caregivers often provide assistance to patients by purchasing and administering analgesics. As a patient's condition declines, the caregiver may assume added responsibilities, including communicating with health care providers and making decisions about the patient's comfort level. Because of this gatekeeper role, caregivers' beliefs about reporting pain and using analgesics are critical to achieving optimal pain control for patients.

Few investigators have examined dyads to determine the relationship between patient and caregiver concerns. Several perspectives pertain to this relationship. First, what is the association between the two sets of concerns? Social influence may induce the patient and the caregiver to share common concerns about reporting pain and using analgesics. For example, if one person in the dyad believes that addiction to analgesics occurs readily, so might the other; this is an issue of association (correlation) between beliefs (Jacobsen, Tulman, & Lowery, 1991).

Second, which of the two persons in a dyad has the higher level of concern is also significant. In a prior study comparing persons with and without cancer, no differences were found with respect to the concerns in question (Ward & Gatwood, 1994). It should be noted, however, that the persons who did not have cancer were not caregivers for an individual with cancer. Having intimate experience with seeing a loved one in pain and interacting with health care providers could result in caregivers having different levels of concern about reporting pain and using analgesics than have been observed in noncaregivers.

Finally, regardless of which person has the higher level of concern, one could consider which half of the dyad exerts a more powerful influence on the patient's behavior. Patients' actions in health care situations are predicted both by their own beliefs and by their significant others' beliefs (Ajzen, 1991; Ajzen & Fishbein, 1980; Triandis, 1977). Whether the patient and caregiver show similarity in beliefs (concerns) may be less critical than the extent to which each person's beliefs influence patient behaviors such as reporting pain and using analgesics.

Based on these possible relationships between concerns with dyads, the specific research questions addressed in this study were (a) What is the strength of association between patient and caregiver concerns?, (b) Who has greater concerns about reporting pain and using analgesics—the patient or the family caregiver?, and (c) Whose concerns are more strongly associated with a patient's hesitancy to report pain and use analgesics?

METHOD

Participants and Setting

Study inclusion criteria were (a) the patient had a diagnosis of cancer, (b) the patient and caregiver were able to read and respond to questionnaire items in English, (c) the patient had been admitted to one of the two participating hospice programs within the past 48 hr, and (d) the patient had an identified primary caregiver at the time of admission. That is, for the purposes of this study, caregivers were identified by the method routinely used at hospice admission—by asking patients to name the person most involved with their care. Of the 65 pairs of patients and caregivers who met the criteria and were invited to join this study, 41 did so, and of those, 35 provided complete data, a 54% response rate. Most people who declined to participate stated that they were too busy or too ill.

The patients ranged in age from 31 to 89 years with a mean *(SD)* age of 69.7 (13.1) years. Of the 35 patients, 16 (46%) were women, 18 (51%) were men, and 1 (3%) did not indicate his or her gender on the questionnaire. Most (91%) of the patients were Caucasian. The most common primary cancer site was lung ($n = 12$), followed by breast ($n = 4$), colon ($n = 4$), pancreas ($n = 4$), and kidney ($n = 3$); a variety of different sites were involved in the other 8 patients. Other demographic data about the patients are presented in Table 1.

Table 1

Demographic Information About the Patients and the Caregivers

	PATIENTS		CAREGIVERS	
	n	%	*n*	%
Marital status				
Married	21	60%	28	80%
Not married	14	40%	7	20%
Education				
< HS	7	20%	1	3%
HS grad	19	54%	16	46%
> HS	8	23%	17	48%
Missing data	1	3%	1	3%
Income				
<$29,000/year	25	71%	18	52%
>$30,000/year	6	17%	17	48%
Missing data	4	12%	—	—

The caregivers ranged in age from 21 to 79 years with a mean *(SD)* age of 56.1 (13.5) years. Nine (26%) of the caregivers were men and 26 (74%) were women. Most (94%) were Caucasian. Their relationships to the patients were as follows: 16 (46%) were spouses, 13 (37%) were children, 3 (9%) were siblings, 1 (3%) was a parent, 1 (3%) was a grandchild, and 1 (3%) was unrelated. Other demographic data about the caregivers are presented in Table 1.

The hospice programs, one in the Midwest and the other on the East Coast, are Medicare-certified home care programs. One of the programs is hospital-based and the other independent. One serves an urban area while the other serves both urban and rural areas.

Measures

Concerns

The Barriers Questionnaire (BQ) measures the eight concerns about reporting pain and using analgesics that were described earlier in this article. It has 27 items—3 items for each of the eight subscales except the side-effects subscale, which has 6 items. Subjects rate the extent to which they agree with each of the items on a scale ranging from *do not agree at all* (0) to *agree very much* (5). Both subscale scores (the mean of the items in a given subscale) and a total score (the mean of all items) are used in analyses. The instructions found at the top of the BQ, which were the same for both patients and caregivers, read as follows: "We are interested in learning more about your attitudes toward the treatment of pain. There are no right or wrong answers; we just want to know what *you* think."

In previous work, internal consistency (alpha) for the BQ Total scale was shown to be very good (alpha = .89); for the subscales alpha ranged from .67 to .91, except for the fatalism subscale for which alpha = .54 (Ward et al., 1993). Alphas in the present study were similar and are reported in Table 2. Test–retest reliability over a 1-week period for 56 persons in a previous

Table 2

Internal Consistency (Alpha) for BQ Subscale and Total Scores for Patients and Caregivers and Correlation Between Patient and Caregiver BQ Scores

| | ALPHA | | |
SUBSCALE	PATIENT	CAREGIVER	CORRELATION PT/CAREGIVER
Fear of addiction	.69	.75	.36
Fatalism about pain relief	.57	.37	.49*
Concern about drug tolerance	.76	.81	.07
Desires to be a good patient	.82	.80	.26
Concern about side effects	.58	.71	.15
Fear of injections	.82	.69	.28
Concern about distracting MD	.74	.70	.03
Concern pain signifies disease progress	.91	.89	.27
BQ total score	.82	.90	.13

*$p < .01$.

study was .90 for the total scale and ranged from .60 to .81 for the subscales (Ward & Gatwood, 1994). Content validity was determined by an expert panel (Ward et al., 1993).

Hesitancy to Report Pain and to Use Analgesics

Patients were asked two questions: "During the past month, have you ever hesitated to take analgesics?" and "During the past month, have you ever hesitated to report pain?" Response options for each item were either *yes* or *no*.

Demographic Information

A short form was used to collect information about age, gender, race, income, marital status, and religious affiliation. In addition, the location of the patient's cancer was ascertained by chart review.

Procedure

Potential participants were given a letter inviting them to join the study by the nurse who admitted them to the hospice program. Within 24 hr, a data collector telephoned them to discuss their interest and eligibility. If they agreed to participate, the data collector scheduled a home visit within an average of 5 days of their admission to the program. It should be emphasized that the person obtaining consent and collecting the data was *not* the nurse providing care. This design decision was based on concern that patients invited by their own nurse might not feel free to decline participation. During the home visit, the data collector asked the patient and the caregiver to complete the BQ and the demographics questionnaire independently, that is, without talking to each other. In most instances, this was done. Three patients, because of weakness, required that the data collector read the questions and record their responses. At the conclusion of the visit, the participants were debriefed about the questionnaire, and the barriers to pain management were discussed and clarified.

RESULTS

In all data analyses, alpha was set at .01. Before addressing the major research questions, analyses were conducted to determine if BQ total scores were associated with demographic variables or with site of data collection, for either the patients or the caregivers. Associations with age, education, and income were examined using Pearson correlations; associations with site (one hospice setting versus the other), gender, caregiver relationship to patient (spouse versus other), and marital status were examined using t tests. For caregivers, none of these variables were related to their BQ total scores. For patients, there was a significant inverse correlation between level of education and BQ total score ($r = -.60, p < .01$). For both caregivers and patients, scores on the BQ did not differ by site.

Patients' and caregivers' total BQ scores were not significantly correlated. Fatalism was the only one of the eight subscales for which the correlation was statistically significant (see Table 2). Even in this instance, the magnitude of the association was not large ($R^2 = .24$) and the subscale involved (fatalism) is the one with the most questionable reliability.

To address the second research question as to whether patients or caregivers have stronger concerns about reporting pain and using analgesics, paired t tests were used to compare their mean BQ subscale and total scores (Table 3). There were no differences between patients and caregivers with respect to total BQ scores. There was, however, one subscale on which the two groups differed: patients had higher scores on the subscale measuring the belief that good patients do not complain about pain. From these analyses one can conclude that, for the most part, the two groups differ very little in the extent to which they have concerns about reporting pain and using analgesics.

To clarify the findings from the correlational analyses and the *t* tests, four possible patterns *could* have been seen in this dyadic data, based on presence versus absence of correlation combined with presence versus absence of mean differences. Of these four possibilities, the pattern that did arise was no correlation and no mean difference, suggesting that, in a given dyad, it was equally possible for either the patient or the caregiver to have greater concerns.

When asked if they had hesitated to report pain, 33 (94%) of the patients said no, and 2 (6%) said yes. Because there was so little variation on this item, no further analyses were pursued. When asked if they had hesitated to use analgesics, 26 (74%) of the patients said no, 8 (23%) said yes, and 1 (3%) did not respond. Patients' mean *(SD)* total BQ scores for those who responded "yes" versus "no" were 1.85 (0.71) and 1.97 (0.87), respectively, a nonsignificant difference. Similarly, caregivers' mean *(SD)* total BQ scores for those patients who responded *yes* versus *no* were 1.73 (0.61) and 1.89 (0.55), respectively; this difference was not significant.

DISCUSSION

These data from patients and caregivers receiving hospice care demonstrate that there is inconsistency regarding which of the pair has greater concerns about reporting pain and using analgesics. That is, in a given pair, either the patient or the caregiver may have greater concerns than the dyadic counterpart. This conclusion may not be intuitively obvious because *t* tests revealed that, on average, patients and caregivers did not differ on concerns. However,

---

Table 3

Mean (SD) BQ Subscale and Total Scores for Patients and Caregivers

SCALE	PATIENT	CAREGIVER	*t*
Fear of addiction	2.34 (1.39)	2.26 (1.18)	−0.35
Fatalism about pain relief	1.29 (1.05)	0.96 (1.01)	−1.80
Concern about drug tolerance	1.39 (1.35)	1.27 (1.25)	−0.41
Desires to be a good patient	1.73 (1.59)	0.83 (1.00)	−3.20*
Concern about side effects	2.50 (1.00)	2.57 (0.83)	0.35
Fear of injections	1.52 (1.27)	1.97 (1.64)	1.50
Concern about distracting MD	1.67 (1.28)	1.06 (1.09)	−2.15
Concern pain signifies disease progress	2.59 (1.39)	2.68 (1.53)	0.32
BQ total score	1.94 (0.85)	1.80 (0.61)	−0.92

*$p < .01$.

when one also considers the results of the correlational analyses (there was no correlation between patient and caregiver concerns), it becomes apparent that within a given dyad either the patient or the caregiver may have greater concerns.

Future investigators and clinicians should carefully consider the contribution of both the patient and the family caregiver in pain management situations. Because there is little association between patient and caregiver concerns, there is a need to assess and intervene with both groups. That is, even though a patient and caregiver are considered to be a unit of care in hospice, their individual needs must be addressed, and similarity between the two should not be presumed. Careful attention, therefore, should be given to assessing the concerns that were examined in this study and intervening with careful explanations for both the patient and the caregiver.

It should be reiterated that, although the patients and caregivers differed in their concerns, both groups did, indeed, *have* concerns. The data are consistent with those from a retrospective study in which charts are examined to determine barriers to optimal pain control in a hospice setting (Morgan, Lindley, & Berry, 1994). The most commonly identified barriers were patient fear/resistance, worry about side effects, and caregiver fear/resistance. Only 21% of the 199 charts that were examined did *not* contain progress notes indicating barriers to pain control.

Another major finding is the lack of association between either patients' or caregivers' concerns and patients' reports of whether they had hesitated to use analgesics in the past week. This finding is not consistent with theoretical propositions that caregiver beliefs will have an impact on patient behavior. Nor is it consistent with past empirical data showing that patients with higher concerns were more hesitant to report pain and more hesitant to use analgesics (Ward & Gatwood, 1994).

There are several differences between the patients in the previous study and those in the present one that might explain this discrepancy. In the prior study, patients were recruited from an ambulatory clinic and were at various stages of illness, including newly diagnosed. In the present study, the patients and caregivers were no longer seeking curative treatment and were likely to perceive death as an imminent possibility. In fact, several caregivers spontaneously observed to the data collector that addiction no longer mattered because the patient was dying. It appears that even though patients and caregivers in a hospice setting *have* misconceptions about using analgesics (e.g., exaggerated fears of addiction), such misconceptions do not affect behaviors related to pain management because anticipated negative outcomes (e.g., addiction) are seen as inconsequential in the face of imminent death.

Similarly, items on the tolerance subscale may have a very different meaning early versus late in the disease. A patient or caregiver may indeed believe that "it is better to save medicine for later in case the pain gets worse," but for persons in hospice care now *is* later. Having entered hospice care, patients and caregivers may see use of analgesic medication as appropriate, not because they have overcome misconceptions, but because those misconceptions become irrelevant at this point in the disease.

This explanation raises a possibility that the impact of misconceptions on pain management changes over the course of the disease, with there being a relatively strong impact early in the disease process and little or no impact later. This scenario is consistent with a common misunderstanding seen among nurses and physicians—many professionals believe that maximum effort to control pain should not be initiated until the patient is near death (VonRoenn, Cleeland, Gonin, Hatfield, & Pandya, 1993).

The relative impact on adequacy of pain management of patients' versus caregivers' beliefs also may be related to the course of the disease. For example, when a patient is relatively independent in meeting his or her own needs, then a caregiver's beliefs about reporting pain and using analgesics may have somewhat less influence over the patient's use of analgesics than if the patient becomes more dependent upon the caregiver. In future research, investigators could explore whether a patient's level of dependence moderates the influence of caregiver attitudes on important outcome variables such as adequacy of pain management.

There are limitations to be considered in interpreting the data in this study. The sample is small and relatively homogeneous, and replication is needed in more diverse samples. Also, although the response rate (54%) was respectable and is similar to that seen in other hospice studies (Curtis & Fernsler, 1989), it was clearly not ideal. Because many patients are admitted to hospice when their disease is far advanced, these debilitated patients and their overwhelmed caregivers are likely to decline to participate in research, which results in study findings that are not representative of such persons. Reliabilities were low for some BQ subscales (particularly fatalism); therefore, results are tentative and attention should be given to testing new items to increase subscale internal consistency.

Another problem in the study is the lack of data about patients' pain (e.g., severity ratings). An attempt was made to gather such data, but the pain scales were placed last in the questionnaire packets (because our primary concern was the BQ data); hence many patients became tired and did not complete them. Because there was so much missing data, those pain ratings that were available were not useable. Had the admitting hospice nurse collected data, this problem could possibly have been avoided but, as mentioned earlier, it could have been construed as coercive to have these nurses obtain consent and gather data.

In conclusion, in a given patient–caregiver dyad, either person may have the greatest concerns about reporting pain and using analgesics. It is, therefore, critical that clinicians attend to both persons with respect to assessment and intervention. Further research is needed to determine whether patient and caregiver concerns change over the course of the illness and whether one versus the other person's concerns have greater impact on the adequacy with which the patient's pain is managed.

REFERENCES

Ajzen, I. (1991). The theory of planned behavior. *Organizational Behavior and Human Decision Processes, 50,* 179-211.

Ajzen, I., & Fishbein, M. (1980). *Understanding attitudes and predicting social behavior.* Englewood Cliffs, NJ: Prentice-Hall.

Berry, P., & Ward, D. (1995). Barriers to pain management in hospice: A study of family caregivers. *The Hospice Journal, 10* (4), 19-33.

Breitbart, W., Passik, S., Rosenfeld, B., McDonald, M., Portenoy, R., & Thaler, H. (1994). Patient-related barriers to pain management in AIDS. Poster presented at the 13th Annual Meeting of the American Pain Society, Miami, FL.

Bruera, E., Macmillan, L., Hanson, J., & MacDonald, R. (1989). The cognitive effects of the administration of narcotic analgesics in patients with cancer pain. *Pain, 39,* 13-16.

Chapman, C.R., & Hill, H.F. (1989). Prolonged morphine self-administration and addiction liability: Evaluation of two theories in a bone marrow transplant unit. *Cancer, 63,* 1636-1644.

Collin, E., Poulain, P., Gauvain-Piquard, A., Petit, G., & Pichard-Leandri, E. (1993). Is disease progression the major factor in morphine "tolerance" in cancer pain treatment? *Pain, 55,* 319-326.

Curtis, A., & Fernsler, J. (1989). Quality of life of oncology hospice patients: A comparison of patient and primary caregiver reports. *Oncology Nursing Forum, 16,* 49-53.

Dar, R., Beach, C., Barden, P., & Cleeland, C. (1992). Cancer pain in the marital system: A study of patients and their spouses. *Journal of Pain and Symptom Management, 7,* 87-93.

Decker, S., & Young, E. (1991). Self-perceived needs of primary caregivers of home-hospice clients. *Journal of Community Health Nursing, 8,* 147-154.

Ferrell, B. R., Ferrell, B.A., Rhiner, M., & Grant, M. (1991). Family factors influencing cancer pain management. *Postgraduate Medical Journal, 67,* (suppl.), s64-s69.

Foley, K.M., & Arbit, E. (1989). Management of cancer pain. In V.T. DeVita, S. Hellman, & S.A. Rosenberg (Eds.), *Principles and practice of oncology* (3rd ed., pp. 2064-2087). Philadelphia: J.B. Lippincott.

Hinds, C. (1985). The needs of families who care for patients with cancer at home: Are we meeting them? *Journal of Advanced Nursing, 10,* 575-581.

Hodes, R. (1989). Cancer patients' needs and concerns when using narcotic analgesics. In C.S. Hill & W.S. Fields (Eds.), *Advances in pain research and therapy, Vol. 11,* (pp. 91-99). New York: Raven Press.

Hull, M. (1989). Family needs and supportive nursing behaviors during terminal cancer: A review. *Oncology Nursing Forum, 16,* 787-792.

Jacobsen, B., Tulman, L., & Lowery, B. (1991). Three sides of the same coin: The analysis of paired data from dyads. *Nursing Research, 40,* 359-363.

Leventhal, H., Meyer, D., & Nerenz, D. (1980). The common-sense representation of illness danger. In S. Rachman (Ed.), *Medical psychology* (Vol. 2., pp. 7-30). New York: Pergamon Press.

Lin, C., & Ward, S. (1995). Patient-related barriers to cancer pain management in Taiwan. *Cancer Nursing, 18,* 16-22.

Longman, A., Atwood, J., Sherman, J., Benedict, J., & Shang, T. (1992). Care needs of home-based cancer patients and their caregivers. *Cancer Nursing, 15,* 182-190.

Morgan, A., Lindley, C., & Berry, J. (1994, Jan/Feb). Assessment of pain and patterns of analgesic use in hospice patients. *The American Journal of Hospice and Palliative Care, 11,* 13-25.

Perry, S., & Heidrich, G. (1982). Management of pain during debridement: A survey of U.S. burn units. *Pain, 13,* 267-280.

Porter, J., & Jick, H. (1980). Addiction rare in patients treated with narcotics. *New England Journal of Medicine, 302,* 123.

Rhymes, J. (1990). Hospice care in America. *Journal of the American Medical Association, 264,* 369-372.

Triandis, H. (1977). *Interpersonal behavior.* Monterey, CA: Brooks/Cole.

Twycross, R. (1994). Opioids. In P. Wall & R. Melzack (Eds.), *Textbook of pain* (pp. 943-962). Edinburgh: Churchill Livingstone.

Ventafridda, V., Tamburini, M., Caraceni, A., DeConno, F., & Naldi, F. (1987). A validation study of the WHO method for cancer pain relief. *Cancer, 59,* 850-856.

VonRoenn, J., Cleeland, C., Gonin, R., Hatfield, A., & Pandya, K. (1993). Physician attitudes and practice in cancer pain management. *Annals of Internal Medicine, 119,* 121-126.

Ward, S. (1993). The common sense model: An organizing framework for knowledge development in nursing. *Scholarly Inquiry for Nursing Practice, 7,* 79-90.

Ward, S., & Gatwood, J. (1994). Concerns about reporting pain and using analgesics: A comparison of persons with and without cancer. *Cancer Nursing, 17,* 200-206.

Ward, S., Goldberg, N., Miller-McCauley, V., Mueller, C., Nolan, A., Pawlik-Plank, D., Robbins, A., Stormoen, D., & Weissman, D. (1993). Patient-related barriers to management of cancer pain. *Pain, 52,* 319-324.

Ward, S., & Hernandez, L. (1994). Patient-related barriers to management of cancer pain in Puerto Rico. *Pain, 58,* 233-238.

Glossary

abstract A brief, comprehensive summary of a study.

accessible population A population that meets the population criteria and is available.

after-only design An experimental design with two randomly assigned groups—a treatment group and a control group. This design differs from the true experiment in that both groups are measured only after the experimental treatment.

after-only nonequivalent control group design A quasiexperimental design similar to the after-only experimental design, but subjects are not randomly assigned to the treatment or control groups.

alternate form reliability Two or more alternate forms of a measure are administered to the same subjects at different times. The scores of the two tests determine the degree of relationship between the measures.

analysis of covariance (ANCOVA) A statistic that measures differences among group means and uses a statistical technique to equate the groups under study in relation to an important variable.

analysis of variance (ANOVA) A statistic that tests whether group means differ from each other, rather than testing each pair of means separately, ANOVA considers the variation among all groups.

animal rights Guidelines used to protect the rights of animals in the conduct of research.

anonymity A research participant's protection in a study so that no one, not even the researcher, can link the subject with the information given.

antecedent variable A variable that affects the dependent variable but occurs before the introduction of the independent variable.

applied research Tests the practical limits of descriptive theories but does not examine the efficacy of actions taken by practitioners.

assent An aspect of informed consent that pertains to protecting the rights of children as research subjects.

assumption A basic principle assumed to be true without the need for scientific proof.

auditability The researcher's development of the research process in a qualitative study that allows a researcher or reader to follow the thinking or conclusions of the researcher.

axial coding A data analysis strategy used the grounded theory method. It requires intense coding around a single theme.

basic research Theoretical or pure research that generates, tests, and expands theories that explain or predict a phenomenon.

beneficence An obligation to do harm and to maximize possible benefits.

benefit Potential positive outcomes of participation in research study.

bias A distortion in the data analysis results.

bracketed A process during which the researcher identifies personal biases about the phenomenon of interest to clarify how personal experience and beliefs may color what is heard and reported.

case study method The study of selected contemporary phenomenon over time to provide an in-depth description of essential dimensions and processes of the phenomenon.

chance error Attributable to fluctuations in subject characteristics that occur at a specific point in time and are often beyond the awareness and control of the examiner. Also called *random error.*

chi-square (χ^2) A nonparametric statistic that is used to determine whether the frequency found in each category is different from the frequency that would be expected by chance.

close-ended item Question that the respondent may answer with only one of a fixed number of choices.

cluster sampling A probability sampling strategy that involves a successive random sampling of units. The units sampled progress from large to small.

computer database Print database that is put on software programs that can be accessed online or on CD-ROM via the computer.

concealment Refers to whether the subjects know that they are being observed.

concept An image or symbolic representation of an abstract idea.

conceptual definition General meaning of a concept.

conceptual literature Published and unpublished non–data-based material, such as reports of theories, concepts, synthesis of research on concepts, or professional issues, some of which underlie reported research, as well as other nonresearch material.

conceptual model A set of interrelated concepts that symbolically represents a phenomenon.

concurrent validity The degree of correlation of two measures of the same concept that are administered at the same time.

confidentiality Assurance that a research participant's identity cannot be linked to the information that was provided to the researcher.

consent *See* **informed consent**.

consistency Data are collected from each subject in the study in exactly the same way or as close to the same way as possible.

constancy Methods and procedures of data collection are the same for all subjects.

constant comparative method A process of continuously comparing data as they are acquired during research with the grounded theory method.

construct An abstraction that is adapted for scientific purpose.

construct replication The use of original methods, such as sampling techniques, instruments, or research design, to study a problem that has been investigated previously.

construct validity The extent to which an instrument is said to measure a theoretical construct or trait.

consumer One who actively uses and applies research findings in nursing practice.

content analysis A technique for the objective, systematic, and quantitative description of communications and documentary evidence.

content validity The degree to which the content of the measure represents the universe of content, or the domain of a given behavior.

contrasted-group approach A method used to assess construct validity. A researcher identifies two groups of individuals who are suspected to have an extremely high or low score on a characteristic. Scores from the groups are obtained and examined for sensitivity to the differences. Also called *known-group approaches.*

control Measures used to hold uniform or constant the conditions under which an investigation occurs.

control group The group in an experimental investigation that does not receive an intervention or treatment; the comparison group.

convenience sampling A nonprobability sampling strategy that uses the most readily accessible persons or objects as subjects in a study.

convergent validity A strategy for assessing construct validity in which two or more tools that theoretically measure the same construct are administered to subjects. If the measures are positively correlated, convergent validity is said to be supported.

correlation The degree of association between two variables.

correlational study A type of nonexperimental research design that examines the relationship between two or more variables.

credibility Steps in qualitative research to ensure accuracy, validity, or soundness of data

criterion-related validity Indicates the degree of relationship between performance on the measure and actual behavior either in the present (concurrent) or in the future (predictive).

critical reading An active interpretation and objective assessment of an article during which the reader is looking for key concepts, ideas, and justifications.

critical thinking The rational examination of ideas, inferences, principles, and conclusions.

critique The process of objectivity and critically evaluating a research report's content for scientific merit and application to practice, theory, or education.

critiquing criteria The criteria used for objectively and critically evaluating a research article.

Cronbach's alpha Test of internal consistency that simultaneously compares each item in a scale to all others.

cross-sectional study A nonexperimental research design that looks at data at one point in time, that is, in the immediate present.

Cumulative Index to Nursing and Allied Health Literature (CINAHL) A print or computerized database; computerized CINAHL is available on CD-ROM and on-line.

data Information systematically collected in the course of a study; the plural of datum.

database A compilation of information about a topic organized in a systematic way.

data-based literature Reports of completed research.

data saturation A point when data collection can cease. It occurs when the information being shared with the researcher becomes repetitive. Ideas conveyed by the participant have been shared before by other participants; inclusion of additional participants does not result in new ideas.

deductive reasoning A logical thought process in which hypotheses are derived from theory; reasoning moves from the general to the particular.

degrees of freedom The number of quantities that are unknown minus the number of independent equations linking these unknowns; a function of the number in the sample.

delimitations Those characteristics that restrict the population to a homogeneous group of subjects.

Delphi technique The technique of gaining expert opinion on a subject. It uses rounds or multiple stages of data collection, with each round using data from the previous round.

dependent variable In experimental studies the presumed effect of the independent or experimental variable on the outcome.

descriptive/exploratory survey A type of nonexperimental research design that collects descriptions of existing phenomena for the purpose of using the data to justify or assess current conditions or to make plans for improvement of conditions.

descriptive statistics Statistical methods used to describe and summarize sample data.

design The plan or blueprint for conduct of a study.

developmental study A type of nonexperimental research design that is concerned not only with the existing status and interrelationship of phenomena but also with changes that take place as a function of time.

direct observation A method for measuring psychological and physiological behaviors for purposes of evaluating change and facilitating recovery.

directional hypothesis Hypothesis that specifies the expected direction of the relationship between the independent and dependent variables.

dissemination The communication of research findings.

divergent validity A strategy for assessing construct validity in which two or more tools that theoretically measure the opposite of the construct are administered to subjects. If the measures are negatively correlated, divergent validity is said to be supported.

domains Symbolic categories that include the smaller categories of an ethnographic study.

downlink A receiver for programs beamed from other agencies that allows a person to participate in telecommunications conferences.

element The most basic unit about which information is collected.

eligibility criteria Those characteristics that restrict the population to a homogeneous group of subjects.

emic view The natives' or insiders' view of the world.

empirical The obtaining of evidence or objective data.

empirical literature A synonym for data-based literature; *see* **data-based literature**.

equivalence Consistency or agreement among observers using the same measurement tool or agreement among alternate forms of a tool.

error variance The extent to which the variance in test scores is attributable to error rather than a true measure of the behaviors.

ethics The theory or discipline dealing with principles of moral values and moral conduct.

ethnographic method A method that scientifically describes cultural groups. The goal of the ethnographer is to understand the natives' view of their world.

ethnography A qualitative research approach designed to produce cultural theory.

etic view An outsider's view of another's world.

evaluation research The use of scientific research methods and procedures to evaluate a program, treatment, practice, or policy outcomes; analytical means are used to document the worth of an activity.

evaluative research The use of scientific research methods and procedures for the purpose of making an evaluation.

ex post facto study A type of nonexperimental research design that examines the relationships among the variables after the variations have occurred.

experiment A scientific investigation in which observations are made and data are collected by means of the characteristics of control, randomization, and manipulation.

experimental design A research design that has the following properties: randomization, control, and manipulation.

experimental group The group in an experimental investigation that receives an intervention or treatment.

external criticism A process used to judge the authenticity of historical data.

external validity The degree to which findings of a study can be generalized to other populations or environments.

extraneous variable Variable that interferes with the operations of the phenomena being studied. Also called *mediating variable*.

face validity A type of content validity that uses an expert's opinion to judge the accuracy of an instrument.

factor analysis A type of validity that uses a statistical procedure for determining the underlying dimensions or components of a variable.

findings Statistical results of a study.

Fisher's exact probability test A test used to compare frequencies when samples are small and expected frequencies are less than six in each cell.

fittingness Answers the questions: Are the findings applicable outside the study situation? Are the results meaningful to the individuals not involved in the research?

frequency distribution Descriptive statistical method for summarizing the occurrences of events under study.

generalizability (generalize) The inferences that the data are representative of similar phenomena in a population beyond the studied sample.

grounded theory Theory that is constructed inductively from a base of observations of the world as it is lived by a selected group of people.

grounded theory method An inductive approach that uses a systematic set of procedures to arrive at theory about basic social processes.

historical research method The systematic compilation of data resulting from evaluation and interpretation of facts regarding people, events, and occurrences of the past.

history The internal validity threat that refers to events outside of the experimental setting that may affect the dependent variable.

homogeneity Similarity of conditions. Also called *internal consistency*.

hypothesis A prediction about the relationship between two or more variables.

hypothesis-testing validity A strategy for assessing construct validity in which the theory or concept underlying a measurement instrument's design is used to develop hypotheses that are tested. Inferences are made based on the findings about whether the rationale underlying the instrument's construction is adequate to explain the findings.

independent variable The antecedent or the variable that has the presumed effect on the dependent variable.

inductive reasoning A logical thought process in which generalizations are developed from specific observations; reasoning moves from particular to the general.

inferential statistics Procedures that combine mathematical processes and logic to test hypotheses about a population with the help of sample data.

informed consent An ethical principle that requires a researcher to obtain the voluntary participation of subjects after informing them of potential benefits and risks.

innovation diffusion Process by which an innovation or research findings are communicated through various channels over time among the members of a profession.

institutional review boards (IRBs) Boards established in agencies to review biomedical and behavioral research involving human subjects within the agency or in programs sponsored by the agency.

instrumentation Changes in the measurement of the variables that may account for changes in the obtained measurement.

integrative research review Synthesis review of the literature on a specific concept or topic.

internal consistency The extent to which items within a scale reflect or measure the same concept.

internal criticism A process of judging the reliability or consistency of information within an historical document.

internal validity The degree to which it can be inferred that the experimental treatment, rather than an uncontrolled condition, resulted in the observed effects.

interrater reliability The consistency of observations between two or more observers; often expressed as a percentage of agreement between raters or observers or a coefficient of agreement that takes into account the element of chance. This usually is used with the direct observation method.

interrelationship/difference studies The classification of a nonexperimental research design that attempts to trace relationships among variables. The four types are *correlational, ex post facto, prediction*, and *developmental*.

interval The level of measurement that provides different levels or gradations in response. The differences or intervals between responses are assumed to be approximately equal.

interval measurement Level used to show rankings of events or objects on a scale with equal intervals between numbers but with an arbitrary zero (e.g., centigrade temperature).

intervening variable A variable that occurs during an experimental or quasiexperimental study that affects the dependent variable.

intervention Deals with whether or not the observer provokes actions from those who are being observed.

interviews A method of data collection in which a data collector questions a subject verbally. Interviews may be face-to-face or performed over the telephone, and they may consist of open-ended or close-ended questions.

item to total correlation The relationship between each of the items on a scale and the total scale.

justice Human subjects should be treated fairly.

key informants Individuals who have special knowledge, status, or communication skills and who are willing to teach the ethnographer about the phenomenon.

Kuder-Richardson (KR-20) coefficient The estimate of homogeneity utilized for instruments that use a dichotomous response pattern.

kurtosis The relative peakness or flatness of a distribution.

level of significance (alpha level) The risk of making a type I error, set by the researcher before the study begins.

levels of measurement Categorization of the precision with which an event can be measured (nominal, ordinal, interval, and ratio).

life context The matrix of human-human-environment relationships emerging over the course of one's life.

Likert scales Lists of statements on which respondents indicate whether they "strongly agree," "agree," "disagree," or "strongly disagree."

limitation Weakness of a study.

linear structural relationships (LISREL) A computer program developed to analyze covariance and the testing of complex causal models.

lived experience In phenomenological research a term used to refer to the focus on living through events and circumstances (prelingual) rather than thinking about these events and circumstances (conceptualized experience).

longitudinal study A nonexperimental research design in which a researcher collects data from the same group at different points in time.

manipulation The provision of some experimental treatment, in one or varying degrees, to some of the subjects in the study.

matching A special sampling strategy used to construct an equivalent comparison sample group by filling it with subjects who are similar to each subject in another sample group in relation to preestablished variables, such as age and gender.

maturation Developmental, biological, or psychological processes that operate within an individual as a function of time and are external to the events of the investigation.

mean A measure of central tendency; the arithmetic average of all scores.

measurement The assignment of numbers to objects or events according to rules.

measures of central tendency Descriptive statistical procedure that describes the average member of a sample (mean, median, and mode).

measures of variability Descriptive statistical procedure that describes how much dispersion there is in sample data.

median A measure of central tendency; the middle score.

mediating variable A variable that is between or occurs between an independent and dependent variable and can produce an indirect effect of the independent variable on the dependent variable.

MEDLINE The print or computerized database of standard medical literature analysis and retrieval system on-line; it is also available on CD-ROM.

metaanalysis A research method that takes the results of multiple studies in a specific area and synthesizes the findings to make conclusions regarding the area of focus.

methodological research The controlled investigation and measurement of the means of gathering and analyzing data.

modal percentage A measure of variability; percent of cases in the mode.

modality The number of peaks in a frequency distribution.

mode A measure of central tendency; most frequent score or result.

mortality The loss of subject from time 1 data collection to time 2 data collection.

multiple analysis of variance (MANOVA) A test used to determine differences in group means; used when there is more than one dependent variable.

multiple regression Measure of the relationship between one interval level dependent variable and several independent variables. Canonical correlation is used when there is more than one dependent variable.

multistage sampling (cluster sampling) Involves a successive random sampling or units (clusters) that programs from large to small and meets sample eligibility criteria.

multitrait-multimethod approach A type of validity that uses more than one method to assess the accuracy of an instrument (e.g., observation and interview of anxiety).

network sampling (snowballing) A strategy used for locating samples difficult to locate. It uses social networks and the fact that friends tend to have characteristics in common; subjects who meet the eligibility criteria are asked for assistance in getting in touch with others who meet the same criteria.

nominal The level of measurement that simply assigns data into categories that are mutually exclusive.

nominal measurement Level used to classify objects or events into categories without any relative ranking (e.g., gender, hair color).

nondirectional hypothesis One that indicates the existence of a relationship between the variables but does not specify the anticipated direction of the relationship.

nonequivalent control group design A quasiexperimental design that is similar to the true experiment, but subjects are not randomly assigned to the treatment or control groups.

nonexperimental research design Research design in which an investigator observes a phenomenon without manipulating the independent variable(s).

nonparametric statistics Statistics that are usually utilized when variables are measured at the nominal or ordinal level because they do not estimate population parameters and involve less restrictive assumptions about the underlying distribution.

nonparametric tests of significance Inferential statistics that make no assumptions about the population distribution.

nonprobability sampling A procedure in which elements are chosen by nonrandom methods.

normal curve A curve that is symmetrical about the mean and unimodal.

null hypothesis A statement that there is no relationship between the variables and that any relationship observed is a function of chance or fluctuations in sampling.

objective Data that are not influenced by anyone who collects the information.

objectivity The use of facts without distortion by personal feelings or bias.

open-ended item Question that the respondent may answer in his or her own words.

operational definition The measurements used to observe or measure a variable; delineates the procedures or operations required to measure a concept.

operationalization The process of translating concepts into observable, measurable phenomena.

ordinal The level of measurement that systematically categorizes data in an ordered or ranked manner. Ordinal measures do not permit a high level of differentiation among subjects.

ordinal measurement Level used to show rankings of events or objects; numbers are not equidistant, and zero is arbitrary (class ranking).

parallel form (reliability) *See* **alternate form (reliability)**.

parameter A characteristic of a population.

parametric statistics Inferential statistics that involve the estimation of at least one parameter, require measurement at the interval level or above, and involve assumptions about the variables being studied. These assumptions usually include the fact that the variable is normally distributed.

path analysis A statistical technique in which the researcher hypothesizes how variables are related and in what order and then tests how strong those relationships or paths are.

Pearson correlation coefficient (Pearson *r*) A statistic that is calculated to reflect the degree of relationship between two interval level variables. Also called *Pearson product moment correlation coefficient*.

percentile A measure of rank; percentage of cases a given score exceeds.

phenomenological method A process of learning and constructing the meaning of human experience through intensive dialogue with persons who are living the experience.

phenomenological research Based on the investigation of the description of experience as it is lived.

phenomenology A qualitative research approach that aims to describe experience as it is lived through, before it is conceptualized.

philosophical research Based on the investigation of the truths and principles of existence, knowledge, and conduct.

physiological measurement The use of specialized equipment to determine physical and biological status of subjects.

population A well-defined set that has certain specified properties.

population validity Generalization of results to other populations.

prediction study A type of nonexperimental research design that attempts to make a forecast or prediction derived from particular phenomena.

predictive validity The degree of correlation between the measure of the concept and some future measure of the same concept.

primary source Scholarly literature that is written by a person(s) who developed the theory or conducted the research. Primary sources include eyewitness accounts of historic events, provided by original documents, films, letters, diaries, records, artifacts, periodicals, or tapes.

print databases Indexes, card catalogues, and abstract reviews. *Print indexes* are used to find journal sources (periodicals) of data-based and conceptual articles on a variety of topics, as well as publications of professional organizations and various governmental agencies.

probability The probability of an event is the event's long-run relative frequency in repeated trials under similar conditions.

probability sampling A procedure that uses some form of random selection when the sample units are chosen.

problem statement An interrogative sentence or statement about the relationship between two or more variables.

process consent In qualitative research the ongoing negotiation with subjects for their participation in a study.

product testing Testing of medical devices.

program A list of instructions in a machine-readable language written so that a computer's hardware can carry out an operation; software.

propositions The linkage of concepts that lays a foundation for the development of methods that test relationships.

prospective study Nonexperimental study that begins with an exploration of assumed causes and then moves forward in time to the presumed effect.

psychometrics The theory and development of measurement instruments.

purposive sampling A nonprobability sampling strategy in which the researcher selects subjects who are considered to be typical of the population.

qualitative measurement The items or observed behaviors are assigned to mutually exclusive categories that are representative of the kinds of behavior exhibited by the subjects.

qualitative research The study of broadly stated questions about human experiences. It is conducted in natural settings and uses descriptive data.

quantitative measurement The assignment of items or behaviors to categories that represent the amount of a possessed characteristic.

quasiexperimental design A study design in which random assignment is not used but the independent variable is manipulated and certain mechanisms of control are used.

questionnaires Paper and pencil instruments designed to gather data from individuals.

quota sampling A nonprobability sampling strategy that identifies the strata of the population and proportionately represents the strata in the sample.

random access memory (RAM) A computer's memory that the user can read or change.

random selection A selection process in which each element of the population has an equal and independent chance of being included in the sample.

randomization A sampling selection procedure in which each person or element in a population has an equal chance of being selected to either the experimental group or the control group.

range A measure of variability; difference between the highest and lowest scores in a set of sample data.

ratio The highest level of measurement that possesses the characteristics of categorizing, ordering, and ranking and also has an absolute or natural zero that has empirical meaning.

ratio measurement Level that ranks the order of events or objects and that has equal intervals and an absolute zero (e.g., height, weight).

reactivity The distortion created when those who are being observed change their behavior because they know that they are being observed.

recommendation Application of a study to practice, theory, and future research.

records or available data Information that is collected from existing materials, such as hospital records, historical documents, or videotapes.

refereed journal or peer-reviewed journal A scholarly journal that has a panel of external and internal reviewers or editors; the panel reviews submitted manuscripts for possible publication. The review panels use the same set of scholarly criteria to judge if the manuscripts are worthy of publication.

reliability The consistency or constancy of a measuring instrument.

replication The repetition of a study that uses different samples and is conducted in different settings.

representative sample A sample whose key characteristics closely approximate those of the population.

research The systematic, logical, and empirical inquiry into the possible relationships among particular phenomena to produce verifiable knowledge.

research base The accumulated knowledge gained from several studies that investigate a similar problem.

research-based practice Nursing practice that is based on research studies; that is, supported by research findings.

research-based protocols Practice standards that are formulated from findings of several studies.

research hypothesis A statement about the expected relationship between the variables; also known as a *scientific hypothesis*.

research literature A synonym for data-based literature.

research problem Presents the question that is to be asked in a research study.

research utilization A systematic method of implementing sound research-based innovations in clinical practice, evaluating the outcome, and sharing the knowledge through the process of research dissemination.

respect for persons People have the right to self-determination and to treatment as autonomous agents; that is, they have the freedom to participate or not participate in research.

retrospective data Data that have been manifested, such as scores on a standard examination.

retrospective study A nonexperimental research design that begins with the phenomenon of interest (dependent variable) in the present and examines its relationship to another variable (independent variable) in the past.

review of the literature An extensive, systematic, and critical review of the most important published scholarly literature on a particular topic. In most cases it is not considered exhaustive.

risk Potential negative outcome(s) of participation in research study.

risk-benefit ratio The extent to which the benefits of the study are maximized and the risks are minimized such that the subjects are protected from harm during the study.

sample A subset of sampling units from a population.

sampling A process in which representative units of a population are selected for study in a research investigation.

sampling error The tendency for statistics to fluctuate from one sample to another.

sampling frame A list of all units of the population.

sampling interval The standard distance between the elements chosen for the sample.

sampling unit The element or set of elements used for selecting the sample.

saturation *See* **data saturation**.

scale A self-report inventory that provides a set of response symbols for each item. A rating or score is assigned to each response.

scholarly literature Refers to published and unpublished data-based and conceptual literature materials found in print and nonprint forms.

scientific approach A logical, orderly, and objective means of generating and testing ideas.

scientific hypothesis The researcher's expectation about the outcome of a study; also known as the *research hypothesis*.

scientific literature A synonym for data-based literature; *see* **data-based literature**.

scientific merit The degree of validity of a study or group of studies.

scientific observation Collecting data about the environment and subjects. Data collection has specific objectives to guide it, is systematically planned and recorded, is checked and controlled, and is related to scientific concepts and theories.

secondary source Scholarly material written by person(s) *other than* the individual who developed the theory or conducted the research. Most are usually published. Often a secondary source represents a response to or a summary and critique of a theorist's or researcher's work. Examples are documents, films, letters, diaries, records, artifacts, periodicals, or tapes that provide a view of the phenomenon from another's perspective.

selection bias The internal validity threat that arises when pretreatment differences between the experimental group and the control group are present.

semiquartile range A measure of variability; range of the middle 50% of the scores. Also known as *semiinterquartile range*.

simple random sampling A probability sampling strategy in which the population is defined, a sampling frame is listed, and a subset from which the sample will be chosen is selected; members randomly selected.

skew Measure of the asymmetry of a set of scores.

snowballing (network sampling) A strategy used for locating samples difficult to locate. It uses social network and the fact that friends tend to have characteristics in common; subjects who meet the eligibility criteria are asked for assistance in getting in touch with others who meet the same criteria.

social desirability The occasion when a subject responds in a manner that he or she believes will please the researcher rather than in an honest manner.

Solomon four-group design An experimental design with four randomly assigned groups— the pretest-posttest intervention group, the pretest-posttest control group, a treatment or intervention group with only posttest measurement, and a control group with only posttest measurement.

split-half reliability An index of the comparison between the scores on one half of a test with those on the other half to determine the consistency in response to items that reflect specific content.

stability An instrument's ability to produce the same results with repeated testing.

standard deviation (SD) A measure of variability; measure of average deviation of scores from the mean.

standard error of the mean The standard deviation of a theoretical distribution of sample means. It indicates the average error in the estimation of the population mean.

statistical hypothesis States that there is no relationship between the independent and dependent variables. The statistical hypothesis also is known as the *null hypothesis*.

statistical reliability An index of the interval consistency of responses to all items of a single form of measure that is administered at one time.

stratified random sampling A probability sampling strategy in which the population is divided into strata or subgroups. An appropriate number of elements from each subgroup are randomly selected based on their proportion in the population.

symbolic interaction A theoretical perspective that holds that the relationship between self and society is an ongoing process of symbolic communication whereby individuals create a social reality.

systematic Data collection carried out in the same manner with all subjects.

systematic error Attributable to lasting characteristics of the subject that do not tend to fluctuate from one time to another. Also called *constant error*.

systematic sampling A probability sampling strategy that involves the selection of subjects randomly drawn from a population list at fixed intervals.

t statistic Commonly used in nursing research; it tests whether two group means are more different than would be expected by chance. Groups may be related or independent.

target population A population or group of individuals that meet the sampling criteria.

test A self-report inventory that provides for one response to each item that the examiner assigns a rating or score. Inferences are made from the total score about the degree to which a subject possess whatever trait, emotion, attitude, or behavior the test is supposed to measure.

testable Variables of proposed study that lend themselves to observation, measurement, and analysis.

testing The effects of taking a pretest on the scores of a posttest.

test-retest reliability Administration of the same instrument twice to the same subjects under the same conditions within a prescribed time interval, with a comparison of the paired scores to determine the stability of the measure.

theoretical framework Theoretical rationale for the development of hypotheses.

theoretical literature A synonym for conceptual literature; *see* **conceptual literature**.

theoretical sampling Used to select experiences that will help the researcher test ideas and gather complete information about developing concepts when using the grounded theory method.

theory Set of interrelated concepts, definitions, and propositions that present a systematic view of phenomena for the purpose of explaining and making predictions about those phenomena.

time series design A quasiexperimental design used to determine trends before and after an experimental treatment. Measurements are taken several times before the introduction of the experimental treatment, the treatment is introduced, and measurements are taken again at specified times afterward.

time-sharing Several users working on one mainframe via terminals at the same time.

true experiment Also known as the *pretest-posttest control group design*. In this design, subjects are randomly assigned to an experimental or control group, pretest measurements are performed, an intervention or treatment occurs in the experimental group, and posttest measurements are performed.

type I error The rejection of a null hypothesis that is actually true.

type II error The acceptance of a null hypothesis that is actually false.

uplink The ability to broadcast conferences so that they can be attended from a distance.

validation sample The sample that provides the initial data for determining the reliability and validity of a measurement tool.

validity Determination of whether a measurement instrument actually measures what it is purported to measure.

variable A defined concept.

web browser Software program used to connect or "read" the World Wide Web (WWW).

World Wide Web (WWW) A conceptual group of servers on the Internet. The Web is multiple hypertext linked together in an Internet network that criss-crosses the whole Internet like a spider web.

Z score Used to compare measurements in standard units; examines the relative distance of the scores from the mean.

Index

A

Abstract
  definition of, 42, 49
  description of, 49
  length of, 49
Accessible population, 250
After-only design
  description of, 181
  diagram of, 180f
After-only nonequivalent control group
      design
  description of, 185-186
  diagram of, 184f
Alpha level; *see* Level of significance
American Nurses Association (ANA) guide-
      lines, 282-284, 283b
America On-Line, 116
Analysis of covariance (ANCOVA), 379
Analysis of linear structural relationships
      (LISREL), 382
Analysis of variance (ANOVA), 378-379
Analysis reading
  critiquing strategies for, 46
  definition of, 45
  strategies, 45
Anecdotes, 315
Animal experiments, legal and ethical
      aspects of, 298-299, 300b
Anonymity
  assurance of, 290
  right to
    description of, 286t
    violation of, 287
Antecedent variables, 179

Assent, 295
Associative relationships, 75, 82
Auditability
  definition of, 463
  qualitative research studies, 237, 238t,
      448t
Available data or records, for collecting data
  advantages and disadvantages, 320
  authenticity issues, 320
  critiquing of, 411t
  description of, 319
Axial coding, 228

B

Baccalaureate-prepared nurses, responsibili-
      ties of
  idea sharing with other nurses, 10
  identification of nursing problems, 10
  promotion of ethical principles, 10
Benefits *vs.* risks, 298
Bias, selection
  definition of, 166
  effect on validity of research design
    external validity, 168
    internal validity, 166
  ways to avoid, in research study, 166
Bracketing, of researcher's perspective, 224

C

Canonical correlation, 382
Case studies, for analysis and critiquing
  qualitative research studies
    conclusions, 464
    data analysis, 451, 452t, 453, 463-464

In pages references, "t" indicates tables; "f" indicates figures; "b" indicates boxes.

Case studies, for analysis and
  critiquing—cont'd
qualitative research studies—cont'd
  data collection, 451, 463
  discussion, 459-460
  findings, 453-459, 464
  implications, 464-465
  method, 462
  overview, 450-451
  purpose, 462
  recommendations, 465
  research approach, 451
  sampling, 462
  statement of phenomenon of interest,
    461-462
  quantitative research studies
  case study 1
    critiquing of
      conclusions, 428
      data analysis, 427-428
      definitions, 424
      external validity, 426
      hypotheses, 424-425
      implications, 428
      independent variables, 425
      instruments, 426-427
      internal validity, 426
      literature view, 424
      problem statement, 423-424
      purpose, 423-424
      recommendations, 428
      reliability, 427
      research approach, 426-427
      research design, 425-426
      sample, 425
      validity, 427
    data analysis, 418
    description of, 413-415
    discussion, 420-421
    experimental interventions, 417-418
    measures, 415-417
    method, 415-418
    procedure, 417
    results, 418, 419t, 420
    sample, 415

Case studies, for analysis and
  critiquing—cont'd
quantitative research studies—cont'd
  case study 2
    conclusion, 436-437
    critiquing of
      analysis of data, 442
      conclusions, 442-443
      definitions, 439
      external validity, 440
      hypotheses and/or research questions,
        440
      implications, 442-443
      instruments, 441
      internal validity, 440
      introduction, 438-439
      methods, 441
      nursing practice application, 443
      problem statement, 439
      purpose, 439
      recommendations, 443
      reliability, 441
      research approach, 441-442
      research design, 440
      review of literature, 439
      sample, 440
      validity, 441-442
    description of, 429
    discussion, 434, 435t, 436
    measures, 433
    methodology, 431-434
    procedure, 434
    results, 434
    review of literature, 430
    subjects, 431-433
    theoretical framework, 430-431
Causal relationships, 75
  experimental designs for testing; see
    Experimental designs
  in nonexperimental designs, 205-206
  time series quasiexperimental design for
    studying, 186-187
CD-ROM, definition of, 100

CD-ROM databases
  CINAHL
    advantages of, 118b
    description of, 118-119
    example of retrieved entry using, 123b
    hints for using, 122b
    structure of, 119
  description of, 117-118
Chance errors; *see* Random errors
Change agents, 478
Chat rooms, for review of literature, 114t-115t, 116
Children, protection of human rights of, 296
Chi-square test, 379
Cluster sampling
  advantages and disadvantages, 260
  principles of, 260
  summary of, 252t
Committee on Public Health Nursing of the National League of Nursing Education (NLNE), 16
Committee on Research and Studies, 17-18
Comparison of Three Wound Dressings in Patients Undergoing Heart Surgery, 499-507
Comprehensive understanding, during critical reading
  definition of, 42
  strategies, 44
Computer database, 110
Computer searches, for review of literature
  critical thinking decision path, 120
  description of, 119
  information necessary for performing, 121, 123
  retrieved information, critical reading of, 123
  search tools, 121, 123
  time lines for, 120-121
Concealment, of observer in observational studies, 313
Concepts
  defining of, 142
  definition of, 139
  purpose of, 139

Concepts—cont'd
  relationship with propositions and hypotheses, 140
Conceptual definition, 87
  examples of, 142b
  purpose of, 142
Conceptual literature, 94
  critiquing of, 126
  nursing journals, 108b
  sources of, 102, 103t
  terms used to describe, 102, 102t
Conceptual model, 140
Concerns about Analgesics Among Patients and Family Caregivers in a Hospice Setting, 537-547
Conclusions, case study evaluations for critiquing
  qualitative research studies, 464-465
  quantitative research studies
    case study 1, 428
    case study 2, 442-443
Concurrent validity, 332-333
Conduct of research
  definition of, 468
  interrelationship with research utilization and research dissemination, 469f
Confidentiality
  assurance of, 290
  right to
    description of, 286t
    violation of, 287
Consent
  definition of, 295
  informed; *see* Informed consent
Consistency, in data collection, 310
Constancy, in data collection, 163
Constant comparative method, 228
Construct validity
  approaches
    contrasted-groups, 336
    convergent, 333-334
    divergent, 334, 336
    factor analytical, 336-337
    hypothesis-testing, 333, 334t
  definition of, 333

Consumer
  definition of, 9
  research
    definition of, 9
    of review of literature
      description of, 96-97
      examples of, 98t
      literature searches, 110
      vs. review of literature for research, 97-99
Content analysis, 316
Content validity
  description of, 331
  example of, 331
  face validity, 332
Contrasted-groups approach, for construct validity, 336
Control
  definition of, 157, 178
  in experimental design, 178
  in research design
    description of, 159
    extraneous variables that affect, methods for controlling
      constancy in data collection, 162
      homogeneous sampling, 161
      manipulation of independent variable, 162
      overview, 159, 161
      randomization, 163
Control group, 162
Convenience sampling
  advantages and disadvantages, 253
  description of, 253
  summary of, 252t
Convergent validity
  description of, 333
  methods for assessing, 334, 335t
  multitrait-multimethod approach for assessing, 334, 336
Correlational studies
  advantages, 199
  disadvantages, 199-200
  misuses of, 200
  objective of, 199

Correlations
  description of, 364-365
  illustration of, 364f
  tests of relationships to determine, 380
Credibility
  definition of, 463
  in qualitative research studies, 237, 238t
Criterion-related validity
  concurrent, 332
  definition of, 332
  predictive, 332
Critical reading
  definition of, 41
  levels of understanding involved in
    analysis, 45-46
    comprehensive, 42, 44
    preliminary, 42
    synthesis, 46-47
Critical thinking, definition of, 40
Critical thinking decision path
  computer searches, 120
  concepts, propositions, and hypotheses, interrelationships of, 140
  data collection methods, 308-309
  decision-driven research utilization, 470-471
  descriptive statistics, 353
  experimental designs, 177
  findings, 391
  hypothesis types, 82-83
  inferential statistics, 370-371
  quantitative research studies *vs.* qualitative research studies, 217
  quasiexperimental design, 177
  reliability, of measurement tools, 339
  results of study, 391
  sampling size and appropriate generalizability, 263
  Stetler model of research utilization, 471
  validity threats, 167
Criticism
  external, 233, 323
  internal, 233, 323
Critiquing, 7
  case studies for; *see* Case studies
  criteria for, 46

Critiquing—cont'd
  data collection methods, 321-324, 410t
  definition of, 44-45
  descriptive statistics, 365-366
  Discussion section, 398-400
  ethical and legal guidelines of research,
        410t
    examples of, 301-302
    guidelines, 301
    methods section in research article, 301-
        302
    vulnerable groups, 302
  evaluation research, 190-191
  experimental designs, 189-191
  external validity, 410t
  hypothesis, 86-88, 409t
  inferential statistics
    criteria, 383
    description of, 383-384
    example of, 384-385
    hypothesis, 383-384
    level of measurement, 384
  internal validity, 410t
  interviews, 322, 411t
  measurement tool
    reliability, 345-346, 411t
    validity, 346-347, 411t
  nonexperimental designs, 210-212
  problem statement, 84-86, 409t
  qualitative research, 240-241, 270
  quasiexperimental designs, 189-191
  questionnaires, 322, 411t
  records or available data, for collecting
        data, 411t
  research articles
    importance of questions, 47-48
    strategies for, 48f
  research design, 169-171, 410t
  research questions, 88, 409t
  Results section, 393-394, 398-400
  review of literature, 124-127, 409t
  sample, 410t
  sample size, 265, 270-271

Critiquing—cont'd
  sampling
    criteria, 268
    human rights protection, 271
    population, 268
    random sampling, 270
    suitability to research design, 270
  theoretical framework, 148-149, 409t
Cronbach's alpha, 343-344, 344b
Cross-sectional studies
  longitudinal studies and, comparison, 203
  objectives of, 202
Cumulative Index to Nursing and Allied
        Health Literature (CINAHL)
  databases of
    CD-ROM
      advantages of, 118B
      description of, 118-119
      example of retrieved entry using, 123b
      hints for using, 122b
      structure of, 119
    description of, 110
  description of, 100

D

Data analysis
  case study evaluations, critiquing of
    qualitative research studies, 463-464
    quantitative research studies
      case study 1, 427-428
      case study 2, 442
  critiquing of, 411t
  description of, 54
  location in research process, 51t
  measurement tools; *see* Measurement tools
  in qualitative research studies, 448t
  statistics; *see* Descriptive statistics; Inferen-
        tial statistics
Data-based literature
  critiquing of, 126
  material for, 105
  nursing journals, 108b
  sources of, 102, 103t, 105
  terms used to describe, 102, 102t

Databases
  CD-ROM
    CINAHL
      advantages of, 118B
      description of, 118-119
      example of retrieved entry using,
        123b
      hints for using, 122b
      structure of, 119
    description of, 117-118
  computer, 110
  print
    commonly used types of, 111b
    elements of, 110
    methods for accessing, 110-111
Data collection
  constancy in, 163
  critical thinking decision path, 308-309
  methods
    case study evaluations, critiquing of
      in qualitative research studies, 462
      quantitative research studies
        case study 1, 426
        case study 2, 441
    critiquing of, 321-324, 410t
    description of, 54
    interviews
      advantages, 318-319
      critiquing of, 322, 411t
      description of, 316
      safeguards for, 319
      vs. questionnaires, 319
    location in research articles, 51t
    new types of, construction of, 320-
      321
    observational
      advantages and disadvantages, 315
      critiquing of, 322
      description of, 312
      ethical considerations, 314
      role of observer in
        concealment, 313
        intervention, 313
        types of, 314f

Data collection—cont'd
  methods—cont'd
    observational—cont'd
      scientific
        advantages, 315
        description of, 312-313
        structured vs. unstructured observations,
          315
      physiological
        advantages and disadvantages, 312
        components needed for, 311
        critiquing of, 322, 410t
        example of, 311
        indications for using, 312
      in qualitative research studies, 448t
      questionnaires
        advantages of, 318
        close-ended items
          description of, 316
          example of, 317b
        critiquing of, 322, 411t
        description of, 316
        example of, 318
        fixed response items, 316
        open-ended items
          description of, 316
          example of, 317b
        scale, 316
        vs. interviews, 319
      records or available data
        advantages and disadvantages, 320
        authenticity issues, 320
        critiquing of, 322
        description of, 319
    objective, 308
    subjective, 308
    variables of interest, measurement of
      conceptual definitions, 309-310
      consistency, 310
      interrater reliability, 310-311
      operational definitions, 309
      selection of variable, 308-309
Data saturation, 218
Debriefing, 314

Deductive reasoning
  definition of, 136
  description of, 137-139
  examples of, 138b
  inherent problems associated with, 138-139
  methods, 146
  research process structure when using, 136b
Delimitations, 249
Dependent variables
  case study evaluations of quantitative research studies, 424
  definition of, 63
  in nonexperimental designs, 211
  in problem statement, 67-68
Descriptive/exploratory surveys
  advantages and disadvantages, 198
  data collection methods, 198
  description of, 197
  for determining differences between variables, 198
  example of, 197-198
  uses of, 197-198
Descriptive statistics
  case study evaluations of quantitative research studies
    case study 1, 427
    case study 2, 442
  correlation, 364-365, 364f
  critical thinking decision path, 353
  critiquing of, 365-366
  definition of, 352
  frequency distribution
    data grouping, 355, 356t
    data presentation, 355, 356f
    description of, 355
  function of, 352
  inferential statistics and, comparison, 370
  level of measurement
    description of, 352
    interval, 354-355
    nominal, 354

Descriptive statistics—cont'd
  level of measurement—cont'd
    ordinal, 354
    ratio, 355
    summary of, 353t
  measures of central tendency
    example of, 357t, 360t
    function of, 357
    mean, 358-359
    median, 358
    mode, 358, 359f
  normal distribution
    description of, 361
    kurtosis, 361-362
    skewness, 361
    symmetry, 359f, 361
  variability measures
    function of, 362-363
    percentile, 363
    range, 363
    semiquartile range, 363
    standard deviation, 363-364
    Z scores, 364
Design, research; *see* Research design
Developmental studies
  cross-sectional, 202
  longitudinal, 203
  overview, 202
Difference studies; *see* Interrelationship/difference studies
Discussion section
  critiquing guidelines, 398-400
  description of, 54
  generalizations, 397-398
  location in research article, 51t
  purpose of, 395, 397
  recommendations; *see* Recommendations
  subjects discussed in, 397
Dissemination
  definition of, 472
  of research information, 26
  research utilization demonstration projects for, 472-473

Divergent validity
  description of, 334
  multitrait-multimethod approach for
      assessing, 334, 336
Doctorally prepared nurses
  research studies by, 11
  responsibilities of, 11
Domains, 231

E

Education, research activities based on level
    of
  associate degree, 9
  baccalaureate degree, 9-10
  doctorate degree, 11
  master's degree, 11
Element, of sample, 250
Eligibility criteria, of population
  definition of, 248-249
  delimitations, 249
  example of, 249
E-mail, 111
Emic view, 229
Equivalence testing, of reliability of mea-
    surement tool
  description of, 344
  interrater reliability, 344-345
  parallel or alternate form, 345
Errors
  inferential statistics
    level of significance, 375
    practical significance vs. statistical signifi-
        cance, 375-376
    type I, 374
    type II, 374
  measurement
    random, 328, 330
    systematic, 328, 330
    variance, 328
  sampling, 372-373
Error variance, 328
Ethical issues
  animal experiments, 298-299, 300b
  critiquing of, 410t

Ethical issues—cont'd
  evolution in nursing research, 282-284
  guidelines, for research
    critiquing of
      examples of, 301-302
      guidelines, 301
      methods section in research article, 301-
          302
      vulnerable groups, 302
    Department of Health and Human
        Services, 281
    dilemmas
      current, 281-282
      future, 281-282
      historical, 276, 277b, 278t-279t, 280b
    National Research Act, 277
    respect for persons, beneficence, and jus-
        tice, 277, 280b
    in United States, 278t-279t
  in observational studies, 314
  in qualitative research
    emergent nature of design, 236-237
    naturalistic settings, 236
    overview, 236t
    researcher as instrument, 237
    researcher-participant interaction, 237
Ethnographic method, for qualitative re-
    search
  data analysis, 231
  data gathering, 230-231
  describing the findings, 231
  history of, 229
  identifying the phenomenon, 229-230
  objectives of, 229
  principles of, 222t
  structuring the study
    researcher's perspective, 230
    research question, 230
    sample selection, 230
Ethnography
  description of, 229
  phenomenon in, 229
Etic view, 229

Evaluation research
  critiquing of, 190-191
  formative, 188
  purposes of, 188
  summative, 188
Experimental designs
  advantages and disadvantages, 182-183
  critical thinking decision path, 177
  critiquing of, 189-191
  internal validity threats, 180-181
  nonexperimental designs and, comparison,
      176
  in quality assurance and evaluation studies,
      189
  setting-based
    field experiments, 181-182
    laboratory experiments, 181-182
  true
    diagram of, 180f
    elements of
      control, 178
      manipulation, 178-179
      randomization, 177
    types of, 177b
      after-only design, 180f, 181
      description of, 179-180
      diagram of, 180f
      Solomon four-group design, 180f, 180-
          181
Experimental group, 162
Exploratory surveys; see Descriptive/
      exploratory surveys
Ex post facto studies
  advantages, 200-201
  disadvantages, 201
  objectives of, 200
  paradigm of, 201t
  principles of, 200
External criticism, 233
External validity, of research design
  case study evaluations of quantitative
      research studies
    case study 1, 426
    case study 2, 440

External validity, of research design—cont'd
  critiquing of, 410t
  definition of, 167
  threats to
    reactivity, 168
    selection, 168
    testing, 168-169
Extraneous variables
  antecedent, 179
  in experimental designs, 179
  intervening, 179
  methods of controlling
    constancy in data collection, 162
    homogeneous sampling, 161
    manipulation of independent variable,
        162
    overview, 159, 161
    randomization, 163

F
Face validity, 332
Factor analysis
  for construct validity, 336-337
  for inferential statistics, 383
Faculty, review of literature use by, 98t
Field experiments, 181-182
File transfer protocol; see FTP
Findings
  critical thinking decision path, 391
  definition of, 390
  Discussion section
    critiquing guidelines, 398-400
    generalizations, 397-398
    purpose of, 395, 397
    recommendations; see Recommendations
    subjects discussed in, 397
  in qualitative research studies
    case study evaluations, 464t
    critiquing, 449t
  Results section, 393b
    critiquing criteria, 393-394, 398-400
    data presentation, 392
    elements of, 390-391
    limitations, 392

Findings—cont'd
  Results section—cont'd
    objectivity of results, 392-393, 393b
    reported statistical results, 391, 392t
    tabular use in, 394t-396t, 394-395
  review of literature, 99
Fisher's exact probability test, 379-380
Fittingness
  definition of, 464
  in qualitative research studies, 237, 238t
Fraud, 297
Frequency distribution
  data grouping, 355, 356t
  data presentation, 355, 356f
  description of, 355
FTP, for transferring text, 113t

G

Generalizations, in *Discussion of the Results*
        section, 397-398
Goldmark report, 16
Goode model, of research utilization,
        478
Gopher search tool, for Internet, 112t
Graduate students, review of literature use
        by, 98t
Ground theory method
  data analysis, 228-229
  data gathering, 227-228
  describing the findings, 229
  development of, 226
  goal of, 226
  identifying the phenomenon, 226
  principles of, 222t
  structuring the study
    researcher's perspective, 227
    research question, 226-227
    sample selection, 227
  symbolic interaction principle of, 226

H

Hawthorne effect, 168, 183, 314
*Healing of Adult Male Survivors of Childhood
    Sexual Abuse,* 509-520

Historical description, of nursing research
  chronological highlights, 13b-15t
  nineteenth century (after 1850), 12, 13b, 16
  twentieth century
    before 1950, 13b-14b, 16-17
    1980s, 19
    1950 through 1980, 14b-15b, 17-19
Historical methods, of qualitative research
  data analysis, 233
  data gathering, 232-233
  describing the findings, 233-234
  fact, probability, and possibility establish-
        ment in, 234b
  goals of, 231
  identifying the phenomenon, 232
  principles of, 223t, 231-232
  structuring the study
    researcher's perspective, 232
    research question, 232
    sample selection, 232
History threat, effect on internal validity of
        research study, 164
Homogeneity
  effect on extraneous variables, 161
  testing, for reliability of measurement tool
    Cronbach's alpha, 343-344, 344b
    description of, 341
    item to total correlations, 342, 342t
    Kuder-Richardson (KR-20) coefficient,
        343
    split-half reliability, 342
Horn model, of research utilization, 478
Human rights
  American Nurses Association classification
        of, 282-284, 283b
  definition of, 284
  protection of
    procedures
      informed consent
        definition of, 285
        form, example of, 291f—292f
        language of, 285
        methods of obtaining, 285
        procedures for, 290

Human rights—cont'd
 protection of—cont'd
  procedures—cont'd
   institutional review board
    code of federal regulations for approv-
     ing research studies, 294b
    description of, 293
    expedited review criteria for, 294
    mechanisms for reviewing research,
     293-294
    responsibilities, 293
    structure of, 293
   vulnerable groups
    children, 296
    elderly, 296
    prisoners, 296
    types of, 294-295
  right to anonymity and confidentiality
   description of, 286t
   violation of, 287
  right to fair treatment, 288t
  right to privacy and dignity, 286t
  right to protection from discomfort and
    harm, 288t
  right to self-determination
   description of, 286t
   violation of, 287
  violations
   right to anonymity and confidentiality, 287
   right to self-determination, 287
   subject selection, 289
Hypothesis; see also Research questions
 case study evaluations of quantitative
   research studies
  case study 1, 424-425
  case study 2, 440
 characteristics of, 74
 critiquing of, 86-88, 409t
 from deductive reasoning, 137
 definition of, 73
 description of, 52
 directional
  advantages of, 78, 80
  definition of, 78
  wording of, 79t-80t

Hypothesis; see also Research
    questions—cont'd
 inferential statistics testing of; see Inferen-
    tial statistics
 interrelationships
  with concepts and propositions, 140
  with problem statement, literature review,
    and theoretical framework, 73f, 77t
 location in research article, 50t
 nondirectional
  definition of, 78
  wording of, 79t-80t
 purpose of, 74
 relationship statement, 74-75
 research
  definition of, 80
  examples of, 79t-80t
  inferential statistics testing of, 371
 and research design, relationship between,
    82
 review of literature, 99
 statistical
  definition of, 81
  examples of, 81t
  inferential statistics testing of, 371
 testability of, 75, 76t, 88
 theory base, 75-76
 variables, critiquing of, 87
 wording of
  directional hypothesis, 79t-80t
  elements, 77
  nondirectional hypothesis, 79t-80t
Hypothesis-generating study, 82-83
Hypothesis-testing validity, 333

I

Implications
 case study evaluations, critiquing of
  qualitative research studies, 464-465
  quantitative research studies
   case study 1, 428
   case study 2, 442-443
 description of, 55
 location in research article, 51t

Independent variables
　case study evaluations of quantitative
　　research studies, 424
　definition of, 67, 162
　in experimental *vs.* nonexperimental
　　designs, 196
　manipulation of, 162
　in problem statement, 67-68
Inductive reasoning
　definition of, 136
　description of, 137
　research process structure when using, 136b
　theory and method, relationship between,
　　146
Inferential statistics
　advanced statistics
　　analysis of linear structural relationships,
　　　382
　　factor analysis, 383
　　path analysis, 382
　case study evaluations of quantitative
　　research studies
　　case study 1, 427-428
　　case study 2, 442
　critical thinking decision path, 370-371
　critiquing of
　　criteria, 383
　　description of, 383-384
　　example of, 384-385
　　hypothesis, 383-384
　　level of measurement, 384
　definition of, 370
　descriptive statistics and, comparison, 370
　errors
　　level of significance, 375
　　practical significance *vs.* statistical signifi-
　　　cance, 375-376
　　type I, 374
　　type II, 374
　hypothesis testing, 370-372
　parameter, 370
　probability
　　definition of, 372
　　principles of, 372
　　sampling error, 372-373

Inferential statistics—cont'd
　purpose of, 370
　random sampling basis for, 370
　statistical significance tests
　　nonparametric
　　　of association, 378t
　　　chi-square, 379
　　　description of, 376
　　　of differences between means, 377t
　　　Fisher's exact probability test, 379-380
　　　types of, 379-380
　　parametric
　　　analysis of covariance, 379
　　　analysis of variance, 378-379
　　　of association, 378t
　　　attributes of, 376
　　　description of, 376
　　　of differences between means, 377t
　　　multiple analysis of variance, 379
　　　t test, 377-378
　　tests of difference
　　　description of, 377-378
　　　nonparametric tests, 379
　　　parametric tests, 378-379
　　tests of relationships
　　　function of, 380
　　　multiple regression, 381-382
　　　Pearson *r*, 380-381
　　vs. practical significance, 375-376
Informed consent
　definition of, 285
　form, example of, 291f-292f
　language of, 285
　methods of obtaining, 285
　procedures for, 290
Institutional review board (IRB), human
　　rights protection by
　code of federal regulations for approving
　　research studies, 294b
　description of, 293
　expedited review criteria for, 294
　mechanisms for reviewing research, 293-
　　294
　responsibilities, 293
　structure of, 293

Instrumentation threats, to internal validity
    of research study, 165-166
Instruments; *see* Data collection, methods;
    Measurement tools
Integrative research review, 473
Internal criticism, 233
Internal validity
  case study evaluations of quantitative re-
      search studies
    case study 1, 426
    case study 2, 440
  critiquing, 410t
  experimental designs, 180-181
  function of, 164
  quasiexperimental designs, 191
  threats to
    history, 164
    instrumentation, 165-166
    maturation, 164-165
    mortality, 166
    overview, 164b
    selection bias, 166
    testing, 165
Internet
  description of, 103, 111
  objectives of, 111
  on-line databases, 111, 112t-113t, 116
  services, 111, 112t-113t
Interrater reliability, 310-311, 344-345
Interrelationship/difference studies
  correlational
    advantages, 199
    disadvantages, 199-200
    misuses of, 200
    objective of, 199
  developmental
    cross-sectional studies, 202
    longitudinal studies, 203
    overview, 202
    prospective studies, 203-204
    retrospective studies, 203-204
  ex post facto
    advantages, 200-201
    disadvantages, 201
    objectives of, 200

Interrelationship/difference studies—cont'd
  ex post facto—cont'd
    paradigm of, 201t
    principles of, 200
  function of, 199
  prediction
    advantages and disadvantages, 202
    examples of, 201-202
    objective of, 201
Interval measurement, 354-355
Intervening variables, 179
Intervention, of observer in observational
    studies, 313
Interviews
  advantages, 318-319
  critiquing of, 322, 411t
  description of, 316
  safeguards for, 319
  vs. questionnaires, 319
Intuition, 134-135
Iowa Model of Research in Practice, 479
Item to total correlations, 342, 342t

J

Journals, nursing, 108b

K

Key informants, 230
Knowledge
  definition of, 134
  sources of
    intuition, 134-135
    overview, 134b
    review of literature, 95
    science/research
      deductive reasoning; see Deductive
          reasoning
      inductive reasoning; see Inductive
          reasoning
    tradition and authority, 135-136
    trial-and-error, 135
Known-groups approach; *see* Contrasted-
    groups approach
Kuder-Richardson (KR-20) coefficient, 343
Kurtosis, 361-362

L

Laboratory experiments, 181-182
Legal issues
  animal experiments, 298-299, 300b
  critiquing of
    examples of, 301-302
    guidelines, 301
    methods section in research article, 301-302
    vulnerable groups, 302
  human rights
    American Nurses Association classifica-
        tion of, 282-284, 283b
    definition of, 284
    protection of
      procedures
        informed consent
          definition of, 285
          form, example of, 291f-292f
          language of, 285
          methods of obtaining, 285
          procedures for, 290
        institutional review board
          code of federal regulations for
            approving research studies, 294b
          description of, 293
          expedited review criteria for, 294
          mechanisms for reviewing research,
            293-294
          responsibilities, 293
          structure of, 293
        vulnerable groups
          children, 296
          elderly, 296
          prisoners, 296
          types of, 294-295
    right to anonymity and confidentiality
      description of, 286t
      violation of, 287
    right to fair treatment, 288t
    right to privacy and dignity, 286t
    right to protection from discomfort and
        harm, 288t
    right to self-determination
      description of, 286t
      violation of, 287

Legal issues—cont'd
  human rights—cont'd
    violations
      right to anonymity and confidentiality, 287
      right to self-determination, 287
      subject selection, 289
Leptokurtic, 362
Level of measurement; see Measurement
    levels
Level of significance, 375
Life context, 216
Likert scale, 316, 343, 343f
ListServ lists, 112t
Literature review; see Review of literature
Lived experience, 225
Longitudinal studies
  advantages and disadvantages, 203
  cross-sectional studies and, comparison, 203
  example of, 203
  objectives of, 203

M

Manipulation
  in experimental design, 178-179
  of independent variable, 162, 178
Master's level-prepared nurses, responsibili-
    ties of, 11
Matching, 262
Maturation
  definition of, 164
  threat to internal validity of research study,
    164-165
Measurement, definition of, 352
Measurement errors
  random, 328, 330
  systematic, 328, 330
  variance, 328
Measurement levels
  description of, 352
  summary of, 353t
Measurement tools
  case study evaluations of quantitative
      research studies
    case study 1, 426-427
    case study 2, 441

Measurement tools—cont'd
reliability
  case study evaluations of quantitative
      research studies
    case study 1, 427
    case study 2, 441
  critical thinking decision path, 339
  critiquing of, 345-346, 411t
  description of, 337
  methods to test
    equivalence
      description of, 344
      interrater reliability, 344-345
      parallel or alternate form, 345
    homogeneity
      Cronbach's alpha, 343-344, 344b
      description of, 341
      item to total correlations, 342, 342t
      Kuder-Richardson (KR-20) coefficient,
          343
      split-half reliability, 342
    overview, 340b
    stability
      description of, 340
      parallel or alternate form, 341
      test-retest reliability, 340-341
  reliability coefficient interpretation, 337,
      339-340
validity
  case study evaluations of quantitative
      research studies
    case study 1, 427
    case study 2, 441
  computer resources for, 329b
  construct
    approaches
      contrasted-groups, 336
      convergent, 333-334
      divergent, 334, 336
      factor analytical, 336-337
      hypothesis-testing, 333, 334t
    definition of, 333
  content
    description of, 331
    example of, 331
    face validity, 332

Measurement tools—cont'd
validity—cont'd
  criterion-related
    concurrent, 332
    definition of, 332
    predictive, 332
  critiquing of, 346-347
  definition of, 331
Measures of central tendency, 352
  example of, 357t, 360t
  function of, 357
  mean, 358-359
  median, 358
  mode, 358, 359f
Measures of variability, 352
  function of, 362-363
  percentile, 363
  range, 363
  semiquartile range, 363
  standard deviation, 363-364
  Z scores, 364
Median, 358
MEDLINE, 117-118
Metaanalysis
  example of, 210
  principles of, 207, 210
Methodological research
  considerations incorporated into, 208t-209t
  example of, 207
  psychometrics, 206-207
  steps involved in, 207
Methods
  data collection
    case study evaluations, critiquing of
      qualitative research studies, 462
      quantitative research studies
        case study 1, 426
        case study 2, 441
    critiquing of, 321-324, 410t
    description of, 54
    interviews
      advantages, 318-319
      critiquing of, 322, 411t
      description of, 316
      safeguards for, 319
      vs. questionnaires, 319

Methods—cont'd
  data collection—cont'd
    location in research articles, 51t
    new types of, construction of, 320-321
    observational
      advantages and disadvantages, 315
      critiquing of, 322
      description of, 312
      ethical considerations, 314
      role of observer in
        concealment, 313
        intervention, 313
        types of, 314f
      scientific
        advantages, 315
        description of, 312-313
      structured *vs.* unstructured observations,
        315
    physiological
      advantages and disadvantages, 312
      components needed for, 311
      critiquing of, 322, 410t
      example of, 311
      indications for using, 312
    in qualitative research studies, 448t
    questionnaires
      advantages of, 318
      close-ended items
        description of, 316
        example of, 317b
      critiquing of, 322, 411t
      description of, 316
      example of, 318
      fixed response items, 316
      open-ended items
        description of, 316
        example of, 317b
      scale, 316
      vs. interviews, 319
    records or available data
      advantages and disadvantages, 320
      authenticity issues, 320
      critiquing of, 322
      description of, 319

Methods—cont'd
  for qualitative research studies
    case study evaluations of, 462
    ethnographic
      data analysis, 231
      data gathering, 230-231
      describing the findings, 231
      history of, 229
      identifying the phenomenon, 229-230
      objectives of, 229
      principles of, 222t
      structuring the study
        researcher's perspective, 230
        research question, 230
        sample selection, 230
    ground theory
      data analysis, 228-229
      data gathering, 227-228
      describing the findings, 229
      development of, 226
      goal of, 226
      identifying the phenomenon, 226
      principles of, 222t
      structuring the study
        researcher's perspective, 227
        research question, 226-227
        sample selection, 227
      symbolic interaction principle of, 226
    historical
      data analysis, 233
      data gathering, 232-233
      describing the findings, 233-234
      fact, probability, and possibility
        establishment in, 234b
      goals of, 231
      identifying the phenomenon, 232
      principles of, 223t, 231-232
      structuring the study
        researcher's perspective, 232
        research question, 232
        sample selection, 232
    phenomenological
      data analysis, 225
      data gathering, 224-225

Methods—cont'd
  for qualitative research studies—cont'd
    phenomenological—cont'd
      describing the findings, 225
      goal of, 221, 223
      identifying the phenomenon, 223
      principles of, 222t
      study structuring
        researcher's perspective, 224
        research question, 224
        sample selection, 224
    in qualitative research studies, 448t
    and theory, relationship between, 146-147
Misconduct, 297
Modality, 358
Mode, 358
Mortality
  definition of, 166
  threat to internal validity of research study,
      166
Multiple analysis of variance (MANOVA),
      379
Multiple regression, 381-382
Multistage sampling
  advantages and disadvantages, 260
  principles of, 260
  summary of, 252t
Multitrait-multimethod approach, for assess-
      ing convergent and divergent valid-
      ity, 334, 336

N

National Institutes of Health, 281
National Research Act, 277
Networking sampling, 262-263, 462
Nightingale, Florence, 12, 13b, 16
Nominal measurement, 354
Nonequivalent control group design
  description of, 184-185
  diagram of, 184f
Nonexperimental designs
  causality of, 205-206
  critiquing of, 210-212
  description of, 196

Nonexperimental designs—cont'd
  descriptive/exploratory surveys
    advantages and disadvantages, 198
    data collection methods, 198
    description of, 197
    for determining differences between
        variables, 198
    example of, 197-198
    uses of, 197-198
  experimental designs and, comparison, 176
  interrelationship/difference studies
    correlational
      advantages, 199
      disadvantages, 199-200
      misuses of, 200
      objective of, 199
    developmental
      cross-sectional studies, 202
      longitudinal studies, 203
      overview, 202
      prospective studies, 203-204
      retrospective studies, 203-204
    ex post facto
      advantages, 200-201
      disadvantages, 201
      objectives of, 200
      paradigm of, 201t
      principles of, 200
    function of, 199
    prediction
      advantages and disadvantages, 202
      examples of, 201-202
      objective of, 201
  metaanalysis
    example of, 210
    principles of, 207, 210
  methodological research
    considerations incorporated into, 208t-
        209t
    example of, 207
    psychometrics, 206-207
    steps involved in, 207
  subjects not analyzed using, 196
  summary of, 196b

Nonparametric tests of statistical
    significance
  of association, 378t
  chi-square, 379
  description of, 376
  of differences between means, 377t
  Fisher's exact probability test, 379-380
  types of, 379-380
Nonprobability sampling
  critiquing of, 269
  elements of, 251
  types of
    convenience
      advantages and disadvantages, 253
      description of, 253
      summary of, 252t
    matching, 262
    networking sampling, 262-263
    purposive
      description of, 255
      indications for using, 255-256
      recruiting of subjects for, 255
      summary of, 252t
    quota
      description of, 254
      strata, 254-255
      summary of, 252t
Normal curve, 361, 362f
Normal distribution
  description of, 361
  kurtosis, 361-362
  skewness, 361
  symmetry, 359f, 361
Null hypothesis
  definition of, 81, 371
  example of, 81t, 371-372
  inferential statistics testing of, 371
  principles of, 371-372
  rejection of, 371-372
Nuremberg code, 277b
Nurses
  research activities of, based on education
    levels
    associate degree, 9
    baccalaureate degree, 9-10

Nurses—cont'd
  research activities of, based on education
    levels—cont'd
    doctorate degree, 11
    master's degree, 11
  role in research process, 9-11
Nursing journals, 108b
Nursing practice, interrelationships
  with education, research, and theory, 7-9,
    94f
  with review of literature, 94f
Nursing research
  future directions (1990s and beyond)
    demographics changes, 24-25
    depth in research, promotion of, 20-22
    doctoral programs, 20
    funding, 24
    health services research, 24, 25b
    information dissemination methods,
      26
    international alliances, 23
    methodological expertise increases, 21
    multiple measures use, 21
    outcome research studies, 22
    public policy changes instituted by
      research, 26
    research designs, 21-22
    research priorities, 23-25, 25b
    research training programs, 22-23
    special interest areas, 25-26
  history of
    chronological highlights, 13b-15t
    nineteenth century (after 1850), 12, 13b,
      16
    twentieth century
      before 1950, 13b-14b, 16-17
      1980s, 19
      1950 through 1980, 14b-15b, 17-19
  significance of
    examples of, 6-7
    utilization in nursing practice, 7
  studies; *see* Research studies
  types of, 12t
Nursing science, qualitative research and,
    220-221

Nursing theory
  definition of, 147
  grand, 148b
  middle-range, 148b
  practice, 148b

O

Objective, definition of, 308
Observational method
  advantages and disadvantages, 315
  critiquing of, 322, 410t
  description of, 312
  ethical considerations, 314
  role of observer in
    concealment, 313
    intervention, 313
    types of, 314f
  scientific
    advantages, 315
    description of, 312-313
  structured *vs.* unstructured observations, 315
On-line databases
  types of, 117b
  via CINAHL direct, 117
  via Internet, 111, 112t-115t, 116
Open coding, 228
Operational definition, 87
  description of, 309
  examples of, 143b
  purpose of, 142-143
Operationalization, 308
Ordinal measurement, 354
Outcome research studies
  advantages of, 22
  proliferation of, 22

P

Parameter
  definition of, 370
  statistic and, differences between, 370
Parameter for the population, 370
Parametric tests of statistical significance
  analysis of covariance, 379
  analysis of variance, 378-379
  of association, 378t

Parametric tests of statistical
      significance—cont'd
  attributes of, 376
  description of, 376
  of differences between means, 377t
  multiple analysis of variance, 379
  t test, 377-378
Path analysis, 382
*Patient Outcomes for the Chronically
      Critically Ill: Special Care Unit Versus
      Intensive Care,* 521-535
Pearson *r,* 380-381
Peer-reviewed journals, 105-106
Percentile, 363
Phenomenological method
  data analysis, 225
  data gathering, 224-225
  describing the findings, 225
  goal of, 221, 223
  identifying the phenomenon, 223
  principles of, 222t
  study structuring
    researcher's perspective, 224
    research question, 224
    sample selection, 224
Phenomenon of interest
  case studies for analysis and critiquing,
      461-462
  ethnographic method, 229-230
  ground-level method, 226
  historical method, 232
  phenomenological method, 223
Physiological method
  advantages and disadvantages, 312
  components needed for, 311
  critiquing of, 322, 410t
  example of, 311
  indications for using, 312
Platykurtic, 362
Population
  critiquing of, 268
  in problem statement, 68, 69t
Posttest-only control group design; *see* After-
      only design

Power analysis, for estimating sample size, 264-265
Practice theory, 148b
Prediction studies
  advantages and disadvantages, 202
  examples of, 201-202
  objective of, 201
Predictive validity, 332
Preliminary reading, strategies for, 42
Primary sources, of literature, 97, 233
  definition of, 106
  nursing journals, 108b
  secondary sources and, comparison, 107t
  sources of, 109t
Print databases
  commonly used types of, 111b
  elements of, 110
  methods for accessing, 110-111
Probability
  definition of, 372
  principles of, 372
  sampling error, 372-373
Probability sampling
  characteristics of, 256
  critiquing of, 269
  elements of, 251
  random selection, 256
  types of
    cluster
      advantages and disadvantages, 260
      principles of, 260
      summary of, 252t
    simple random
      advantages, 256, 258
      description of, 256
      disadvantages, 258
      random numbers, 257f
      summary of, 252t
    stratified random
      advantages and disadvantages, 259-260
      criteria for selecting, 258-259
      principles of, 258
      subject selection, 259f
      summary of, 252t

Probability sampling—cont'd
  types of—cont'd
    systematic
      advantages and disadvantages, 261-262
      critiquing, 262
      definition of, 260-261
      population considerations, 261
      sampling interval, 261
      summary of, 252t
Problem solving, using trial-and-error method, 135
Problem statement; *see also* Research problem
  case study evaluations of quantitative research studies
    case study 1, 423-424
    case study 2, 439
  components
    example of use of, 69, 70t, 71
    population, 68
    testability, 68-69, 71
    variables, 67-68
  critiquing of, 84-86, 409t
  forms of
    declarative, 66t
    interrogative, 66t
  interrelationship with literature review, theoretical framework, and hypothesis, 73f, 77t
  in published research, 71-72
  refined *vs.* unrefined, 70t-71t
  review of literature, 99
Product testing, 298, 299t
Propositions
  definition of, 139
  relationship with concepts and hypotheses, 140
Prospective studies
  examples of, 204
  objectives of, 204
Psychometrics, 206-207
Purpose statement
  case study evaluations, critiquing of
    qualitative research studies, 462
    quantitative research studies
      case study 1, 423-424
      case study 2, 439

Purpose statement—cont'd
  description of, 52, 71
  examples of, 72b
  function of, 72
  location in research article, 50t
  in qualitative research studies, 448t
Purposive sampling
  description of, 255
  indications for using, 255-256
  recruiting of subjects for, 255
  summary of, 252t

Q

Qualitative research studies
  auditability, 237, 238t, 448t
  case study for analysis and critiquing
    critique of
      conclusions, 464
      data analysis, 463-464
      data collection, 463
      findings, 464
      implications, 464-465
      method, 462
      purpose, 462
      recommendations, 465
      sampling, 462
      statement of phenomenon of interest,
        461-462
    data analysis, 451, 452t, 453
    data collection, 451
    discussion, 459-460
    findings, 453-459
    overview, 450-451
    research approach, 451
  case study methodology, 234-236
  credibility, 237, 238t
  critiquing of, 240-241, 270, 448t-449t
  data, computer management of, 238, 240
  description of, 216
  ethical concerns
    emergent nature of design, 236-237
    naturalistic settings, 236
    overview, 236t
    researcher as instrument, 237
    researcher-participant interaction, 237

Qualitative research studies—cont'd
  fittingness, 237, 238t
  methods
    case study evaluations of, 462
    ethnographic
      data analysis, 231
      data gathering, 230-231
      describing the findings, 231
      history of, 229
      identifying the phenomenon, 229-230
      objectives of, 229
      principles of, 222t
      structuring the study
        researcher's perspective, 230
        research question, 230
        sample selection, 230
    ground theory
      data analysis, 228-229
      data gathering, 227-228
      describing the findings, 229
      development of, 226
      goal of, 226
      identifying the phenomenon, 226
      principles of, 222t
      structuring the study
        researcher's perspective, 227
        research question, 226-227
        sample selection, 227
      symbolic interaction principle of, 226
    historical
      data analysis, 233
      data gathering, 232-233
      describing the findings, 233-234
      fact, probability, and possibility estab-
        lishment in, 234b
      goals of, 231
      identifying the phenomenon, 232
      principles of, 223t, 231-232
      structuring the study
        researcher's perspective, 232
        research question, 232
        sample selection, 232
    phenomenological
      data analysis, 225
      data gathering, 224-225

Qualitative research studies—cont'd
  methods—cont'd
    phenomenological—cont'd
      describing the findings, 225
      goal of, 221, 223
      identifying the phenomenon, 223
      principles of, 222t
      structuring the study
        researcher's perspective, 224
        research question, 224
        sample selection, 224
  nursing methodology, 234, 235t
  nursing practice applications, 447, 449
  nursing science and, 220-221
  quantitative research and, comparison
    beliefs, 216, 218
    critical thinking decision path, 217
    life context, 216
    research activities, 218
    research questions, 218, 219t, 220
  research instrument development and, 449
  research questions *vs.* hypotheses, 84
  review of literature use for, 96t
  scientific rigor criteria, 237, 238t
  sections of, 448t-449t
  stylistic considerations, 446-447
  theory development using, 221
  triangulation
    description of, 237
    sequential, 237-238, 239t
    simultaneous, 237-238, 239t
    types of, 240t
Quantitative research studies
  case studies for analysis and critiquing
    case study 1
      critiquing of
        analysis of data, 427-428
        conclusions, 428
        definitions, 424
        external validity, 426
        hypotheses, 424-425
        implications, 428
        independent variables, 425
        instruments, 426-427
        internal validity, 426

Quantitative research studies—cont'd
  case studies for analysis and
      critiquing—cont'd
    case study 1—cont'd
      critiquing of—cont'd
        literature view, 424
        problem statement, 423-424
        purpose, 423-424
        recommendations, 428
        reliability, 427
        research approach, 426-427
        research design, 425-426
        sample, 425
        validity, 427
      data analysis, 418
      description of, 413-415
      discussion, 420-421
      experimental interventions, 417-418
      measures, 415-417
      method, 415-418
      procedure, 417
      results, 418, 419t, 420
      sample, 415
    case study 2
      conclusion, 436-437
      critiquing of
        analysis of data, 442
        conclusions, 442-443
        definitions, 439
        external validity, 440
        hypotheses and/or research questions, 440
        implications, 442-443
        instruments, 441
        internal validity, 440
        introduction, 438-439
        methods, 441
        nursing practice application, 443
        problem statement, 439
        purpose, 439
        recommendations, 443
        reliability, 441
        research approach, 441-442
        research design, 440
        review of literature, 439
        sample, 440
        validity, 441-442

Quantitative research studies—cont'd
  case studies for analysis and
      critiquing—cont'd
    case study 2—cont'd
      description of, 429
      discussion, 434, 435t, 436
      measures, 433
      methodology, 431-434
      procedure, 434
      results, 434
      review of literature, 430
      subjects, 431-433
      theoretical framework, 430-431
  qualitative research studies and,
      comparison
    beliefs, 216, 218
    critical thinking decision path, 217
    life context, 216
    research activities, 218
    research questions, 218, 219t, 220
  review of literature use for, 96t
Quasiexperimental designs
  advantages and disadvantages, 187-188
  critical thinking decision path, 177
  critiquing of, 189-191
  description of, 183
  internal validity threats, 191
  nonexperimental designs and, comparison,
      176
  in quality assurance and evaluation studies,
      189
  types of
    after-only nonequivalent control group
        design
      description of, 185-186
      diagram of, 184f
    diagrams, 184f
    nonequivalent control group design
      description of, 184-185
      diagram of, 184f
    time series design
      description of, 186-187
      diagram of, 184f
  vs. experimental designs, 183

Questionnaires
  advantages of, 318
  close-ended items
    description of, 316
    example of, 317b
  critiquing of, 322, 411t
  description of, 316
  example of, 318
  fixed response items, 316
  open-ended items
    description of, 316
    example of, 317b
  scale, 316
  vs. interviews, 319
Questions, research
  critiquing of, 88, 409t
  description of, 52, 82-83
  example of, 83
  location in research article, 50t
  vs. research problem, 84
Quota sampling
  description of, 254
  strata, 254-255
  summary of, 252t

R

Random errors, 328, 330
Randomization, 163, 177
Range, 363
Ratio measurement, 355
Reactivity, 314
  definition of, 168
  threat to external validity of research
      design, 168
Reasoning; see Deductive reasoning; Induc-
      tive reasoning
Recommendations
  case study evaluations, critiquing of
    qualitative research studies, 464-465
    quantitative research studies
      case study 1, 428
      case study 2, 443
  critiquing of, 411t-412t
  description of, 55

Recommendations—cont'd
  in *Discussion* section, 398, 399b, 411t-412t
  location in research article, 51t
Records or available data, for collecting data
  advantages and disadvantages, 320
  authenticity issues, 320
  critiquing of, 411t
  description of, 319
Refereed journals, 105-106
References, in research article
  description of, 55
  location of, 51t
Relational statements, 136
Relationship statement, of hypothesis, 74-75
Reliability
  description of, 54
  location in research articles, 51t
  of measurement tool
    case study evaluations of quantitative
      research studies
      case study 1, 427
      case study 2, 441
    critical thinking decision path, 339
    critiquing of, 345-346
    description of, 337
    methods to test
      equivalence
        description of, 344
        interrater reliability, 344-345
        parallel or alternate form, 345
      homogeneity
        Cronbach's alpha, 343-344, 344b
        description of, 341
        item to total correlations, 342, 342t
        Kuder-Richardson (KR-20) coefficient,
          343
        split-half reliability, 342
      overview, 340b
      stability
        description of, 340
        parallel or alternate form, 341
        test-retest reliability, 340-341
    reliability coefficient interpretation, 337,
      339-340

Research
  applied, 11
  basic, 11
  examples of, 36-37
  interrelationships
    with review of literature, 94f
    with theory, education, and practice, 7-9,
      94f
  in qualitative *vs.* quantitative research
    processes, 218
  and theory, relationship between, 144-146
Research approach
  case study evaluations of quantitative re-
    search studies
    case study 1, 426-427
    case study 2, 441-442
  data collection methods; *see* Data
    collection, methods
Research articles
  examples of
    *Comparison of Three Wound Dressings in
      Patients Undergoing Heart Surgery,*
      499-507
    *Concerns about Analgesics Among Patients
      and Family Caregivers in a Hospice
      Setting,* 537-547
    *Healing of Adult Male Survivors of Child-
      hood Sexual Abuse,* 509-520
    *Patient Outcomes for the Chronically Criti-
      cally Ill: Special Care Unit Versus In-
      tensive Care,* 521-535
  organization and format of, 48-49
  research process steps in, 50t-51t
  stylistic considerations, 408
Research-based practice
  characteristics of, 20
  in research utilization
    description of, 484
    example of, 485b-486b
Research-based protocols, 468
Research consumer
  definition of, 9
  of review of literature
    description of, 96-97
    examples of, 98t

Research consumer—cont'd
 of review of literature—cont'd
  literature searches, 110
  vs. review of literature for research, 97-99
Research design
 accuracy of, 158
 case study evaluations of quantitative research studies
  case study 1, 425-426
  case study 2, 440
 components of, 157
 control
  description of, 159
  extraneous variables that affect, methods
    for controlling
   constancy in data collection, 162
   homogeneous sampling, 161
   manipulation of independent variable, 162
   overview, 159, 161
   randomization, 163
  critiquing of, 169-171, 410t
 experimental; *see* Experimental designs
 external validity
  case study evaluations of quantitative
    research studies
   case study 1, 426
   case study 2, 440
  definition of, 167
  threats to
   reactivity, 168
   selection, 168
   testing, 168-169
 feasibility of, 159, 160t
 and hypothesis, relationship between, 82
 internal validity
  case study evaluations of quantitative re-
    search studies
   case study 1, 426
   case study 2, 440
  function of, 164
  threats to
   history, 164
   instrumentation, 165-166
   maturation, 164-165
   mortality, 166

Research design—cont'd
 internal validity—cont'd
  threats to—cont'd
   overview, 164b
   selection bias, 166
   testing, 165
  interrelationships with problem statement,
    literature review, theoretical frame-
    work, and hypothesis, 156f
  location in research article, 50t
  nonexperimental; *see* Nonexperimental de-
    signs
  problem conceptualization, objectivity in,
    157-158
  purpose of, 157
  qualitative *vs.* quantitative, 53
  quantitative control and flexibility, 163
  quasiexperimental; *see* Quasiexperimental
    designs
  review of literature, 99
  types of, 52-53
Research dissemination, 26
 definition of, 472
 interrelationship with conduct of research
   and research utilization, 469f
 research utilization demonstration projects
   for, 472-473
Research hypothesis
 definition of, 80-81
 examples of, 79t-80t
 inferential statistics testing of, 371
Research problem; *see also* Problem
   statement
 conceptualization of, objectivity in, 157-
   158
 critiquing of, 84-86
 description of, 51
 development of
  criteria for
   feasibility, 65
   problem area, 63
   review of literature, 63
   significance to nursing, 65
  potential sources of research ideas
   gaps in literature, 62t
   practical experience, 61t

Research problem; *see also* Problem
       statement—cont'd
  development of—cont'd
    potential sources of research ideas—cont'd
      scientific literature appraisal, 61t
      untested theory, 62t
      schematic, 64f
    placement in research articles, 50t
Research process
  role of nurse in, 9-11
  steps involved in
    communicating results, 55
    data analysis, 54
    data collection methods, 54
    discussion, 54
    hypothesis/research question, 52
    implications, 55
    instruments, 54
    location in research article, 50t-51t
    purpose, 52
    recommendations, 55
    references, 55
    research design, 52-53
    research problem, 51
    results, 54
    review of literature, 52
    sampling, 53
    theoretical framework, 52
    validity and reliability, 54
Research questions
  critiquing of, 88, 409t
  description of, 52, 82-83
  example of, 83
  location in research article, 50t
  vs. research problem, 84
Research studies
  case study evaluations of quantitative re-
       search studies
    case study 1
      article, 413-421
      critiquing of
        analysis of data, 427-428
        conclusions, 428
        definitions, 424
        external validity, 426

Research studies—cont'd
  case study evaluations of quantitative re-
       search studies—cont'd
    case study 1—cont'd
      critiquing of—cont'd
        hypotheses, 424-425
        implications, 428
        independent variables, 425
        instruments, 426-427
        internal validity, 426
        literature view, 424
        problem statement, 423-424
        purpose, 423-424
        recommendations, 428
        reliability, 427
        research approach, 426-427
        research design, 425-426
        sample, 425
        validity, 427
      data analysis, 418
      discussion, 420-421
      experimental interventions, 417-418
      measures, 415-417
      method, 415-418
      procedure, 417
      results, 418, 419t, 420
      sample, 415
    case study 2
      conclusion, 436-437
      critiquing of
        analysis of data, 442
        conclusions, 442-443
        definitions, 439
        external validity, 440
        hypotheses and/or research questions,
             440
        implications, 442-443
        instruments, 441
        internal validity, 440
        introduction, 438-439
        methods, 441
        nursing practice application, 443
        problem statement, 439
        purpose, 439
        recommendations, 443

Research studies—cont'd
  case study evaluations of quantitative re-
      search studies—cont'd
    case study 2—cont'd
      critiquing of—cont'd
        reliability, 441
        research approach, 441-442
        research design, 440
        review of literature, 439
        sample, 440
        validity, 441-442
      description of, 429
      discussion, 434, 435t, 436
      measures, 433
      methodology, 431-434
      procedure, 434
      results, 434
      review of literature, 430
      subjects, 431-433
      theoretical framework, 430-431
  content sections of, 409t-412t
  design of; see Research design
  examples of; see Research articles, examples
      of
Research utilization
  conceptual driven, 468
  conduct of research and, comparison,
      468
  criteria for evaluating success of, 494,
      494b
  decision-driven
    critical thinking decision path, 470-471
    description of, 468-469
  definition of, 6, 468
  demonstration projects of
    CURN, 472
    Nursing Child Assessment Satellite Train-
        ing, 472-473
    Western Interstate Commission for
        Higher Education in Nursing, 472
  future directions, 494-495
  historical perspective, 471
  implementation of
    options for, 493b
    overview, 491

Research utilization—cont'd
  implementation of—cont'd
    requirements for
      access to human resources, 492
      access to information, 492
      organizational commitment, 492-493
  interrelationship with conduct of research
      and research dissemination, 469f
  models
    Goode, 478
    Horn, 478
    Iowa Model of Research in Practice, 479
    Stetler
      critical thinking decision path, 471
      description of, 473
      phases of, 473, 477
      refinement of, 474b-477b
  steps of
    critique of studies
      description of, 482
      resources for, 482
    evaluation
      amount of data needed, 490-491
      data collection, 490
      elements of, 488
      feedback, 491
      outcome data, 489-490
      process questions, 489, 490b
      purpose of, 488
      steps involved in, 489b
    literature retrieval, 481-482
    practice changes
      decision to make, 483-484
      implementation of
        core group approach, 487-488
        role of nurse manager in, 487
        steps involved in, 487
    research-based practice
      description of, 484
      example of, 485b-486b
    synthesis of research findings, 483
    topic selection
      criteria for, 480b
      knowledge-focused, 480
      problem-focused, 479-480
      tool for, 481f

Resources, for review of literature
  CD-ROM databases
    CINAHL, 118B, 118-119
    description of, 117-118
  on-line databases
    types of, 117b
    via CINAHL direct, 117
    via Internet, 111, 112t-115t, 116
  print databases, 110-111
Results section
  critiquing criteria, 393-394, 398-400
  data presentation, 392
  description of, 54
  elements of, 390-391
  limitations, 392
  location in research article, 51t
  objectivity of results, 392-393, 393b
  in qualitative studies, 393b
  in quantitative studies, 393b
  reported statistical results, 391, 392t
  tabular use in, 394t-396t, 394-395
Retrospective studies
  example of, 204
  objectives of, 204
Review of literature
  case study evaluations of quantitative
      research studies
    case study 1, 424
    case study 2, 439
  computer searches for
    critical thinking decision path, 120
    description of, 119
    information necessary for performing,
        121, 123
    retrieved information, critical reading of,
        123
    search tools, 121, 123
    time lines for, 120-121
  critiquing of, 124-127, 409t
  description of, 52
  effect on research design
    accuracy, 158
    problem conceptualization, 157-158
  format, 123-124

Review of literature—cont'd
  interrelationships
    with problem statement, theoretical frame-
        work, and hypothesis, 73f, 77t
    with theory, research, education, and
        nursing practice, 94f
  literature search, steps and strategies, 101t
  location in research article, 50t
  perspectives
    consumer of research, 100-101
    researcher's, 99-100
  primary sources, 97
    definition of, 106
    nursing journals, 108b
    secondary sources and, comparison, 107t
    sources of, 109t
  purposes of
    knowledge base acquisition, 95
    overall, 95, 95b
    research
      consumer of, 96-97
      description of, 95-96
    for quantitative study
      conductor of research perspective,
          99-100
      description of, 139
    research conduct *vs.* consumer of research,
        comparison of, 97-99
    in research problem development, 63
  resources
    CD-ROM databases
      CINAHL, 118B, 118-119
      description of, 117-118
    on-line databases
      types of, 117b
      via CINAHL direct, 117
      via Internet, 111, 112t-115t, 116
    print databases, 110-111
  scholarly literature
    conceptual
      critiquing of, 126
      nursing journals, 108b
      sources of, 102, 103t
      terms used to describe, 102, 102t

Review of literature—cont'd
  scholarly literature—cont'd
    data-based
      critiquing of, 126
      material for, 105
      nursing journals, 108b
      sources of, 102, 103t, 105
      terms used to describe, 102, 102t
    definition of, 94
    refereed journals, 105-106
    sources of, 102-103
    theoretical material, examples of, 103-105
  secondary sources
    considerations for using, 106
    definition of, 106
    nursing journals, 108b
    primary sources and, comparison, 107t
    reasons for using, 106
    in refereed journals, 107
    sources of, 109t
  theoretical framework critique using, 149
Right to anonymity and confidentiality
  description of, 286t
  violation of, 287
Right to fair treatment, 288t
Right to personal privacy, 284
Right to privacy and dignity, 286t
Right to protection from discomfort and
    harm, 288t
Right to self-determination
  description of, 286t
  violation of, 287
Risks vs. benefits, 298

S
Sample
  case study evaluations, critiquing of
    quantitative research studies
      case study 1, 425
      case study 2, 440
    in quantitative research studies
      case study 1, 415
      case study 2, 440
  critiquing, 410t
  definition of, 250
  representative, 251

Sample size
  critiquing of, 265, 270-271
  data saturation considerations, 264
  factors that determine, 263-264
  population considerations, 264
  power analysis for estimating, 264-265
Sample statistic, 370
Sampling
  case study evaluations in qualitative
      research studies, 462
  concepts, population
    accessible, 250
    composition, 248
    definition of, 248
    eligibility criteria, 248-249
    target, 250
  critiquing of
    criteria, 268
    human rights protection, 271
    population, 268
    random sampling, 270
    suitability to research design, 270
  definition of, 248, 250
  description of, 53
  knowledge derived from, 248
  location in research article, 50t
  nonprobability
    elements of, 251
    types of
      convenience
        advantages and disadvantages,
          253
        description of, 253
        summary of, 252t
      matching, 262
      networking sampling, 262-263
      purposive
        description of, 255
        indications for using, 255-256
        recruiting of subjects for, 255
        summary of, 252t
      quota
        description of, 254
        strata, 254-255
        summary of, 252t

Sampling—cont'd
  probability
    characteristics of, 256
    elements of, 251
    random selection, 256
    types of
      cluster
        advantages and disadvantages, 260
        principles of, 260
        summary of, 252t
      simple random
        advantages, 256, 258
        description of, 256
        disadvantages, 258
        random numbers, 257f
        summary of, 252t
      stratified random
        advantages and disadvantages, 259-260
        criteria for selecting, 258-259
        principles of, 258
        subject selection, 259f
        summary of, 252t
      systematic
        advantages and disadvantages,
          261-262
        critiquing, 262
        definition of, 260-261
        population considerations, 261
        sampling interval, 261
        summary of, 252t
  procedures
    organization of, 266
    summary of, 266f
    target population, 266-267
  purpose of, 251
  in qualitative research studies, 448t
Sampling distribution of the means, 361
Sampling error, 372-373
Sampling frame, 256
Sampling unit, 250
Scale, of questionnaires, 316
Scholarly literature, 94
  conceptual
    critiquing of, 126
    nursing journals, 108b

Scholarly literature—cont'd
  conceptual—cont'd
    sources of, 102, 103t
    terms used to describe, 102, 102t
  data-based
    critiquing of, 126
    material for, 105
    nursing journals, 108b
    sources of, 102, 103t, 105
    terms used to describe, 102, 102t
  definition of, 94
  refereed journals, 105-106
  sources of, 102-103
  theoretical material, examples of, 103-105
Scientific fraud, 297
Scientific hypothesis; see Research hypothesis
Scientific misconduct, 297
Scientific observation
  advantages, 315
  description of, 312-313
Secondary sources, of literature, 233
  considerations for using, 106
  definition of, 106
  nursing journals, 108b
  primary sources and, comparison, 107t
  reasons for using, 106
  in refereed journals, 107
  sources of, 109t
Selection bias
  definition of, 166
  effect on validity of research design
    external validity, 168
    internal validity, 166
  ways to avoid, in research study, 166
Semiquartile range, 363
Simple random sampling
  advantages, 256, 258
  description of, 256
  disadvantages, 258
  random numbers, 257f
  summary of, 252t
Skewness, of distribution
  description of, 361
  illustration of, 362f
Skilled reading, 42

Skimming
  definition of, 42
  illustration of, 43f-44f
Snowballing; *see* Networking sampling
Solomon four-group design
  description of, 180-181
  diagram of, 180f
Split-half reliability, 342
Stability testing, of reliability of measure-
      ment tool
  description of, 340
  parallel or alternate form, 341
  test-retest reliability, 340-341
Standard deviation (SD), 363-364
Standard error of the mean, 373
Statement of purpose; *see* Purpose statement
Statistical hypothesis
  definition of, 81
  example of, 81t, 371-372
  inferential statistics testing of, 371
Statistical significance tests
  nonparametric
    of association, 378t
    chi-square, 379
    description of, 376
    of differences between means, 377t
    Fisher's exact probability test, 379-380
    types of, 379-380
  parametric
    analysis of covariance, 379
    analysis of variance, 378-379
    of association, 378t
    attributes of, 376
    description of, 376
    of differences between means, 377t
    multiple analysis of variance, 379
    t test, 377-378
  tests of difference
    description of, 377-378
    nonparametric tests, 379
    parametric tests, 378-379
  tests of relationships
    function of, 380
    multiple regression, 381-382
    Pearson *r*, 380-381

Statistics
  descriptive
    correlation, 364-365, 364f
    critical thinking decision path, 353
    critiquing of, 365-366
    definition of, 352
    frequency distribution
      data presentation, 355, 356f
      description of, 355
    function of, 352
    inferential statistics and, comparison, 370
    level of measurement
      description of, 352
      interval, 354-355
      nominal, 354
      ordinal, 354
      ratio, 355
      summary of, 353t
    measures of central tendency
      example of, 357t, 360t
      function of, 357
      mean, 358-359
      median, 358
      mode, 358, 359f
    normal distribution
      description of, 361
      kurtosis, 361-362
      skewness, 361
      symmetry, 359f, 361
    variability measures
      function of, 362-363
      percentile, 363
      range, 363
      semiquartile range, 363
      standard deviation, 363-364
      Z scores, 364
  inferential
    advanced statistics
      analysis of linear structural relationships,
        382
      factor analysis, 383
      path analysis, 382
    case study evaluations in quantitative
        research studies
      case study 1, 427-428
      case study 2, 442

Statistics—cont'd
  inferential—cont'd
    critical thinking decision path, 370-371
    critiquing of
      criteria, 383
      description of, 383-384
      example of, 384-385
      hypothesis, 383-384
      level of measurement, 384
    definition of, 370
    descriptive statistics and, comparison, 370
    errors
      level of significance, 375
      practical significance *vs.* statistical signif-
        icance, 375-376
      type I, 374
      type II, 374
    hypothesis testing, 370-372
    parameter, 370
    probability
      definition of, 372
      principles of, 372
      sampling error, 372-373
    purpose of, 370
    random sampling basis for, 370
    statistical significance tests
      nonparametric
        of association, 378t
        chi-square, 379
        description of, 376
        of differences between means, 377t
        Fisher's exact probability test, 379-380
        types of, 379-380
      parametric
        analysis of covariance, 379
        analysis of variance, 378-379
        of association, 378t
        attributes of, 376
        description of, 376
        of differences between means, 377t
        multiple analysis of variance, 379
        t test, 377-378
      tests of difference
        description of, 377-378
        nonparametric tests, 379
        parametric tests, 378-379

Statistics—cont'd
  inferential—cont'd
    statistical significance tests—cont'd
      tests of relationships
        function of, 380
        multiple regression, 381-382
        Pearson *r*, 380-381
      vs. practical significance, 375-376
Stetler model, of research utilization, 98
  critical thinking decision path, 471
  description of, 473
  phases of, 473, 477
  refinement of, 474b-477b
Stratified random sampling
  advantages and disadvantages, 259-260
  criteria for selecting, 258-259
  principles of, 258
  subject selection, 259f
  summary of, 252t
Students; *see* Graduate students; Undergraduate students
Subjective, definition of, 308
Surveys; *see* Descriptive/exploratory surveys
Symbolic interaction, 226
Symmetry, of distribution
  description of, 361
  illustration of, 359f
Synthesis reading
  definition of, 46
  strategies, 47
Systematic error, 330
Systematic sampling
  advantages and disadvantages, 261-262
  critiquing, 262
  definition of, 260-261
  population considerations, 261
  sampling interval, 261
  summary of, 252t

T

Target population, 250
Telnet services, 112t-113t
Testability
  of hypothesis, 75, 76t, 88
  of problem statement, 68-69, 69t, 71

Testing
  definition of, 165
  effect on validity of research design
    external validity, 168-169
    internal validity, 165
Test-retest reliability, of research instrument,
    340-341
Tests of difference, in inferential statistics
  description of, 377-378
  nonparametric tests, 379
  parametric tests, 378-379
Tests of relationships, in inferential statistics
  function of, 380
  multiple regression, 381-382
  Pearson r, 380-381
Theoretical framework
  critiquing of, 148-149, 409t
  description of, 52
  effect on research design
    accuracy, 158
    problem conceptualization, 157-158
  function of, 141, 146
  importance in research process, 146
  interrelationship with problem statement,
      literature review, and hypothesis,
      73f, 77t
  location in research article, 50t
  review of literature, 99
Theoretical material, examples of, 103-105
Theoretical sampling, 228
Theory
  definition of, 140
  development of, using qualitative research,
      221
  effect on decision making, 145
  function of, 140
  generation of, using inductive processes,
      140
  interrelationships
    with education, practice, and research, 7-
        9, 94f
    with review of literature, 94f
  and method, relationship between, 146-
      147

Theory—cont'd
  modification of existing, using deductive
      processes, 140
  nursing
    definition of, 147
    grand, 148b
    middle-range, 148b
    practice, 148b
  and research, relationship between, 144-
      146
  untested, 60
Time series design, of quasiexperimental de-
    signs
  description of, 186-187
  diagram of, 184f
Tools, for measurement; see Measurement
    tools
Tradition and authority, as sources of knowl-
    edge, 135-136
Trial-and-error knowledge, 135
Triangulation, of qualitative research
  description of, 237
  sequential, 237-238, 239t
  simultaneous, 237-238, 239t
  types of, 240t
t tests
  description of, 376
  in parametric testing, 378
  purpose of, 378

U

Unauthorized research, 297-298
Undergraduate students, review of literature
    use by, 98t, 110
Unethical research studies, 278t-279t
Utilization, research
  conceptual driven, 468
  conduct of research and, comparison, 468
  criteria for evaluating success of, 494, 494b
  decision-driven
    critical thinking decision path, 470-471
    description of, 468-469
  definition of, 6, 468

Utilization, research—cont'd
  demonstration projects of
    CURN, 472
    Nursing Child Assessment Satellite Train-
      ing, 472-473
    Western Interstate Commission for
      Higher Education in Nursing,
      472
  future directions, 494-495
  historical perspective, 471
  implementation of
    options for, 493b
    overview, 491
    requirements for
      access to human resources, 492
      access to information, 492
      organizational commitment,
        492-493
  interrelationship with conduct of research
      and research dissemination, 469f
  models
    Goode, 478
    Horn, 478
    Iowa Model of Research in Practice,
      479
    Stetler
      critical thinking decision path, 471
      description of, 473
      phases of, 473, 477
      refinement of, 474b-477b
  steps of
    critique of studies
      description of, 482
      resources for, 482
    evaluation
      amount of data needed, 490-491
      data collection, 490
      elements of, 488
      feedback, 491
      outcome data, 489-490
      process questions, 489, 490b
      purpose of, 488
      steps involved in, 489b
    literature retrieval, 481-482

Utilization, research—cont'd
  steps of—cont'd
    practice changes
      decision to make, 483-484
      implementation of
        core group approach, 487-488
        role of nurse manager in, 487
        steps involved in, 487
    research-based practice
      description of, 484
      example of, 485b-486b
    synthesis of research findings, 483
    topic selection
      criteria for, 480b
      knowledge-focused, 480
      problem-focused, 479-480
      tool for, 481f

V
Validity
  of measurement tools
    case study evaluations of quantitative re-
      search studies
      case study 1, 427
      case study 2, 441-442
    computer resources for, 329b
    construct validity
      approaches
        contrasted-groups, 336
        convergent, 333-334
        divergent, 334, 336
        factor analytical, 336-337
        hypothesis-testing, 333, 334t
      definition of, 333
    content validity
      description of, 331
      example of, 331
      face validity, 332
    criterion-related validity
      concurrent, 332
      definition of, 332
      predictive, 332
    critiquing of, 346-347
    definition of, 331

Validity—cont'd
 of research design
  description of, 54
  external
   case study evaluations of quantitative
     research studies
    case study 1, 426
    case study 2, 440
   critiquing of, 410t
   definition of, 167
   threats to
    reactivity, 168
    selection, 168
    testing, 168-169
  internal
   case study evaluations of quantitative
     research studies
    case study 1, 426
    case study 2, 440
   critiquing, 410t
   experimental designs, 180-181
   function of, 164
   quasiexperimental designs, 191
   threats to
    history, 164
    instrumentation, 165-166
    maturation, 164-165
    mortality, 166
    overview, 164b
    selection bias, 166
    testing, 165
  location in research articles, 51t
Variability measures, of descriptive statistics
 function of, 362-363
 percentile, 363
 range, 363
 semiquartile range, 363
 standard deviation, 363-364
 Z scores, 364
Variables
 defining of, 143
 definition of, 67
 dependent
  case study evaluations of quantitative re-
    search studies, 424
  definition of, 63

Variables—cont'd
 dependent—cont'd
  in nonexperimental designs, 211
  in problem statement, 67-68
 extraneous; see Extraneous variables
 of hypothesis, critiquing of, 87
 independent
  case study evaluations of quantitative re-
    search studies, 424
  definition of, 67, 162
  in experimental vs. nonexperimental de-
    signs, 196
  manipulation of, 162
  in problem statement, 67-68
 in problem statement, 67-68, 69t
Vulnerable groups
 future priorities for, 24
 protection of human rights of
  children, 296
  elderly, 296
  prisoners, 296
  types of, 294-295

W

Web browser, 116
Western Interstate Commission for Higher
      Education in Nursing (WICHEN),
      472
Wording, of hypothesis
 critiquing of, 87
 directional hypothesis, 79t-80t
 elements, 77
 nondirectional hypothesis, 79t-80t
World Wide Web (WWW)
 description of, 103
 web sites for literature review, 114t-115t,
      116

Z

Z scores, 364